Medical-Surgical Nursing

Decision Making in Clinical Nursing™ Series

Baird:
Decision Making in Oncology Nursing

Baumann, Johnston, Antai-Otong:
Decision Making in Psychiatric and Psychosocial Nursing

Drain:
Decision Making in Postanesthesia Nursing

Gorzeman, Bowdoin:
Decision Making in Medical-Surgical Nursing

Knor:
Decision Making in Obstetrical Nursing

Mancini:
Decision Making in Emergency Nursing

Murphy:
Decision Making in Pediatric Nursing

Wells:
Decision Making in Perioperative Nursing

Williams:
Decision Making in Critical Care Nursing

DECISION MAKING IN

Medical-Surgical Nursing

Joy Gorzeman, RN, MSN

Director, Institute of Professional Development
Manatee Community College
Bradenton, Florida

Carol Bowdoin, RN, MSN, CCRN

Instructor, Department of Nursing
Manatee Community College
Bradenton, Florida

B.C. Decker • Toronto • Philadelphia

Publisher

B.C. Decker Inc
3228 South Service Road
Burlington, Ontario L7N 3H8

B.C. Decker Inc
320 Walnut Street
Suite 400
Philadelphia, Pennsylvania 19106

Sales and Distribution

United States and Puerto Rico
The C.V. Mosby Company
11830 Westline Industrial Drive
Saint Louis, Missouri 63146

Canada
McAinsh & Co. Ltd.
2760 Old Leslie Street
Willowdale, Ontario M2K 2X5

Australia
McGraw-Hill Book Company Australia Pty. Ltd.
4 Barcoo Street
Roseville East 2069
New South Wales, Australia

Brazil
Editora McGraw-Hill do Brasil, Ltda.
rua Tabapua, 1.105, Itaim-Bibi
Sao Paulo, S.P. Brasil

Colombia
Interamericana/McGraw-Hill de Colombia, S.A.
Apartado Aereo 81078
Bogota, D.E. Colombia

Europe
McGraw-Hill Book Company GmbH
Lademannbogen 136
D-2000 Hamburg 63
West Germany

France
MEDSI/McGraw-Hill
6, avenue Daniel Lesueur
75007 Paris, France

Hong Kong and China
McGraw-Hill Book Company
Suite 618, Ocean Centre
5 Canton Road
Tsimshatsui, Kowloon
Hong Kong

India
Tata McGraw-Hill Publishing Company, Ltd.
12/4 Asaf Ali Road, 3rd Floor
New Delhi 110002, India

Indonesia
P.O. Box 122/JAT
Jakarta, 1300 Indonesia

Italy
McGraw-Hill Libri Italia, s.r.l.
Piazza Emilia, 5
I-20129 Milano MI
Italy

Japan
Igaku-Shoin Ltd.
Tokyo International P.O. Box 5063
1-28-36 Hongo, Bunkyo-ku,
Tokyo 113, Japan

Korea
C.P.O. Box 10583
Seoul, Korea

Malaysia
No. 8 Jalan SS 7/6B
Kelana Jaya
47301 Petaling Jaya
Selangor, Malaysia

Mexico
Interamericana/McGraw-Hill de Mexico, S.A. de C.V.
Cedro 512, Colonia Atlampa
(Apartado Postal 26370)
06450 Mexico, D.F., Mexico

New Zealand
McGraw-Hill Book Co. New Zealand Ltd.
5 Joval Place, Wiri
Manukau City, New Zealand

Panama
Editorial McGraw-Hill Latinoamericana, S.A.
Apartado Postal 2036
Zona Libre de Colon
Colon, Republica de Panama

Portugal
Editora McGraw-Hill de Portugal, Ltda.
Rua Rosa Damasceno 11A-B
1900 Lisboa, Portugal

South Africa
Libriger Book Distributors
Warehouse Number 8
"Die Ou Looiery"
Tannery Road
Hamilton, Bloemfontein 9300

Southeast Asia
McGraw-Hill Book Co.
348 Jalan Boon Lay
Jurong, Singapore 2261

Spain
McGraw-Hill/Interamericana de Espana, S.A.
Manuel Ferrero, 13
28020 Madrid, Spain

Taiwan
P.O. Box 87-601
Taipei, Taiwan

Thailand
632/5 Phaholyothin Road
Sapan Kwai
Bangkok 10400
Thailand

United Kingdom, Middle East and Africa
McGraw-Hill Book Company (U.K.) Ltd.
Shoppenhangers Road
Maidenhead, Berkshire
SL6 2QL England

Venezuela
McGraw-Hill/Interamericana, C.A.
2da. calle Bello Monte
(entre avenida Casanova y Sabana Grande)
Apartado Aereo 50785
Caracas 1050, Venezuela

NOTICE

The authors and publisher have made every effort to ensure that the patient care recommended herein, including choice of drugs and drug dosages, is in accord with the accepted standards and practice at the time of publication. However, since research and regulation constantly change clinical standards, the reader is urged to check the product information sheet included in the package of each drug, which includes recommended doses, warnings, and contraindications. This is particularly important with new or infrequently used drugs. The authors, editors, and publisher disclaim responsibility for any adverse effects resulting directly or indirectly from the use of algorithms, any undetected text errors, or misinterpretation of this information.

Decision Making in Medical-Surgical Nursing

ISBN 1–55664–120–6

Library of Congress catalog card number: 89–50932

10 9 8 7 6 5 4 3 2 1

To our families,
our colleagues,
and all aspiring nurses

CONTRIBUTORS

CAROL BOWDOIN, RN, MSN, CCRN

Instructor, Department of Nursing, Manatee Community College, Bradenton, Florida; Former Instructor, College of Nursing, University of Alabama at Huntsville, Huntsville, Alabama

CARLA K. CALLOWAY, RN, BSN, CCRN

Senior Research Nurse, The University of Texas Southwestern Medical Center, Dallas, Texas

SUSAN CAULEY, RN, BSN

Assistant Director of Nursing, Surgical Specialties, Parkland Memorial Hospital, Dallas, Texas

MARSHA CLOAK, RN, MS

Oncology Nurse Consultant, Georgetown University Hospital, Washington, D.C.

MICHELLE CORNISH, RN, BSN, CEN

Assistant Unit Manager, Emergency Department, Tri-City Medical Center, Oceanside, California

CINDY DREW, RN, MS

Instructor, Department of Nursing, Manatee Community College, Bradenton, Florida

PAMELA Y. DONNELLY, RN, MSN

Staff Nurse, Labor and Delivery, Parkland Memorial Hospital, Dallas, Texas

KENDRA ELLIS, RN, CCRN

Staff Development Educator, Specialty Care Area, John Peter Smith Hospital, Fort Worth, Texas

MICHELE GANN, RN, BSN, CCRN

Head Nurse, Intensive Care Unit, Doctor's Hospital, Dallas, Texas

BONITA M. GARVEY, RN, BSN

Staff Nurse, Sarasota Memorial Hospital, Sarasota, Florida; Graduate Student, MPH, University of South Florida, Tampa, Florida

KATHY GILLILAND, BSN, CNRN

Clinical Specialist, Neurology/Neurosurgery, Holmes Regional Medical Center, Melbourne, Florida

JOY GORZEMAN, RN, MSN

Director, Institute of Professional Development, Manatee Community College, Bradenton, Florida; Former Nursing Education Coordinator, Parkland Memorial Hospital, Dallas, Texas

BARBARA GREAUX, RN, MS

Professor, Department of Nursing, Manatee Community College, Bradenton, Florida

HAZEL HARRIS, RN, BSN

Head Nurse, Orthopedics, Parkland Memorial Hospital, Dallas, Texas

LESLIE C. HUSSEY, RN, PhD

Patient Education Coordinator, Parkland Memorial Hospital, Dallas, Texas

BARBARA KALO, RNC, BSN

Quality Assurance Coordinator, Special Care Units, Parkland Memorial Hospital, Dallas, Texas

ROSEMARY KELLER, RN, MS

Assistant Professor, Department of Nursing, Manatee Community College, Bradenton, Florida

CHRIS KIRSCH, RN, MS

Associate Professor, Department of Nursing, Manatee Community College, Bradenton, Florida

MICHELE KONNICK, RN, MS

Professional Development Educator, University of Chicago Hospitals, Chicago, Illinois

JEAN OSWALD KONRADY, RN, MS, ARNP, CDE

Clinical Diabetes Educator, Sarasota Memorial Hospital, Sarasota, Florida

MANJA LEE, RN, BSN

Operating Room Internship Instructor, Parkland Memorial Hospital, Dallas, Texas

CECILE A. LENGACHER, RN, PhD

Assistant Dean, Undergraduate Studies, College of Nursing, University of South Florida, Tampa, Florida

LAURA LUECKE, RN, BSN, CCRN

Critical Care Nurse Educator, Parkland Memorial Hospital, Dallas, Texas

DAVID L. LYBARGER, RNC, MSN

Family Nurse Practitioner, University Medical Center, Lebanon, Tennessee

MARY E. MANCINI, RN, MSN, CNA

Vice President, Nursing Administration, Parkland Memorial Hospital, Dallas, Texas

MARY BETH MARDJETKO, RN, MN

Clinical Manager, Hematology/Oncology, University of Chicago Hospitals, Chicago, Illinois

MARY LINDELL MARQUIS, RN, MS

Instructor, Department of Nursing, Manatee Community College, Bradenton, Florida

WILLIAM B. MARSHALL, RN, MS, CCRN

Instructor, College of Nursing, University of Oklahoma, Oklahoma City, Oklahoma

NINA McINTOSH, RN, BSN

Administrative Assistant, Outpatient Services, Parkland Memorial Hospital, Dallas, Texas

JAN METRO-EMMERT, RN, MSN

Associate Professor, Department of Nursing, Manatee Community College, Bradenton, Florida

SUSAN NUSSLE, RN, BSN, CCRN

Renal Nurse Educator, Parkland Memorial Hospital, Dallas, Texas

KAREN O'BRIEN, RN, BSN

Director, Emergency Services, Tri-City Medical Center, Ocean City, California

PAULA K. OVENS, RN, MS

Nurse Recruiter, Parkland Memorial Hospital, Dallas, Texas

LESLIE RACH, RN, BSN

Head Nurse, General Surgery, Parkland Memorial Hospital, Dallas, Texas

MARY K. ROBERTS, RN, BSN, CCRN

Graduate Student, MSN, The University of Texas at Arlington, Arlington, Texas

GAIL SHORES, RN, BSN

Medical Case Manager, Intracorp, Dallas, Texas

SUSAN J. SMITH, PhD, RN

Assistant Professor, College of Nursing, University of Arkansas for Medical Sciences, Little Rock, Arkansas

ROBERT STEELE, MHS, CRNA, ARNP

Staff Nurse Anesthetist, Tri-City Hospital, Dallas, Texas

LYNNE TIER, RN, MSN

Assistant Professor, Department of Nursing, Manatee Community College, Bradenton, Florida

KATHLEEN H. TOTO, RN, MSN, CCRN

Nurse Internship Instructor, Parkland Memorial Hospital, Dallas, Texas

LINDA WELD, RN, MSN

Clinical Specialist, RHD Hospital, Dallas, Texas

NANCY A. YOUNG, RN, MSN

Former Instructor, Intercollegiate Center for Nursing Education, Washington State University, Spokane, Washington

DIANE M. ZINTAK, RN, MSN

Clinical Director, Medical-Surgical, Lutheran General Hospital—Lincoln Park, Chicago, Illinois

PREFACE

Medical-surgical nursing represents the largest segment of nursing. General floor nursing has changed over the years, presenting many challenges. Medical-surgical nurses care for patients with physical, emotional, and spiritual needs resulting from a broad spectrum of diseases and therapies. During a patient's hospitalization, these nurses interact with other nursing specialists and health care providers to develop and carry out a plan of care while managing six to twelve acutely ill patients. This book is for you—to be a quick reference, a guide in clinical decision making, and a resource for updating nursing knowledge.

A few words of thanks are in order to all of those who have supported and assisted us during the course of this project: to Beth Mancini for introducing Joy to the Decision Making series and opening the door to a dream, and to Walter Bailey for the opportunity to author and edit; to Agnes McIvor, Dana Dreibelbis, and Amy Gewirtzman for sharing their talent, support, and encouragement; to Kathy Grey for her excellent illustrations which truly enhance this book; and to all the staff nurses who saved rhythm strips and offered suggestions. Special thanks are due to Dan Bowdoin for patiently typing our manuscripts and revisions. His diligence greatly facilitated the completion of this project. We appreciate all of our friends, colleagues, and students who have been so interested and patient when we have had that "far-away gaze." A special acknowledgment is due to our contributors who have given so much of their time and expertise without which this book would not have been possible. Words cannot express our thanks to our husbands, Jack and Dan, and our children, Angela, David, and Elizabeth, who understood our many working days, evenings, and weekends, and helped us at home so we could devote the time needed to this project.

Joy Gorzeman, RN, MSN
Carol Bowdoin, RN, MSN, CCRN

CONTENTS

CARDIOVASCULAR SURGERIES

RESPIRATORY SYSTEM

REPRODUCTIVE AND GENITOURINARY SYSTEMS

FEMALE

REPRODUCTIVE AND GENITOURINARY SURGERIES (FEMALE)

MALE

REPRODUCTIVE AND GENITOURINARY SURGERIES (MALE)

RENAL SYSTEM

EAR, NOSE, and THROAT

Ear, Nose, and Throat Surgery and Procedure

SPECIAL CONSIDERATIONS

INTRODUCTION

Decision Making in Medical-Surgical Nursing is meant to be used for quick reference. It is our intent that this book will be beneficial to all nurses regardless of experience. Each chapter and accompanying algorithm, or decision tree, may serve as an individual reference, as on-the-spot refreshing for a unit in-service, or as a review for the nurse returning to practice. Clinical instructors and nurse educators may find the trees valuable in teaching critical thinking to orientees and nursing students.

The decision tree, the focal point of each chapter, demonstrates the thought process the nurse should review for each medical-surgical patient. Narrative is added to provide detail and the theory behind the actions. The tree is keyed with letters that steer the reader to the corresponding sections in the text. Boxes around components of the tree indicate independent or interdependent nursing actions at most institutions.

The philosophy behind the decision trees can be conceptualized as a structure for clinical decision making. The steps of the nursing process—assessment, diagnosis, planning, implementation, and evaluation of care—can be followed in each tree. Each tree begins with a diagnosis for which the patient has been admitted or which could be a secondary complication or condition in addition to an admitting diagnosis.

A. Assessment includes a nursing history, holistic assessment—physical, emotional, social, and spiritual—and diagnostic tests. Although the nursing assessment complements the medical assessment, many independent nursing plans and actions result from the nursing assessment.

B. The nursing assessment leads to the development of the nursing diagnoses (Appendix A).

C. The nursing diagnoses are the basis for the development of the individualized care plan.

D. The physical aspects of care as well as the psychosocial and emotional support of the patient and family are highlighted throughout the tree.

E. The outcome of each action is evaluated.

F. If unsuccessful, the plan is reassessed and revisions are made.

G. If the outcome is successful, implementation is continued and the patient is ultimately discharged. Each tree emphasizes the instructions, referrals, and follow-up plans essential to providing comprehensive care.

The contributors to this text are clinically active in major health care institutions, and the information in the algorithms is current in relation to methods used in those institutions. To the best of our knowledge, this information is accurate and reflects currently accepted practice. The nurse should consider the process presented here as a guide. Individual agency policies as well as the patient's clinical condition must be considered in relation to the use of these decision trees.

References

Guzzetta CE. Developing a nursing data base prototype from the unitary person framework. In: Guzzetta CE, Banton SD, Pinkey LA, Sherer AP, Seifert PC. Clinical assessment tools for use with nursing diagnoses. St. Louis: CV Mosby, 1989:6–22.

McFarland GK, McFarland EA. Nursing diagnosis and intervention. St. Louis: CV Mosby, 1988.

The NURSING PROCESS

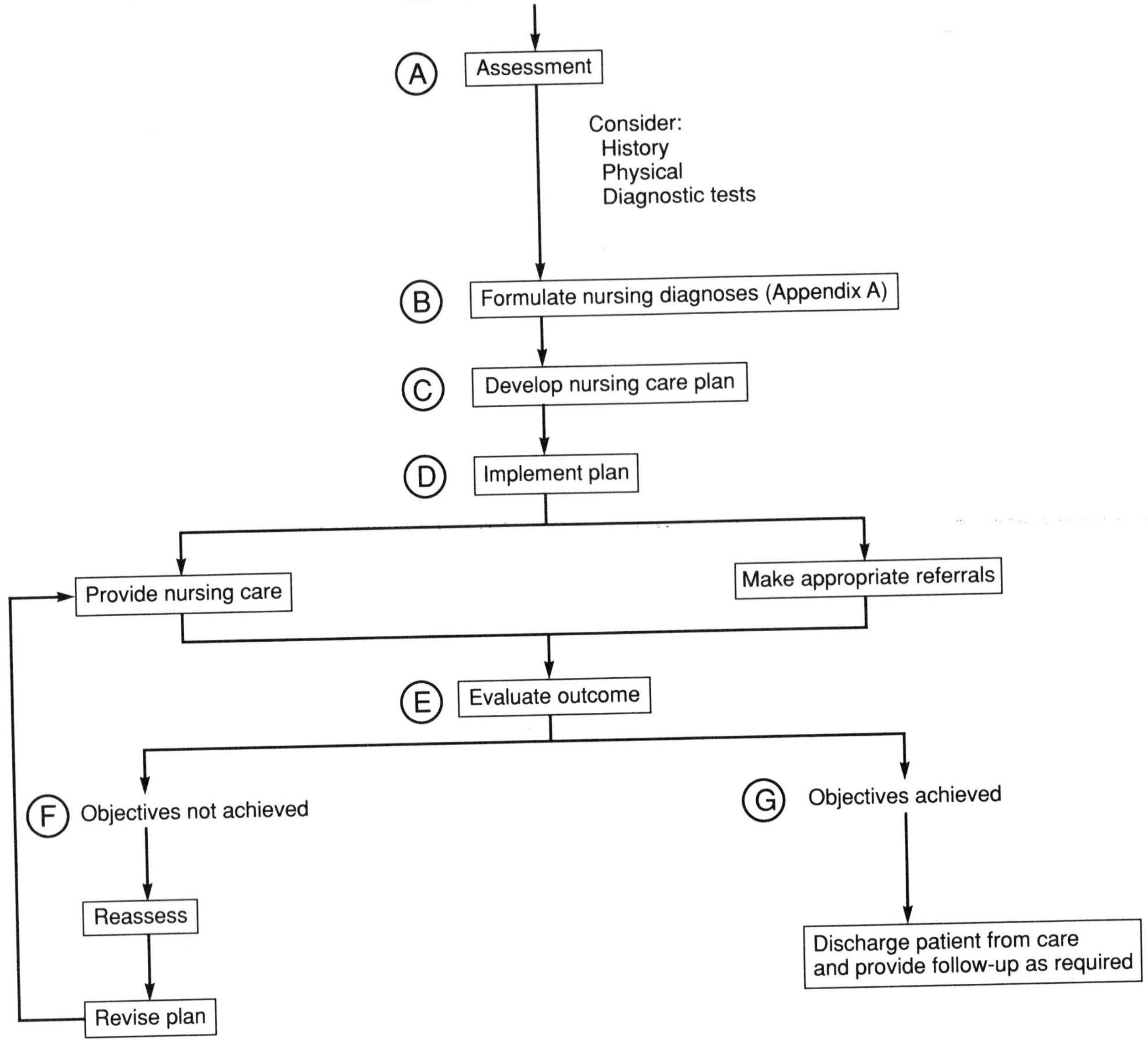

THE SURGICAL EXPERIENCE

The Preoperative Phase
The Postoperative Phase

THE PREOPERATIVE PHASE

Joy Gorzeman

Patients undergo surgery for one of four reasons: (1) diagnosis and/or exploration—as in a biopsy or laparotomy, (2) cure—removal or repair of a diseased organ or tissue, (3) palliation—relief of symptoms, or (4) cosmesis. Some surgeries are performed as emergencies, whereas elective surgeries may be scheduled months in advance or may be optional.

A. Whether the surgical procedure is emergency or elective, surgery always has a physical and emotional impact on the patient. General effects of surgery include (1) increased anxiety, (2) lowered defense against infection, (3) blood loss, and (4) organ function disturbance. In some instances body image may be affected and/or lifestyle may change. Depending on the degree of risk to the patient, surgeries are categorized as major or minor. Age, nutritional status, health history, medications, attitude, economic status, and the nature and extent of the illness all affect the risk and must be included in the nursing assessment. In the health care system today, many minor surgeries are done through day surgery units where a patient is admitted, has surgery, and is discharged all in one day. Even in this setting, the phases and considerations of the surgical experience are the same.

B. The perioperative experience includes three phases: preoperative, intraoperative, and postoperative. The preoperative phase prepares the patient for surgery. Laboratory tests are done. Radiologic studies and other tests or treatments may be done to assess the patient's general condition.

C. The patient needs to sign an operative consent form before surgery can be performed. It is the physician's legal responsibility to explain the surgical procedure and the risks, benefits, and possible complications involved. The nurse must be certain the operative permit is signed and on the chart before the patient is released to the operating room (OR).

D. Another preparation for surgery is the skin prep. The skin is cleansed with an antiseptic soap and the hair is removed. Some surgical procedures also require bowel preparation. All patients will be NPO (nothing by mouth) before surgery to decrease the risk of aspiration.

E. One of the most important aspects of the preoperative phase is patient and family teaching. This is the time to explain to the patient what to expect: the tests and procedures that will be done, an approximation of the time schedule for surgery, any special technology or monitoring devices that might be anticipated, and where the family can wait for updates regarding the patient's progress. The time spent preparing the patient and answering questions is important to decrease stress and to establish rapport.

F. This is also the time to instruct patients and have them practice coughing and deep breathing so that when they are uncomfortable and groggy after surgery, they will have been instructed about the importance of these activities. Surgery is different for each individual, so teaching should be tailored to incorporate the patient's knowledge, educational level, anxiety level, culture, religion, and individual concerns.

G. A couple of hours before surgery, the patient is given sedation and medication to decrease secretions. The chart should be completed and the operative checklist done. This documentation is turned over to the operating room personnel when they transfer the patient to the OR. It is important to allow the family time with the patient before surgery.

H. While the patient is in surgery, the bed linen is changed. Equipment such as an emesis basin, suction, and oxygen is prepared at the bedside.

References

Long B, Greig J. Perioperative nursing. In: Phipps W, Long B, Woods N, eds. Medical-surgical nursing concepts and clinical practice. St. Louis: CV Mosby, 1987.

Luckmann J, Sorensen KC. Medical-surgical nursing. 3rd ed. Philadelphia: WB Saunders, 1987.

Yocum C. Pre- and postoperative nursing care. In: Hincker E, Malasanos L, eds. The Little, Brown manual of medical-surgical nursing. Boston: Little, Brown, 1983.

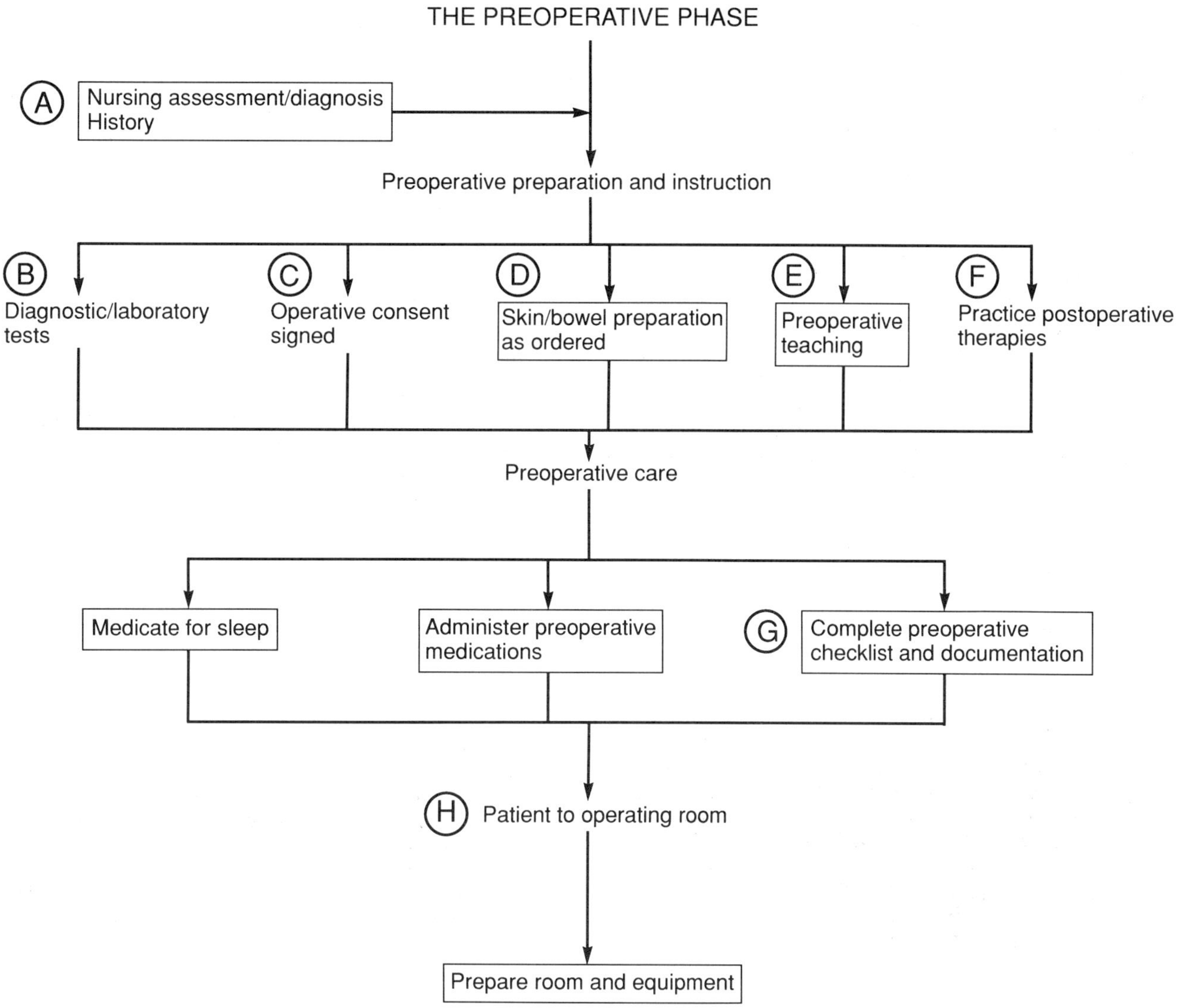
THE PREOPERATIVE PHASE
A
Nursing assessment/diagnosis
History
Preoperative preparation and instruction
B
Diagnostic/laboratory tests
C
Operative consent signed
D
Skin/bowel preparation as ordered
E
Preoperative teaching
F
Practice postoperative therapies
Preoperative care
Medicate for sleep
Administer preoperative medications
G
Complete preoperative checklist and documentation
H
Patient to operating room
Prepare room and equipment

THE POSTOPERATIVE PHASE

Joy Gorzeman

A. The goal of the postoperative phase is to enable the patient to recover as quickly as possible from surgery and return home to resume a productive life. Nursing care involves the promotion of healing and the prevention of complications. The patient usually spends about 2 hours in the recovery room. If there are no complications, the patient is returned to the unit, and the recovery room nurse gives a verbal report which includes the type of anesthesia that was administered. The unit nurse receiving the patient reviews the doctor's orders and does a baseline assessment. It is important to note skin color and temperature. The patient should be awake and oriented. The dressing should be checked for drainage and the amount noted in the record. Intravenous lines should be checked at the needle site, the drip rate calculated, and the amount of fluid left in the bag recorded. Other lines and/or tubes must be checked for patency and connected to suction if appropriate. Patients should be assessed for the presence of pain. They should be positioned for comfort with side rails up and the call bell within easy reach.

B. All data from the assessment must be accurately documented in the patient's record. The family should be advised of the patient's progress. This is a good time to develop appropriate nursing diagnoses and an initial plan of care.

C. The remaining postoperative period is one of observation and maintenance of systems, with progress depending on the type of surgery and the patient's response. Healing is affected by the patient's age, nutritional status, circulation status, and general health condition. Coughing, deep breathing, and position changes help maintain ventilation. Early ambulation and elastic stockings help to maintain circulation. Intake and output should be monitored until the fluid and electrolyte balance and nutritional status are stable. Elimination should also be monitored. If the patient is constipated, a laxative may relieve the discomfort.

D. No matter how minor the surgery, there is always the possibility of postoperative complications. The most common complications are hemorrhage, shock (p 70), phlebitis and thrombophlebitis, pulmonary embolism (p 116), wound infection, paralytic ileus, urinary retention and infection, and venous thrombus in the lower extremities.

E. The nurse must be cognizant of signs and symptoms, such as prolonged fever, that indicate possible problems. Appropriate treatment measures should be initiated and the physician notified.

F. If there are no complications, the patient is discharged with instructions regarding diet and activity, depending on the type of surgery performed. Heavy lifting, pushing, and pulling should be avoided for 6 weeks. The patient is advised of the importance of follow-up visits. Referral to community resources should be made if appropriate.

References

Long B, Greig J. Perioperative nursing. In: Phipps W, Long B, Woods N, eds. Medical-surgical nursing concepts and clinical practice. St. Louis: CV Mosby, 1987.

Luckmann J, Sorensen KC. Medical-surgical nursing. 3rd ed. Philadelphia: WB Saunders, 1987.

Yocum C. Pre- and postoperative nursing care. In: Hincker E, Malasanos L, eds. The Little, Brown manual of medical-surgical nursing. Boston: Little, Brown, 1983.

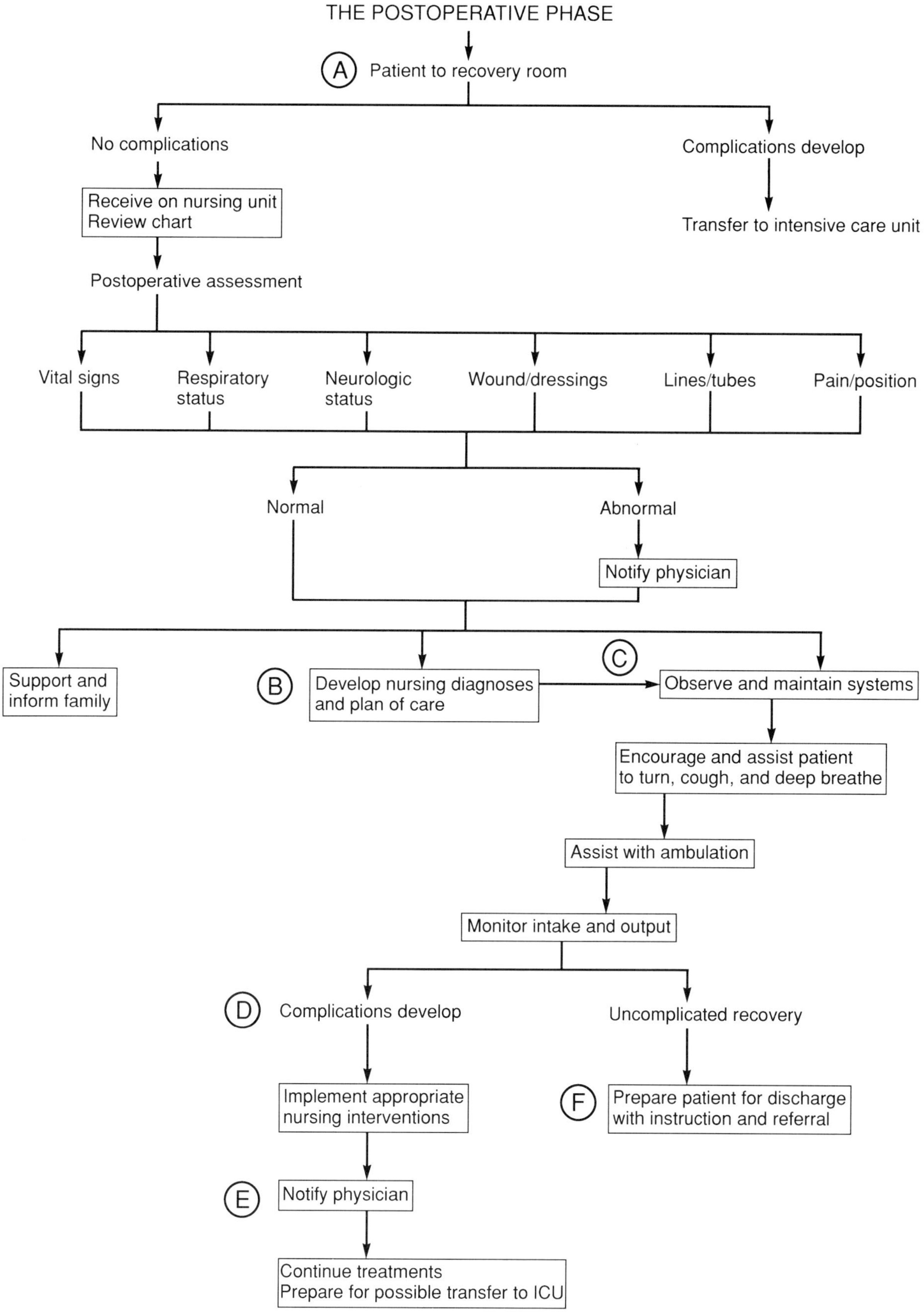
THE POSTOPERATIVE PHASE
A
Patient to recovery room
No complications
Complications develop
Receive on nursing unit
Review chart
Transfer to intensive care unit
Postoperative assessment
Vital signs
Respiratory status
Neurologic status
Wound/dressings
Lines/tubes
Pain/position
Normal
Abnormal
Notify physician
Support and inform family
B
Develop nursing diagnoses and plan of care
C
Observe and maintain systems
Encourage and assist patient to turn, cough, and deep breathe
Assist with ambulation
Monitor intake and output
D
Complications develop
Uncomplicated recovery
Implement appropriate nursing interventions
F
Prepare patient for discharge with instruction and referral
E
Notify physician
Continue treatments
Prepare for possible transfer to ICU

NEUROLOGIC SYSTEM

BRAIN ABSCESS

Joy Gorzeman

A. A brain abscess is a rare occurrence in which there is a localized collection of pus within the brain. The majority of brain abscesses follow a recent sinus or ear infection, making prompt treatment of these conditions of utmost importance to prevent abscess formation. Other causes of brain abscess include intracranial trauma and infections spread from other organs such as the lungs. The organisms that most commonly cause a brain abscess are staphylococci and streptococci. These organisms cause an inflammatory reaction that results in localized edema. The area usually becomes encapsulated, but the infection may spread through a weakened portion of the capsule. Mortality from brain abscess is high.

B. Early clinical manifestations of a brain abscess include headache, drowsiness, and transient confusion. Fever may be present. As intracranial pressure increases, the headache becomes more severe and is not relieved by medication, and the patient may experience seizures. Specific focal and neurologic manifestations, such as weakness in arm or leg, visual impairment, and papilledema, depend on the location of the abscess. A subnormal temperature is of importance to the nursing assessment as it may indicate a thick-walled abscess that has developed over time. In some patients progression of symptoms is rapid and ends in death, while for others progression is slower.

C. Diagnosis of brain abscess may be confirmed by examination of the cerebrospinal fluid, a brain scan, and a computerized tomographic (CT) scan. Other studies may include skull films and electroencephalography (EEGs). A complete blood count (CBC) with differential may reveal leukocytosis, which indicates an infectious process. It is important that the focus of the infection be identified.

D. Nursing care is supportive and requires ongoing assessment for signs of increased intracranial pressure. Seizure precautions must be taken, and anticonvulsants may be ordered. Depending on the level of confusion, safety measures should be implemented. Emergency airway equipment should be at the bedside. Surgery is the only successful form of treatment for a brain abscess, and residual disability is to be expected. The abscess may be drained through burr holes and antibiotics instilled, or the patient may undergo a craniotomy (p 42) to have the abscess excised. The goal is to remove the entire abscess in its capsule, although that is not always possible. Large doses of antibiotics are given both pre- and postoperatively.

E. Patient and family teaching should include the possibility of residual symptoms and need for rehabilitation. Neurologic deficits after surgery may include hemiparesis, seizures, visual deficits, cranial nerve palsies, and learning disorders in children and adolescents. Nurses should emphasize safety measures and compliance with the medication regimen. Referral to community agencies is also recommended.

References

Brunner LS, Suddarth DS. The Lippincott manual of nursing practice. 4th ed. Philadelphia: JB Lippincott, 1986.

Luckmann J, Sorensen KC. Medical-surgical nursing. 3rd ed. Philadelphia: WB Saunders, 1987.

Thompson J, McFarland G, Hirsch J, Tucker S, Bruers A. Clinical nursing. St. Louis: CV Mosby, 1986.

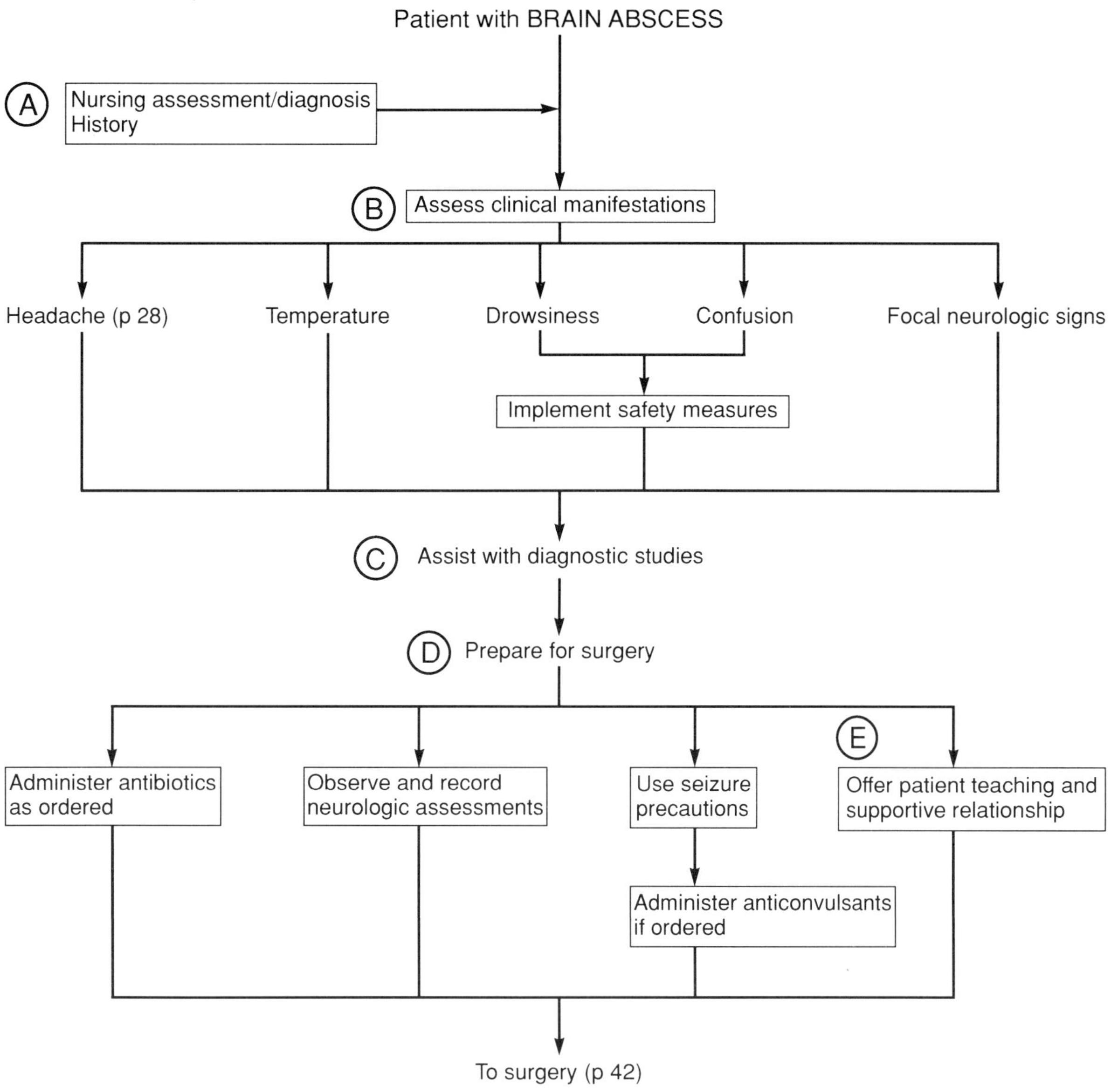
Patient with BRAIN ABSCESS
A
Nursing assessment/diagnosis
History
B
Assess clinical manifestations
Headache (p 28)
Temperature
Drowsiness
Confusion
Focal neurologic signs
Implement safety measures
C
Assist with diagnostic studies
D
Prepare for surgery
E
Administer antibiotics as ordered
Observe and record neurologic assessments
Use seizure precautions
Offer patient teaching and supportive relationship
Administer anticonvulsants if ordered
To surgery (p 42)

GUILLAIN-BARRÉ SYNDROME

Barbara Kalo

Guillain-Barré syndrome or infectious polyneuritis is an acute inflammation of the peripheral and cranial nerves and ganglia. The cause is unknown, but is thought to be an allergic or immunologic reaction preceded by an infection. The syndrome is not prevalent in one particular sex and affects adults of all ages. Signs and symptoms may range from minor to severe weakness.

A. The initial nursing assessment includes a history of the onset of symptoms and the course they have taken. Part of the history will include a previous infection. A sudden onset of flaccid weakness with paresthesia, beginning in the lower extremities and progressing upward, is indicative of Guillain-Barré syndrome. It is thought that the antibodies produced when an infection occurs leads to demyelination. Determine if the symptoms occurred and progressed in an ascending pattern.

B. Continual monitoring and assessment of the clinical manifestations is necessary. Muscle weakness varies widely in severity and usually begins in the lower extremities with symmetric distribution. As the weakness ascends, monitor and assess the patient's respirations and ability to swallow. Distal paresthesia, or abnormal sensations with heightened sensitivity and pain with any sensation, is another common symptom. The patient may have neuropathic or radicular pain, resulting in difficulty in chewing, swallowing, and talking. Loss of sensation and sphincter disturbances of bladder and rectum may also be present.

C. There is no conclusive diagnostic test to confirm the diagnosis of Guillain-Barré, but several tests can exclude other diseases, such as myasthenia gravis (p 18), poliomyelitis (p 36), botulism, and tick paralysis. Electromyography (EMG) and nerve conduction velocity studies show muscles that are weak from denervation or neuromuscular block, and nerve conduction velocity is reduced. EMG patterns also show repetitive firing of the same motor unit. Repeated lumbar punctures may be necessary throughout the course of the disease. The cerebrospinal fluid protein level may be normal at onset, but rises as the disease progresses. An elevated protein level with a normal pressure and cell count is characteristic of Guillain-Barré syndrome. Explain the studies to alleviate the patient's fears and ensure cooperation.

D. Supportive nursing care and close observation of the symptoms are indicated to prevent or treat complications. Some complications that may be seen are respiratory failure, vascular collapse, pulmonary emboli (p 116), hypertension (pp 80,124), and cardiac arrhythmias (p 52). Respiratory distress is paramount and may necessitate a tracheostomy and/or ventilator support. Notify the physician if the patient begins shallow breathing or irregular or labored breathing. Arterial blood gas (ABG) determinations and pulmonary function tests are performed. Frequent suctioning is necessary if the patient needs a tracheostomy or endotracheal tube.

E. Monitor vital signs frequently to detect development of a complication or worsening of the disease.

F. The neurologic status requires close observation to detect spinal cord involvement. Motor loss is greater than sensory loss in Guillain-Barré syndrome.

G. Well-balanced nutritious meals should be provided for proper functioning of every body system. Report weight loss to the physician to prevent wasting of muscles and decreasing strength of extremities. When a patient has difficulty chewing and/or swallowing, tube feedings and intravenous (IV) fluids are instituted.

H. Impaired physical mobility and poor nutritional status may lead to skin breakdown. Frequent turning, repositioning, and keeping the patient's skin clean and dry are important aspects of care. Assess the body's pressure points for redness when repositioning the patient.

I. Range of motion exercises and physical therapy are necessary to prevent contractures, strengthen muscles, and maintain joint flexion. Report overexertion to the physician, because this increases the demyelination and extends the paralysis. Too rigorous exercise may dislocate a weak joint and may also burn more calories than are taken in.

J. Recovery is usually spontaneous and occurs within 6 to 18 months. Care after discharge includes physical therapy, possibly speech therapy, and continued visits with vocational and psychiatric counselors. Rehabilitation is a slow process; approximately one patient in 10 is left with muscle weakness.

References

Brunner LS, Suddarth DS. The Lippincott manual of nursing practice. 4th ed. Philadelphia: JB Lippincott, 1986.

Brunner LS, Suddarth DS, eds. Textbook of medical-surgical nursing. 6th ed. Philadelphia: JB Lippincott, 1988.

Crabbe RA. Neurologic problems: Guillain-Barré syndrome. In: Goldberg K, ed. Nurse review. Springhouse, PA: Springhouse Corporation, 1986: 104–106.

Samonds RJ. Guillain-Barré syndrome: helping the patient in the acute stage. Nursing 80 1980; 10(8):35–41.

Thompson JM, McFarland GK, Hirsch JE, Tucker SM, Bowers AC. Clinical nursing. St. Louis: CV Mosby, 1986.

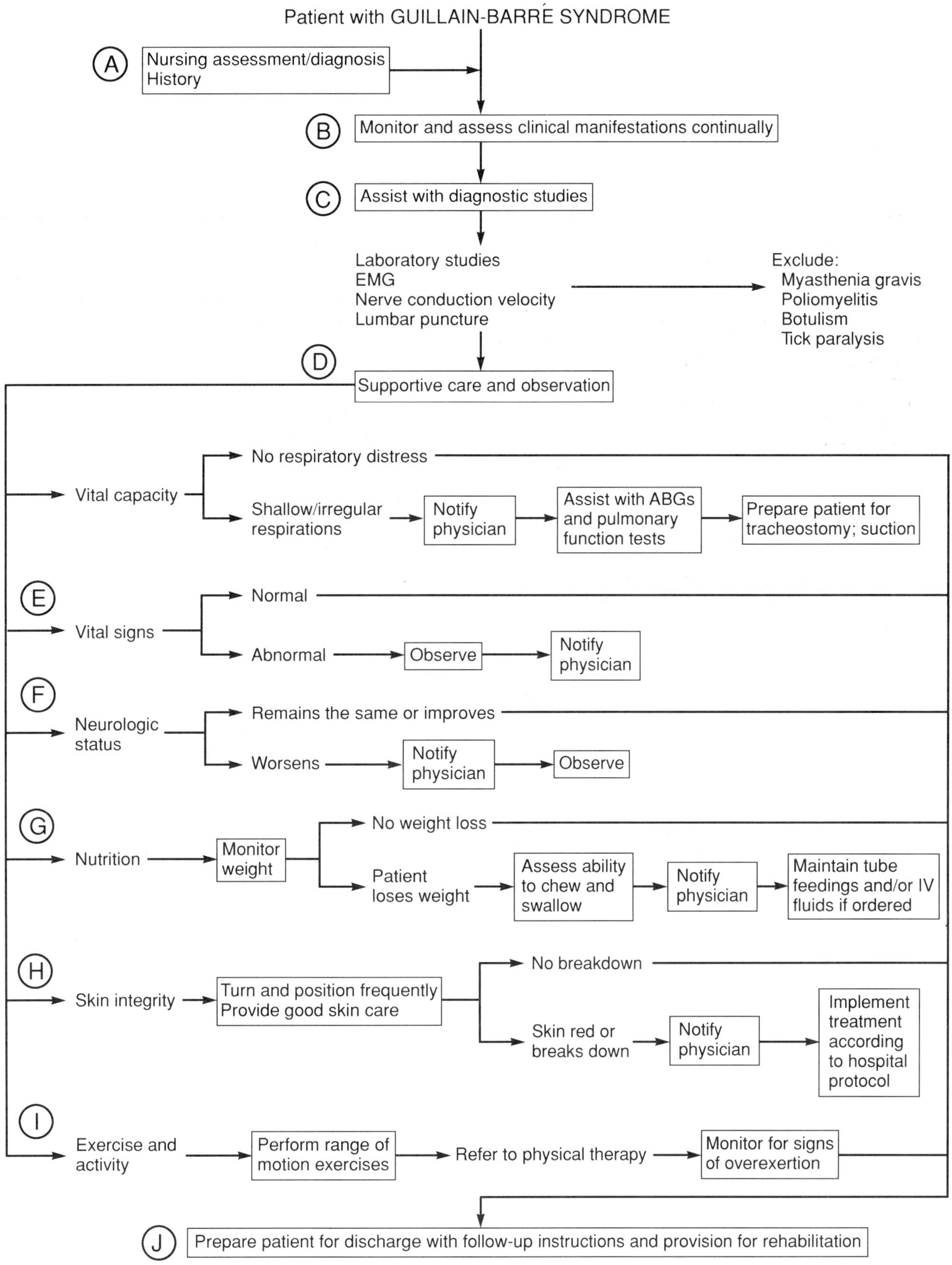
Patient with GUILLAIN-BARRÉ SYNDROME
A
Nursing assessment/diagnosis
History
B
Monitor and assess clinical manifestations continually
C
Assist with diagnostic studies
Laboratory studies
EMG
Nerve conduction velocity
Lumbar puncture
Exclude:
Myasthenia gravis
Poliomyelitis
Botulism
Tick paralysis
D
Supportive care and observation
Vital capacity
No respiratory distress
Shallow/irregular respirations
Notify physician
Assist with ABGs and pulmonary function tests
Prepare patient for tracheostomy; suction
E
Vital signs
Normal
Abnormal
Observe
Notify physician
F
Neurologic status
Remains the same or improves
Worsens
Notify physician
Observe
G
Nutrition
Monitor weight
No weight loss
Patient loses weight
Assess ability to chew and swallow
Notify physician
Maintain tube feedings and/or IV fluids if ordered
H
Skin integrity
Turn and position frequently
Provide good skin care
No breakdown
Skin red or breaks down
Notify physician
Implement treatment according to hospital protocol
I
Exercise and activity
Perform range of motion exercises
Refer to physical therapy
Monitor for signs of overexertion
J
Prepare patient for discharge with follow-up instructions and provision for rehabilitation

TRIGEMINAL NEURALGIA

Barbara Kalo

Trigeminal neuralgia (tic douloureux) is a nerve disorder affecting the fifth cranial nerve. The trigeminal nerve is both a sensory and motor nerve, but only the sensory branches (maxillary and mandibular) are involved in this disorder. The cause of trigeminal neuralgia is unknown, but it is thought that (1) the nerve is compressed by blood vessels, (2) demyelinating plaques occur, or (3) herpesvirus may be the responsible factor. This disorder affects 2 percent of the population, usually at 50 to 60 years of age, and is more common in women. The patient experiences sudden, severe attacks of facial pain, twitching, grimacing, and frequent blinking and tearing of the eye. The attacks occur without warning in one or more branches of the trigeminal nerve, usually unilaterally, and pain radiates from the angle of the jaw.

A. Assessing the nature of attacks, triggering factors, and pain management techniques is indicated. The sudden attacks last 2 to 3 minutes and recurrences are unpredictable. The remissions decrease as the patient ages. Because the nerve disorder affects one's entire lifestyle, it is important to assess the nutritional status, hygiene, and behavior of the patient.

B. Diganostic tests such as a computerized tomographic (CT) scan and arteriography may be done to rule out disorders of the brain and vascular problems. Explain the diagnostic procedures to alleviate the patient's fears.

C. The drugs most frequently used are the antiepileptic drugs Dilantin and Tegretol. They help to relieve the pain and delay the attacks. One of the concerns in administering narcotics is the possibility of addiction.

D. Providing comfort involves environmental management to decrease the triggering stimuli. A room free of drafts with an even, moderate temperature is preferable. Usually, the patient prefers self-care, especially for personal hygiene, because the ministrations of others may trigger an attack.

E. As the disorder progresses and the attacks become more frequent, the patient may consent to surgical intervention. Two of the most common operations are percutaneous radiofrequency rhizotomy and microvascular decompression. Nursing care is the same as for the patient with a craniotomy (p 42).

F. When the symptoms are relieved and a specific plan of treatment is devised, the patient is discharged with instructions regarding low doses of medications and the side effects. Keeping the environmental stimuli at moderate levels is advised.

References

Brunner LS, Suddarth DS. The Lippincott manual of nursing practice. 4th ed. Philadelphia: JB Lippincott, 1986.

Brunner LS, Suddarth DS, eds. Textbook of medical-surgical nursing. 6th ed. Philadelphia: JB Lippincott, 1988.

Krupp MA, Chatton MJ, Werdegar D, eds. Current medical diagnosis and treatment. Los Altos, CA: Lange, 1985.

Lewis SM, Collier IC. Medical-surgical nursing: assessment and management of clinical problems. New York: McGraw-Hill, 1983.

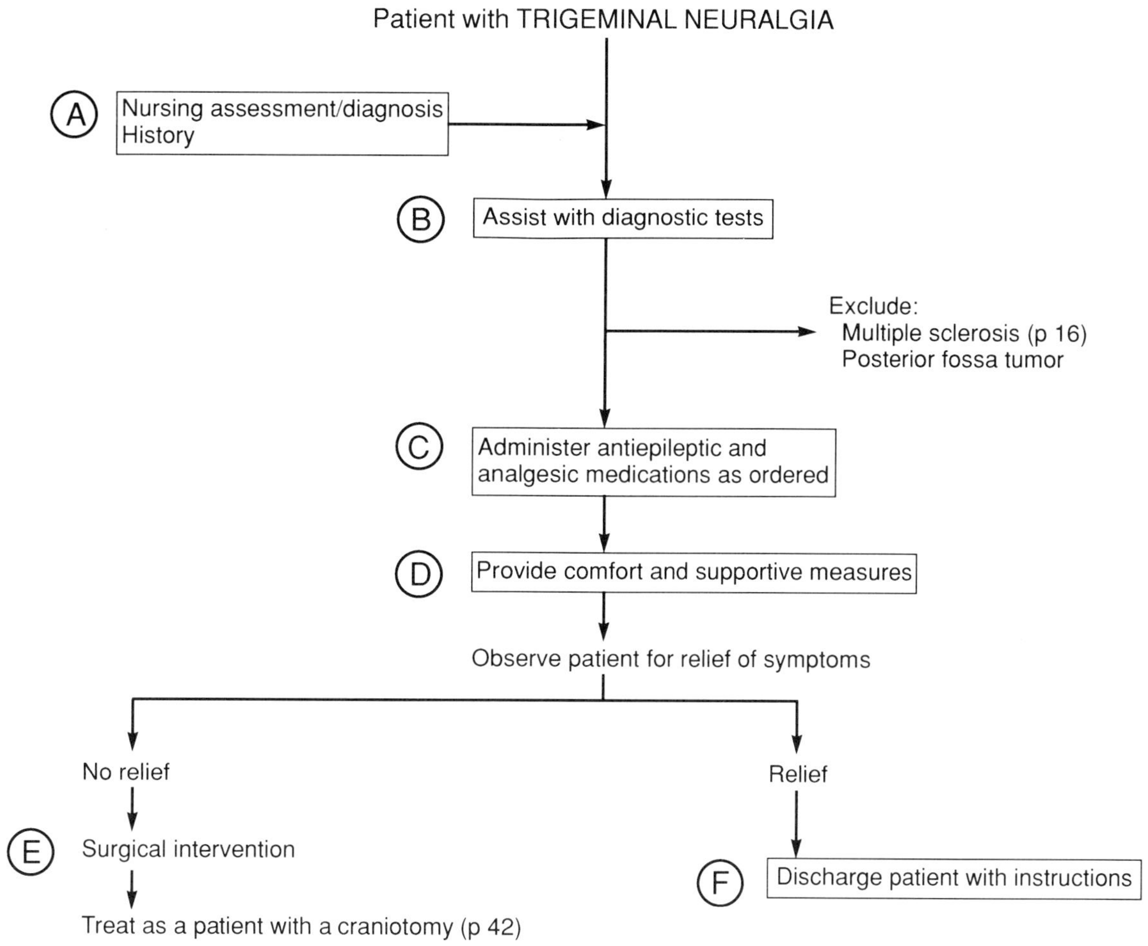

Patient with TRIGEMINAL NEURALGIA
A
Nursing assessment/diagnosis
History
B
Assist with diagnostic tests
Exclude:
Multiple sclerosis (p 16)
Posterior fossa tumor
C
Administer antiepileptic and analgesic medications as ordered
D
Provide comfort and supportive measures
Observe patient for relief of symptoms
No relief
E
Surgical intervention
Treat as a patient with a craniotomy (p 42)
Relief
F
Discharge patient with instructions

AMYOTROPHIC LATERAL SCLEROSIS

Kathy Gilliland

Amyotrophic lateral sclerosis (ALS, Lou Gehrig's disease) is a progressive degenerative disease with a prognosis of death 3 to 5 years after onset. There are three primary types of motor neuron disease that are classified according to the signs and symptoms. One type may be dominant, but manifestations of the others complicate the disease process. The degenerative process affects the motor neurons of the cerebral hemispheres, the brain stem, and the motor fiber tracts of the lateral and ventral spinal cord. The disease is sparing of the sensory neurons and fiber tracts.

A. The etiology of ALS is unknown; however, theories of cause remain under investigation, namely autoimmune disease, slow viral infection, vitamin deficiencies, enzyme abnormality, and genetic predisposition. ALS is more common in men and is usually seen in patients in their 50s.

B. The majority of patients diagnosed with ALS have few presenting symptoms. Patients may complain of dropping things and feeling awkward with fine motor skills. Many times minor afflictions are bothersome and not investigated until they become disabling. Progressive bulbar palsies involving the motor nuclei of the midbrain, pons, and medulla manifest associated tongue-tiring when talking, dysarthria, difficulty swallowing, facial muscle twitching, and facial muscle atrophy. Signs of primary lateral sclerosis include slow progressive hemiparesis with spasticity, hyperactive deep tendon reflexes (DTRs), and emotional lability. Progressive muscular atrophies present with symmetric upper extremity muscle wasting beginning at digits, decreased or absent DTRs, and generalized fasciculations. While exaggerated reflexes and muscle wasting are part of the progression of ALS, any of the manifestations of these motor neuron diseases may also be seen.

C. Diagnostic findings are based on history, neurologic examination, and laboratory studies. Enzyme levels usually reveal continuous elevation of serum creatine phosphokinase (CPK) and aldolase in 60 to 75 percent of all reported cases. Serum creatine levels are greatly increased. Electromyography (EMG) shows widespread fasciculations, patterns of denervation, and muscle wasting and atrophy. Peripheral nerve biopsies are almost always normal; however, muscle biopsies show atrophic muscle fibers. Cerebrospinal fluid is usually normal. Myelography (p 240) also shows no abnormalities but may be done to rule out treatable degenerative processes.

D. There remains no proven treatment, and care is centered on supportive and symptomatic measures. Antispasmodic drug therapy gives temporary assistance in patients with bulbar weakness and spasticity. Surgical therapy may include neurectomy to control effects of drug therapy and decrease spastic movements.

E. Patients with ALS are usually admitted to the hospital twice—once for diagnosis and again as the disease is at its final stage. Supportive care to maintain function and promote quality of life is the most important factor in dealing with the person with ALS. Patients should remain as active as possible. Splints and braces may be needed to assist with functioning as weakness increases due to paralysis and/or spasticity and mobility is impaired. ALS patients need assistance specifically related to impaired ability to chew and swallow and potential aspiration. Suction should be available. The patient may have involuntary outbursts of laughing or crying. Communication may become difficult. Alternative methods of communication may need to be developed. Families need caring support during this time. As the disease progresses, patients and families need to be advised about the potential development of respiratory failure. If the patient decides not to use a ventilator, a "living will" may be considered. Advise patient and family of support groups, such as the ALS Society of America and the Muscular Dystrophy Association.

References

American Association of Neuroscience Nursing. Core curriculum. Park Ridge, IL: AANN, 1980:511.

Luckmann J, Sorensen KC. Medical-surgical nursing: a psychophysiologic approach. 3rd ed. Philadelphia: WB Saunders, 1987.

Mulder DW, ed. The diagnosis and treatment of ALS. Boston: Houghton Mifflin, 1980.

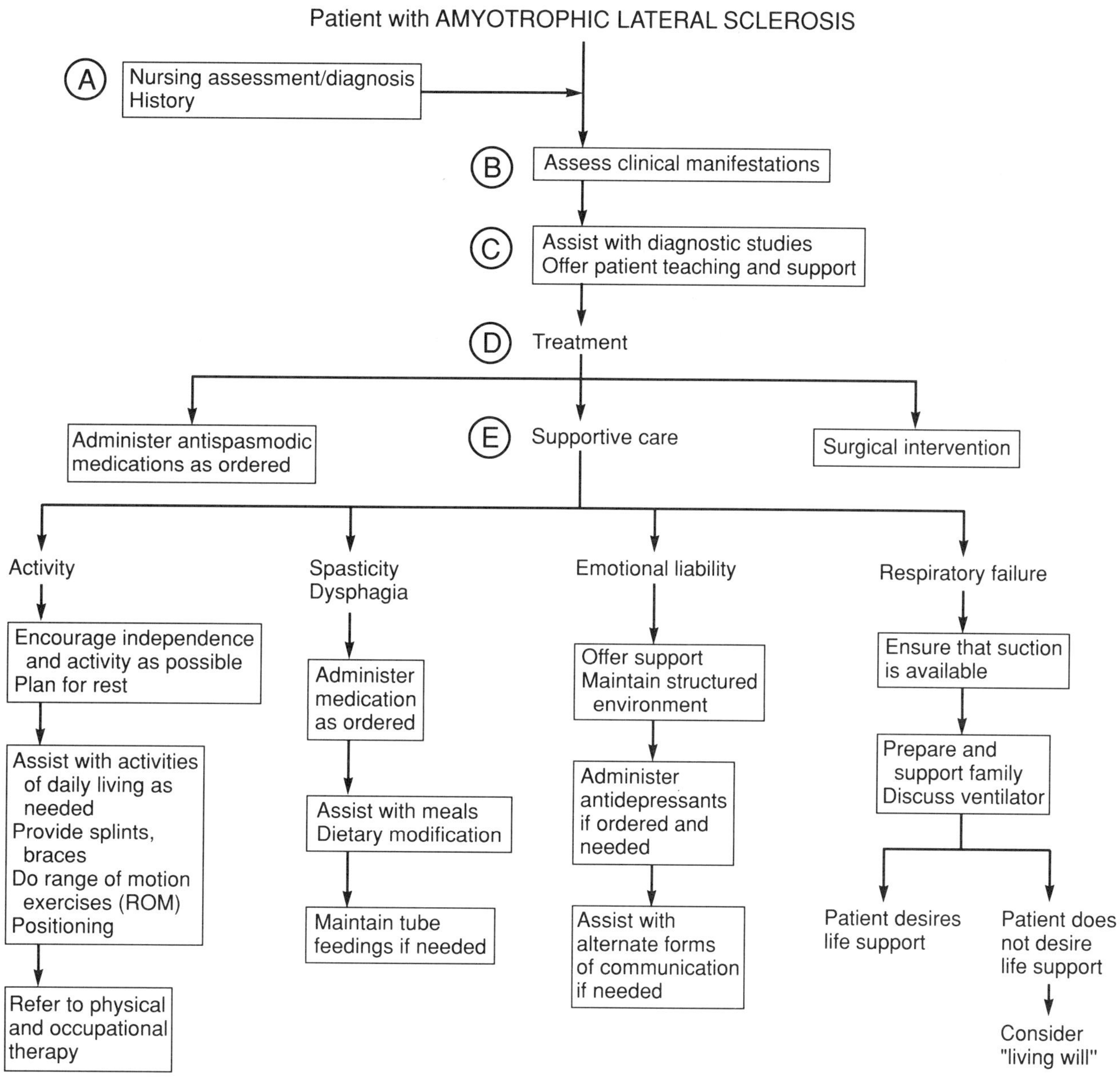
Patient with AMYOTROPHIC LATERAL SCLEROSIS
A
Nursing assessment/diagnosis
History
B
Assess clinical manifestations
C
Assist with diagnostic studies
Offer patient teaching and support
D
Treatment
Administer antispasmodic medications as ordered
E
Supportive care
Surgical intervention
Activity
Encourage independence and activity as possible
Plan for rest
Assist with activities of daily living as needed
Provide splints, braces
Do range of motion exercises (ROM)
Positioning
Refer to physical and occupational therapy
Spasticity
Dysphagia
Administer medication as ordered
Assist with meals
Dietary modification
Maintain tube feedings if needed
Emotional liability
Offer support
Maintain structured environment
Administer antidepressants if ordered and needed
Assist with alternate forms of communication if needed
Respiratory failure
Ensure that suction is available
Prepare and support family
Discuss ventilator
Patient desires life support
Patient does not desire life support
Consider "living will"

MULTIPLE SCLEROSIS

Joy Gorzeman

Multiple sclerosis (MS) is a demyelinating disorder of the central nervous system. The destruction of the fatty and protein material that ensheaths certain nerve fibers in the main spinal cord occurs in patches and results in disordered transmission of nerve impulses. MS is a chronic illness and the most common cause of progressive neurologic disability.

A. Although the cause of most demyelinating disorders is not known, current evidence suggests that an autoimmune basis along with genetic and geographic factors are related to MS. The incidence of MS is highest in cool, temperate climates. MS affects women almost twice as often as men, with the usual age of onset between 20 and 40 years. The onset of MS varies: symptoms may develop quickly or over several months. Lesions of MS are scattered throughout the brain and spinal cord, so signs and symptoms vary and are related to the location and areas of demyelinization.

B. Early signs and symptoms include weakness, sensory disturbances, paresthesias in one or more limbs, visual disturbances, unsteady gait, and incoordination. Most patients who have had MS for many years exhibit Charcot's triad: (1) nystagmus, (2) intention tremor, and (3) scanning speech (slow enunciation and hesitation before a word or syllable). Other clinical manifestations include emotional lability and bladder dysfunction, such as neurogenic bladder, retention, and incontinence. MS patients are often depressed and irritable. Extensive involvement of the white matter of the frontal lobes may cause them to be euphoric. In the late stages of the disease, most MS patients experience partial or complete paralysis of the lower extremities and become totally debilitated.

C. Diagnosis of MS is usually made on clinical presentation. If further testing is necessary, cerebrospinal fluid (CSF) examination may be helpful. Usually, the gamma globulin content is elevated.

D. The clinical course of MS is characterized by remissions and exacerbations, which may be precipitated by infection, trauma, and pregnancy. As the disease progresses, the remissions become shorter and the exacerbations more severe. The usual duration of the disease is about 20 years. There is no cure for MS. Care is basically symptomatic and individual. The patient should stay as active and functional as possible. The goal is to relieve the patient's symptoms and offer support during acute episodes and remissions, and to assist in the management of chronic neurologic disabilities. In general, the MS patient should avoid overwork and fatigue. A regular daily schedule of activity that includes rest and relaxation should be established. A well-balanced diet and plenty of fresh air and sunshine are advised. The MS patient should maintain social contacts and remain active as long as possible.

E. It is extremely important to involve the patient's family and to help them understand the stresses of MS and problems associated with the illness. Support groups, such as the National Multiple Sclerosis Society, are available.

References

Berkow R, ed. The Merck manual. 19th ed. Rahway, NJ: Merck, Sharp and Dohme, 1981.

Brunner LS, Suddarth DS. The Lippincott manual of nursing practice. 4th ed. Philadelphia: JB Lippincott, 1986.

Luckmann J, Sorensen KC. Medical-surgical nursing. 3rd ed. WB Saunders, 1987.

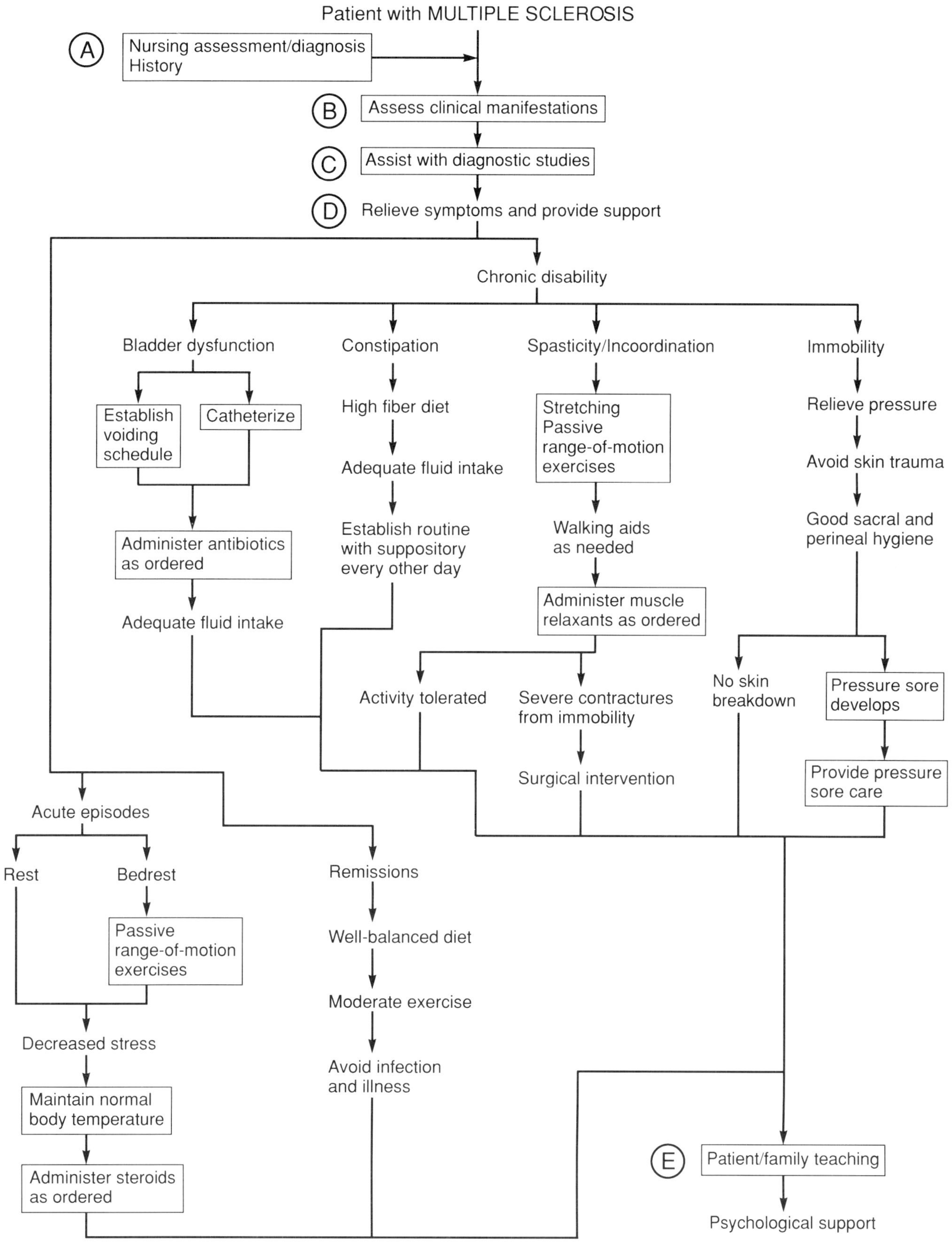
Patient with MULTIPLE SCLEROSIS
A
Nursing assessment/diagnosis
History
B
Assess clinical manifestations
C
Assist with diagnostic studies
D
Relieve symptoms and provide support
Chronic disability
Bladder dysfunction
Establish voiding schedule
Catheterize
Administer antibiotics as ordered
Adequate fluid intake
Constipation
High fiber diet
Adequate fluid intake
Establish routine with suppository every other day
Spasticity/Incoordination
Stretching
Passive range-of-motion exercises
Walking aids as needed
Administer muscle relaxants as ordered
Activity tolerated
Severe contractures from immobility
Surgical intervention
Immobility
Relieve pressure
Avoid skin trauma
Good sacral and perineal hygiene
No skin breakdown
Pressure sore develops
Provide pressure sore care
Acute episodes
Rest
Bedrest
Passive range-of-motion exercises
Decreased stress
Maintain normal body temperature
Administer steroids as ordered
Remissions
Well-balanced diet
Moderate exercise
Avoid infection and illness
E
Patient/family teaching
Psychological support

MYASTHENIA GRAVIS

William B. Marshall
Carol Bowdoin

Myasthenia gravis is characterized by easy fatigability of voluntary muscles, especially the facial, ocular, lingual, and swallowing muscles. Activities precipitate weakness, and as the condition worsens, lesser amounts of activity are required to bring about muscle weakness. The muscles usually regain strength after rest.

A. The exact etiology of myasthenia gravis is unknown, but the following factors have been known to precipitate a crisis: alcohol intake (p 402), menses, influenza virus (p 118), anxiety, psychological stress, and medications such as barbiturates, narcotics, quinidine, procainamide, and some tranquilizers. There is evidence that myasthenia gravis is an autoimmune disorder, and it may be accompanied by a thymoma. The disease is characterized by remissions and exacerbations. It is most common in people between 20 and 30 years of age.

B. Clinical manifestations are caused by muscle weakness. The development of symptoms is insidious, and progression of the disease is slow. Nursing assessment focuses on voluntary muscles, respiratory muscles, and dysfunctional cranial nerves that may cause ptosis, diplopia, dysmasesis, and dysphagia.

C. Ocular muscles are the first involved. Resting the eye by patching bilaterally may prevent headaches or disorientation brought about by double vision.

D. Dysmasesis (difficulty chewing) and dysphagia (difficulty swallowing) develop as myasthenia gravis progresses. Voice rest and soft or pureed foods may need to be instituted. A weighted feeding tube (such as the Dobhoff or Entriflex) may be placed instead of the standard nasogastric tube.

E. Chewing, swallowing, and handling saliva may become difficult, creating a danger of aspiration. A tonsil suction setup should be at the bedside.

F. Rest to decrease fatigue is an important nursing measure. Passive exercises will maintain muscle tone without increasing weakness.

G. Respiratory effort may also be compromised, leading to decreased vital capacity and dyspnea. Respiratory complications are a frequent cause of death in these patients, warranting close nursing observation.

H. Vital capacity (VC) can be measured at the bedside with a spirometer. Normal VC for an average 70-kg male is approximately 1,000 ml. A baseline VC is essential to monitor trends. Decreasing VC may be noted before anxiety, dyspnea, or arterial blood gas (ABG) changes are noted.

I. Position changes have been shown to help stabilize or even increase VC.

J. Obtain ABGs to monitor both acid-base balance and oxygenation of tissues. With a diminished respiratory effort hypoventilation will occur, increasing the $PaCO_2$ to greater than 45 mm Hg (normal 35–45 mm Hg), and pH will decrease to less than 7.35 (normal 7.35 to 7.45). PaO_2 may drop below 80 mm Hg (normal 80 to 100 mm Hg), and oxygen saturation (O_2 Sat) may be below 95 percent (normal 95 to 100 percent).

K. Oxygen therapy may be instituted, with the goal of keeping the PaO_2 above 80 mm Hg and the oxygen saturation above 95 percent, as measured by the ABGs.

L. Endotracheal intubation may become necessary in the unstable patient. The nurse should be prepared to assist with intubation and mechanical ventilation. Familiarity with laryngoscope, endotracheal tube, and Ambu Bag before the need for intubation is paramount. The patient will be transferred to the ICU for further care.

M. Diagnosis of myasthenia gravis is confirmed with the intravenous (IV) administration of Tensilon (edrophonium chloride) 2 mg. Within 45 seconds there should be a change in muscle strength. If no change occurs after 1 minute, another 3 to 5 mg of Tensilon may be given and repeated again after another minute, for a total dosage of 10 mg. If muscle strength increases, myasthenic crisis is diagnosed. A longer-acting anticholinesterase medication should be instituted. If muscle strength decreases, cholinergic crisis is diagnosed. All anticholinesterase medications should be withheld. The effects of Tensilon last approximately 5 minutes. Respiratory depression caused by Tensilon can be reversed by the administration of atropine, 1 mg IV. Equipment to facilitate suctioning and endotracheal intubation should be at the bedside prior to administering Tensilon.

N. Upon stabilization and regulation of medications, the patient is prepared for discharge. Teaching includes specific instructions for anticholinesterase medications; avoidance of over-the-counter drugs; use of a Medic Alert tag; need to avoid alcohol, tobacco, and prolonged exposure to heat, cold, or other stressors; activity and rest guidelines; and symptoms of progression or recurrence that should be reported to the physician.

References

Campbell VG. Neurologic system. In: Thompson JM, McFarland GK, Hirsch JE, Tucker SM, Bowers AC, eds. Clinical nursing. St. Louis: CV Mosby, 1986:343–345.

Noroian EL. Myasthenia gravis. A nursing perspective. J Neurosci Nurs 1986; 18:74.

Price SA, Wilson LM. Pathophysiology: clinical concepts of disease processes. New York: McGraw-Hill, 1986.

Slonim NB, Hamilton LH. Respiratory physiology. St. Louis: CV Mosby, 1981.

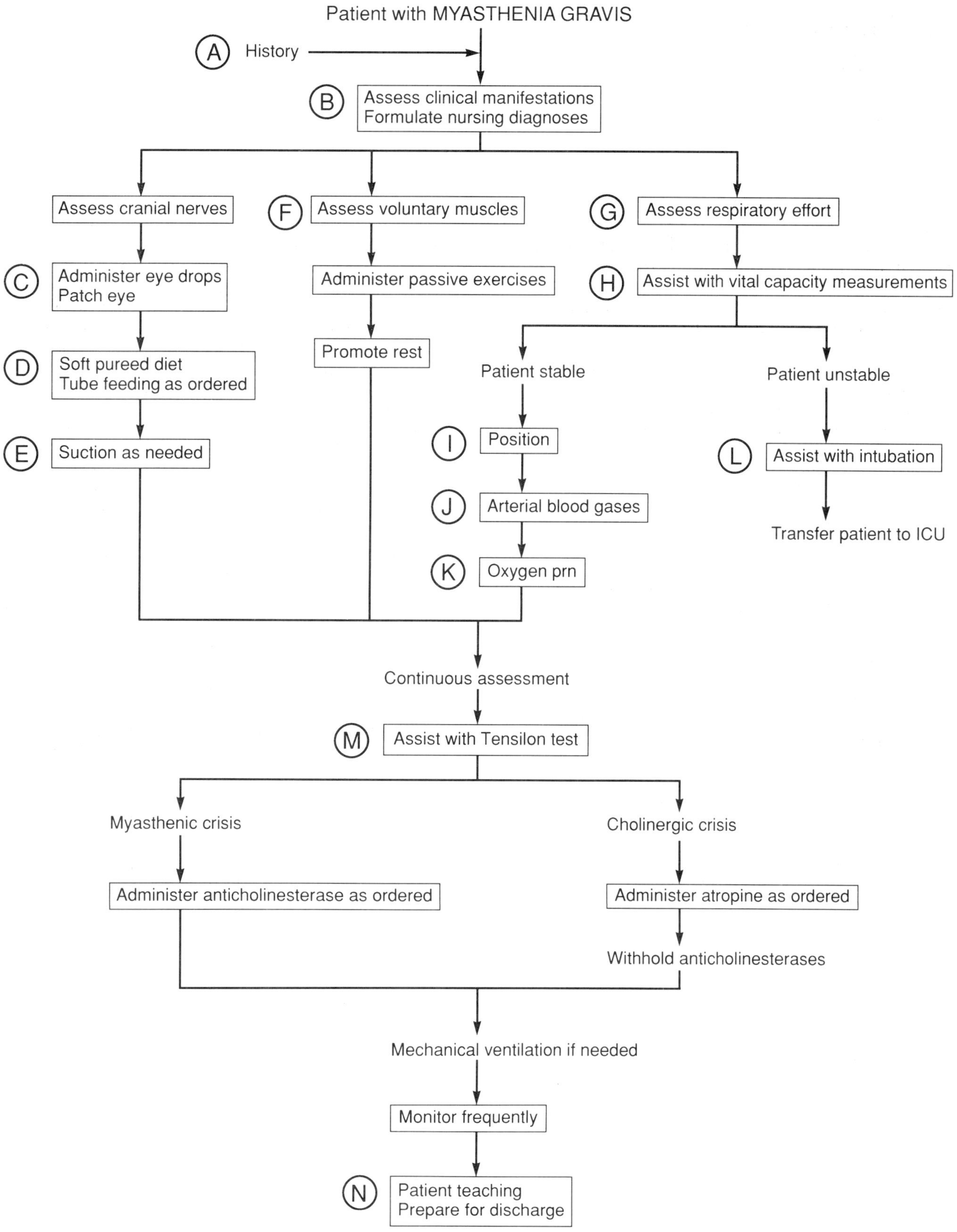
Patient with MYASTHENIA GRAVIS
A
History
B
Assess clinical manifestations
Formulate nursing diagnoses
Assess cranial nerves
F
Assess voluntary muscles
G
Assess respiratory effort
C
Administer eye drops
Patch eye
Administer passive exercises
H
Assist with vital capacity measurements
D
Soft pureed diet
Tube feeding as ordered
Promote rest
Patient stable
Patient unstable
E
Suction as needed
I
Position
L
Assist with intubation
J
Arterial blood gases
Transfer patient to ICU
K
Oxygen prn
Continuous assessment
M
Assist with Tensilon test
Myasthenic crisis
Cholinergic crisis
Administer anticholinesterase as ordered
Administer atropine as ordered
Withhold anticholinesterases
Mechanical ventilation if needed
Monitor frequently
N
Patient teaching
Prepare for discharge

CEREBRAL ANEURYSM

Diane M. Zintak

A cerebral aneurysm is a localized dilatation of an artery resulting from a weakness in the arterial wall. It may remain silent, it may dilate causing pressure on adjacent areas, or it may rupture and result in subarachnoid hemorrhage, with a 28 percent immediate mortality rate. Usually an aneurysm causes no symptoms until it bursts.

A. Typically the onset is explosive with a sudden, severe generalized headache (p 28), nausea and vomiting, and some degree of loss of consciousness. As blood accumulates in the subarachnoid space, meningeal irritation causes neck stiffness, pain down the back and into the legs, temperature elevation, restlessness, confusion, visual disturbances, cranial nerve dysfunction, and seizures (p 30). More specific symptoms will be determined by the exact location of the aneurysm.

B. Because *rupture of a cerebral aneurysm is a life-threatening situation,* carefully evaluate the patient and maintain airway, breathing, and circulation (ABCs) as necessary. Immediately insert an intravenous (IV) line so that emergency drugs can be administered as ordered.

C. Once the patient's condition has stabilized, the highest priority is to identify and control increased intracranial pressure (ICP). The patient must be continually monitored for symptoms of increased ICP, which include a change in level of consciousness, elevation of systolic blood pressure, widening pulse pressure, a slowing pulse rate, impaired pupillary reflex, and changes in motor or sensory function. ICP monitoring can be directly accomplished by ventriculostomy and introduction of a cannula attached to a pressure transducer. A drainage bag can also be attached and used to drain excess fluid, if necessary. Other measures such as fluid restriction and the use of steroids and osmotic diuretics can aid in the control of increased ICP.

D. The patient remains in danger of two life-threatening complications: rebleeding and vasospasm. After the initial bleed a clot seals over the rupture and reinforces the aneurysm. However, as the clot undergoes the natural lytic process, most commonly occurring from the third to eleventh day, chances of rebleeding from the same site arise. In addition, arterial vasospasm, a severe constriction or narrowing of vessels adjacent to the ruptured aneurysm, always is a potential threat. This vasospasm can cause ischemia or infarction of the cerebral tissue supplied by the vessel. Both rebleeding and vasospasm are characterized by deterioration in neurologic function with an alteration in level of consciousness and an increase in the severity of headache. Therefore, diligent assessment of the patient's neurologic status and vital signs will aid in the identification of these two complications.

E. Since hemorrhage can recur any time after the initial bleed, aneurysm precautions must be taken to minimize this risk. The patient is placed in a calm, quiet environment with dim lights and decreased stimuli so that blood pressure stays low. The head of the bed should be elevated 30 degrees to promote drainage. All basic care should be performed for the patient to prevent exertion that would raise blood pressure. The patient should be turned and encouraged to deep breathe, but warned not to cough or sneeze, as this would increase ICP. Stool softeners are given to avoid straining. The patient may be sedated to decrease restlessness, but since it is essential to be able to assess the patient's neurologic status, oversedation must be avoided. Visitors are generally limited unless they promote a calming effect on the patient. Lastly, seizure precautions are initiated, as seizure activity frequently occurs after an aneurysm bleed.

F. A lumbar puncture that reveals bloody spinal fluid is indicative of an aneurysm bleeding into the subarachnoid space, but it cannot reveal the location. Cerebral arteriography will pinpoint the exact location of the aneurysm and will therefore contribute to the definitive treatment plan. In addition, computed tomography (CT), magnetic resonance imaging (MRI), skull films, electroencephalography (EEG), and/or a brain scan may also be done.

G. As surgical intervention for the patient with a ruptured aneurysm is often delayed until after the patient's initial injury has stabilized, medical management is frequently initiated. Steroids and osmotic diuretics are given carefully to maintain blood pressure at a level so as not to burst the wall of an already weakened aneurysm. However, blood pressure must not be allowed to drop so low that inadequate perfusion of the brain results in hypoxic damage. An antifibrinolytic drug (Amicar) is given to prevent rebleeding by minimizing destruction of the clot that formed over the initial rupture. Phenobarbital is frequently given, for both its sedative and anticonvulsant effects.

H. For aneurysm patients, surgical intervention is the only sure method to prevent a rebleed. The main procedures used, depending on the location and type of aneurysm, are clipping, wrapping, ligation, embolization, or gradual clamping.

References

Bruenig KA. Ruptured cerebral aneurysm. In: Williams S, McVan B, eds. Coping with neurologic problems proficiently. 2nd ed. Springhouse, PA: Springhouse Corporation, 1984:71–80.

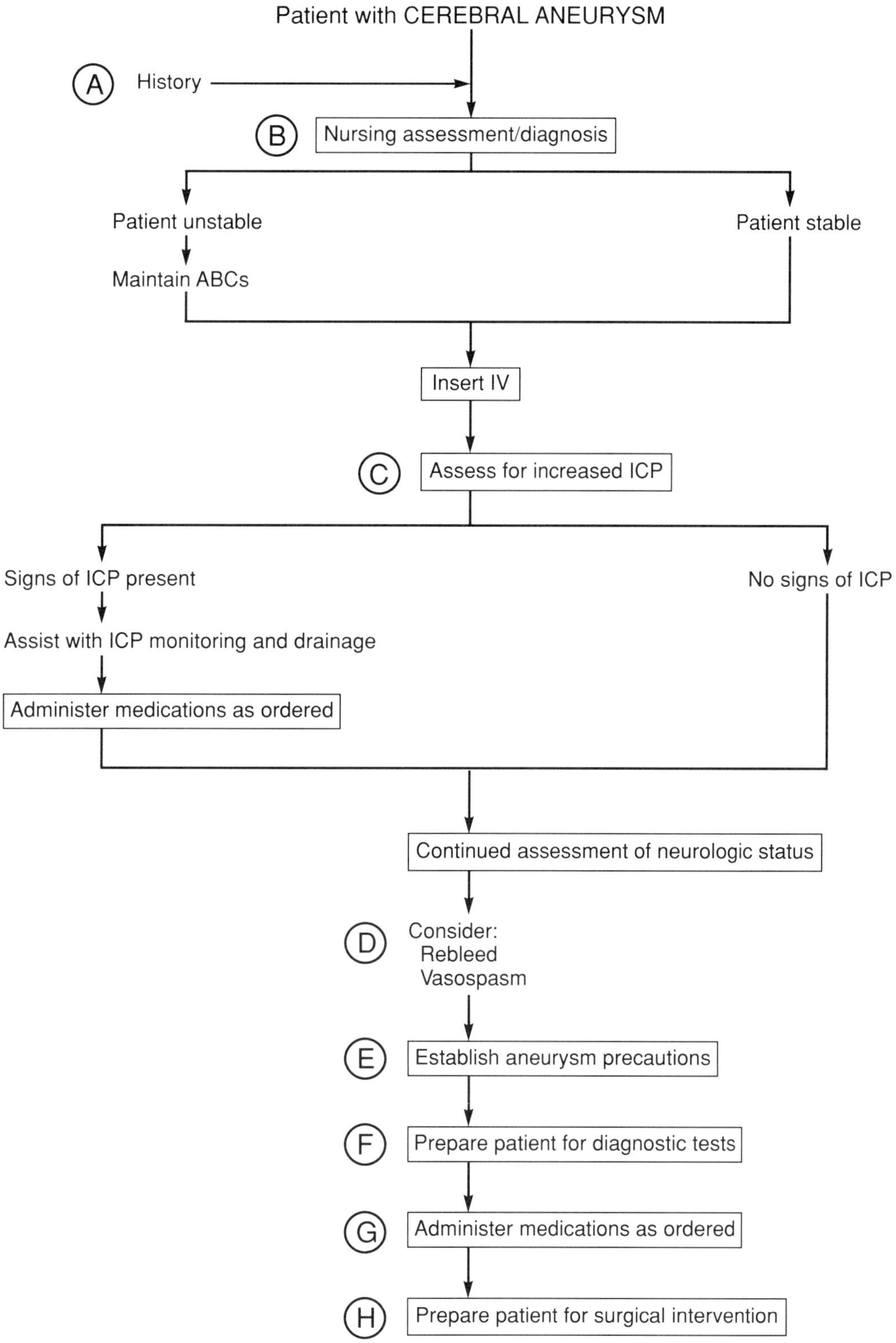

Bubb DI. Neurologic problems. Oradell, NJ: Medical Economics Books, 1984:118–122.

Hartshorn JC. Aneurysm! Keeping your patient alive until surgery. RN 1984; 47:30–33.

Raimond J, Taylor JW. Neurological emergencies: effective nursing care. Rockville, MD: Aspen, 1986:255–260.

Thompson J, MacFarland G, Hirsch J, Tucker S, Bowers A. Clinical nursing. St. Louis: CV Mosby Company, 1986.

STROKE

Diane M. Zintak

Stroke, or cerebrovascular accident (CVA), occurs when rupture or obstruction of an artery sharply reduces blood supply to a portion of the brain, resulting in ischemia of the area of the brain normally perfused by the damaged vessels (see Fig. 1). The specific signs and symptoms of a stroke are determined by the area and extent of the damage.

A. During the initial 24 to 48 hours after a stroke, frequent, thorough patient assessment is essential. Begin with an evaluation of vital signs, especially blood pressure, as hypertension (p 80) is the main factor that may predispose an individual to stroke. A careful assessment of neurologic status (p 42) including level of consciousness, pupil size and reaction to light, response to stimulation, and motor and sensory function must be completed, making special note of the type, location, and degree of any deficits. This will provide the baseline for assessing the patient's subsequent progress.

B. The patient or family should be questioned about the history, onset, and duration of any current symptoms, as well as any presence of weakness, tingling, numbness, dizziness, fainting, or speech or visual disturbances that have occurred in the past. The patient should also be evaluated for the presence of any predisposing factors such as diabetes mellitus (p 176), obesity, elevated serum cholesterol levels, cigarette smoking, use of oral contraceptives, heart disease, and sedentary lifestyle.

C. A transient ischemic attack (TIA) produces a focal neurologic deficit caused by localized cerebral ischemia that resolves before tissue necrosis occurs. The most frequent symptoms are visual disturbances, tingling or numbness in arms or feet, dizziness, or falling. These symptoms can last from a few minutes to hours and generally resolve completely within 24 hours. Such attacks are often a prelude to a stroke and can be experienced any number of times.

D. Symptoms similar to those of a TIA, but possibly more severe, may last for up to 2 weeks, after which the patient may recover completely. This is known as a reversible ischemic neurologic deficit (RIND) and occurs when collateral circulation makes up the oxygen deficit to tissues before necrosis occurs. A computed tomographic (CT) scan will reveal small areas of cerebral infarction.

E. The stroke-in-evolution, whether thrombotic, embolic, or hemorrhagic in origin, is an *emergency* leading to motor and sensory deficits that develop and worsen over hours or days, culminating in a cerebral infarction. This can be a *life-threatening situation*. Therefore, immediate stroke treatment aims to restore circulation to the patient's brain as quickly as possible while trying to minimize complications.

F. Ensure that the patient has a clear functioning airway. The patient's decreased level of consciousness, altered gag and swallow reflexes, or inability to control secretions can cause him to aspirate or develop other respiratory problems. Position the patient on his side or in a high Fowler's position to promote lung expansion and drainage of secretions. Have suction equipment available for emergency use. Keep in mind that patients whose respiratory centers have been damaged may need to be intubated.

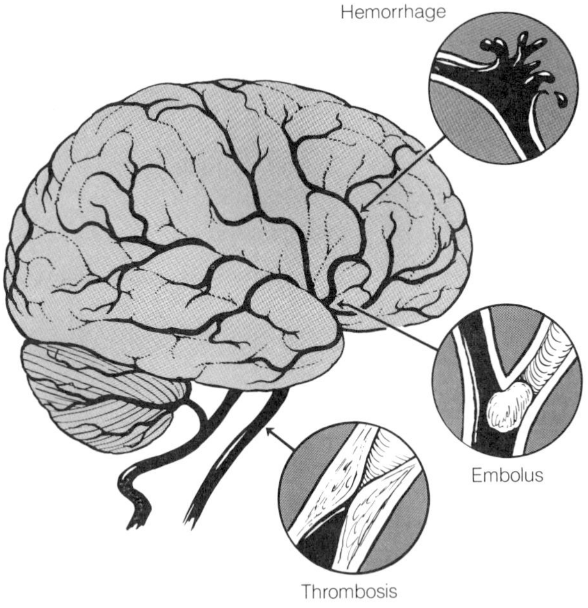

Figure 1 Causes of stroke.

G. Patients are generally given supplemental oxygen therapy to compensate for reduced cerebral perfusion. Arterial blood gas measurements should be frequently evaluated for effectiveness of oxygenation.

H. Assess the patient's hemodynamic status. If the patient's blood pressure is elevated, raise the head of the bed at least 30 degrees. This will reduce intracranial pressure (ICP) and reduce the tendency to hemorrhage. In addition, antihypertensive medication, frequently intravenous (IV) nitroprusside, will be given to bring the blood pressure down. However, this must be carefully done, as too great a drop in blood pressure can increase ischemia by reducing cerebral perfusion. If the blood pressure is low, lay the patient flat to increase cerebral perfusion. The physician may order volume expanders or other medications to stabilize blood pressure.

I. The patient's neurologic status must be carefully monitored to assess the progress of the stroke and to observe for increased ICP, which may cause supratentorial herniation and death. Deterioration in the level of consciousness, decreased response to stimuli, pupillary changes, along with increasing systolic blood pressure, widening pulse pressure, slowing pulse rate, and altered breathing patterns are all significant indicators of rising ICP. Steroids and osmotic diuretics such as mannitol are generally given to help reduce cerebral edema.

J. Because strokes can precipitate seizure activity, especially during their early stages, implement seizure

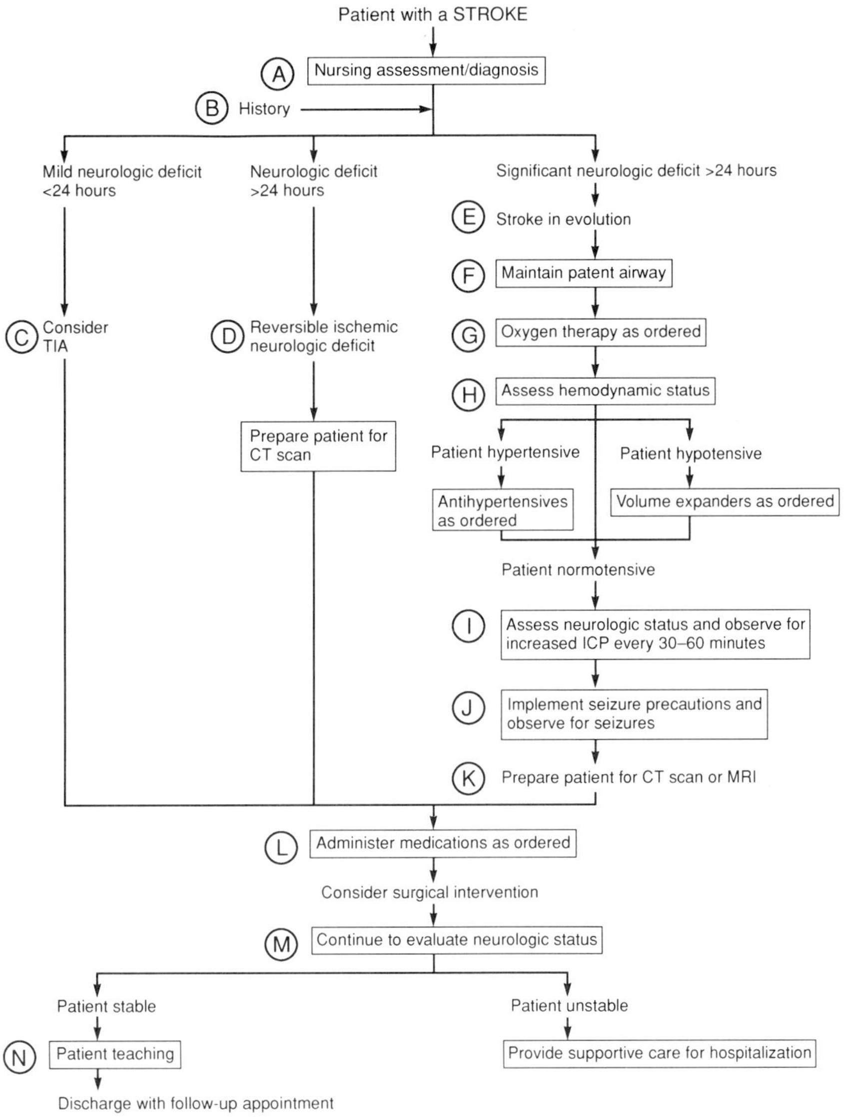

precautions and observe the patient for any signs of seizure activity (p 30). The physician may prophylactically order anticonvulsant medications such as phenytoin or phenobarbital.

K. CT scan or magnetic resonance imaging (MRI) will assist in the diagnosis and determination of the extent of the stroke. In addition, cerebral angiography, lumbar puncture, brain scan, or electroencephalography may be done.

L. Medical management for the patient with a stroke begins with aspirin and dipyridamole (Persantine) for mild symptoms. These drugs impede platelet aggregation and allow the body's natural fibrinolytic factors to break down obstructions that have already formed. Patients with more severe symptoms receive IV heparin therapy initially, and then progress to oral warfarin (Coumadin).

M. The patient may be evaluated as a surgical candidate for either carotid endarterectomy (p 90) or extracranial-intracranial bypass surgery, depending on the location and extent of the injury.

N. Before being discharged, patients should be taught about predisposing risk factors for stroke and given appropriate suggestions for lifestyle modification. Stress the importance of blood pressure control through medication compliance, diet modifications, and weight loss. Teach about low-cholesterol foods and the role cholesterol plays in stroke development. Discuss an exercise plan and a program to quit smoking, if necessary, along with stress management techniques and principles. Provide the patient with resources in the community that may be called on for follow-up and assistance.

References

Bubb DI. Neurologic problems. Oradell, NJ: Medical Economics Books, 1984:110–122.

Conway B. Carini and Owen's neurological and neurosurgical nursing. 8th ed. St. Louis: CV Mosby, 1986:609–620.

Gary R, Jerimer BJ, Hickey A. Stroke: how to contain the damage. RN 1986; 49:36–41.

Raimond J, Taylor JW. Neurological emergencies: effective nursing care. Rockville, MD: Aspen, 1986:251–268.

PARKINSON'S DISEASE

Kathy Gilliland

Parkinson's disease (paralysis agitans) is a chronic degeneration of the basal ganglia. The etiology of Parkinsonism is not entirely clear, but current research has shown that there is a reduction in the amount of the neurotransmitter dopamine and chemical imbalances between the acetylcholine and dopaminergic systems that impair the transmission of impulses from nerve cell to muscle cell. Parkinson's disease is one of the most common neurologic diseases in persons over 30 years of age and is most often seen in patients in their 60s. The extent of the disease process may be mild, with involvement of one side of the body, or it may be fully developed, with severe bilateral involvement requiring confinement to a bed or wheelchair.

A. Persons with Parkinson's disease usually have tremors of the arms and legs at rest and reduced body movements. Many exhibit masklike facial expressions, with the inability to express emotions. Parkinson's disease is progressively disabling, accelerating until there is impaired cardiovascular and respiratory function, depression, and mild intellectual and mental changes.

B. The diagnosis is based on the history and presenting physical signs and symptoms. Clinical manifestations include emotional lability, autonomic dysfunction, impaired mobility, decreased functional ability, cogwheel rigidity, and tremors often with "pill-rolling" movement of the thumb and finger.

C. Diagnostic screening includes analysis of homovanillic acid (HVA), a metabolite of dopamine, which is performed on urine and cerebrospinal fluid.

D. There is no known treatment to stop the degeneration caused by Parkinson's disease. Drug therapy (levodopa) provides a substance that increases available chemicals needed for nerve impulse transmission and prevents dopamine turnover. Generally there is a good initial response to drug therapy programs, but usually a gradual decline in effectiveness is noted. In this case a "drug holiday" is undertaken—medications are stopped. During these periods symptoms accelerate. Medicines are returned slowly to reach near-preholiday functioning. Medication therapy must be carefully supervised because of toxic side effects, such as nausea, vomiting, anxiety, confusion, and postural hypotension. Levodopa may be contraindicated in patients with peptic ulcers, asthma, renal disease, or severe cardiovascular or pulmonary disease.

E. Severe cases that do not respond to drug therapy may be considered for thalamotomy, a surgical procedure that may alleviate some of the symptoms; however, it is not without devastating physical and emotional effects.

F. Physical therapy programs are important to maintain normal muscle tone and maximize levels of activity.

G. Quality of life is a major focus in the management of the person with Parkinson's disease. The causes of death relate to the complications of immobility, such as pulmonary embolism (p 116), pneumonia (p 104), and urinary tract infection. Sudden withdrawal of medication may precipitate a *Parkinsonian crisis.* This is rare, but requires *immediate intervention* to provide respiratory and cardiac support. Crisis should be suspected with severe exacerbation of tremor and rigidity accompanied by anxiety, tachycardia, and sweating.

H. Assistance with activities of daily living and the management of drug effects is important. A supportive relationship with emphasis on emotional caring and acceptance can provide an environment of personal importance despite physical and mental changes. Exercise, rest, and activity should be planned appropriately.

I. Dischage planning includes providing for in-home assistance, physical therapy, dietary requirements (meals-on-wheels), health aids (e.g., walkers), restrictions regarding medications, and referral to community support groups for patients and families.

References

American Association of Neuroscience Nursing. Core curriculum. Park Ridge, IL: AANN, 1980:485–493.

Garrett E. Parkinsonism: forgotten considerations in medical treatment and nursing care. J Neurosurg Nurs 1982; 14: 13–18.

Luckmann J, Sorensen KC. Medical-surgical nursing: a psychophysiologic approach. 3rd ed. Philadelphia: WB Saunders, 1987.

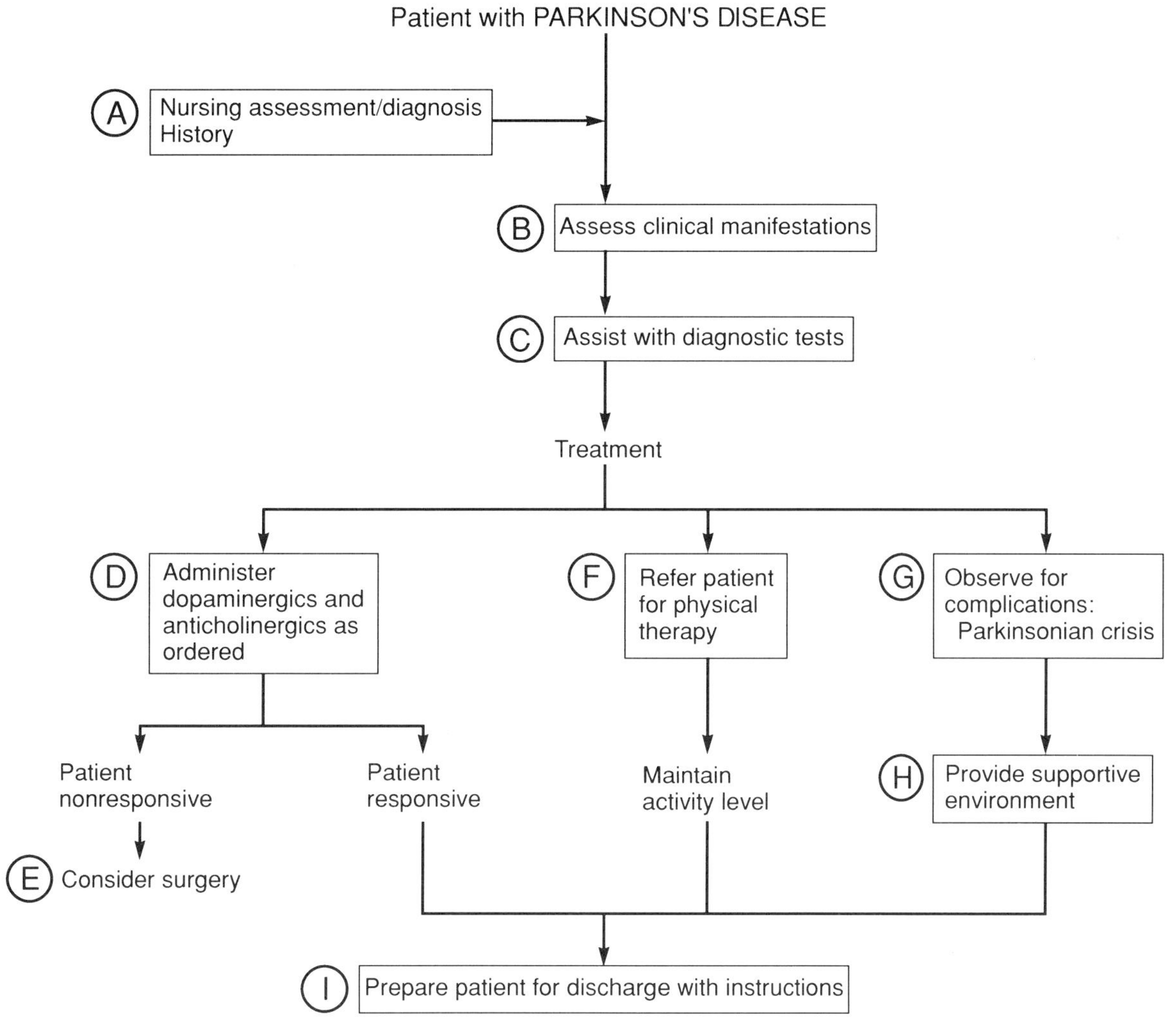
Patient with PARKINSON'S DISEASE
A
Nursing assessment/diagnosis
History
B
Assess clinical manifestations
C
Assist with diagnostic tests
Treatment
D
Administer dopaminergics and anticholinergics as ordered
F
Refer patient for physical therapy
G
Observe for complications:
Parkinsonian crisis
Patient nonresponsive
Patient responsive
Maintain activity level
H
Provide supportive environment
E
Consider surgery
I
Prepare patient for discharge with instructions

SPINAL CORD INJURY

Linda Weld

Injury to the spinal cord is usually the result of trauma that causes edema and possible cord compression or severance. The majority of patients with spinal cord injuries are young males involved in motor vehicle accidents. The symptoms range from no neurologic deficit to quadriplegia, depending on the location and severity of the injury. The spinal cord responds to injury with an inflammatory response and edema formation. The spinal cord is enclosed by bone which may cause the edema to move up the column and cause damage above the level of the anatomic injury. Because of this edema formation, the exact extent of the injury cannot be determined for several days. If the lesion is major, the nurse must consider the physiologic and psychological impact on the patient and family. Many of these patients require lengthy rehabilitation and may never return to their previous level of functioning.

A. The nursing assessment must include the location and severity of the injury: the higher the lesion, the more severe the symptoms. In general, complete cervical lesions cause quadriplegia and thoracic lesions cause some type of paraplegia. Incomplete lesions can cause a wide variety of sensory and motor deficits. An open airway must be maintained, and the patient must be immobilized, usually on a specialized bed that assists turning and maintains proper alignment. Because of edema formation, the nurse must frequently assess the patient for changes in neurological status.

B. Spinal cord injury affects all the nerves exiting or entering the cord. These include nerves performing sensory and motor functions as well as nerves of the autonomic nervous system. The patient may exhibit symptoms in almost every body system. Initially the patient is in spinal shock, which causes flaccid paralysis, arterial and venous vasodilation, bradycardia, absent reflexes, and loss of temperature control below the level of the lesion.

C. Spinal shock lasts from 3 days to 3 months; the end of this phase is manifested by the return of reflexes and spastic paralysis. At this time patients with an injury at the thoracic level or higher may experience an excessive autonomic nervous system response to stimuli, known as autonomic hyperreflexia (dysreflexia). Signs and symptoms of dysreflexia include severe hypertension, bradycardia, headache, and diaphoresis. This is an *emergency situation* and the nurse must take immediate action. The head of the bed should be elevated, the physician must be notified, and stimuli producing the reaction must be eliminated. Possible stimuli include bladder distention, bowel impaction, painful stimuli below the level of the lesion, and digital stimulation. If removing the stimuli does not lower the blood pressure, the physician may order medication.

D. The patient with a spinal cord injury requires considerable emotional support through the phases of acceptance of the injury and its future implications. This support also needs to include the family.

E. Some patients with spinal cord injuries may benefit from surgical intervention, such as laminectomy with fusion (p 46) or Harrington rod insertion to stabilize the spinal column.

F. After the extent of injury is determined and the patient is stabilized, he or she is transferred to a rehabilitation unit. The rehabilitation program includes bowel and bladder training; activities of daily living; sexual activity; care of stabilization devices, such as a halo jacket; and skin care.

References

Lewis SM, Collier IC. Medical-surgical nursing: assessment and management of clinical problems. New York: McGraw-Hill, 1983.

Nikas DL. The critically ill neurosurgical patient. New York: Churchill Livingstone, 1982.

Shoemaker WC, Thompson WL, Holbrook PR. The society of critical care medicine: textbook of critical care. Philadelphia: WB Saunders, 1984.

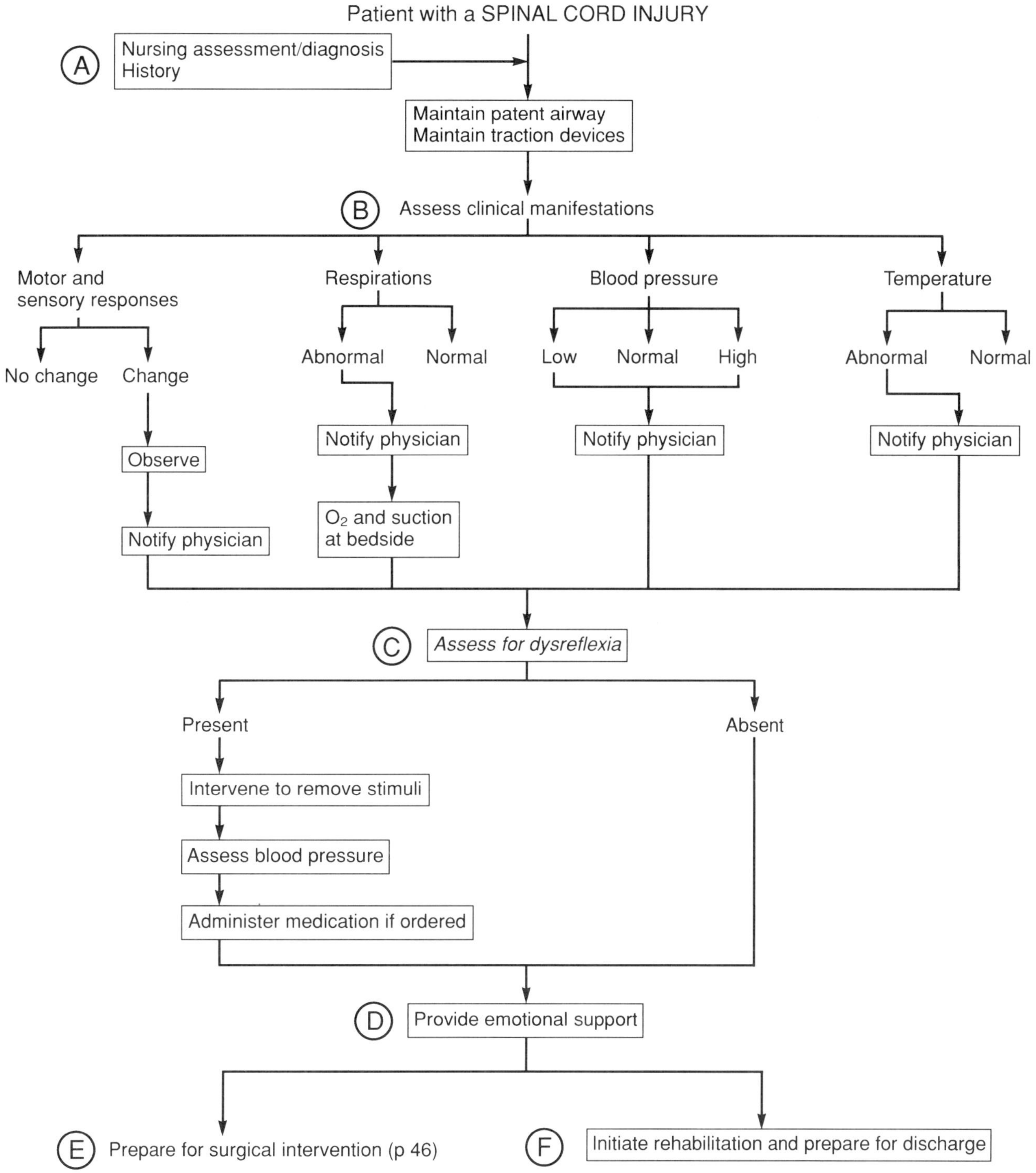
Patient with a SPINAL CORD INJURY
A
Nursing assessment/diagnosis
History
Maintain patent airway
Maintain traction devices
B
Assess clinical manifestations
Motor and sensory responses
No change
Change
Observe
Notify physician
Respirations
Abnormal
Normal
Notify physician
O_2 and suction at bedside
Blood pressure
Low
Normal
High
Notify physician
Temperature
Abnormal
Normal
Notify physician
C
Assess for dysreflexia
Present
Intervene to remove stimuli
Assess blood pressure
Administer medication if ordered
Absent
D
Provide emotional support
E
Prepare for surgical intervention (p 46)
F
Initiate rehabilitation and prepare for discharge

HEADACHE

Kathy Gilliland

Headache is one of the most common symptoms experienced by the general population. Several million persons seek medical advice because of headaches in the United States yearly. Headaches are symptoms that occur as a result of benign and/or pathologic conditions. Differential diagnoses pertinent in patients presenting with headaches include intracranial mass (p 38), central nervous system (CNS) infection, meningitis (p 32), cerebral artery disease (p 20), minor head injury, and stroke (p 22).

A. Throughout the assessment, identification of the associated symptoms and contributing factors is important. These include onset, frequency, duration, triggering mechanisms, and physical disturbances. Familial history of headaches may be important and can identify preexisting or contributing conditions such as diabetes (p 176), hypertension (p 80), allergy, menstrual patterns, past or recent drug use, and concurrent illness.

B. Clinical manifestations of headaches vary according to type, etiology, and precipitating symptoms. Subjective reports of associated symptoms include steady or intermittent burning; throbbing or stretching type of pain; aching of neck and scalp muscles; visual disturbances; partial or whole flushing of the face; dizziness; tinnitus; diaphoresis; eye pain; and twitching. Dietary habits, lifestyle and exercise patterns, stress levels, triggering events, medication or drug use, and pain relief should be documented.

C. Diagnosis and treatment are based on history, triggering events, and the completion of neurodiagnostic studies to rule out structural disease processes. Diagnostic studies include serum metabolic screens, electroencephalogram (EEG), brain scan, allergy testing, and cerebrospinal fluid (CSF) screening.

D. Pathologic headaches require immediate intervention, which may include surgery (p 42).

E. Benign headaches usually fall into one of two major categories—tension headaches or migraine headaches. Migraine headaches are usually a syndrome caused by vascular spasm. A prodromal period occurs as intracranial vasoconstriction and the headache as extracranial vasodilation. Migraine headaches are three times as prevalent in women as in men and are usually experienced between ages 10 and 30. Tension headaches involve muscular contractions about the head, face, and neck. They are generally seen in persons experiencing stressful life events. The pain of these headaches generally lasts from 6 to 12 hours and is not particularly disabling, but is constantly annoying.

F. Treatments are supportive, based on the type of headache identified, and generally include medication, biofeedback, behavior therapy, psychotherapy, and avoidance of triggers. Comfort measures such as massage or heat may help. Vasoconstrictors such as Midrin (Isometheptene mucate) and ergotamine are helpful in vascular headaches. Common prophylactic medications such as Sansert (methysergide maleate) and Bellergal (belladonna alkaloid) have been successful in reducing the frequency or abating the headache in its early stages.

G. Dietary instruction and avoidance of food products like red wine, chocolate, hot dogs, cheeses, or others containing tyramine, nitrites, and glutamate may be helpful.

H. Biofeedback in conjunction with other measures can assist in active changes and adaptation.

I. If headaches are secondary, the primary stimulus should be removed or treated. Assisting patients with analysis of their lifestyle may help them identify areas where modification could relieve headaches. Patient education emphasizes treatment measures, medication use, and lifestyle changes.

References

Campbell VC. Neurologic system (headaches). In: Thompson JM, McFarland GK, Hirsch JE, Tucker SM, Bowers AC. Clinical nursing. St. Louis: CV Mosby, 1986:394–399.

Daroff RB, Whitney CM. Treatment of vascular headaches. Headache 1987; 26:470–472.

Saper JR. Headache disorders, current concepts, and treatment strategies. PSG, 1983.

Whitney CM, Daroff RB. An approach to migraine. J Neurol Nurs 1988; 20:284–289.

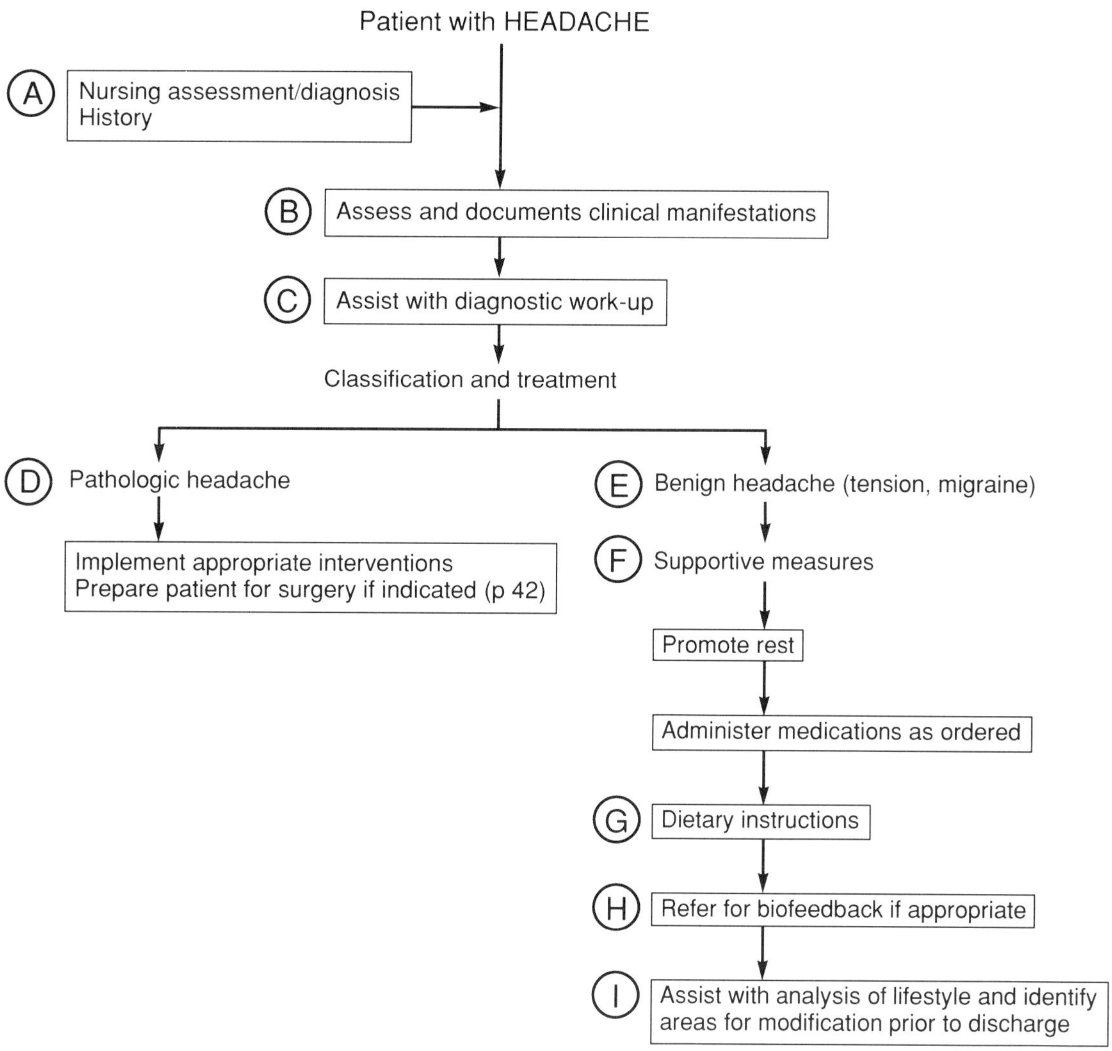
Patient with HEADACHE
A
Nursing assessment/diagnosis
History
B
Assess and documents clinical manifestations
C
Assist with diagnostic work-up
Classification and treatment
D
Pathologic headache
Implement appropriate interventions
Prepare patient for surgery if indicated (p 42)
E
Benign headache (tension, migraine)
F
Supportive measures
Promote rest
Administer medications as ordered
G
Dietary instructions
H
Refer for biofeedback if appropriate
I
Assist with analysis of lifestyle and identify areas for modification prior to discharge

SEIZURES

Karen O'Brien

A seizure is a sudden pathologic alteration in brain activity that causes changes in body and behavior function. Seizures frequently occur after head trauma. Tumors or space-occupying lesions may cause seizures at any age, but the incidence of neoplastic disease is higher in adults; often focal seizures are the initial symptoms of these diseases (p 38). Metabolic disorders (pp 182, 192), drug and alcohol withdrawal (pp 402, 405), diabetes (p 176), renal failure (p 318), vascular disorders (p 22, 80), and acute or inflammatory illness (p 32) may precipitate seizure activity. Often a patient is admitted to a medical-surgical unit for diagnostic studies and observation after experiencing a seizure. An epileptic patient may be admitted to a medical-surgical unit because of another illness or condition, and have a seizure.

A. The history should include extensive questioning about seizure history, known seizure disorders, drug and alcohol intake, other medications, recent injury, and chronic illness.

B. Controlled epileptics admitted for other problems need to be observed for seizures, because illness or change in routine may initiate a seizure. Appropriate precautions should be taken, but the patient's need for dignity and independence also must be considered.

C. A first-time seizure or one that seems secondary to another condition requires aggressive diagnostic testing because of the wide variety of possible causes. Computer tomography or a magnetic resonance imaging scan is performed to rule out neoplasm, cerebral bleeding, or cerebral vascular disorders. Cerebral arteriography may also be necessary to confirm diagnosis. Initial laboratory testing should include, but is not limited to, a complete blood count, electrolytes, and liver and renal function tests. Toxicology and alcohol levels may also be helpful. Electroencephalography (EEG) is done to support the clinical diagnosis. An EEG may help classify the seizure and may indicate prognosis. Lumbar punctures are done to rule out infectious diseases.

D. Treatment of seizure activity depends on the cause and is planned on an individual basis. Some patients may be managed through treatment of the underlying cause. Most are placed on an anticonvulsant medication. The dosage of the selected drug is increased until seizure activity is controlled, blood levels reach the upper limit of the therapeutic range, or side effects prevent further progression. Frequently, patients are controlled with a 1-g loading dose of Dilantin followed by a maintenance dose of 300 mg daily. Additional drug combinations may be added as needed. Occasionally, surgical management is attempted if seizures cannot be controlled by anticonvulsant agents. Administering medications on schedule is crucial to maintaining a therapeutic blood level.

E. The patient's safety is foremost. For patients at high risk for seizure, siderails should be raised at all times and padded. A suction setup should be maintained at the bedside, and the bed should be placed in a low position. Patients should be instructed to call for help and lie down if they experience an aura.

F. Management of a seizure should be directed toward protecting the patient. Provide privacy by closing the door or pulling the curtain and keep the area clear.

G. Maintain a reliable route for administration of anticonvulsant drugs.

H. Frequent suctioning in the postictal stage is usually required to prevent aspiration.

I. Depending on the type of seizure, the patient may be confused afterward. Offer reassurance and a calm, quiet environment.

J. Monitor patient activity on a regular basis. If a seizure is witnessed, document the onset of how and where the seizure began, type of movements and body parts involved, pupillary change or a conjugate gaze, incontinence, duration of seizure activity, behavior after the seizure, neurologic deficits, and number of seizures.

K. Teaching and rehabilitation must begin before discharge. Patients must be taught to identify and avoid activities that could be life-threatening should seizures occur (e.g., swimming alone, water sports, and driving). The importance of compliance with medications on a long-term basis must be stressed. Family and friends should be taught what to do should seizures occur. Life-style should be normalized as much as possible. Patients should be knowledgeable about their condition and share this with others. Referral to the Epilepsy Foundation of America may be helpful.

References

Friedman D. Taking the scare out of caring for seizure patients. Nursing 88 1988;18:2, 53–59.

Hickey J. The clinical practice of neurological and neurosurgical nursing. Philadelphia: JB Lippincott, 1981:409–431.

Mancini M. Decision making in emergency nursing. Toronto: BC Decker, 1987.

Mills J, Ho M, Salber P, Trunkey D. Current emergency diagnosis and treatment. Los Altos, CA: Lange, 1985:97–101, 104.

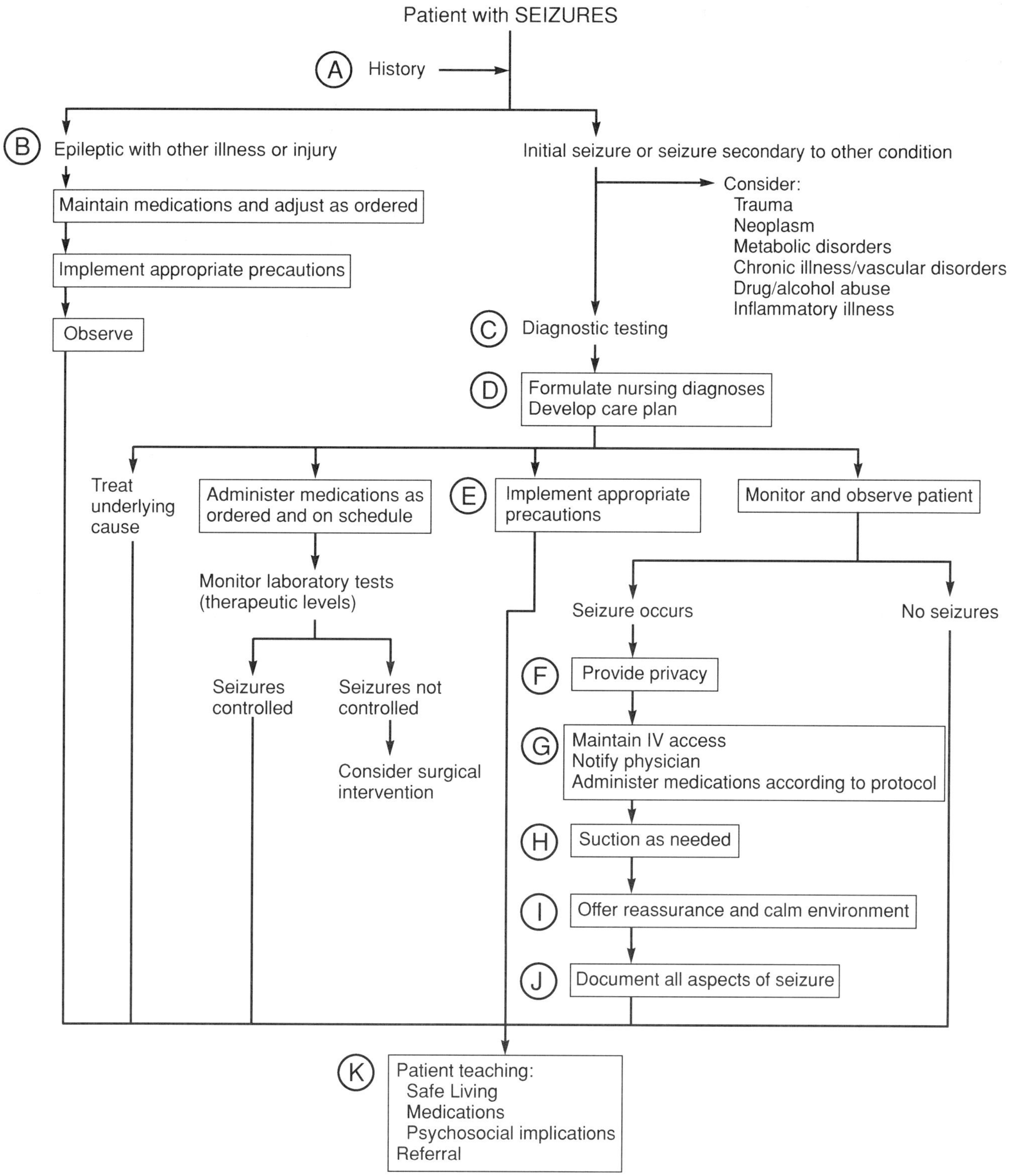
Patient with SEIZURES
A
History
B
Epileptic with other illness or injury
Maintain medications and adjust as ordered
Implement appropriate precautions
Observe
Initial seizure or seizure secondary to other condition
Consider:
Trauma
Neoplasm
Metabolic disorders
Chronic illness/vascular disorders
Drug/alcohol abuse
Inflammatory illness
C
Diagnostic testing
D
Formulate nursing diagnoses
Develop care plan
Treat underlying cause
Administer medications as ordered and on schedule
Monitor laboratory tests (therapeutic levels)
Seizures controlled
Seizures not controlled
Consider surgical intervention
E
Implement appropriate precautions
Monitor and observe patient
Seizure occurs
No seizures
F
Provide privacy
G
Maintain IV access
Notify physician
Administer medications according to protocol
H
Suction as needed
I
Offer reassurance and calm environment
J
Document all aspects of seizure
K
Patient teaching:
Safe Living
Medications
Psychosocial implications
Referral

MENINGITIS AND ENCEPHALITIS

Nina McIntosh

Meningitis is an inflammation of the meninges covering the brain and spinal cord, resulting from acute meningeal infection, caused by the invasion of bacteria, viruses, fungi, or parasitic worms into the tissues. The organisms usually gain entry to the central nervous system through the upper respiratory tract, but may also enter by direct extension from penetrating wounds of the skull. Encephalitis is an inflammation of the tissues of the brain and spinal cord and is frequently accompanied by signs of systemic infection. Like meningitis, encephalitis may result from a variety of causes, including viruses, bacteria, and chemicals. The majority of viruses producing encephalitis as a primary focal infection are transmitted by mosquitoes.

A. All patients with meningitis or encephalitis should be observed closely for manifestations of increased intracranial pressure (ICP). A baseline of neurologic function should be established immediately upon admission. The history may reveal a respiratory infection or "flu" prior to onset. Any patient with a basal skull fracture or penetrating injury to the head should be observed for signs of meningitis. Mumps and measles viruses can cause both meningitis and encephalitis. Early onset of back and leg aches and sore throat are common manifestations following mumps and measles immunizations.

B. Severe headache with photophobia accompanied by fever of 39° to 41°C are primary clues to meningitis. Signs of meningeal irritation, such as nuchal rigidity (stiff neck) and flexion rigidity of the leg muscles, are seen. Other common manifestations of meningitis and encephalitis are general irritability, anorexia, nausea and vomiting, malaise, confusion, and in some cases seizures (p 30). Petechiae on lower extremities and trunk may occur. Although the manifestations of encephalitis resemble those of meningitis, they usually have a more gradual onset.

C. The patient with meningitis or encephalitis is usually acutely ill. Specific diagnosis depends on laboratory data not usually available until after recovery. Thus, isolation is recommended for all patients during the febrile period. Enteric precautions are indicated until enteroviral disease is excluded. Use of universal precautions is recommended for all blood and body secretions. The fever may be resistant to aspirin. Therefore, other means must be attempted to lower the temperature.

D. Headache pain and neck pain secondary to movement require attention. Codeine provides some relief without undue sedation for most patients. Assist the patient to a position of comfort, often curled up with head slightly extended. Keeping the room darkened and placing a cool cloth over the eyes relieves the discomfort of photophobia. Every attempt should be made to minimize environmental stimuli and the resulting exaggerated perception. A familiar person at the bedside has a calming effect.

E. If seizures (p 30) occur, appropriate observations should be made and protective measures taken. Anticonvulsant medications are given as ordered.

F. Assess the patient frequently for dehydration and adequacy of intake. Antiemetics may be indicated to prevent episodes of increased ICP during vomiting.

G. The skin needs to be protected from excessive drying or injury.

H. Rapid diagnosis is crucial; the patient is usually in a crisis state when health care is sought. Diagnostic measures include lumbar puncture and analysis of cerebrospinal fluid to determine viral versus bacterial causative agents. Blood cultures may also be drawn to attempt to isolate the causative agent. Blood chemistries help to differentiate bacterial from viral infections. Computerized tomographic (CT) scan, skull films, and/or electroencephalography (EEG) may be done to determine changes in ICP as well as the degree of brain involvement.

I. In nonbacterial cases of encephalitis and meningitis, medical and nursing care and management are primarily symptomatic and supportive.

J. Penicillin and ampicillin are the drugs of choice for bacterial infections, with chloramphenicol used for persons allergic to penicillin. Nafcillin can be used for gram-negative organisms. These drugs are effective because of their ability to penetrate the blood-brain barrier. Close contacts should be informed of the possibility they may contract meningitis and should be alert for signs and symptoms. Patients remain on category-specific isolation until the causative organisms are identified.

K. Early treatment *is* essential, because some forms of viral encephalitis may cause irreversible changes in the central nervous system that result in death. Untreated bacterial meningitis can also be fatal. Most often, with treatment, symptoms subside within 4 days to 2 weeks and the patient is discharged.

L. Possible residual effects from encephalitis or meningitis include dementia, epilepsy, deafness, hemiplegia, paralysis, and hydrocephalus. Patients and families should be informed of the need for periodic evaluation and long-term physical therapy and of potential resources to help them cope. Vision, hearing, cognitive skills, and motor-sensory abilities should be assessed for deficiencies, with appropriate referrals made.

References

Benenson AS, ed. Control of communicable diseases in man. 13th ed. Washington, DC: The American Public Health Association, 1981:217–228.

Lewis SM, Collier IC. Medical-surgical nursing: assessment and management of clinical problems. New York: McGraw-Hill, 1983.

Moriarty M. Jay's alive. Do we owe him an apology? (case study). RN 1987; 50(5):38–41.

Swisher C, Williams A. Herpes encephalitis: a nursing challenge. J Neurosurg Nurs 1981; 13(1):34–37.

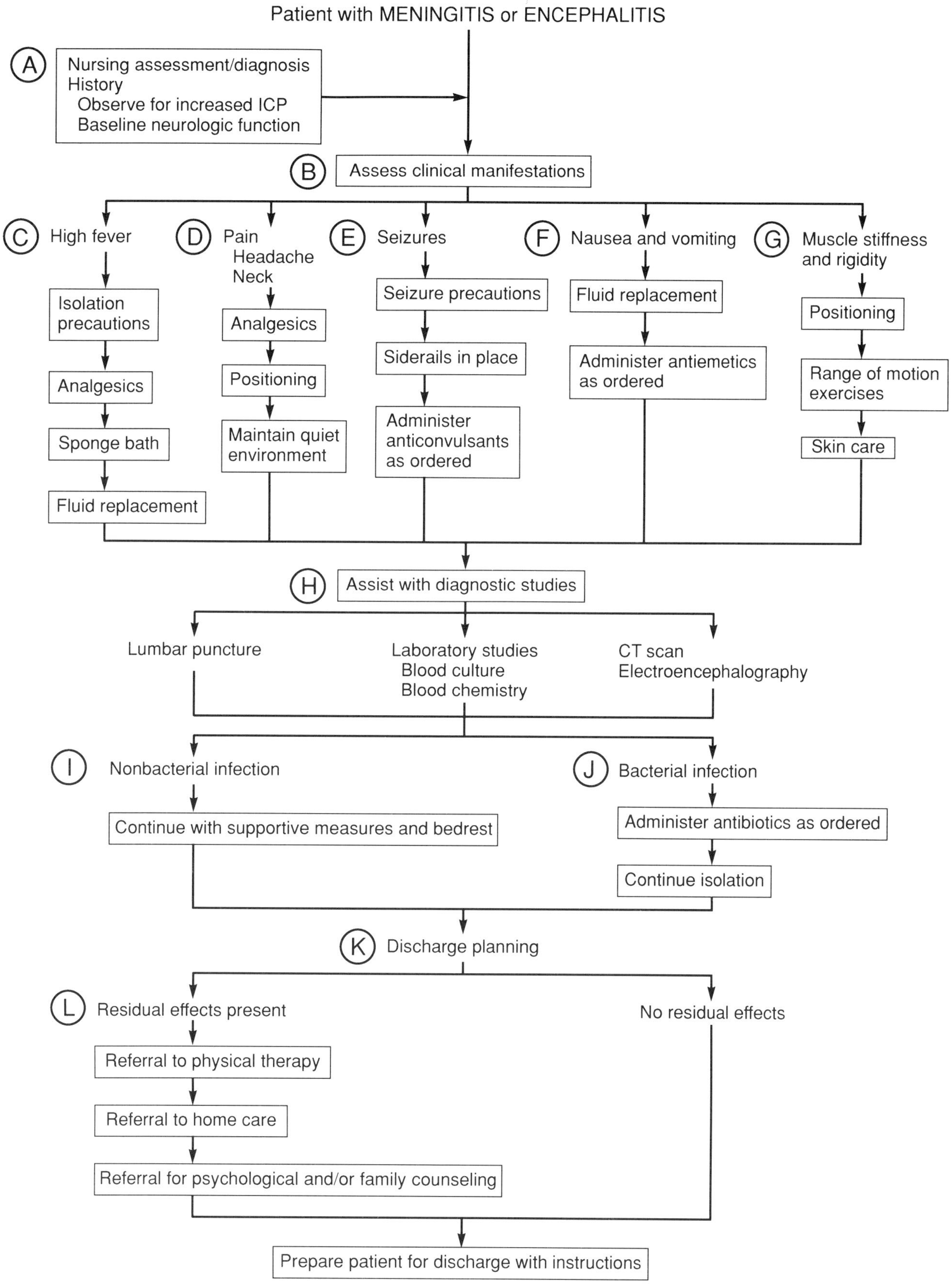
Patient with MENINGITIS or ENCEPHALITIS
A
Nursing assessment/diagnosis
History
Observe for increased ICP
Baseline neurologic function
B
Assess clinical manifestations
C
High fever
Isolation precautions
Analgesics
Sponge bath
Fluid replacement
D
Pain
Headache
Neck
Analgesics
Positioning
Maintain quiet environment
E
Seizures
Seizure precautions
Siderails in place
Administer anticonvulsants as ordered
F
Nausea and vomiting
Fluid replacement
Administer antiemetics as ordered
G
Muscle stiffness and rigidity
Positioning
Range of motion exercises
Skin care
H
Assist with diagnostic studies
Lumbar puncture
Laboratory studies
Blood culture
Blood chemistry
CT scan
Electroencephalography
I
Nonbacterial infection
Continue with supportive measures and bedrest
J
Bacterial infection
Administer antibiotics as ordered
Continue isolation
K
Discharge planning
L
Residual effects present
Referral to physical therapy
Referral to home care
Referral for psychological and/or family counseling
No residual effects
Prepare patient for discharge with instructions

TETANUS

Nina McIntosh

Tetanus is an acute disease caused by *Clostridium tetani* (tetanus bacillus) spores, which are introduced into the body when an injury becomes contaminated with soil, street dust, or animal or human feces. Bacilli gain entry into the body through traumatic or purulent wounds that provide an appropriate low-oxygen environment. The incubation period is 2 days to 3 weeks, with symptoms frequently appearing after the original wound is healed. The toxin reaches the central nervous system (CNS) and binds with CNS tissue and spinal motor ganglia. There, it interferes with the release of an inhibitory transmitter and induces hyperexcitability of motor neurons, resulting in tonic rigidity and spasms of facial, cervical, masseter, respiratory, abdominal, and extremity muscles. The lay term for this condition is lockjaw.

A. Tetanus-prone wounds are those that have been invaded by soil or feces or those involving a severe traumatic injury. However, tetanus may develop from an insignificant wound. Suspect tetanus in wounds originating from compound fractures, gunshot, burns, foreign bodies, punctures, abortions, human and animal bites, dirty hypodermic needles, and in purulent lesions and wounds neglected for more than 24 hours.

B. Care of the tetanus-prone patient depends on the immunization status (Table 1), nature and age of the wound, and circumstances surrounding the injury. All individuals should receive active immunity against tetanus during childhood with a booster every 10 years.

TABLE 1 Immunizations for the Tetanus-Prone Patient

Immunization Status	*Clean Minor Wound*	*Clean Large Wound*	*Dirty Wound*
Immunized (initial immunization DPT and booster ≤10 years)	N/A	N/A	TIG
Immunized; Booster >10 years	TT	TT	TIG
Unimmunized	Initial dose TT; repeat × 2 at 4-wk intervals	TT & TIG*	TT & TIG*
Unable to determine immunization status	TIG	TIG	TIG

* Use different sites and separate syringes
TT = tetanus toxoid
TIG = tetanus immunoglobulin-human

Note: Equine antitoxin (horse serum) is rarely used because of risk of serum sickness; if used, it must *always* be preceded by careful skin testing.

(Table developed by Carol Bowdoin.)

Tetanus immune globulin (TIG-human) is given in the presence of "dirty wounds" or indeterminate immunization status, in order to neutralize the exotoxin produced by the tetanus bacillus. Tetanus toxoid (TT) is given if a year has passed since the patient's last booster. Wounds must be thoroughly cleansed to include removal of foreign debris and debridement of nonviable tissue. Prophylactic antibiotics may be ordered.

C. The clinical manifestations of tetanus include a prickly sensation in the jaw muscles, stimulating excessive yawning early in the disease. Within 24 hours the jaw muscles become tender and stiff, and dysphagia and generalized tonic spasms are present. As the disease progresses, the neck, back, and extremity muscles become progressively rigid. Laryngeal and respiratory spasms cause apnea and anoxia. Airway maintenance is a primary priority. Patients should be placed in a quiet semidark room. The slightest noise, jarring motion, or bright light can set off a convulsion. Muscle relaxants such as diazepam (Valium) and sedatives are given to manage reflex spasms and prevent seizures. The nurse should start and keep open an intravenous line for medications.

D. Patients who develop respiratory complications need to be monitored in the ICU. Tetanic spasms of the larynx, pharynx, and respiratory muscles may occur during convulsions, leading to hypoxia, aspiration, and death. *Immediate intubation and mechanical ventilation is necessary.*

E. If there are no complications, the patient is discharged with specific instructions for wound care. The patient should receive a written record of immunizations given and be encouraged to complete an active immunization schedule. The patient may also need referral for outpatient physiotherapy.

References

Brunner LS, Suddarth DS. The Lippincott manual of nursing practice. 4th ed. Philadelphia: JB Lippincott, 1986.

Lewis SM, Collier IC. Medical-surgical nursing: assessment and management of clinical problems. New York: McGraw-Hill, 1983.

Thompson JM, McFarland GK, Hirsch JE, Tucker SM, Bowers AC. Clinical nursing. St. Louis: CV Mosby, 1986.

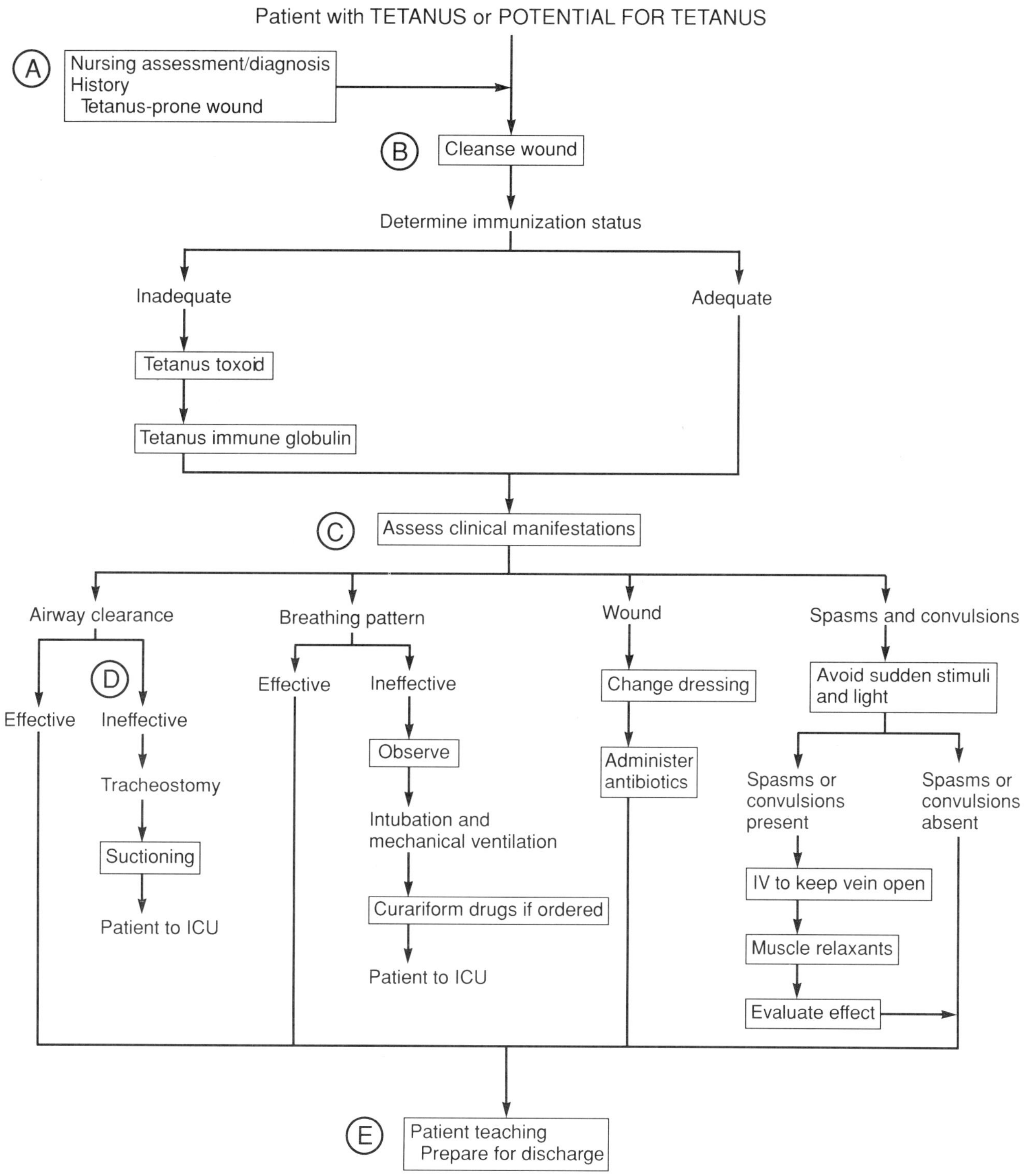
Patient with TETANUS or POTENTIAL FOR TETANUS
A
Nursing assessment/diagnosis
History
Tetanus-prone wound
B
Cleanse wound
Determine immunization status
Inadequate
Adequate
Tetanus toxoid
Tetanus immune globulin
C
Assess clinical manifestations
Airway clearance
Breathing pattern
Wound
Spasms and convulsions
Effective
D
Ineffective
Tracheostomy
Suctioning
Patient to ICU
Effective
Ineffective
Observe
Intubation and mechanical ventilation
Curariform drugs if ordered
Patient to ICU
Change dressing
Administer antibiotics
Avoid sudden stimuli and light
Spasms or convulsions present
Spasms or convulsions absent
IV to keep vein open
Muscle relaxants
Evaluate effect
E
Patient teaching
Prepare for discharge

POLIOMYELITIS

Joy Gorzeman

Acute poliomyelitis ("polio," infantile paralysis) is a viral infection characterized by the destruction of motor cells in the spinal cord (spinal form) and/or brain stem (bulbar or spinal-bulbar form). It is caused by one of three types of poliovirus that spreads from the gastrointestinal tract to the nervous system. In the 1950s, the number of polio cases was markedly reduced worldwide because of mass immunization. However, failure to keep up with immunizations has resulted in an increase in the number of reported polio cases over the last several years.

A. Factors such as recent tonsillectomy, tooth extraction, diphtheria-tetanus-pertussis vaccine (DTP) injections, pregnancy, and physical exhaustion are predisposing to poliomyelitis.

B. Poliomyelitis is categorized into two types: paralytic and nonparalytic. Symptoms of nonparalytic poliomyelitis include headache, lethargy, anorexia, vomiting, and fever, followed by muscle pain and stiffness. Patients with paralytic poliomyelitis experience these same symptoms for about 1 week. Then they usually experience loss of deep tendon reflexes and demonstrate positive Kernig's sign (reflex contraction and pain in the hamstring muscle when straightening the leg after flexing the thigh to the body), and positive Brudzinski's sign (when the patient's neck is flexed on the chest, flexion of the knees and hips is produced, and when the lower extremity on one side is passively flexed, similar movement is seen on the opposite extremity). These symptoms are followed by weakening of muscles and paralysis in about 1 to 2 days.

C. Since the symptoms of poliomyelitis are similar to those of meningitis, isolation of the virus from cultures of the throat or feces is needed to confirm the diagnosis. Poliomyelitis is also frequently confused with Guillain-Barré syndrome. However, in Guillain-Barré syndrome patients, there is usually no fever, muscle weakness is symmetric, sensory findings are present, and the cerebrospinal fluid (CSF) protein is markedly elevated with a normal cell count. Asymmetric flaccid limb paralysis during a febrile illness in a child or young adult almost always indicates poliomyelitis. In addition, the CSF protein is slightly elevated, and the cell count is elevated.

D. Treatment for poliomyelitis is primarily supportive. The milder, nonparalytic forms of polio respond to bedrest.

E. Muscle pain may be relieved with moist hot-pack applications and pain medication.

F. Antipyretics for fever also promote comfort.

G. The patient should rest on a firm bed, and a footboard should be used to prevent footdrop.

H. The patient with poliomyelitis should be in enteric isolation, since the virus is spread via saliva, vomitus, and feces.

I. Patients with nonparalytic poliomyelitis experience complete recovery. More than half of patients with paralytic poliomyelitis recover without residual paralysis. However, approximately 25 percent of patients with paralytic poliomyelitis suffer severe permanent disability, and 25 percent have mild disability.

J. The most common complication of poliomyelitis is respiratory failure, which is caused by paralysis of the respiratory muscles as a result of spinal cord involvement or damage to the respiratory center in the medulla. These patients must be placed on artificial ventilation. A tracheostomy may be required to keep the airway clear. Patients placed on the respirator *before* serious respiratory paralysis develops have a better chance of recovery.

K. For women, it may be noted that polio does not affect menstruation or fertility. Pregnancy and delivery may be difficult, depending on the severity and type of disability. The most important aspect of care for a patient with permanent disability from poliomyelitis is physical therapy and rehabilitation. This is a long process and both the patient and family need a lot of support. Some recent reports have indicated that patients who experienced poliomyelitis in the 1950s are at risk of recurrence. These people are encouraged to avoid fatigue and stress.

References

Brunner LS, Suddarth DS. The Lippincott manual of nursing practice. 4th ed. Philadelphia: JB Lippincott, 1986.

Luckmann J, Sorensen KC. Medical-surgical nursing. 3rd ed. Philadelphia: WB Saunders, 1987.

Thompson J, McFarland G, Hirsch J, Tucker S, Bowers A. Clinical nursing. St. Louis: CV Mosby, 1986.

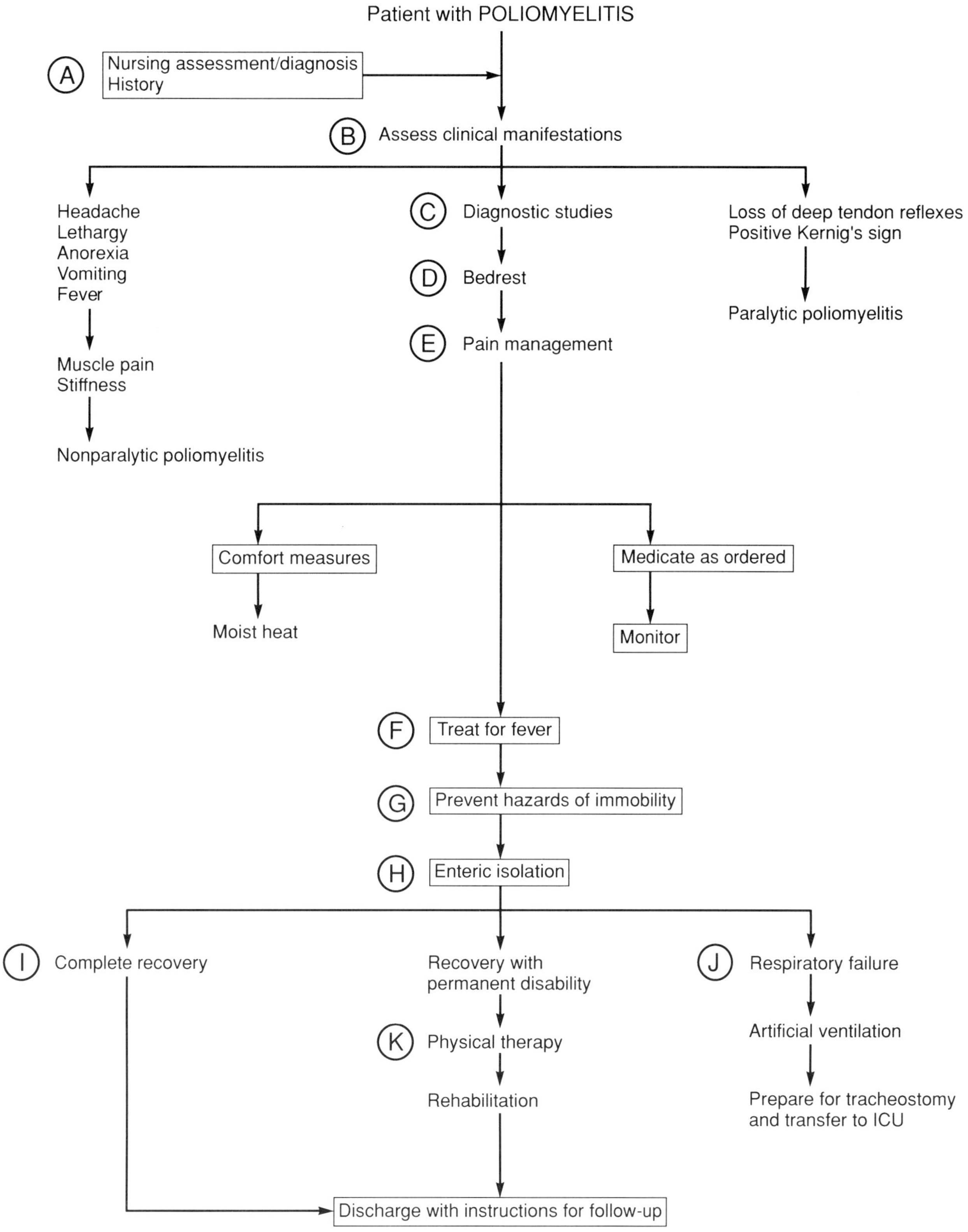
Patient with POLIOMYELITIS
A
Nursing assessment/diagnosis
History
B
Assess clinical manifestations
Headache
Lethargy
Anorexia
Vomiting
Fever
Muscle pain
Stiffness
Nonparalytic poliomyelitis
C
Diagnostic studies
D
Bedrest
E
Pain management
Loss of deep tendon reflexes
Positive Kernig's sign
Paralytic poliomyelitis
Comfort measures
Moist heat
Medicate as ordered
Monitor
F
Treat for fever
G
Prevent hazards of immobility
H
Enteric isolation
I
Complete recovery
Recovery with
permanent disability
K
Physical therapy
Rehabilitation
J
Respiratory failure
Artificial ventilation
Prepare for tracheostomy
and transfer to ICU
Discharge with instructions for follow-up

INTRACRANIAL TUMOR

Kathy Gilliland

An estimated 15,000 brain tumors occur annually in the United States. Abnormal tissue growth invades normal brain tissue and by mechanical displacement and altered metabolism causes compression and cell damage. Altered neurologic function occurs, and as the tumor increases in size, compression of brain structures produces increased intracranial pressure (IICP). IICP causes progressive motor and sensory impairment and obstruction of cerebrospinal fluid. If pressure is unrelieved, infarction or herniation can lead to respiratory and/or cardiac arrest.

A. Signs and symptoms of brain tumors occur in different degrees depending on the type, location, and size of the tumor. Brain tumors can occur at any age and affect the sexes equally. Tumors are classified according to location and tissue type. A single specific cause of brain tumors is unknown; however, several theories are under investigation. It is thought that viral infections, stress, trauma, cell abnormalities, and environmental toxins are contributing factors. Some, such as von Recklinghausen's tumors, are inherited.

B. Patients may complain of generalized or localized headaches (p 28), visual disturbances, memory loss, personality changes, seizures (p 30), and motor-sensory impairment. A differential diagnosis is necessary because of the variety of disorders (e.g., headaches, central nervous system infections, cerebrovascular accident, arteriovenous malformation, and seizure disorder) that may mimic or mask a brain tumor. The initial plan of care focuses on assessment, pain management (p 406), and patient safety.

C. A complete diagnostic work-up is necessary to confirm brain tumor and identify specific tumor characteristics (location, size, suspected histology, prognosis, surgical approach). Skull radiographs identify bony involvement; cerebral angiography confirms vessel incorporation; computed tomography provides confirmed location, structural involvement, and tissue invasion; bone scans identify metastatic disease, electroencephalography identifies areas of abnormal or impaired electrical activity of brain tissue, and cerebral blood flow studies pinpoint deficient areas of circulation. Because brain tumors carry a high morbidity and mortality, early diagnosis is the key to recovery.

D. Patients undergoing complete work-ups need ongoing support and specific diagnostic education. Throughout the diagnostic period, continuous neurologic assessment, assistance with activities of daily living, pain control, and emotional support should be considered.

E. Treatment is instituted from medical and surgical modalities. Surgical resection of brain tumors attempts removal of the total tumor mass without impairment of adjacent structures. Nonoperative treatment encompasses short- and long-term medical therapies.

F. Corticosteroids assist in decreasing cerebral edema resulting from cell invasion, destruction, and mechanical compression. Prednisone is given for metastatic brain tumors.

G. Chemotherapy is usually reserved for palliative treatment measures, but may be used in conjunction with tumor resection and radiation. The selection of specific agents is dependent on tumor type, projected prognosis, age, and function of the patient. Care of the patient receiving chemotherapy is discussed on p 408.

H. Postoperative radiation attempts to destroy tumor cells by damaging DNA molecules. Radiation may also be used when the location of the tumor in or near vital structures makes surgery difficult. The effects of radiotherapy are directly related to the number of treatments and the cumulative amount of radiation.

I. After the tumor is confirmed, care is directed toward managing the effects of treatment, supporting altered self-perceptions, and managing pain and seizure activities (p 30).

J. Recovery from intracranial tumors is usually a long process and includes rehabilitation and/or referral to support organizations. Family members or other support persons should be included in discharge planning.

References

American Association of Neuroscience Nursing. Core curriculum. Park Ridge, IL: AANN, 1980:355–361.

Belcher AE. Neoplasia. In: Thompson J, McFarland GK, Hirsch JE, Tucker SM, Bowers AC. Clinical nursing. St. Louis: CV Mosby, 1986:1442–1443.

Burgess KE. Neurological disturbance in a patient with an intracranial neoplasm: sources and implications for nursing care. J Neurol Nurs 1983; 15:237–242.

Heckey J. The clinical practice of neurological and neurosurgical nursing. Philadelphia: JB Lippincott, 1981.

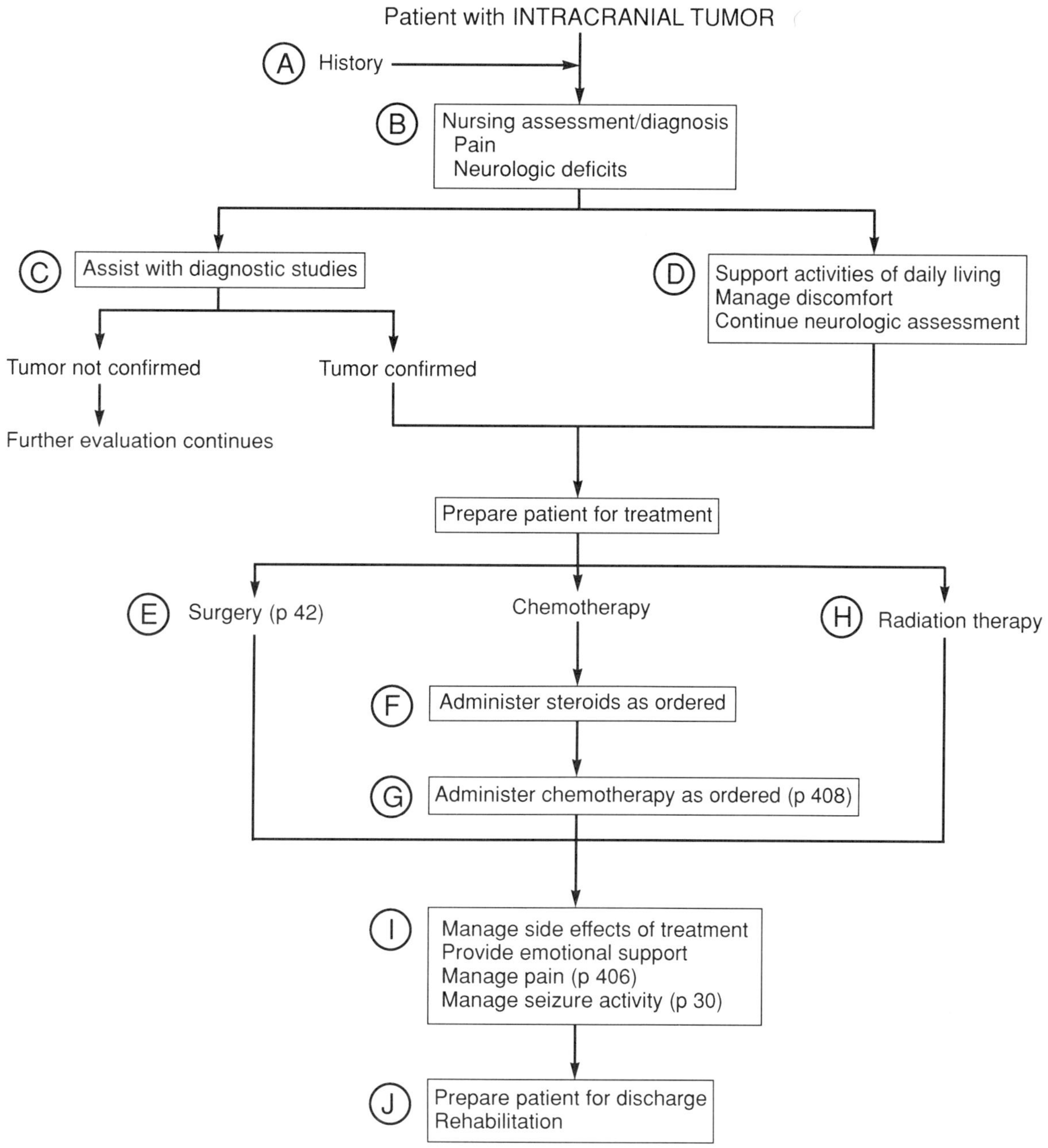
Patient with INTRACRANIAL TUMOR
A History
B Nursing assessment/diagnosis
Pain
Neurologic deficits
C Assist with diagnostic studies
Tumor not confirmed
Further evaluation continues
Tumor confirmed
D Support activities of daily living
Manage discomfort
Continue neurologic assessment
Prepare patient for treatment
E Surgery (p 42)
Chemotherapy
H Radiation therapy
F Administer steroids as ordered
G Administer chemotherapy as ordered (p 408)
I Manage side effects of treatment
Provide emotional support
Manage pain (p 406)
Manage seizure activity (p 30)
J Prepare patient for discharge
Rehabilitation

SPINAL CORD TUMOR

Kathy Gilliland

Spinal tumors comprise approximately $\frac{1}{2}$ to 1 percent of all tumors occurring in the general population. These tumors are classified according to location, type, and extent of tissue involvement (Table 1). Most spinal tumors are benign unless they arise from primary sources such as the lung (p 122), kidney, gastrointestinal tract, or breast. Tumors of the spine and/or spinal cord are more commonly found in the thoracic area, but cervical and lumbar area lesions are also found.

TABLE 1 Tumor Classification

Classification	*Characteristics*
Extradural	(Approximately 50% of total) Arise in the vertebral bones, the extradural space, or in the paraspinal tissue Usually have an abrupt onset due to compression forces.
Intradural	Contained within or below the dural meningeal layer. Two basic types.
Extramedullary	Usually benign, located within the dural layer but without spinal cord involvement
Intramedullary	Contained within the spinal cord tissue. Often with diffuse involvement of multiple fiber tracts resulting in chronic progressive changes Can be associated with low-grade malignancy or metastasis

A. Signs and symptoms are related to the area and extent of involvement. The parameters affected are the degree of spinal instability, the level of pain, the existing motor and/or sensory impairment, and the loss of sphincter control. These effects correspond with the degree of bony erosion, compression of the spinal cord, and tissue invasion. The onset and progression of neurologic impairment is commonly proportional to the growth rate and the particulate make-up of the tumor (hard versus soft). Generally, slow-growing tumors permit the spinal cord to adjust to the invasion and/or compression, and as a result the deficits seen with this type of tumor have a nonspecific onset and are usually less severe. Fast-growing tumors, such as malignant lesions, have a more abrupt onset and usually present with notable deficits.

B. Pain that can be localized to the affected area is caused by compression, bony destruction, stress on the dural structures and nerve roots, and edema. Motor and sensory impairment can be identified with the myotomal and sensory dermatome patterns. Bladder and bowel sphincter weakness is assessed by noting current function compared with previous habits. Lesions producing sphincter involvement are usually bilateral in nature and present with urinary retention, overflow, constipation, and/or fecal impaction.

C. Nursing care initially focuses on assisting the patient with the activities of daily living (ADLs) altered by neurologic deficits.

D. The diagnosis of spinal tumor is made by a complete neurologic examination and neuroradiologic diagnostic procedures such as spinal radiology, electromyography (EMG), myelography (p 240), bone scan, lumbar puncture, angiography, and magnetic resonance imaging (MRI).

E. Patient support is required throughout this phase and is best implemented through pre- and postprocedure teaching with reinforcement and discussion of the patient-physician communications.

F. Medical and/or surgical interventions are employed in the treatment of spinal tumors. Surgical decompression and tumor resection is accomplished with spinal laminectomy or vertebrectomy and is frequently followed by spinal fusion.

G. Nursing care during the treatment period centers on general postoperative care (see laminectomy care, p 46) and is related to the types of procedures employed as well as the degree of neurologic deficit present (pain, motor and sensory impairment, sphincter disturbance). The nursing care plan addresses assessment of motor and sensory function (compared with baseline); pain control; bowel and bladder training and maintenance; positioning and range of motion; and use of orthoses, i.e., TLSO (thoracic lumbosacral orthosis), cervical collar, or halo jacket.

H. Medical management is employed for metastatic lesions and involves radiation and chemotherapy (p 408). It is believed that spinal metastasis occurs as a late involvement and is associated with a short overall survival. Death in these cases is usually attributed to associated complications, e.g., pulmonary obstruction or renal failure (p 210).

I. Discharge planning includes referral to rehabilitation support groups to assist with long-term deficits. Regular follow-ups are necessary to avoid secondary complications.

References

American Association of Neuroscience Nursing. Core curriculum. Park Ridge, IL: AANN, 1980:378–388.

Hickey J. The clinical practice of neurological and neurosurgical nursing. Philadelphia: JB Lippincott, 1980.

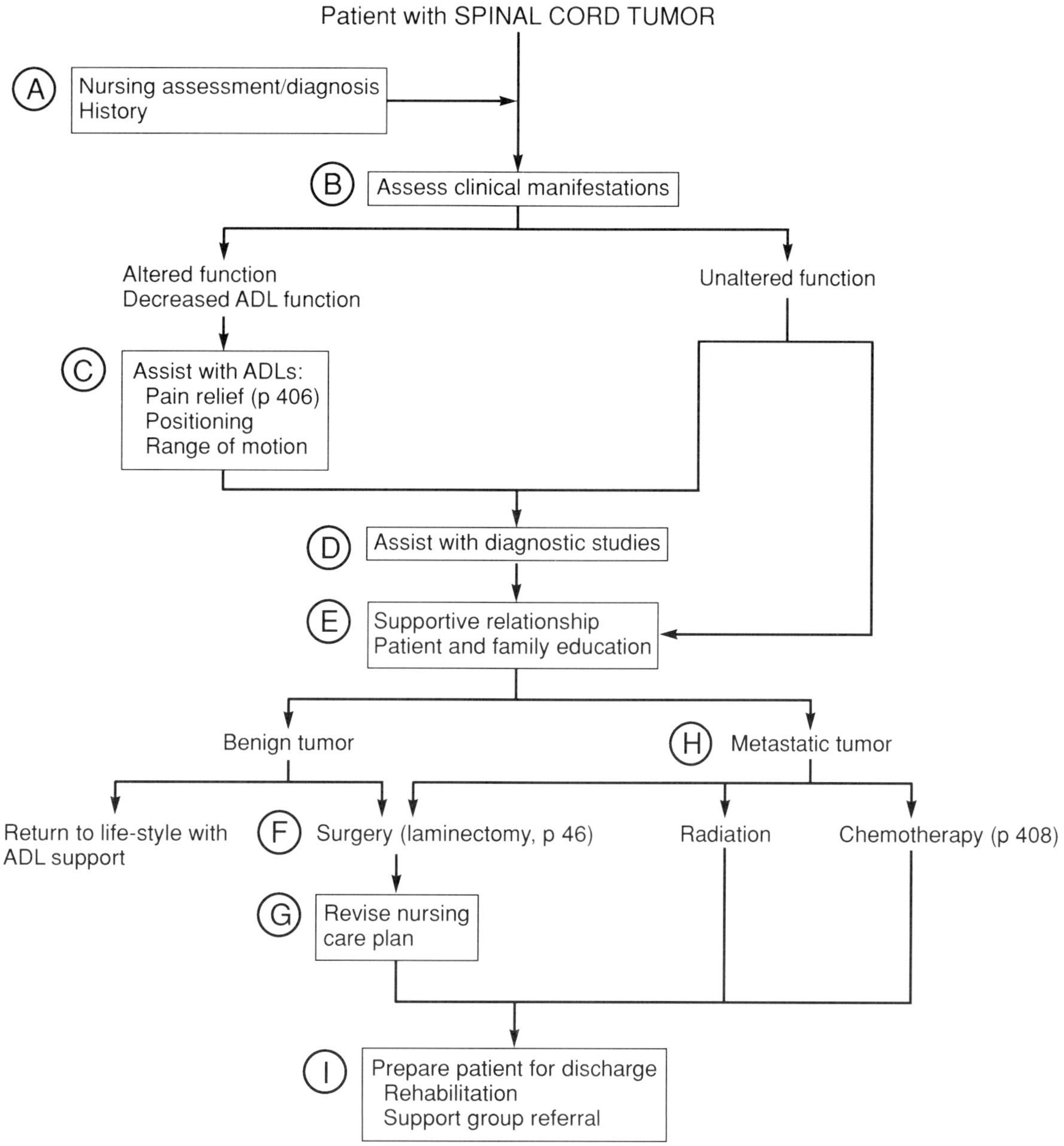
Patient with SPINAL CORD TUMOR
A
Nursing assessment/diagnosis
History
B
Assess clinical manifestations
Altered function
Decreased ADL function
Unaltered function
C
Assist with ADLs:
Pain relief (p 406)
Positioning
Range of motion
D
Assist with diagnostic studies
E
Supportive relationship
Patient and family education
Benign tumor
H
Metastatic tumor
Return to life-style with
ADL support
F
Surgery (laminectomy, p 46)
Radiation
Chemotherapy (p 408)
G
Revise nursing
care plan
I
Prepare patient for discharge
Rehabilitation
Support group referral

CRANIOTOMY

Joy Gorzeman
Carol Bowdoin

A craniotomy is a surgical opening through the skull. It is the method for gaining access to intracranial structures for the removal of a tumor (p 36), abscess (p 6), or blood clot, to relieve pressure or to stop hemorrhage (p 20) (Fig. 1).

A. Unless the procedure is an emergency, patients scheduled for a craniotomy have generally been through many examinations and diagnostic studies. These patients are usually in the hospital being treated for the clinical manifestations that caused them to seek medical help and diagnosis initially (such as headaches). Treatments are maintained during the preoperative phase.

B. In neurologic surgeries it is especially important that a preoperative baseline neurologic and physiologic assessment be completed and recorded, in order to make postoperative comparisons. Other preoperative care is similar to that for general surgery (p 2). Care should include patient and family teaching, checking the operative permit, and performing a skull prep according to orders. The nurse should be sensitive to the patient's concerns regarding the change in body image resulting from shaving the scalp. The use of a scarf, wig, or other headpiece may be suggested to allay the patient's anxiety. Enemas should be avoided because of the increased intracranial pressure (ICP) caused by straining. Preoperative medications may also vary in neurologic patients. Narcotics are rarely ordered because they depress cerebral function. Steroids may be given to decrease brain edema. A Foley catheter is inserted before surgery so that urine output can be monitored throughout the long surgical procedure. An orientation to the neurologic ICU should be included if intensive care is anticipated postoperatively.

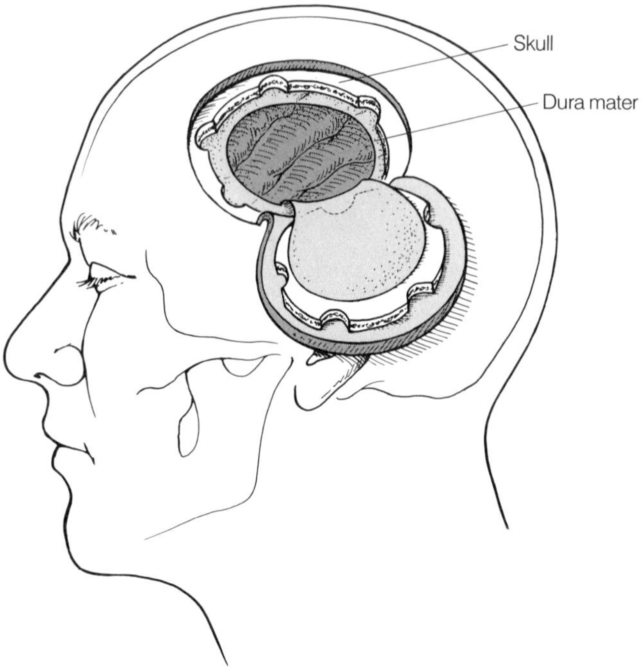

Figure 1 Craniotomy

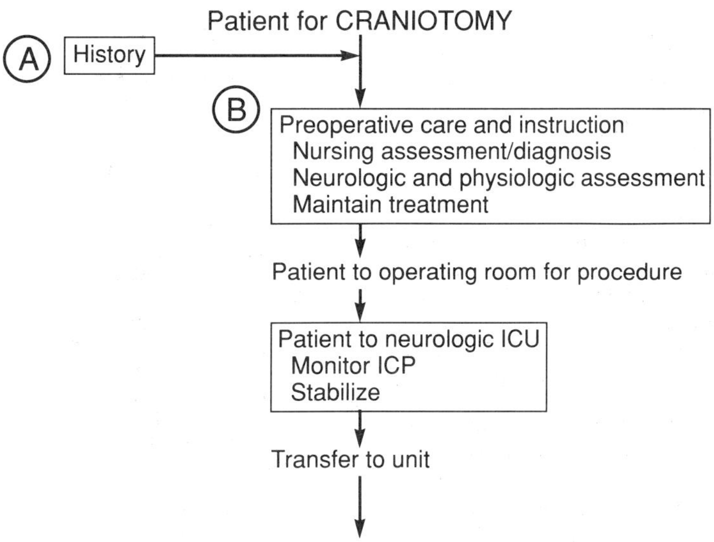
Patient for CRANIOTOMY
A
History
B
Preoperative care and instruction
Nursing assessment/diagnosis
Neurologic and physiologic assessment
Maintain treatment
Patient to operating room for procedure
Patient to neurologic ICU
Monitor ICP
Stabilize
Transfer to unit

(Cont'd on p 45)

C. Postoperative nursing care for the craniotomy patient during the intensive care period focuses on observation for life-threatening complications such as increased ICP via invasive ICP monitoring devices. Upon stabilization, the patient is transferred to the nursing unit.

D. Since even mild hypoxia increases swelling of the brain, it is of utmost importance to maintain an adequate airway in the craniotomy patient. Monitoring of arterial blood gases is important. The unconscious patient should be positioned in a lateral position to promote drainage. Coughing is contraindicated because it increases ICP. Suctioning also increases ICP and extreme caution must be taken if suctioning is necessary.

E. It is important to assess the patient's vital signs and level of consciousness frequently. A neurologic assessment tool should be used to document and record findings, as changes may indicate increased ICP (Table 1). In addition, an increased temperature and/or pulse and respiratory rate should cause the nurse to suspect infection.

F. The dressing should be checked regularly and reinforced as necessary. Wet dressings may promote absorption of pathogens and increase the risk of meningitis (p 30). Yellow drainage should be reported to the physician, since it may indicate loss of cerebrospinal fluid. It is not unusual for the physician to remove the dressings on the first postoperative day. At this point, the wound is observed to be sure it is clean and dry. Hydrogen peroxide may be used to clean the incisional area. Report any bulging since that is a sign of increased ICP or fluid accumulation.

G. It is common for craniotomy patients to experience a severe headache for 24 to 48 hours postoperatively. Codeine, aspirin, or acetaminophen is the drug of choice; central nervous system depressants are avoided. An ice bag on the head may help. Other comfort measures include maintaining a quiet environment and avoiding sudden, jarring movements.

H. Fluid intake and output must be accurately recorded. Intravenous fluids must be run slowly as rapid administration raises ICP. Fluids by mouth may be resumed when the patient is conscious and has a stable neurologic status. Urine output should be monitored and any abnormalities must be reported. Specifically, patients who have undergone hypophysectomy (pituitary surgery) must be observed for diabetes insipidus (p 178). Constipation should be avoided, since straining also increases ICP.

I. Depending on the location of the lesion, some craniotomy patients may be allowed out of bed on the third postoperative day. Activity should begin slowly and the patient must be observed for signs of increased ICP. Complaints of dizziness or drop in blood pressure should stop ambulation, and the patient should rest several hours before activity is tried again.

J. Craniotomy patients and their families require a great deal of emotional support. The recovery process is long and often involves adaptation to a change in body image.

TABLE 1 Neurological Assessment Tool*

Focus of Assessment	*Rating*
Orientation	
Time, place, person	x3
2 of 3	x2
1 of 3	x1
Not oriented	0
Level of consciousness	
Eye-opening response	
With purpose/spontaneous	4
To voice/command	3
To painful stimuli	2
No opening/response	1
Verbal response	
Oriented x3	5
Disoriented/confused	4
Inappropriate	3
Groans, grunts	2
No response	1
Motor response	
Obeys commands	6
Localizes pain	5
Withdraws from pain	4
Flexes to pain	3
Extends to pain	2
Flaccid	1
Pupils	
Reaction	
Brisk	B
Sluggish	S
Absent	A
Equality	
Equal	=
Left larger	L > R
Right larger	R > L
Size	1–8 mm

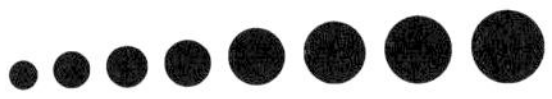

1 2 3 4 5 6 7 8

Limb movement	
Normal	5
Weak (mild or severe)	4
Spastic flexion of arms	3
Extension	2
No response	1
Untestable	U

* Eye-opening, verbal, and motor responses are adapted from the Glasgow Coma Scale. The highest possible rating is 15; scores of 7 or less indicate coma.

References

Brunner LS, Suddarth DS. The Lippincott manual of nursing practice. 4th ed. Philadelphia: JB Lippincott, 1986.

Luckmann J, Sorensen KC. Medical-surgical nursing. 3rd ed. WB Saunders, 1987.

Phipps WJ, Long BC, Woods NF. Medical surgical nursing concepts and clinical practice. St. Louis: CV Mosby, 1987.

Stevens SA, Becker KL. Neurologic assessment. Part 1. Nursing 1988; 18(9): 53–61.

Patient for CRANIOTOMY

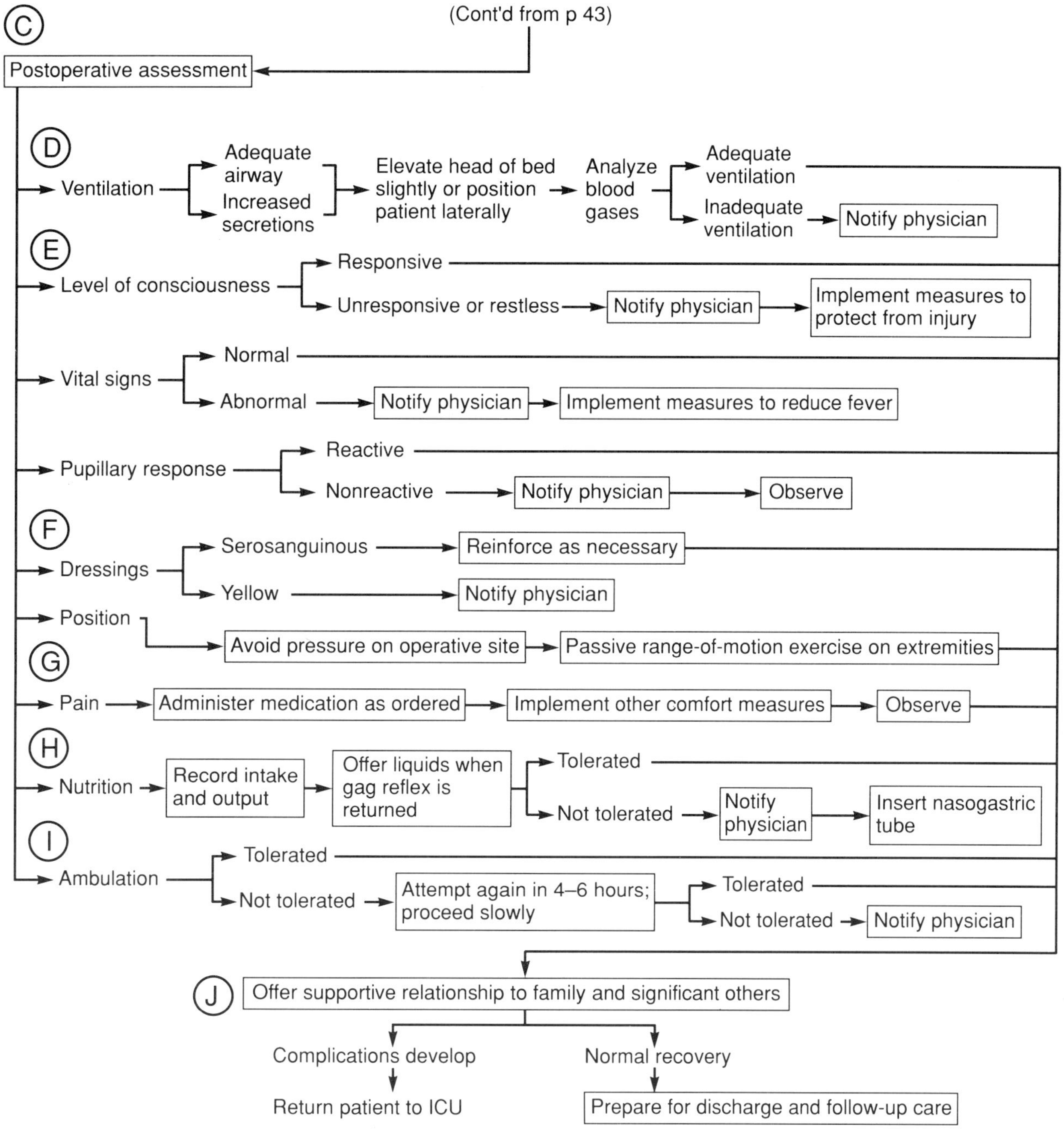

LAMINECTOMY AND SPINAL FUSION

Joy Gorzeman

Laminectomy is a surgical procedure performed when a patient has a herniated, ruptured, or prolapsed intervertebral disc (Fig. 1). The posterior arch of vertebra is removed, exposing the spinal cord. The portion of the nucleus pulposus that is protruding or ruptured is removed from the intervertebral disc (Fig. 2). Depending on the patient's history, previous treatment, type of injury, and the extent of damage (neurologic deficit), a spinal fusion may be done. This procedure involves the removal of a piece or pieces of bone from another area of the body (usually the iliac crest) and the grafting of these pieces onto the vertebrae. Once the graft "takes," a bony union is formed and causes stiffness in that area. Usually, ruptured, prolapsed, or herniated intervertebral discs occur at the fourth or fifth intervertebral spaces in the lumbar spine because of the intense wear and tear in that area. Less frequently, herniation of a disc occurs in the cervical region.

A. Unless the laminectomy/spinal fusion is the direct result of serious injury, the patient usually has a long history of back pain. Probably several more conservative methods of treatment have been tried, such as bedrest, pain medication, steroid injections, and/or use of a transcutaneous electrical nerve stimulation (TENS) unit, without success. The patient will have been through a complete evaluation involving diagnostic tests, such as electromyography, discography, computerized tomographic (CT) scan, and/or myelography (p 240). The psychological impact of chronic pain (p 406) must be considered when caring for a patient undergoing back surgery.

B. Preoperative nursing care includes promoting comfort if the patient is experiencing pain, patient teaching, emotional support, and physical preparation. Patient teaching should include expectations after surgery. The patient should practice deep breathing and log rolling. Demonstrate any equipment the patient will be using, such as a special bed or a TENS unit. Reassure the patient that medication will be given for pain after surgery. Physical preparation includes a prepackaged enema and a Betadine or cleansing shower. Routine laboratory and x-ray studies are also done.

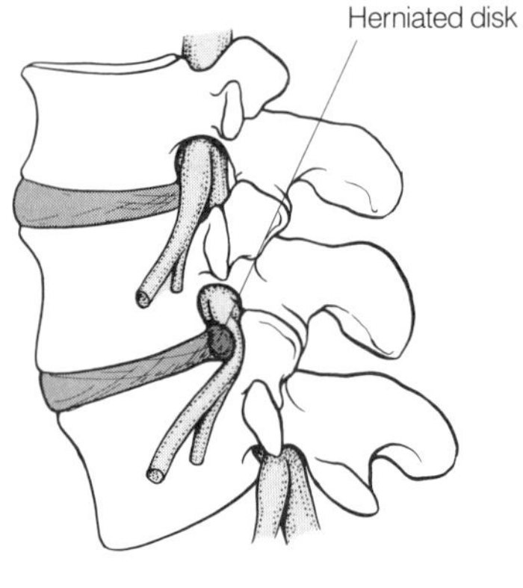

Figure 1 Herniated disk between L4 and L5, lateral view.

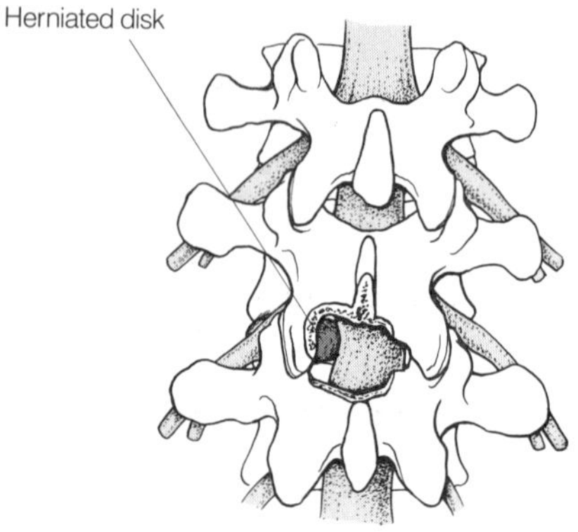

Figure 2 Laminectomy: Posterior arch removed to relieve compression.

C. Postoperative nursing care is directed at preventing complications or further injury and providing opportunity for the wound/graft to heal. Routine postoperative procedures such as vital signs and assessment are done. Assessment of the patient with a laminectomy/spinal fusion includes motor function, sensation, color, and temperature of the lower extremities. When evaluating numbness and tingling, it is important to know whether these sensations were present before surgery. Worsening of any of these conditions may indicate nerve root injury, spinal cord edema, or hemorrhage and must be reported to the physician immediately. The patient with cervical laminectomy/spinal fusion requires frequent neurologic checks. This patient may experience respiratory difficulty, since it is hard to cough and eliminate respiratory secretions.

D. Observe the dressing for cerebrospinal fluid leakage or bleeding. Patients with spinal fusions may have two dressings, one at the graft site. Oozing is not common following a laminectomy and should be reported. There may be some oozing after a spinal fusion. When changing the dressing, observe the wound for infection.

E. Administer pain medication as needed. Encourage the patient to cough and breathe deeply. Assist him in turning (log rolling) according to the doctor's orders. The spine must be in correct alignment at all times. Twisting and bending must be avoided. The call bell should be within reach so that the patient doesn't have to strain. Gentle neck and back rubs help stimulate circulation.

F. Check the patient's bladder for distention. Straining should be avoided; encourage fluids and assist with diet selections high in roughage to avoid constipation.

G. The timing of ambulation depends on the type of procedure and the physician. The trend is toward earlier ambulation. If the patient has had a spinal fusion, he needs to wear a brace or corset when walking.

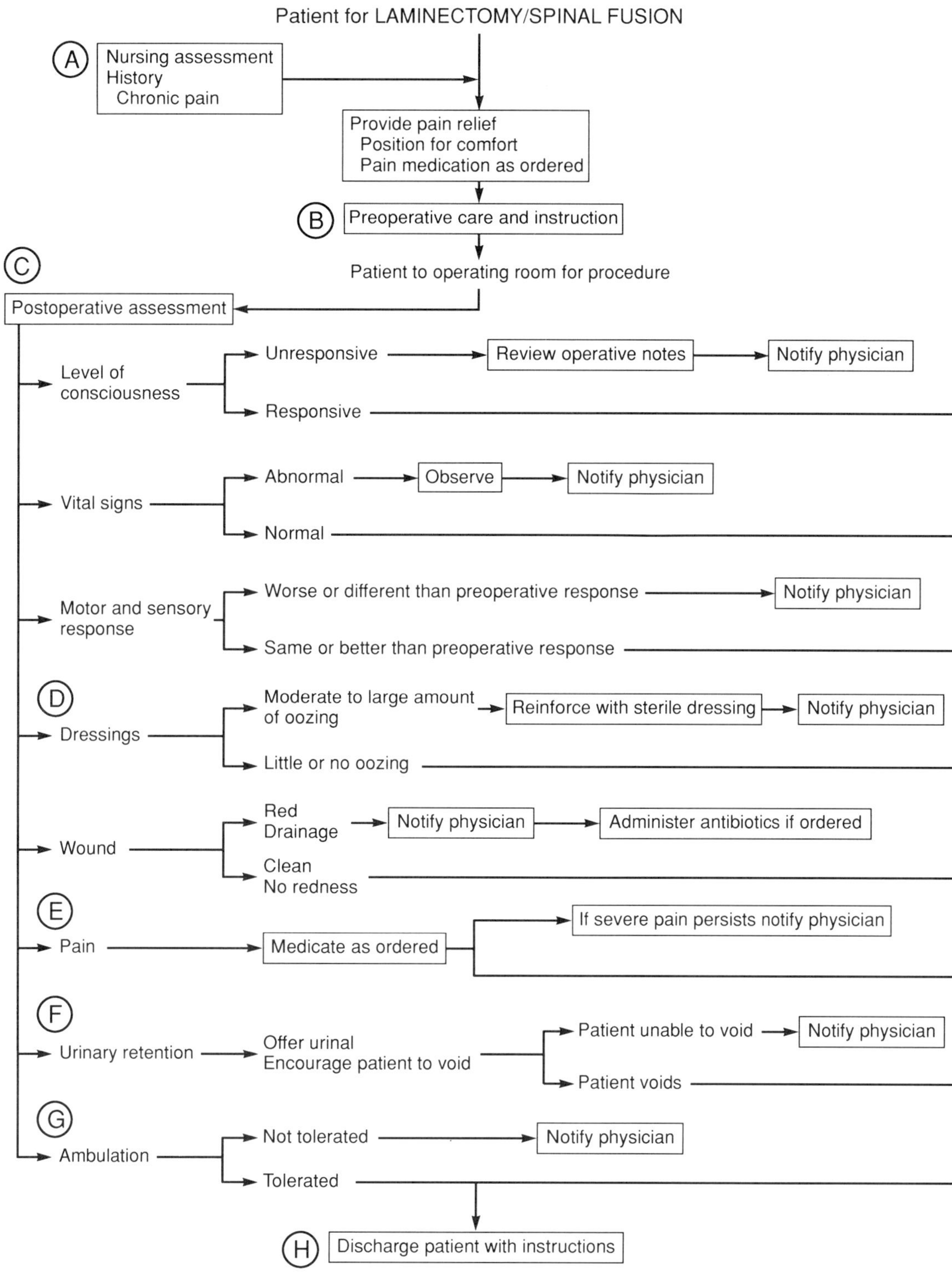

H. If there are no complications, the patient is discharged with specific instructions. He should avoid strain on the spine, which would preclude such activities as climbing stairs, driving the car, and sexual intercourse, for about 6 weeks. He should do exercises as taught by the physical therapist. Walking is better than standing; the patient needs to be alert when walking in order to avoid falling. He should sit for only about 30 minutes at a time. Heavy lifting should be avoided for 3 to 6 months.

References

Brunner LS, Suddarth DS. The Lippincott manual of nursing practice. 4th ed. Philadelphia: JB Lippincott, 1986.

Luckmann J, Sorensen KC. Medical-surgical nursing. 3rd ed. Philadelphia: WB Saunders, 1987.

Mims BC. Current trends in the diagnosis and treatment of low back pain. RN 1985; 48(5):26–32.

CARDIOVASCULAR SYSTEM

CHEST PAIN

Carla K. Calloway

The single biggest cause of significant chest pain is ischemic heart disease. However, ischemic heart disease usually does not occur until the cross-sectional area of a major coronary artery is reduced by 50 to 75 percent. Therefore, one must consider the many other causes of chest pain, including cardiovascular disease, pulmonary disease, musculoskeletal pain, and gastrointestinal pain (Fig. 1). In the patient with cardiovascular disease (p 66), myocardial infarction (MI), angina pectoris, unstable angina, Prinzmetal's angina, valvular disease (p 72), dissecting aortic aneurysm, acute pericarditis (p 76), congenital abnormalities, and arrhythmia and conduction defects (p 52) must be considered. In the patient with pulmonary disease, consideration should be given to pulmonary embolus (p 116), pneumonia (p 104), pneumothorax or hemothorax (p 110), and pleurisy (p 106). Musculoskeletal-related chest pain may be caused by muscle cramps or rib fractures. Gastrointestinal-related chest pain may be caused by esophageal reflux, esophagitis, cholecystitis (p 160), hiatal hernia, or peptic ulcer disease (p 130).

A. The initial assessment and history should attempt to distinguish between minor causes of chest pain and those that are potentially life-threatening. The history should include a definition of the chest pain. The nurse should determine the location of pain, severity, and whether it is dull or sharp, intermittent or continuous, increased by deep inspiration or cough, induced by activity or trauma, or relieved by position. Consider also any recent or associated symptoms with the pain. Assess the patient for dyspnea and labored breathing. Identify any cardiac risk factors; the more risk factors present, the greater the chance a person has heart disease. These factors include heredity, male sex, cigarette smoking, elevated blood cholesterol, hypertension, and diabetes. Obesity, lack of exercise, and stress are also contributing factors. Diagnosis begins with differentiating the chest pain as cardiac-related or due to some other cause. Diagnosis and treatment are based on the history, physical assessment, and diagnostic studies (which include electrocardiography [ECG], chest film, and cardiac enzyme studies).

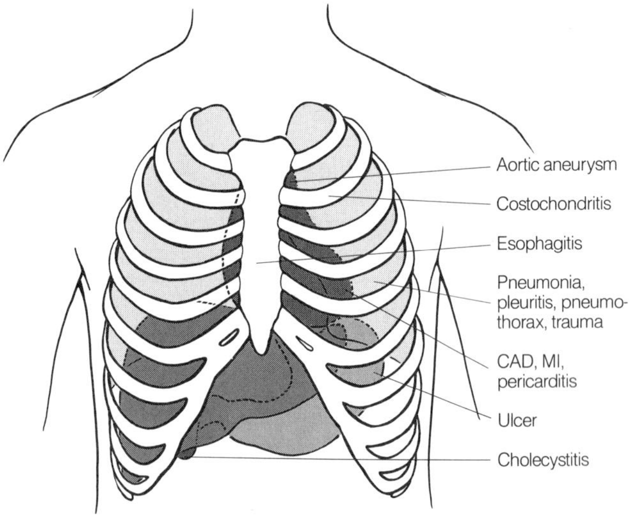

Figure 1 Sources of chest pain.

B. ECG monitoring with a single lead helps to identify arrhythmias; however, other changes (e.g., ischemia, infarction, hypertrophy, bundle branch blocks) may only be appreciated by a 12-Lead ECG (p 54). It is most important to obtain the ECG while the patient is experiencing chest pain. Ischemic changes may appear *only* during this time. It is also important to obtain an ECG as soon as possible, not only for differential purposes, but also to document evolutional changes in the setting of MI. While looking for new changes, it is helpful to compare the most recent ECG with a previous one.

C. The chest radiograph helps identify infiltrates or consolidation, which could occur with pneumonia (p 104); abnormalities in the pleural space, such as pneumothorax or hemothorax (p 110); or bony abnormalities, such as rib fractures. An enlarged heart or pericardial sac (p 76) could be due to any number of acute or chronic causes.

D. Cardiac enzymes should also be studied soon after the onset of chest pain in order to document any elevation. Repeat measurements, at 6- to 8-hour intervals over the next 2 to 3 days, will indicate the extent of damage in the setting of a cardiac event.

E. Nursing care of the patient with chest pain is directed at immediate nursing assessment and interventions and assisting with a differential diagnosis. Preventing complications and further injury is important; therefore, the patient should be kept on bedrest until further evaluation can be done. The nurse should offer emotional support and reassurance to the patient while the cause of pain is being determined. The call bell should be within easy reach. All procedures and diagnostic tests should be explained to allay anxiety. Patients should be told that they can help by reporting any change in the character of their pain or other symptoms they may experience. Once a differential diagnosis has been made, nursing care can be focused on managing specific problems related to the etiology, e.g., MI (p 66), pulmonary embolism (p 104), pericarditis (p 76), or pneumonia (p 104).

F. Discharge instructions depend on the cause of the chest pain. The patient should, however, be taught how to prevent or reduce the risk of a recurrence of chest pain and what to do if the pain does recur. Prevention of recurrence may include instructions regarding medications, activity levels, reduction of risk factors, and changes in dietary habits.

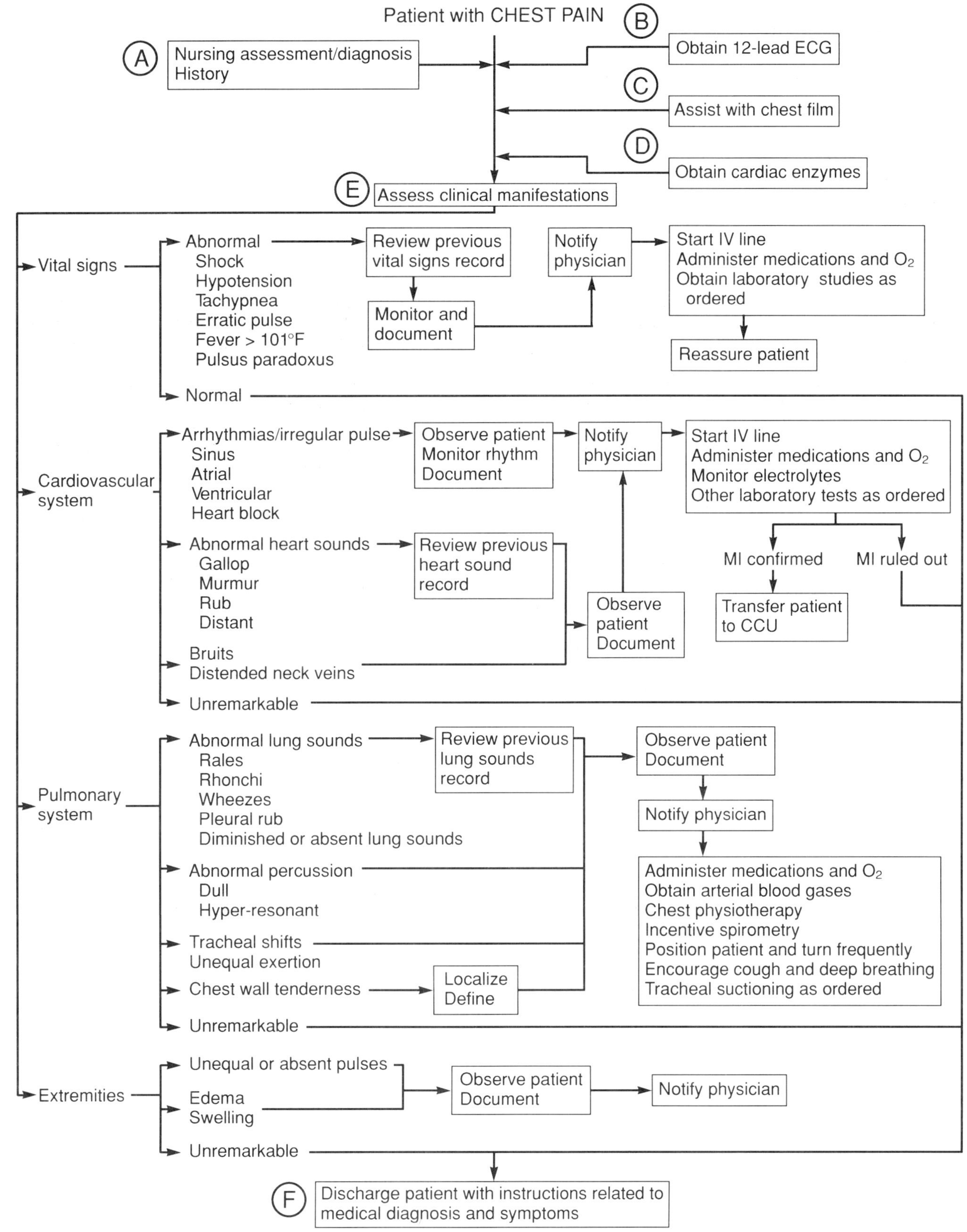

References

Handerhan B. Action stat: chest pain. Nursing 89; 19(6):33.

May HL. Emergency medicine. New York: John Wiley, 1984.

Mills J, Ho MT, Salber PR, Trunkey DD. Current emergency diagnosis and treatment. 2nd ed. Los Altos, CA: Lange, 1985.

Smith CE. Assessing chest pain quickly and accurately. Nursing 88 1988; 18(5): 52–59.

AN INTRODUCTION TO CARDIAC ARRHYTHMIAS

Kendra Ellis
Carol Bowdoin

An alteration in the normal rhythm of the heart is often called an arrhythmia, dysrhythmia, or ectopic rhythm.

A. Arrhythmias may be caused by underlying cardiac disease, metabolic disorders, electrolyte imbalances, drug intoxication, or congenital defects that result in conduction abnormalities. Occasionally ectopic rhythms are normal variations; however, they may be a warning of a potentially life-threatening situation. The ability to recognize arrhythmias, assess the cause, and intervene appropriately is of utmost importance.

B. An arrhythmia causes concern when cardiac output is decreased, affecting perfusion to the heart, brain, and kidneys. The patient experiencing arrhythmias may complain of symptoms such as irregular heartbeat, pausing, palpitations, and/or dizziness and should be assessed for hemodynamic consequences. Change in heart rate or irregular pulse, drop in blood pressure, decrease in sensorium, low urine output, and cool skin indicate a decrease in perfusion to the major organs. Angina may also accompany decreased perfusion to the heart. These conditions warrant further evaluation with electrocardiography (ECG).

C. A few "ECG basics" are necessary to utilize the algorithms in the following chapters effectively. The basic conduction system consists of the sinoatrial (SA) node, atrioventricular (AV) node, bundle of His, and Purkinje fibers (Fig. 1). The SA node is the primary pacemaker, with the AV node and Purkinje-ventricular system serving as "escape" pacemakers should the SA node fail. As an electrical impulse travels through the conduction system, depolarization and repolarization of the cardiac muscle occurs. This is seen as a waveform on the ECG monitor in the familiar PQRST complex (Fig. 2) and depicts one cardiac cycle.

The ECG is a graphic representation of the impulses produced by the heart. The first deflection is the P wave, representing atrial depolarization. The spiked wave is the QRS complex, representing ventricular depolarization. The T wave is the last wave, representing ventricular repolarization. In lead II, the most common monitoring lead, these waveforms appear upright or positive. "Rhythm strips" are 6-second printed records of the cardiac rhythm used for routine monitoring. A 12-lead ECG is a diagnostic method for assessing the heart in several planes to detect conduction and ischemic abnormalities. The 12-lead ECG is indicated in the patient with questionable arrhythmias and chest pain (p 50). Figure 3 shows a normal 12-lead ECG. ECG changes indicating ischemia, injury and necrosis (infarction) of cardiac muscle are depicted in Figure 4.

Interpretation is best accomplished in a systematic manner. Five components are analyzed: rate (atrial and ventricular), rhythm, P-R interval, QRS duration, and P wave configuration. The rate can be determined by counting the number of complexes P (atrial), QRS (ventricular) within 6 seconds (between two sets of marks) and multiplying this number by 10. To determine rhythm, measure the distance between two consecutive complexes (P to P, R to R), comparing the determined distance to the rest of the complexes. If the distance is maintained at regular intervals, the rhythm is considered regular. The P-R interval is measured from the beginning of the P wave to the beginning of the QRS complex. This interval indicates the time an impulse takes to travel from the SA node to the ventricles. The normal range is 0.12 to 0.20 second or 3 to 5 small squares. The QRS duration represents the time taken for an impulse to travel through the ventricles. It is measured from the beginning of the complex to the end. The normal range is 0.06 to 0.10 second or 1.5 to 2.5 squares. P wave configuration should be noted as being a positive or negative deflection. The ECG strip should be examined to determine that every QRS complex is preceded by a P wave.

D. All newly detected arrhythmias and those producing hemodynamic consequences should be documented and immediately reported to the physician for intervention. Protocols for the treatment of life-threatening arrhythmias should be established and followed according to agency policy. Many institutions use Advanced Cardiac Life Support (ACLS) guidelines for policy development. Nurses should thoroughly familiarize themselves with their agency's policies and procedures.

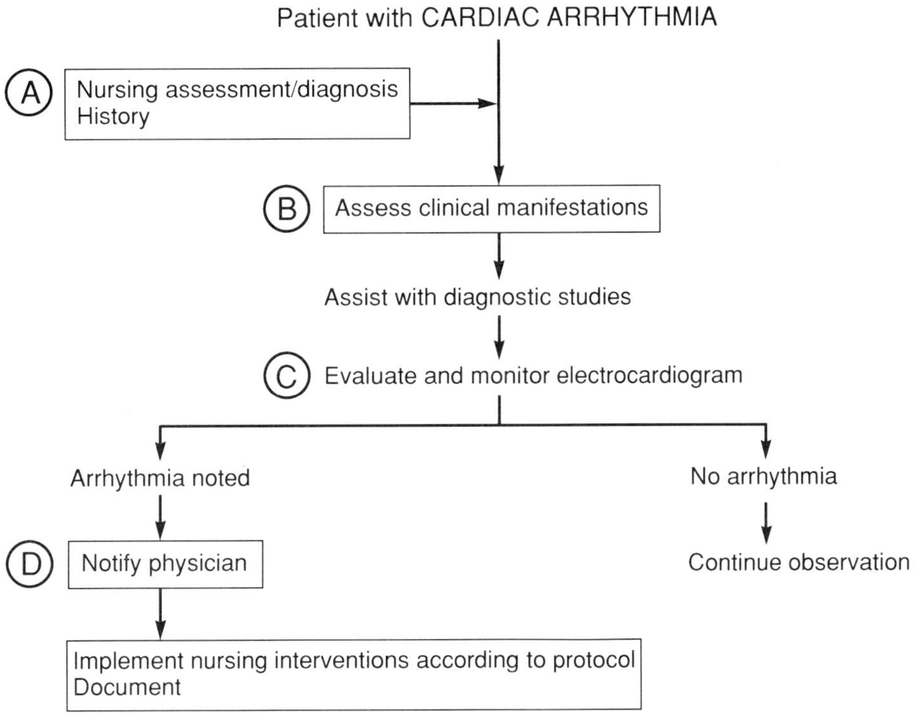

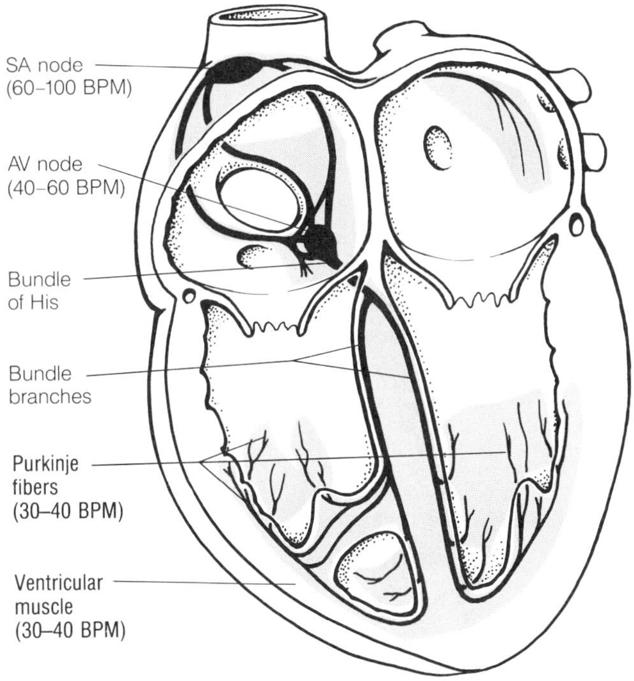

Figure 1 The conduction system consisting of (*1*) SA node with an intrinsic rate of 60 to 100 BPM, (*2*) AV node, rate 40 to 60 BPM, (*3*) bundle of His, (*4*) bundle branches, (*5*) Purkinje fibers, and (*6*) Ventricles, rate 30–40 BPM.

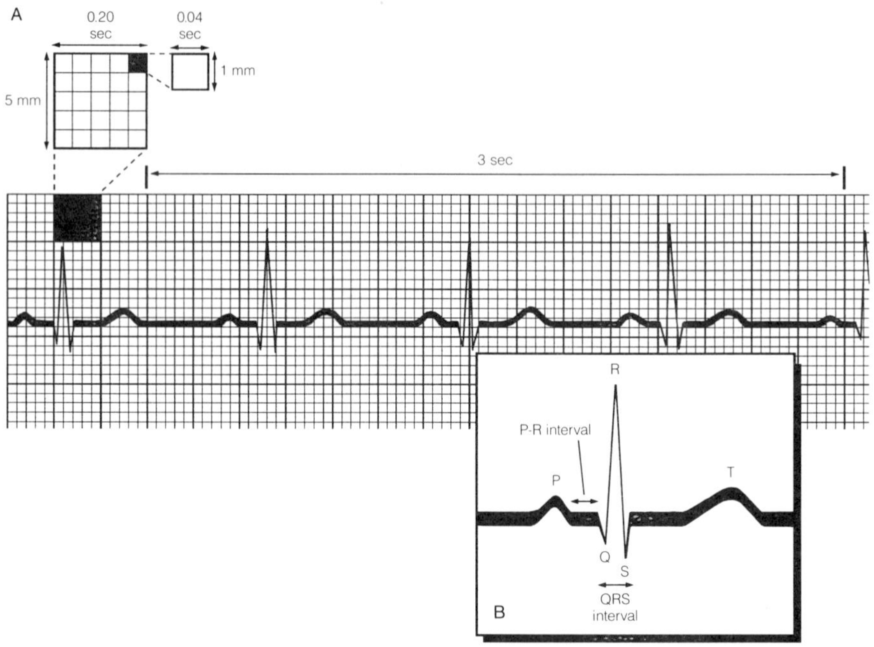

Figure 2 Basic components of 6-second rhythm strip in relation to a cardiac rhythm. (*A*) Blocks measure time and amplitude; (B) PQRST complex: P, atrial depolarization; P-R interval, impulse travels to ventricles, normal = 0.12–0.20 sec; QRS, ventricular depolarization, normal = 0.06–0.10 sec; T, ventricular repolarization.

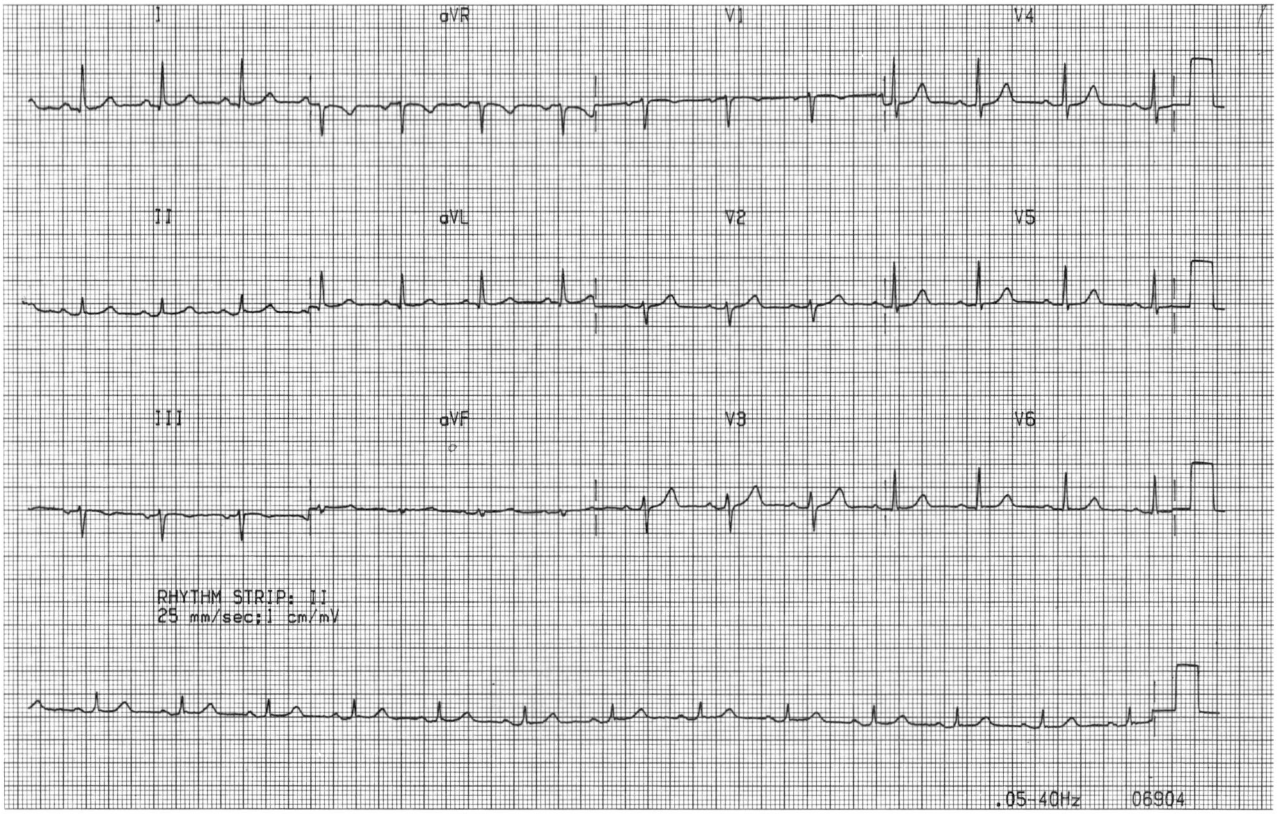

Figure 3 Normal 12-lead ECG. Leads view various surfaces of the heart: I and AVL, lateral surface; II, III, and AVF, inferior surface; V1–V6, anterior surface; AVR, mirror lead. PQRST complexes are positive in leads I, II, AVL, and V4–6. Complexes may be positive or biphasic in leads III and AVF. V1–V3 will show "R wave progression" (size of R will grow more positive). AVR will be negative.

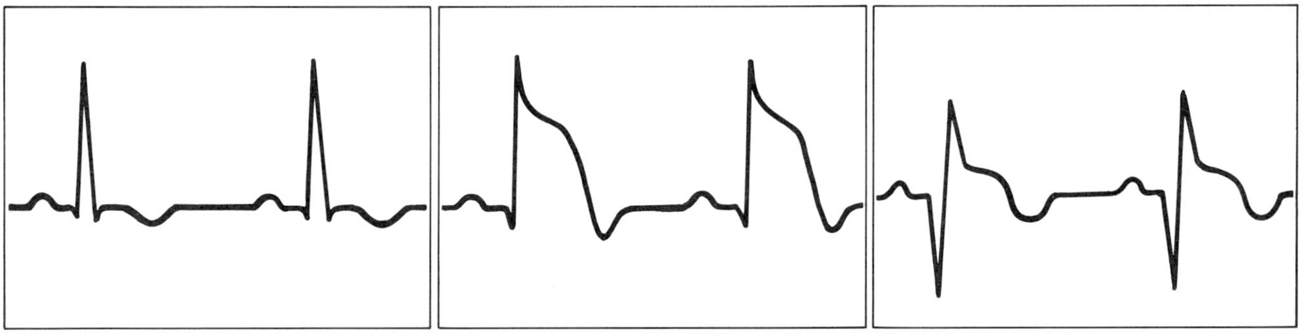

Ischemia A Injury B Infarction C

Figure 4 ECG changes indicating (*A*) ischemia, (*B*) injury, and (*C*) infarction that occur with decreased perfusion to the myocardium.

References

Bowdoin C. Alterations in cardiac rhythms. In: Bullock B, Rosenthal P, eds. Pathophysiology: adaptations and alterations in function. Boston: Scott, Foresman, 1988.

Kenner C, Guzetta C, Dossey B. Critical care nursing. Boston: Little, Brown, 1981.

Norsen L, Telfair M, Wagner A. Detecting dysrhythmias. Nursing 1986; 16(11):34–42.

SINUS RHYTHMS

Kendra Ellis

Sinus arrhythmias usually result from changes in the automaticity of the SA node. These changes may be caused by pathologic states, the effects of pharmacologic agents, or physiologic compensatory mechanisms. Arrhythmias most commonly detected by the nurse in both adult and pediatric populations are those that arise from the sinoatrial (SA) node. Normal P waves indicate sinus activity. The P-R and QRS intervals remain within normal limits. Aberrations occur in the rate or rhythm of the impulses generated by the SA node. These arrhythmias are generally benign, and treatment is directed at correcting the underlying cause.

Sinus tachycardia, sinus bradycardia, and sinus arrhythmia, the arrhythmias most often associated with changes in ventricular rate or rhythm without changes in the P, P-R, or QRS intervals, are discussed in this chapter. Sinoatrial block is discussed under "Heart Block" (p 58). Arrhythmias originating from the SA node are often asymptomatic and are discovered during routine physical examination, surgery, or treatment for another disorder. Each should be monitored, evaluated, and treated symptomatically.

A. Normal sinus rhythm (NSR) is the rhythm produced by the normally functioning conduction system. NSR is characterized by a rate of 60 to 100 beats per minute with a regular rhythm (Fig. 1A).

B. Sinus tachycardia (Fig. 1B) is caused by increased automaticity in the SA node, producing a ventricular rate greater than 100 beats per minute. Causes include fever, anxiety, pain, hypoxia, hypovolemia, and drugs (i.e., caffeine, nicotine, and aminophylline). The rapid heart rate increases myocardial oxygen demand, placing patients with a history of coronary artery disease (CAD) (p 66) at risk. This is clinically significant in the patient experiencing a myocardial infarction (MI) because infarction size may be increased.

C. Sinus bradycardia (Fig. 1C) is due to decreased automaticity in the SA node, producing a rate of 50 beats per minute or less. The causes include increased vagal tone, athletic conditioning, sleep, increased intracranial pressure, inferior MI, and drugs (i.e., digitalis, morphine, and Inderal). It is important to assess hemodynamic stability. Bradycardia may allow other pacemakers in the heart to fire an impulse, resulting in "breakthrough" arrhythmias. Hemodynamically, the slow rate may produce a "symptomatic" reduction in cardiac output. In some cases, a slow heart rate lowers myocardial oxygen demands, which may be beneficial after an MI. Sinus bradycardia is treated when the patient experiences dizziness, hypotension, and/or loss of consciousness. Atropine, 0.5 mg to 1.0 mg, is given intravenously if the patient is hemodynamically unstable. Atropine increases the heart rate by altering vagal effects on the SA node.

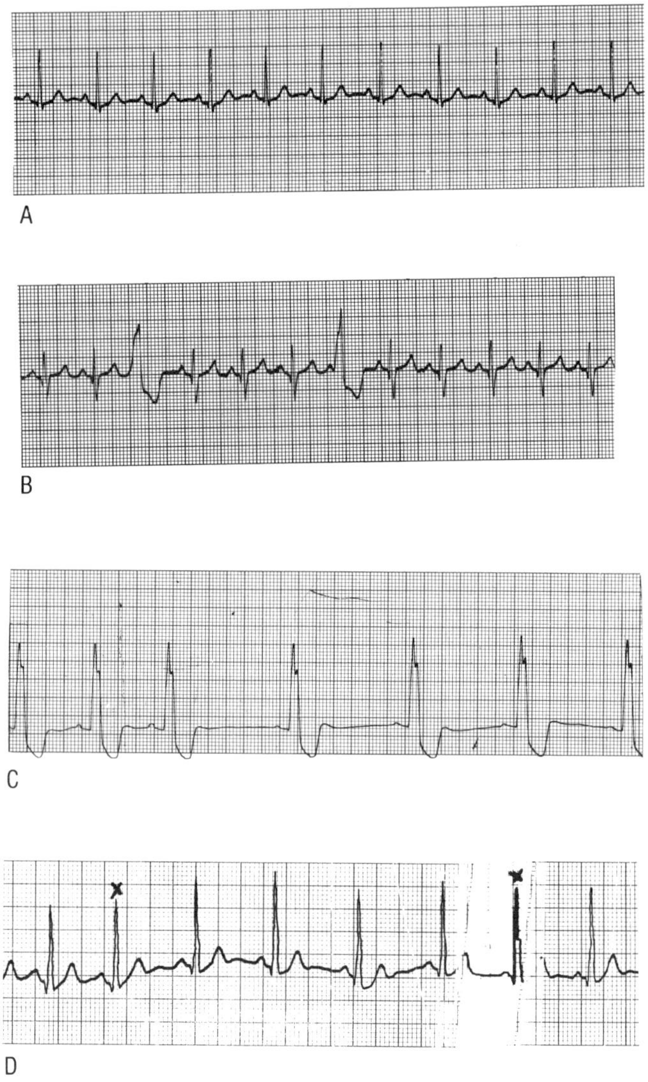

Figure 1 *A.* Normal sinus rhythm. *B.* Sinus tachycardia. *C.* Sinus bradycardia with Bundle Branch Block configuration. *D.* Sinus arrhythmia: Heart rate varies from 96 to 84 with respiratory cycle at x's.

D. Sinus arrhythmia is the most common sinus rhythm disturbance. It is caused by physiologic factors that influence vagal tone. In the patient with sinus arrhythmia, the heart rate varies with the respiratory cycle, increasing with inhalation and decreasing with exhalation. The PQRS complexes and intervals remain normal (p 53). This arrhythmia is clinically significant only when the ventricular rate slows enough to allow ectopic beats to escape.

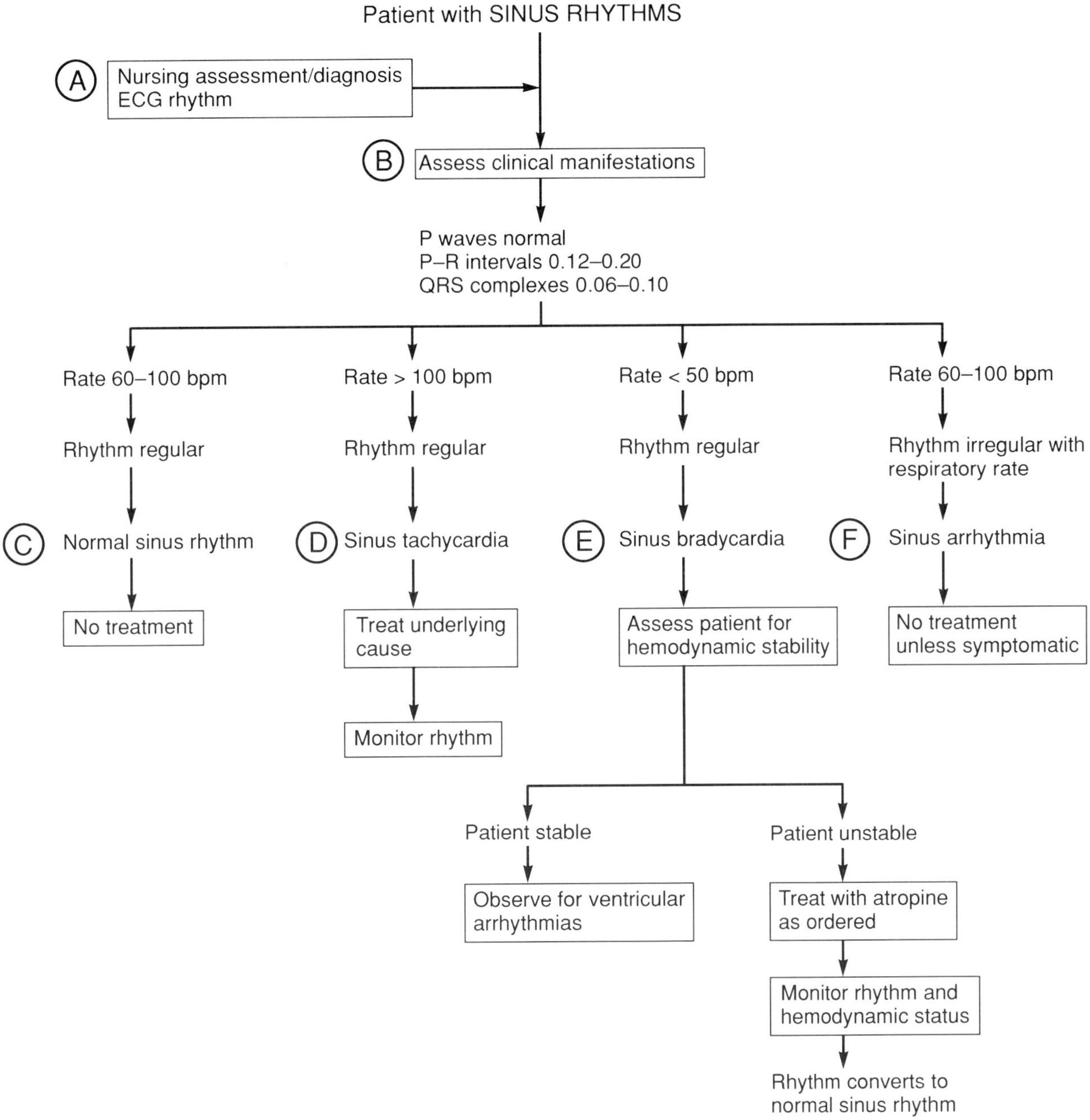

References

Bowdoin C. Alterations in cardiac rhythms. In: Bullock BL, Rosenthal PP. Pathophysiology: adaptations in function. 2nd ed. Glenview, IL: Scott Foresman/Little, Brown, 1988:281–303.

Conover MB. Pocket guide to electrocardiography. St. Louis: CV Mosby, 1986.

Sweetwood HM. Clinical electrocardiography for nurses. Rockville, MD: Aspen, 1983.

HEART BLOCK

Kendra Ellis
Carol Bowdoin

Heart block occurs when an impulse is initiated but is delayed or blocked within the electrical pathways. The delayed impulse results in a prolonged conduction period, because the blocked impulse causes a loss of conduction. There are several degrees of heart block that differ in the amount of block present, where the block occurs, and the seriousness of the block.

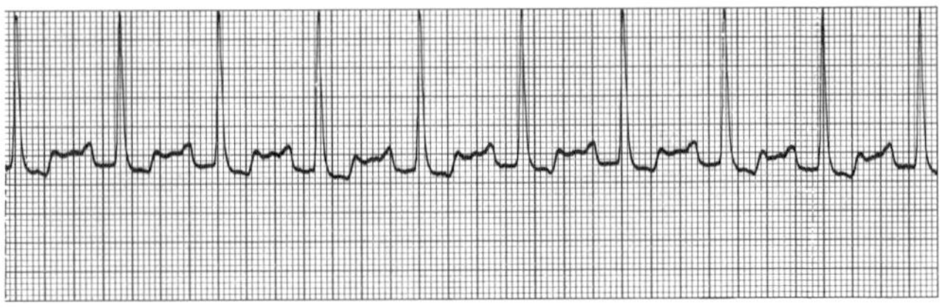

Figure 1 First-degree heart block.

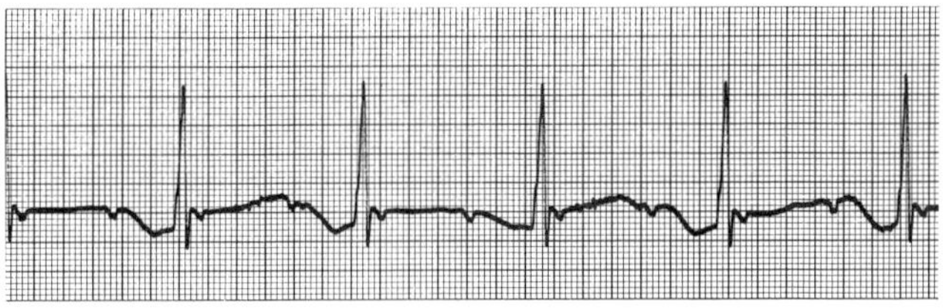

Figure 2 Mobitz type II second-degree heart block.

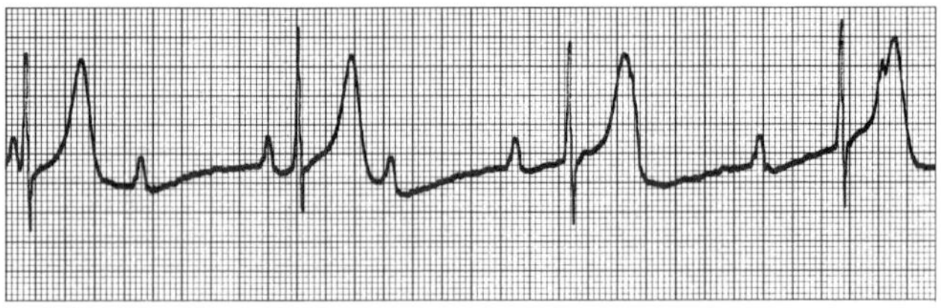

Figure 3 Third-degree heart block.

A. Patients may present with slowed, irregular heart rate, complaints of dizziness, transient giddiness, fainting, fatigue, and/or sense of "impending doom." The physician should be notified and a 12-lead ECG done stat. Sudden onset of second- or third-degree heart attack can be life-threatening and require immediate transfer to CCU for continuous monitoring and treatment.

B. Patients and families require constant reassurance and thorough explanations of procedures during evaluation of clinical symptoms.

C. In first-degree heart block, a delay is present in conduction from the atria to the ventricles. The sinoatrial (SA) node remains the pacemaker, and the impulse follows the normal conduction pathways. Every initiated impulse is conducted or every P wave is followed by a QRS complex (Fig. 1). The delay in conduction results in a prolonged P-R interval (greater than 0.20 second). The causes of first-degree heart block are digitalis toxicity, ischemia of the atrioventricular (AV) node, and degenerative changes associated with aging. This rhythm indicates an underlying problem but does not produce symptoms. The risk occurs when a higher, more dangerous block develops.

D. The Mobitz type I second-degree heart block is also called Wenckebach. The P-R interval has increasing length until a P wave is not followed by a QRS complex, because damage results in delays in conduction until impulses are no longer transmitted. This period of nontransmission allows the AV tissue to rest and the next beat to be conducted with the original P-R interval. The causes of Wenckebach include an inferior myocardial infarction (MI), digitalis toxicity, and ischemia of the AV node. This rhythm may cause a slowing of the heart rate, allowing a decrease in cardiac output. Usually it is transient in nature and resolves when edema and/or ischemia to the AV node abates.

E. The Mobitz type II second-degree heart block (Fig. 2) is caused by intermittent block in the ventricular conduction system. This block occurs lower in the ventricles. It causes an intermittent loss of conduction. Every P wave is not followed by a QRS, but the interval remains fixed. Mobitz II second-degree heart block is caused by chronic lesions in the conduction system. It is the more serious of the two second-degree heart blocks because of the area of damage and its chronic nature. Almost all patients with a Mobitz II require a pacemaker. This block may convert to a third-degree block.

F. The third-degree heart block is the most serious. It involves a complete block of the impulse from the atria to the ventricles. As a result, the atria and ventricles beat separately at their own inherent rates. There is no relationship between the P waves and the QRS complexes (Fig. 3). The causes include an acute MI, myocarditis, and tumors involving the heart. Third-degree heart block is frequently associated with a decrease in cardiac output and perfusion, which needs to be treated, if the patient is symptomatic, with a continuous infusion of Isuprel. Isuprel is a pure beta stimulant, increasing the heart's contractility. A pacemaker (p 84) will need to be permanently inserted.

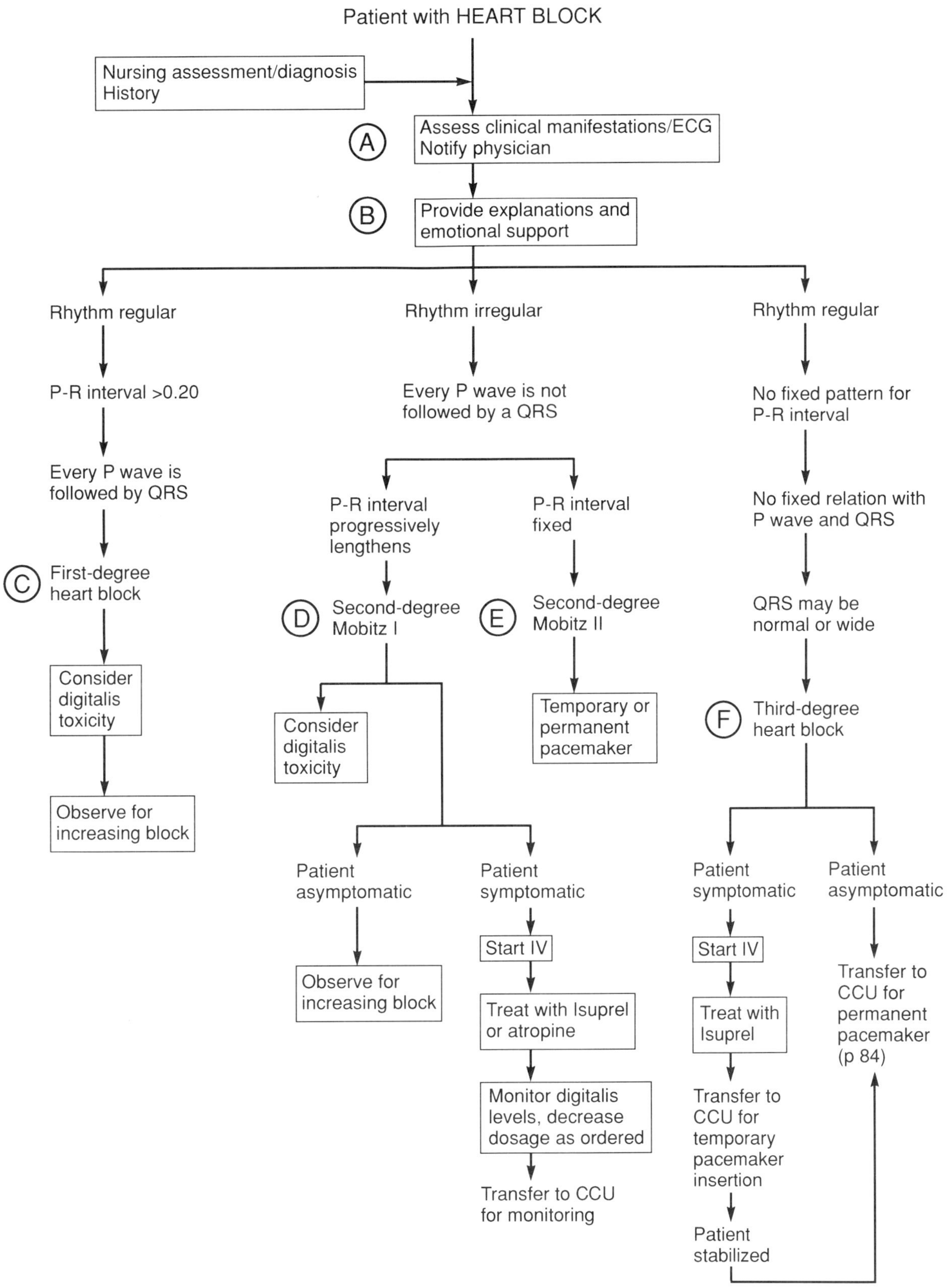

References

Bowdoin C. Alterations in cardiac rhythms. In: Bullock BL, Rosenthal PP. Pathophysiology: adaptations and alterations in function. 2nd ed. Glenview, IL: Scott Foresman/Little, Brown; 1988:291–303.

Kenner C, Guzzetta C, Dossey B. Critical care nursing. Boston: Little, Brown, 1986.

Norsen L. Detecting dysrhythmias. Nursing 1986; 16(11):34–42.

ATRIAL ARRHYTHMIAS

Kendra Ellis

A. In atrial arrhythmias, the patient may complain of palpitations, syncope, or a fluttering sensation in the chest. An electrocardiogram (ECG) reveals a rhythm in which the atrial arrhythmias are caused by impulses originating in the atria, but not from the sinoatrial (SA) node. They are due to an irritable (ectopic) focus. Often the ectopic focus "escapes" into the sinus rhythm or may take over the rhythm when the SA node is not able to produce an impulse or impulses at the normal rate. The P wave may appear different in configuration from the normal sinus P wave, and the atrial and ventricular rates vary. Often the patient has a long history of cardiac disease. A thorough review of medications with patient compliance patterns must be included in the assessment.

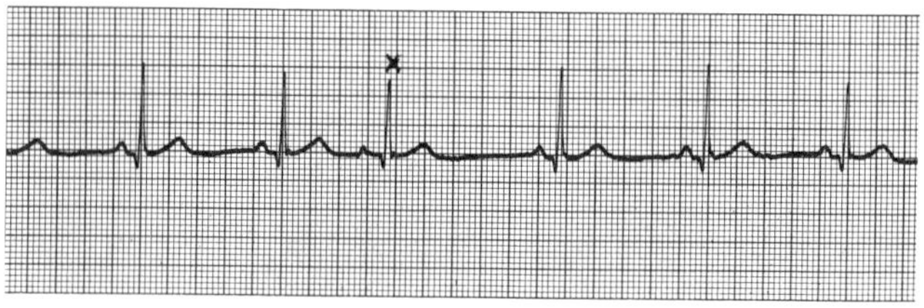

Figure 1 Normal sinus rhythm with a premature atrial contraction (at x).

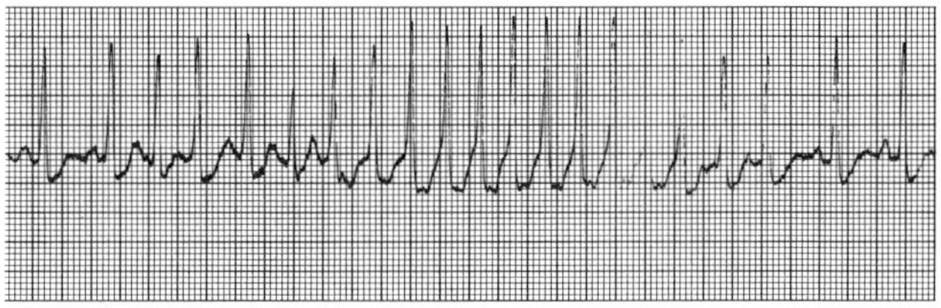

Figure 2 Sinus tachycardia with a burst of paroxysmal atrial tachycardia.

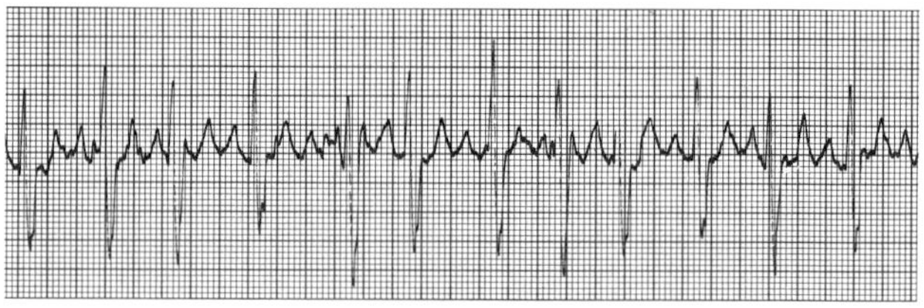

Figure 3 Atrial flutter with varying degrees of block.

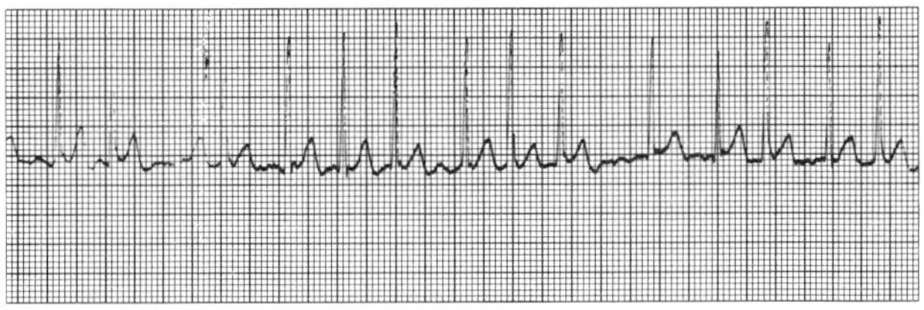

Figure 4 Atrial fibrillation.

B. Premature atrial contractions (PACs) (Fig. 1) are ectopic beats that occur before the next expected sinus beat. They can occur in a normal heart as well as a diseased heart. They are considered benign but may precipitate more serious atrial arrhythmias. They are caused by stress, fever, caffeine, nicotine, myocardial infarction (MI), or electrolyte disturbances. They are usually just identified and observed. Increasing frequency of PACs is an indication of increased atrial irritability and should be evaluated, as it may be a precursor to paroxysmal atrial tachycardia.

C. Paroxysmal atrial tachycardia (PAT) (Fig. 2) is caused by an irritable focus in the atria, which takes over as a pacemaker. This usually occurs suddenly, but may be preceded by PACs. The increased rate results in increased myocardial oxygen consumption, which would be insignificant in a healthy person, but if the patient is having an MI, it will increase the infarction size. Causes of PAT include emotional stress, nicotine, caffeine, MI, hyperventilation, and hypoxia.

D. The physician may perform vagal stimulation to decrease the rate. This is not a nursing function. It includes carotid massage, Valsalva maneuvers, supraorbital pressure, and submersion of the patient's face in ice water.

E. Atrial flutter (Fig. 3) occurs when an atrial ectopic focus takes over at a rate of 250 to 350 beats per minute. It can be identified by its classic "sawtooth" P waves. The atrioventricular (AV) node blocks the conduction of most of the impulses, allowing for a regular, slower ventricular rate. The patient may experience palpitations, angina, or dyspnea because of the rapid rate. Causes include MI, ischemia to the SA node, valvular heart disease (p 72), and postoperative cardiac surgery (p 92).

F. Atrial fibrillation (Fig. 4) is a rapid-firing ectopic focus that does not allow time for the atria to contract. The atrial wall quivers or fibrillates. The AV node allows some impulses through to initiate ventricular contraction. The ventricular response is irregular, resulting in an irregular rhythm. The loss of the atrial contraction causes a decrease in cardiac output. This may cause the patient to experience angina, syncope, or dyspnea. Thrombi may form in the fibrillating atria, resulting in the patient being at high risk for pulmonary (p 116), cerebral (p 20), and peripheral emboli. The causes of atrial fibrillation include infection, hypoxia, valvular heart disease (p 72), MI, ischemia of the SA node, and atrial infarction.

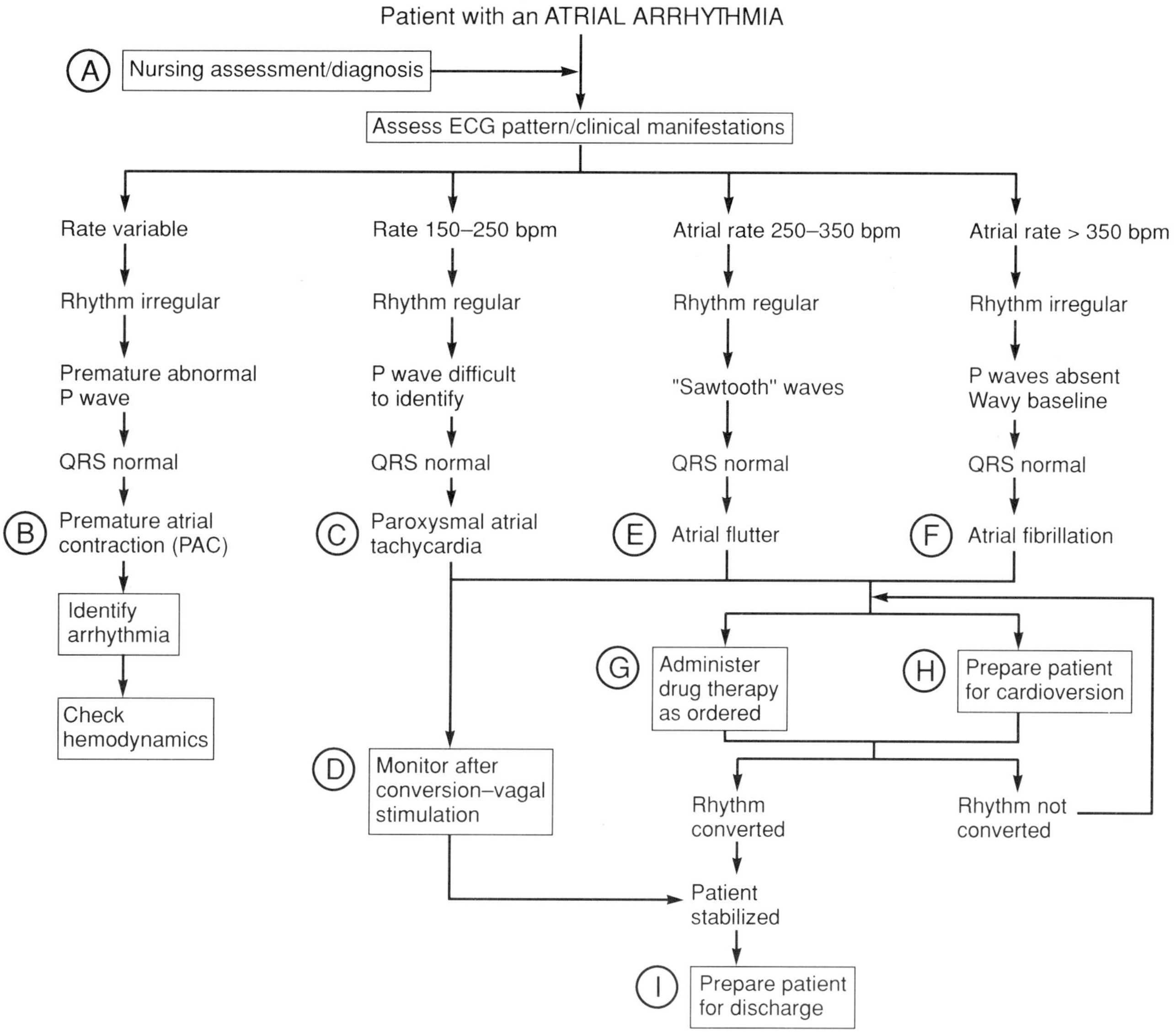

G. Drug therapy is sometimes used for rapid atrial arrhythmias in stable patients. This includes digitalis, Inderal, quinidine, and verapamil. These drugs work on the heart by decreasing the automaticity and the speed of conduction through the electrical pathways.

H. Cardioversion is performed when the patient is unstable or unresponsive to medical treatment. The synchronized mode is used to prevent discharge on the T wave, which could result in ventricular fibrillation or asystole (p 64). Resuscitation equipment should be on hand and an intravenous access in place as a precaution. Cardioversion is started with 75 to 100 joules. If no response is noted, it can be increased to 200 to 360 joules.

I. After conversion by pharmacologic or electrical means, the patient's medication regimen is adjusted. Following observation and stabilization the patient is discharged with instructions about follow-up office visits and strict adherance to medication therapy. Referrals to home health may be necessary for routine follow-up for elderly clients living alone.

References

Conover MB. Pocket Guide to electrocardiography. St. Louis: CV Mosby, 1986.

Kenner C, Guzzetta C, Dossey B. Critical care nursing. Boston: Little, Brown, 1986.

Norsen L. Detecting dysrhythmias: Nursing 1986; 16(11): 34–42.

JUNCTIONAL ARRHYTHMIAS

Kendra Ellis

Junctional arrhythmias originate in the junction of the atrioventricular (AV) node and bundle of His. A junctional rhythm may take over the heart's rhythm when impulses from the sinoatrial (SA) node are blocked or unable to be initiated. Usually this is a transient condition, abating when the cause (ischemia, edema, or decreased automaticity) is resolved. The P waves are usually inverted and may be found before, during, or after the QRS complex. This is caused by abnormal retrograde conduction through the atria. The conduction from the AV node to the ventricles is usually normal.

A. Premature junctional contractions (PJCs) (Fig. 1) are electrical impulses that arise in the AV node, superceding the SA node. The beat occurs before the next expected sinus beat. They are caused by an increased automaticity in the AV node. The causes include ischemia to the AV node, anxiety, and hypoxia. PJCs are usually insignificant and do not require treatment. If the patient is hemodynamically unstable, drug therapy includes quinidine, Inderal, or digoxin.

B. A junctional rhythm is considered an "escape" rhythm, because the AV node takes over as the primary pacemaker. Conduction through the atria is abnormal, while conduction through the ventricles is normal. The rate is 40 to 60 beats per minute, because of the intrinsic rate of the AV node. The causes include increased vagal stimulation, ischemia to the SA node, and digitalis toxicity. This slow rate may allow for breakthrough arrhythmias to occur in the ventricles.

C. Vagal stimulation, i.e., Valsalva maneuver, can cause the AV node to fail, resulting in the loss of a pacemaker. Patients should be instructed not to strain with their bowel movements.

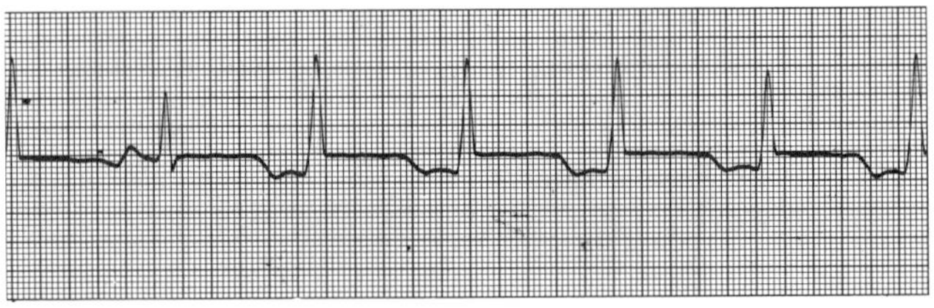

Figure 1 Junctional arrhythmia with premature junctional contractions.

D. Patients receiving digoxin need to be monitored for therapeutic drug levels. Potassium supplements are given to prevent digitalis toxicity.

E. The patient who is hemodynamically unstable is treated with atropine or Isuprel. Central venous pressure (CVP) and continuous ECG monitoring may be indicated.

F. Junctional arrhythmias are relatively benign. The goals of treatment are to treat the underlying causes, monitor hemodynamic status, and support the patient until sinus rhythm returns.

References

Bowdoin C. Alterations in cardiac rhythms. In: Bullock B, Rosenthal P, eds. Pathophysiology: adaptations and alterations in function. Boston: Scott Foresman, 1988.

Kenner C, Guzetta C, Dossey B. Critical care nursing. Boston: Little, Brown, 1981.

Norsen L, Telfair M, Wagner A. Detecting dysrhythmias. Nursing 1986; 16(11): 34–42.

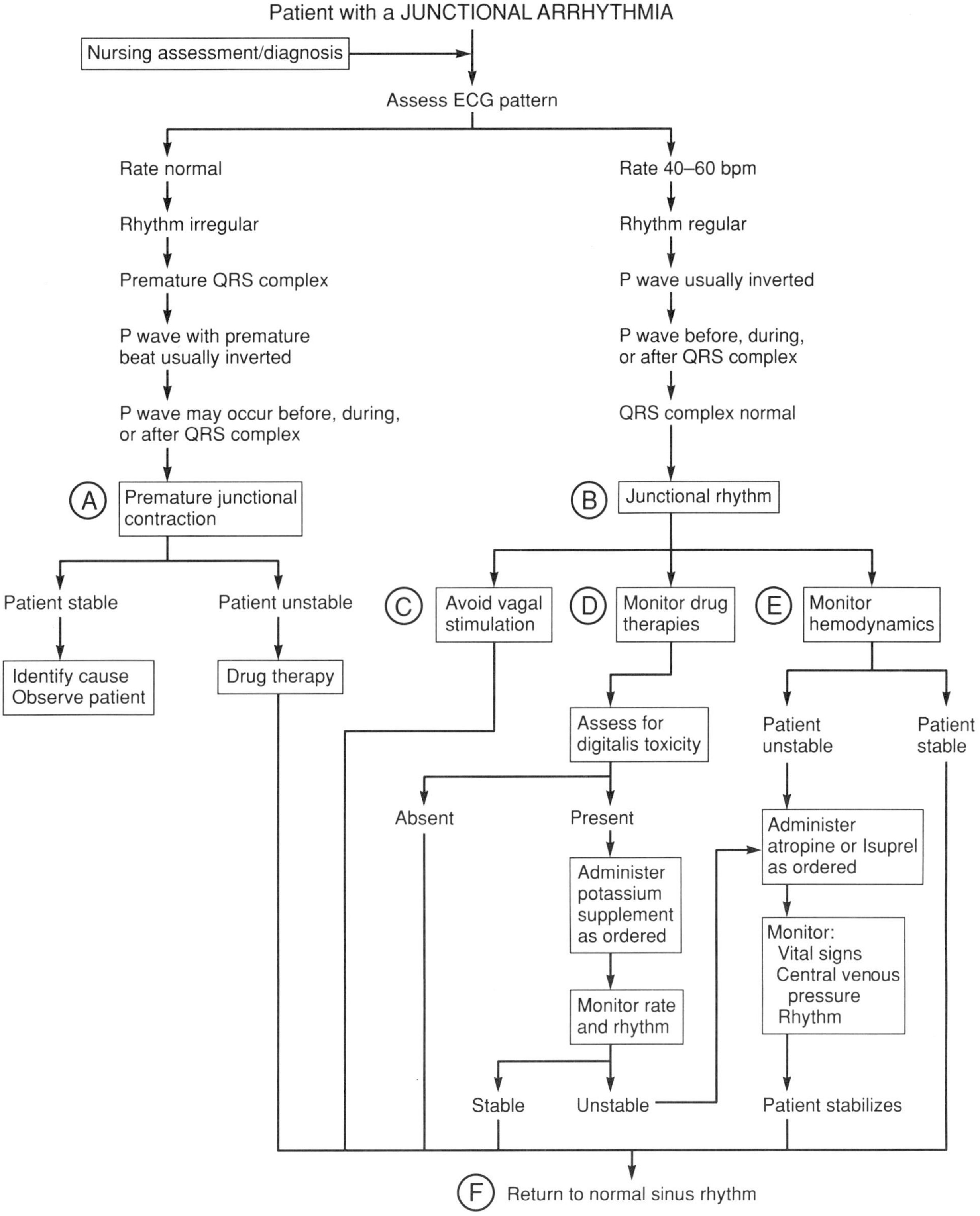
Patient with a JUNCTIONAL ARRHYTHMIA
Nursing assessment/diagnosis
Assess ECG pattern
Rate normal
Rhythm irregular
Premature QRS complex
P wave with premature beat usually inverted
P wave may occur before, during, or after QRS complex
A
Premature junctional contraction
Patient stable
Identify cause
Observe patient
Patient unstable
Drug therapy
Rate 40–60 bpm
Rhythm regular
P wave usually inverted
P wave before, during, or after QRS complex
QRS complex normal
B
Junctional rhythm
C
Avoid vagal stimulation
D
Monitor drug therapies
Assess for digitalis toxicity
Absent
Present
Administer potassium supplement as ordered
Monitor rate and rhythm
Stable
Unstable
E
Monitor hemodynamics
Patient unstable
Patient stable
Administer atropine or Isuprel as ordered
Monitor:
Vital signs
Central venous pressure
Rhythm
Patient stabilizes
F
Return to normal sinus rhythm

VENTRICULAR ARRHYTHMIAS

Kendra Ellis

Ventricular arrhythmias, the most dangerous of the arrhythmias, can result in sudden death. Ventricular ectopy is caused by an irritable focus in the ventricles, usually due to ischemia. These arrhythmias need to be recognized and treated immediately.

A. A premature ventricular contraction (PVC) is a beat that originates in the ventricles, with a compensatory pulse prior to the expected sinus beat. The causes include hypoxia, hypokalemia (p 200), myocardial infarction (MI), digitalis toxicity, and anxiety. The treatment includes treating the underlying cause and administering antiarrhythmic drugs, i.e., lidocaine, bretylium, and procainamide. These drugs are given by intravenous bolus, followed by a continuous infusion to maintain therapeutic drug levels.

B. An isolated PVC is frequently experienced by healthy people and is considered benign. However, there are five circumstances when a PVC is considered malignant and needs to be treated. These include more than five PVCs occurring in a minute, multiform PVCs (varying in size and shape), two or more PVCs in a row, a PVC falling on or near the T wave, and PVCs that occur every other beat (called bigeminy). Any of these patterns is dangerous and may precipitate lethal ventricular arrhythmias. Immediate action according to agency protocol is necessary.

C. Ventricular tachycardia (V-tach; Fig. 1) is defined as three or more PVCs in succession. The impulse originates in the ventricular conduction system. It is potentially life threatening, and immediate action needs to be taken. The causes of V-tach include MI, digitalis toxicity, hypoxia, acidosis, and hypokalemia. V-tach causes the heart to become ineffective as a pump. The patient may or may not have a pulse. This results in hypotension and loss of consciousness.

D. Ventricular fibrillation (V-fib; Fig. 2) results in cardiopulmonary arrest. It is a chaotic ventricular rhythm caused by multiple foci in the ventricles attempting to become the pacemaker. The heart is unable to respond to any of the electrical stimuli, so the ventricles quiver without contracting. This results in complete loss of circulation to the body. The major cause of V-fib is acute MI. V-fib is the number one cause of sudden death in patients with MI.

E. Emergency treatment of a patient with V-tach or V-fib includes quickly assessing for a carotid pulse and respirations. If the patient has a pulse with V-tach, the hemodynamic status is assessed. Patients in V-tach with a pulse are cardioverted with the synchronized mode to prevent discharge on the T wave. The patient who does not have a pulse is treated as V-fib. Cardiopulmonary resuscitation (CPR) is started immediately. The patient is defibrillated with 200 to 360 joules. Defibrillation is performed in succession, increasing the joules each time. The antiarrhythmic drugs lidocaine and bretylium are given. If the sinus rhythm returns, the patient is maintained on a continuous antiarrhythmic drug infusion, monitored closely, and moved to CCU.

F. Asystole is the absence of electrical activity in the ventricles (Fig. 3). It is also called ventricular standstill. There is no depolarization of the ventricles, resulting in a total absence of cardiac output. Clinical death occurs instantaneously. CPR must be initiated immediately. The drugs administered include epinephrine and atropine. CPR is discontinued if the patient converts to a sinus rhythm.

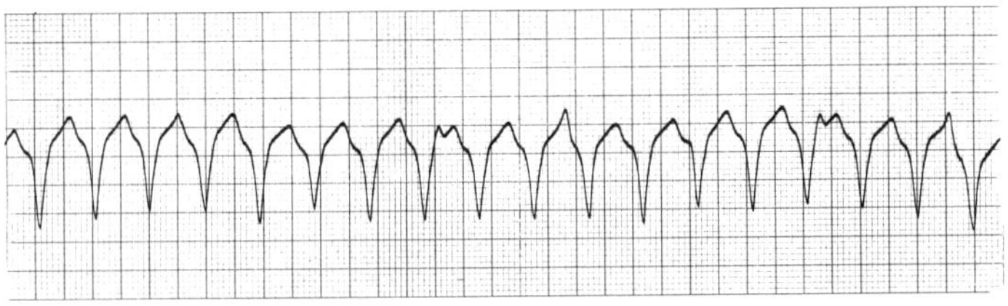

Figure 1 Ventricular tachycardia.

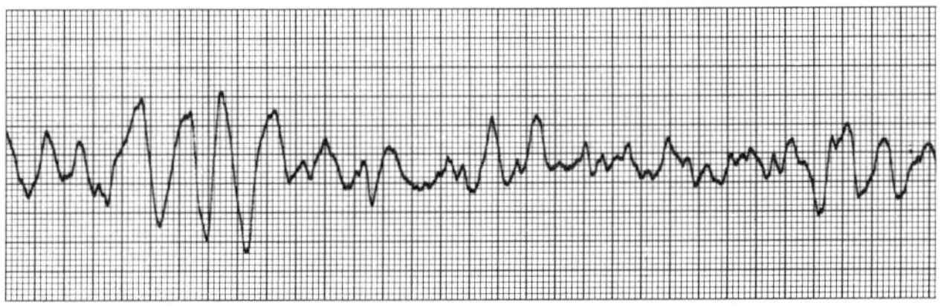

Figure 2 Ventricular fibrillation.

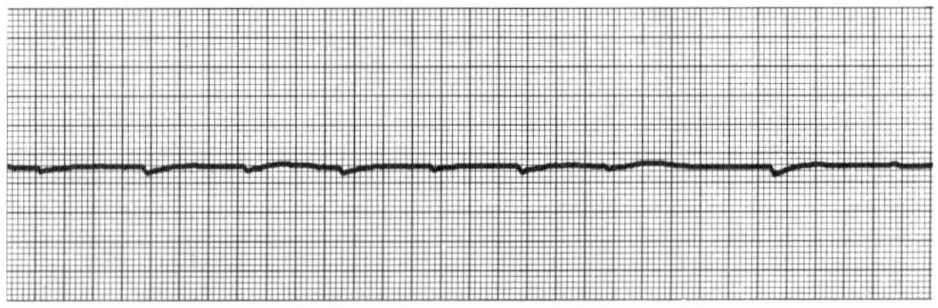

Figure 3 Asystole.

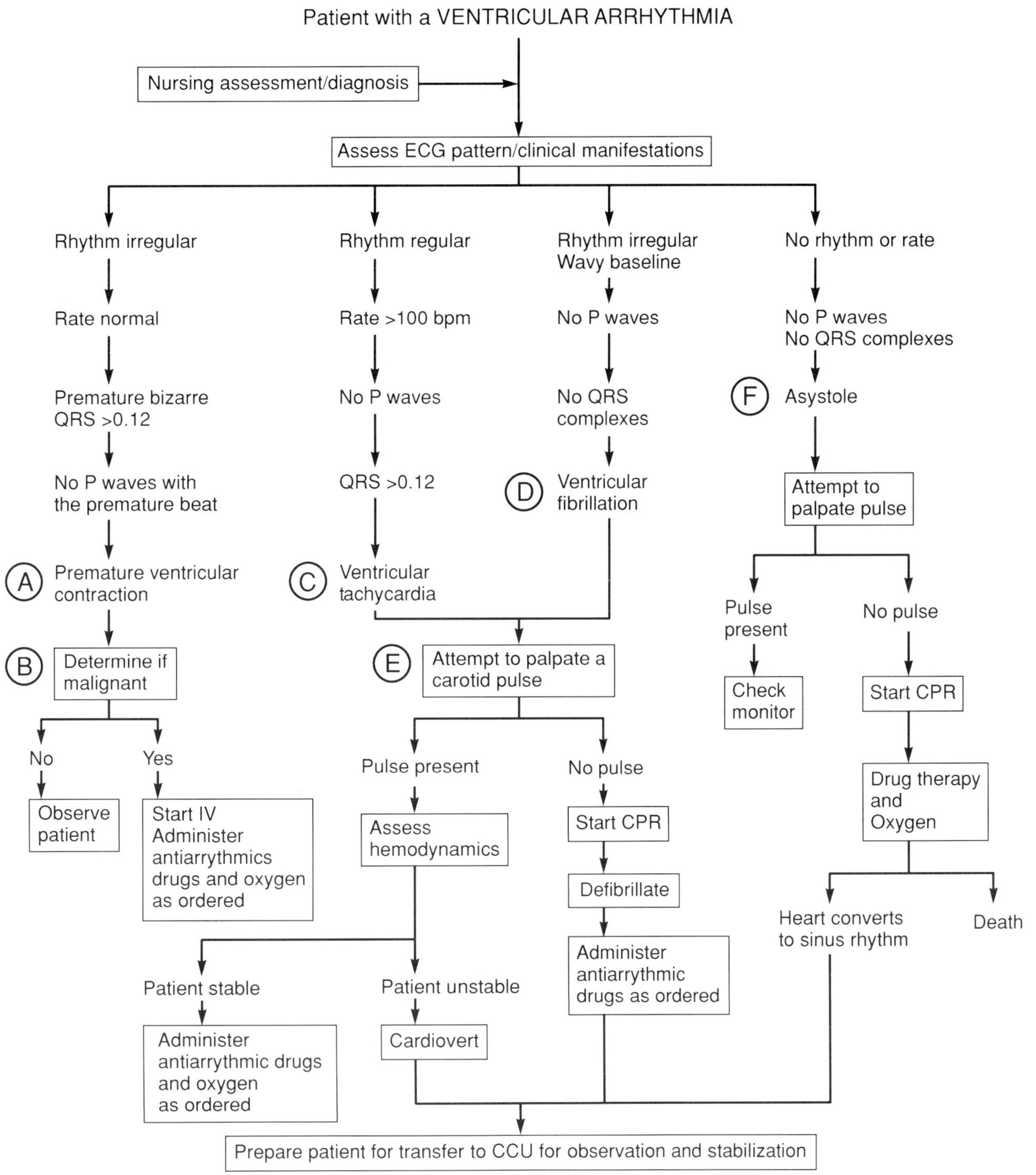

References

Bowdoin C. Alterations in cardiac rhythms. In: Bullock B, Rosenthal P, eds. Pathophysiology: adaptations and alterations in function. Boston: Scott Foresman, 1988.

Kenner C, Guzetta C, Dossey B. Critical care nursing. Boston: Little, Brown, 1981.

Norsen L, Telfair M, Wagner A. Detecting dysrhythmias. Nursing 1986; 16(11):34–42.

CORONARY ARTERY DISEASE

Mary E. Mancini

A. Coronary artery disease (CAD) ranks among the leading causes of death in the United States. Syndromes include stable angina pectoris, unstable angina pectoris, variant angina (Prinzmetal's angina), and acute myocardial infarction. History is of the utmost importance in distinguishing the various types of CAD. A description of the chest pain and investigation of precipitating factors are key points. A history of diabetes, hypertension, obesity, hyperlipidemia, or a family history of CAD may predispose the patient to CAD.

B. The nursing assessment should include a complete cardiac and respiratory assessment as well as the recording of all facets of the patient's activities that precede or precipitate the pain. Location, radiation, character, and duration of pain should also be noted.

C. The patient should be considered unstable if there is a progressive increase in frequency, intensity, or duration of pain. Objectives for managing the unstable patient include reducing the workload of the heart, thereby reducing myocardial oxygen demand; relieving pain; and preventing myocardial infarction. Patients should be monitored for development of congestive heart failure and arrhythmias.

D. The electrocardiogram (ECG) may show transient ST segment shifts or T wave changes that indicate decreased myocardial oxygen delivery and myocardial ischemia; Q waves indicating myocardial infarctions (ECG changes are normally seen within 2 to 12 hours, but may take as long as 72 to 96 hours), or arrhythmias related to ischemia or infarction (p 55).

E. Laboratory tests may include cardiac isoenzymes, electrolytes, and complete blood counts to differentiate other causes of pain.

F. The patient should be monitored continuously and stabilized. Unstable patients should be transferred to the coronary care unit (CCU) for further evaluation and treatment of occurring chest pain. Information and emotional support are essential to assist the patient and family to cope.

G. Instruct the stable patient and/or significant other that chest discomfort or pain can occur any time an activity increases heart rate or blood pressure and therefore increases myocardial demand. Moderation is to be encouraged. Activities such as sudden exertion, extremes of temperature, emotional stress, or overeating should be avoided. All medications should be carefully reviewed. Instructions related to effective use of nitroglycerin and beta-blockers must be given in detail. *If pain becomes more intense, different in character, or persists for more than 20 minutes, the patient should be alerted to request assistance in getting to the nearest hospital for evaluation.*

References

Brunner LS, Suddarth DS. The Lippincott manual of nursing practice. 3rd ed. Philadelphia: JB Lippincott, 1982:284–290.

Forshee T. Track down the what, where, when and how of chest pain. Nursing 1986; 16(5):34–42.

Gliss CL, Sparacino PS, Gortner SR. Leading to the treatment of coronary artery disease: implications for nursing care. Heart Lung 1985; 14:350–356.

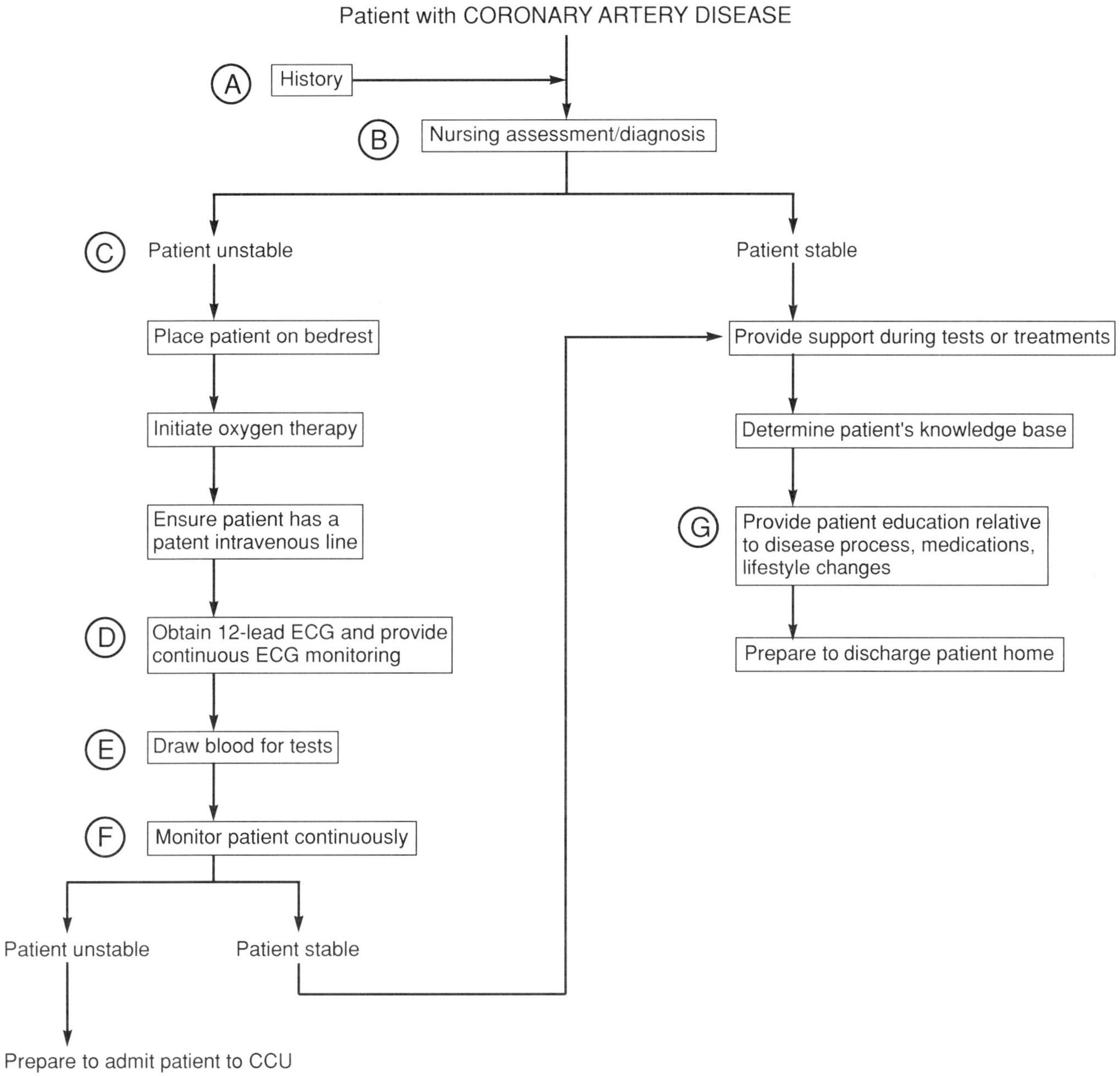
Patient with CORONARY ARTERY DISEASE
A
History
B
Nursing assessment/diagnosis
C
Patient unstable
Patient stable
Place patient on bedrest
Provide support during tests or treatments
Initiate oxygen therapy
Determine patient's knowledge base
Ensure patient has a patent intravenous line
G
Provide patient education relative to disease process, medications, lifestyle changes
Prepare to discharge patient home
D
Obtain 12-lead ECG and provide continuous ECG monitoring
E
Draw blood for tests
F
Monitor patient continuously
Patient unstable
Patient stable
Prepare to admit patient to CCU

CONGESTIVE HEART FAILURE

Mary E. Mancini
Kathleen H. Toto

A. Congestive heart failure is a clinical syndrome, not a definitive diagnosis. A complete patient history helps to determine the etiology of the heart failure. The history should include the onset of the illness, precipitating factors, medications, and whether this is a new onset or an exacerbation of chronic congestive heart failure. It is important to identify the etiology of heart failure, such as myocardial weakness or inflammation (as with coronary artery disease, congestive cardiomyopathy, and drugs) and excessive workload on the heart (as with hypertension, valvular disease, and hypertrophic cardiomyopathy). Factors that may precipitate heart failure include myocardial infarction; infection; anemia; thyrotoxicosis and pregnancy; arrhythmias; physical, dietary, environmental, and emotional excesses; new-onset hypertension; endocarditis and myocarditis; and pulmonary embolism.

B. The nursing assessment should include complete cardiovascular and respiratory assessment. The presence or absence of peripheral edema, and S_3 heart sound, rales, rhonchi, wheezing, jugular vein distention, and shortness of breath should be noted.

C. Hemodynamic instability in congestive heart failure is due to severe pump failure. The patient is hypotensive and may be in acute respiratory distress. Supplemental oxygen or ventilatory support may be necessary to maintain an arterial oxygen saturation greater than 90 percent. Diuretics are given intravenously to reduce preload, decrease the work of the heart, and improve oxygenation. Dobutamine may be given intravenously for severe heart failure as inotropic therapy; other inotropic drugs that may be given include digitalis, dopamine, and amrinone.

D. An intravenous infusion of 5 percent dextrose in water at a keep-vein-open rate should be maintained. Normal saline is rarely indicated for the patient in heart failure.

E. A 12-lead electrocardiogram should be obtained to rule out myocardial infarction or arrhythmias as the cause of congestive heart failure.

F. Continuous electrocardiographic monitoring is helpful in detecting arrhythmias during treatment.

G. Laboratory tests include serum and urine electrolyte levels, blood urea nitrogen level, a complete blood count, arterial blood gas levels, urinalysis, and cardiac enzyme levels.

H. The urine output should also be assessed. If the patient is unable to void, a Foley catheter should be inserted.

I. If the patient is hemodynamically stable, the treatment includes diuretics to decrease preload and digitalis to enhance myocardial contractility. Close attention should be given to the serum potassium level during diuretic and digitalis treatment. Hypokalemia potentiates the effect of digitalis, and arrhythmias may develop as a result of digitalis toxicity, such as ventricular bigeminy, heart block, and junctional tachycardia.

J. The patient may demonstrate severe anxiety due to hypoxia. Both the patient and family need support and explanations as to what to expect.

K. The hemodynamically unstable patient in congestive failure should be admitted to the coronary care unit for placement of a pulmonary artery balloon flotation catheter. Once this is in place, a better understanding of the patient's hemodynamics (cardiac output, preload, and afterload) can be obtained. Vasodilator therapy improves the cardiac output in patients with an increased afterload. Intravenous afterload-reducing drugs include nitroprusside and phentolamine.

L. The patient may be sent home with oral doses of prazosin, minoxidil, captopril, enalapril, or hydralazine.

References

McCauley K, Burke KG. Your detailed guide to drugs for C.H.F. Nursing 1984; 14(5):47–50.

Toto H. Congestive heart failure. In: Mancini ME. Decision making in emergency nursing. Toronto: BC Decker, 1987:106–107.

Van Parys E. Assessing the failing state of the heart. Nursing 1987; 17(2):42–49.

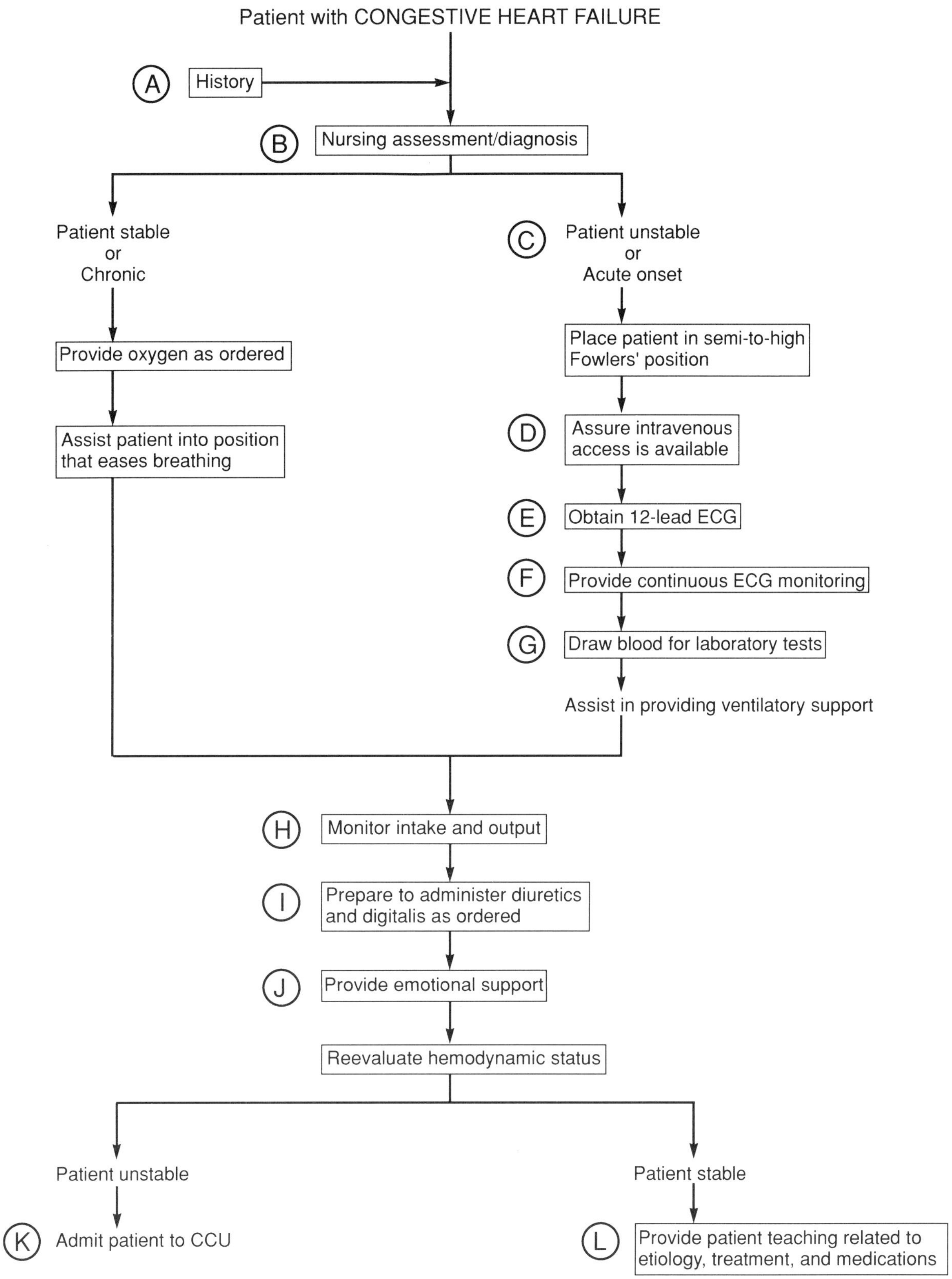
Patient with CONGESTIVE HEART FAILURE
A
History
B
Nursing assessment/diagnosis
Patient stable
or
Chronic
C
Patient unstable
or
Acute onset
Provide oxygen as ordered
Assist patient into position
that eases breathing
Place patient in semi-to-high
Fowlers' position
D
Assure intravenous
access is available
E
Obtain 12-lead ECG
F
Provide continuous ECG monitoring
G
Draw blood for laboratory tests
Assist in providing ventilatory support
H
Monitor intake and output
I
Prepare to administer diuretics
and digitalis as ordered
J
Provide emotional support
Reevaluate hemodynamic status
Patient unstable
Patient stable
K
Admit patient to CCU
L
Provide patient teaching related to
etiology, treatment, and medications

SHOCK

Marsha Cloak

Shock is a state of inadequate tissue perfusion and oxygen delivery, resulting in impaired cellular metabolism, cellular hypoxia, and vital organ damage. Shock can be classified into four categories (Table 1). In most shock states the initial hemodynamic alteration is a reduction in cardiac output caused by a decrease in circulatory blood volume and impairment of cardiac pumping.

A. Patients at risk for shock are those with a recent history of trauma, burns (p 248), hemorrhage, infection, myocardial infarction, cardiac failure (p 68), pulmonary edema (p 114), and cardiac tamponade (p 74).

B. Clinical findings vary with the severity and stage of shock. Compensated shock attempts to restore homeostasis by a number of compensatory negative feedback mechanisms. Clinical manifestations of compensated shock include decreased arterial pulse pressure; increased diastolic pressure; slightly increased or unchanged systolic pressure; tachycardia; weak thready peripheral pulses; decreased central venous pressure and pulmonary capillary wedge pressure; tachypnea; cold, clammy, pale skin; respiratory alkalosis; oliguria; restlessness; anxiety; insatiable thirst; decreased urine sodium; and increased urine osmolarity. As shock progresses to a decompensated state, clinical findings include hypotension, anuria, hypothermia, diaphoresis, lethargy, confusion, obtundation, and metabolic acidosis.

C. Serial arterial blood gases (ABGs) and chest films evaluate ventilatory function. Serial hematocrit, electrolyte, and acid-base studies are needed to determine fluid and electrolyte therapy. Obtain cultures in septic shock. Continuous monitoring should include respiration rate, level of consciousness, hourly urine outputs, and temperature. Hemodynamic monitoring should include blood pressure, heart rate, and central venous pressure (CVP).

D. Shock requires immediate intervention while a determination of the underlying cause is being made. Depending on the etiology and stage of shock, treatment may vary to include (1) initial resuscitation and supportive measures, (2) fluid and pharmacologic therapy, and (3) definitive therapy to treat the underlying cause.

E. If respirations are adequate, supplemental oxygen is given at 8 to 10 L per minute. Endotracheal intubation may be needed to maintain PaO_2 and CO_2 levels. Correction of acid-base disturbances and arrhythmias is a main concern.

F. Pain should be relieved with small doses of a narcotic analgesic such as morphine sulfate or meperidine.

G. For all types of shock, parenteral fluid administration is essential. Establish two large-bore lines to facilitate rapid administration of fluid. Careful monitoring is essential to decrease risk of pulmonary edema (p 114).

H. Failure of fluid therapy to increase cardiac output and perfusion necessitates the use of vasoconstrictors and inotropic drugs such as dopamine and norepinephrine. Dosages should be carefully titrated to maintain a minimum systolic pressure of 80 to 90 mm Hg and diastolic pressure of 60 to 70 mm Hg.

I. Diuretics furosemide and mannitol may be used if urine output remains less than 50 cc per hour after stabilization of volume and blood pressure. The smallest effective dose to maintain renal function and prevent secondary hypovolemia should be given.

J. Further deterioration may necessitate transfer of the patient to the ICU for treatment requiring invasive monitoring, cardiac pacing, intra-aortic balloon counterpulsation or mechanical ventilation.

K. Patient survival depends on the underlying disease process and its response to treatment. Prognosis is affected by complications such as myocardial infarction, adult respiratory distress syndrome (p 96), disseminated intravascular coagulation (p 348), or cardiopulmonary arrest.

L. For the patient in septic shock, broad-spectrum antibiotics must be started immediately. Large doses of steroids may be of benefit to patients with gram-negative sepsis. In the cardiogenic shock patient, ventricular rate must be controlled. Therapy may include agents such as digitalis for rapid rates, isoproterenol or atropine for slow rates, or cardiac pacing.

M. Throughout the aggressive management of shock, provision of emotional support to the patient and family is essential. After the patient has been stabilized, patient education should be initiated. Initially, discuss the variables that caused shock and the rationale for immediate treatments. As the patient's condition improves, discuss rehabilitation with the patient and family.

TABLE 1 Classification of Shock

Classification	*Etiology*	*Example*
Cardiogenic	Cardiac muscle contractility or electrical dysfunction	Biventricular failure Myocardial infarction
Hypovolemic	Decreased intravascular blood volume	Hemorrhage
Obstructive	Mechanical impediment to central blood flow	Pulmonary embolus
Distributive	Vasomotor and microcirculatory dysfunction	Neurogenic, septic (endotoxic) and anaphylactic shock states

References

Dale DC, Petersdorf RG. Septic shock. In: Harrison's principles of internal medicine. 11th ed. New York: McGraw-Hill, 1987.

Prough DS, Johnston WE, Royster RL, Beamer WC. Recent advances in critical care pharmacology. Part III: Treatment of shock. Hosp Formulary, 1985; 20(1):40–52.

Rice V. The clinical continuum of septic shock. Crit Care Nurse 1984; 4(5):86–109.

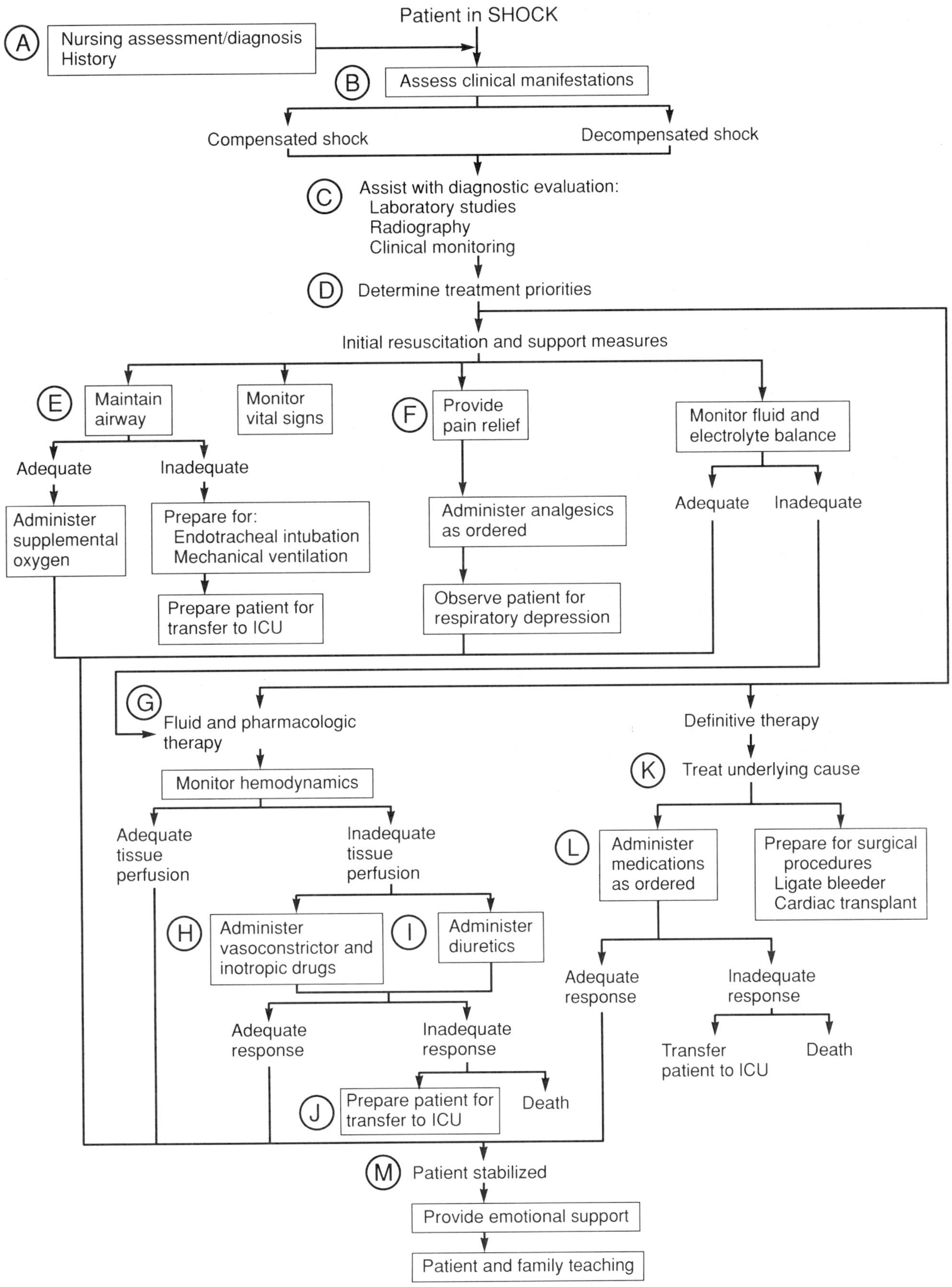
Patient in SHOCK
A
Nursing assessment/diagnosis
History
B
Assess clinical manifestations
Compensated shock
Decompensated shock
C
Assist with diagnostic evaluation:
Laboratory studies
Radiography
Clinical monitoring
D
Determine treatment priorities
Initial resuscitation and support measures
E
Maintain airway
Monitor vital signs
F
Provide pain relief
Monitor fluid and electrolyte balance
Adequate
Inadequate
Administer supplemental oxygen
Prepare for:
Endotracheal intubation
Mechanical ventilation
Prepare patient for transfer to ICU
Administer analgesics as ordered
Observe patient for respiratory depression
Adequate
Inadequate
G
Fluid and pharmacologic therapy
Monitor hemodynamics
Adequate tissue perfusion
Inadequate tissue perfusion
H
Administer vasoconstrictor and inotropic drugs
I
Administer diuretics
Adequate response
Inadequate response
J
Prepare patient for transfer to ICU
Death
Definitive therapy
K
Treat underlying cause
L
Administer medications as ordered
Prepare for surgical procedures
Ligate bleeder
Cardiac transplant
Adequate response
Inadequate response
Transfer patient to ICU
Death
M
Patient stabilized
Provide emotional support
Patient and family teaching

VALVULAR HEART DISEASE

Linda Weld
Michele Gann

Valvular heart disease is a condition that may affect any one or combination of the four heart valves. The valves may fail to open (stenosis) or close (insufficiency) properly, thus affecting normal blood flow through the heart. These conditions may be either congenital or acquired. Causes of acquired valvular dysfunctions include rheumatic heart disease, endocarditis, ischemia, and trauma. The treatment of valvular heart disease depends greatly on the patient's condition, diagnostic findings, and physician recommendations. Even though patients exhibit similar signs and symptoms, treatment for each patient may be vastly different because of the specific valve damaged and its prognostic implications.

A. The majority of patients present with either signs of congestive heart failure or activity intolerance. The nurse must take a detailed history of the patient's signs and symptoms to determine a baseline. These patients are frequently admitted multiple times for treatment, and the nurse should compare present status with that on previous admissions. The history should include medications, since these patients may be taking a wide variety of medications.

B. The clinical manifestations of these conditions include but are not limited to the ones listed on the decision tree. Other signs and symptoms include syncope, palpitations, arrhythmias (p 60), activity intolerance, dyspnea, and ascites.

C. Congestive heart failure, although often present in these patients, is a condition in and of itself (p 68).

D. Diagnostic studies include electrocardiography, echocardiography, chest film, nuclear cardiac scans, and cardiac catheterization (p 82). Other tests may be ordered to determine the effects of low cardiac output on other organs.

E. The physician determines when and if surgical intervention would be beneficial, based on the patient's symptoms and diagnostic tests. Surgical interventions could include commissurotomy or valve replacement. The general postoperative care of these patients is similar to that for open heart bypass (p 92).

F. Discharge instructions should include diet, medication instructions, and activity. The patient must have an understanding of the importance of prophylactic antibiotic therapy prior to any invasive or dental procedure. If appropriate, special emphasis should be placed on the side effects of anticoagulant therapy.

References

Guzzetta CE, Dossey BM. Cardiovascular nursing: bodymind tapestry. St. Louis: CV Mosby, 1984.
Kenner CV, Guzzetta CE, Dossey BM. Critical care nursing: body-mind-spirit, 2nd ed. Boston: Little, Brown, 1985.
Lewis SM, Collier IC. Medical surgical nursing: assessment and management of clinical problems. New York: McGraw-Hill, 1983.

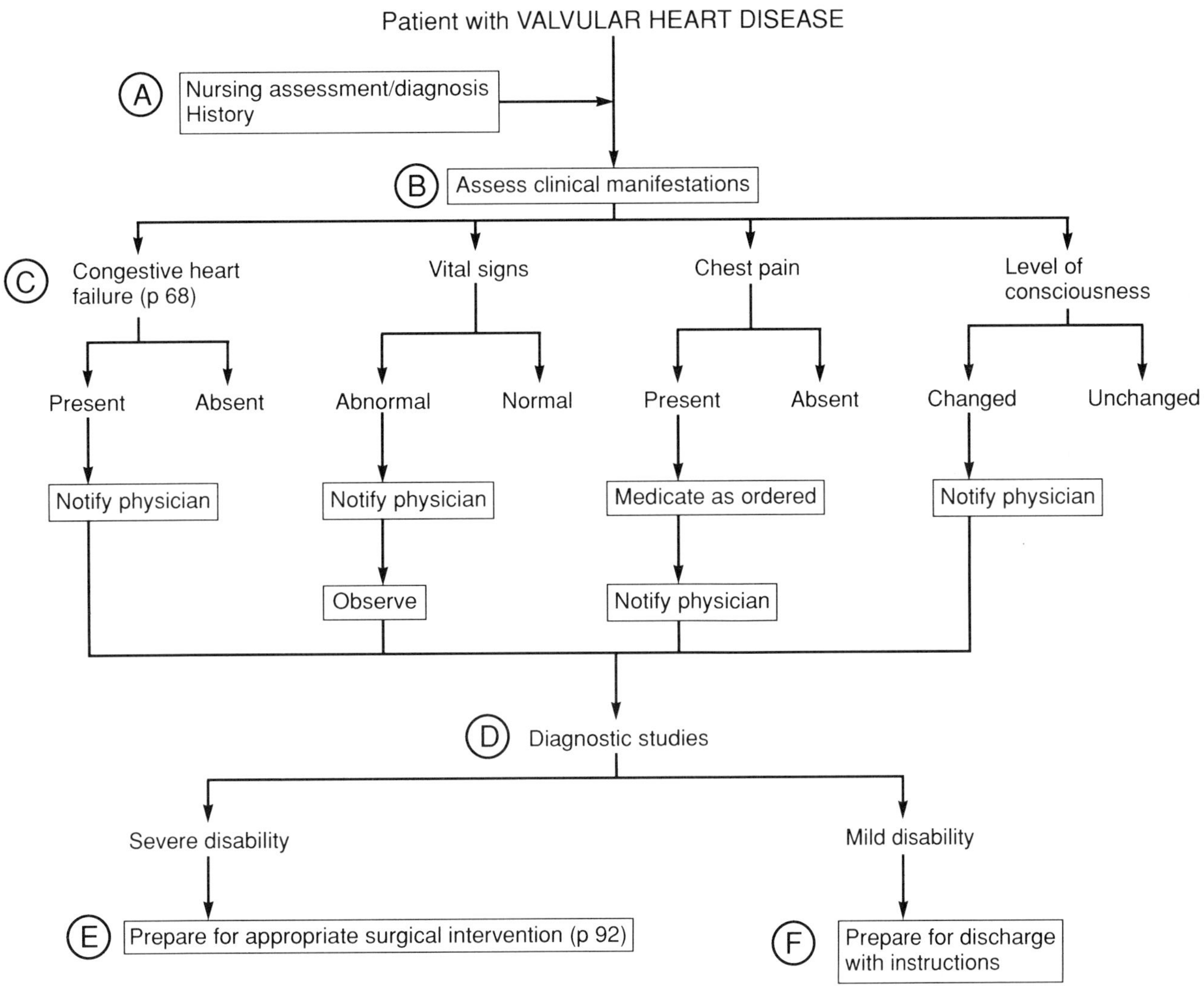
Patient with VALVULAR HEART DISEASE
A
Nursing assessment/diagnosis
History
B
Assess clinical manifestations
C
Congestive heart failure (p 68)
Vital signs
Chest pain
Level of consciousness
Present
Absent
Abnormal
Normal
Present
Absent
Changed
Unchanged
Notify physician
Notify physician
Medicate as ordered
Notify physician
Observe
Notify physician
D
Diagnostic studies
Severe disability
Mild disability
E
Prepare for appropriate surgical intervention (p 92)
F
Prepare for discharge with instructions

CARDIAC TAMPONADE

Michele Gann

A small amount of fluid is normally present in the pericardial sac. Cardiac tamponade occurs when the accumulated fluid in the sac restricts venous return. The amount of fluid capable of restricting venous return is dependent upon the rate of accumulation. Common causes of cardiac tamponade are (1) bleeding into the sac as a result of trauma or anticoagulant therapy, (2) malignancy, (3) infection, (4) uremia, and (5) idiopathic pericarditis. *Cardiac tamponade is a medical emergency.*

A. Common signs and symptoms of cardiac tamponade include hypotension, increased central venous pressure, decreased pulse pressure, tachycardia, muffled heart sounds, jugular vein distention on inspiration, and pulsus paradoxus (Fig. 1). (Pulsus paradoxus is a decrease of more than 10 mm Hg in systolic blood pressure during normal inspiration. It is assessed by having the patient breathe normally, inflating the blood pressure cuff to 20 mm Hg above patient's normal systolic pressure, then deflating the cuff slowly until the Karotkoff sounds are heard only on expiration. Continue deflating the cuff until sounds are heard on both inspiration and expiration. The difference between the two levels determines whether pulsus paradoxus exists.) This phenomenon is also seen in patients with congestive heart failure, hypovolemia, chronic obstructive pulmonary disease, and some cardiomyopathies. Another common symptom of tamponade is anxiety.

B. Possible diagnostic tests include chest film, electrocardiography, and echocardiography.

C. Pericardiocentesis is performed to evacuate clots or fluid from the pericardial sac. Usual equipment includes a large-bore cardiac needle and a 50- to 60-ml syringe. The patient should be monitored before, during, and after the procedure. Complications include arrhythmias, laceration of the coronary artery, and pneumothorax (p 110).

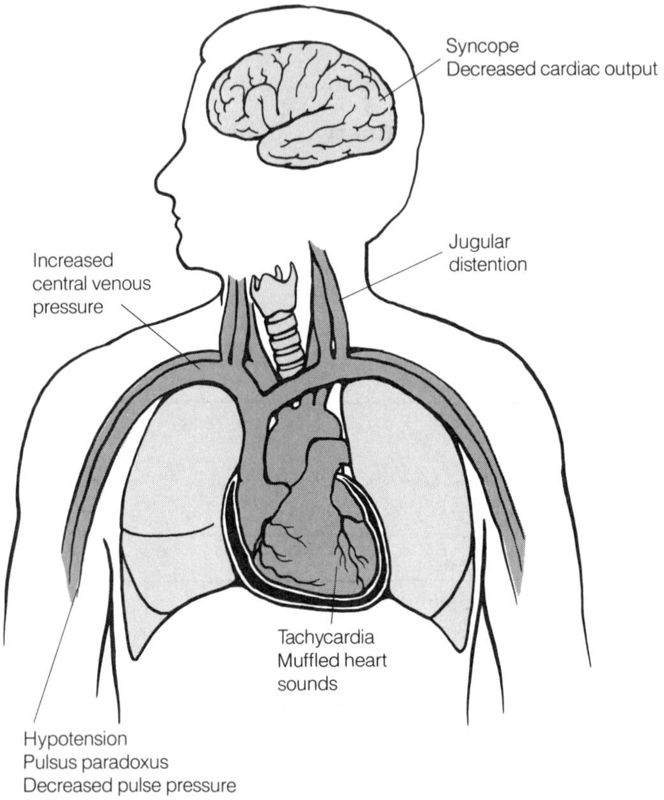

Figure 1 Signs and symptoms of cardiac tamponade.

References

Guzzetta CE, Dossey BM. Cardiovascular nursing: bodymind tapestry. St. Louis: CV Mosby, 1984.

Kenner CV, Guzzetta CE, Dossey BM. Critical care nursing: body-mind-spirit, 2nd ed. Boston: Little, Brown, 1985.

Lewis SM, Collier IC. Medical-surgical nursing: assessment and management of clinical problems. New York: McGraw-Hill, 1983.

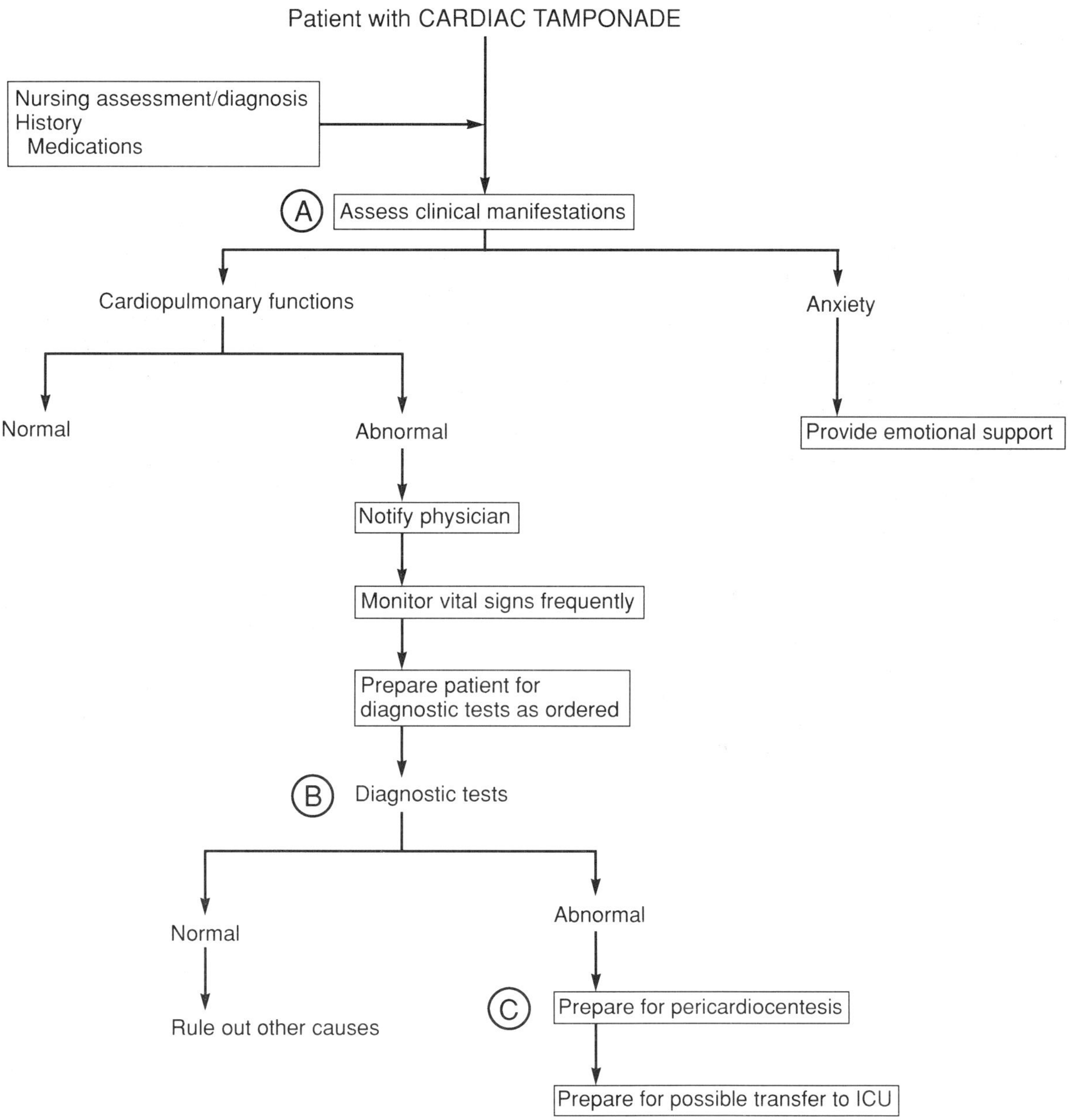
Patient with CARDIAC TAMPONADE
Nursing assessment/diagnosis
History
Medications
A
Assess clinical manifestations
Cardiopulmonary functions
Anxiety
Normal
Abnormal
Provide emotional support
Notify physician
Monitor vital signs frequently
Prepare patient for diagnostic tests as ordered
B
Diagnostic tests
Normal
Abnormal
Rule out other causes
C
Prepare for pericardiocentesis
Prepare for possible transfer to ICU

PERICARDITIS

Laura Luecke
Carol Bowdoin

The pericardium is the fibroserous sac that surrounds the heart and protects the heart chambers from friction. The endocardium is the inner layer that lines the heart cavities and aids in the formation of valves. Pericarditis is an inflammation of the pericardium, which may result in compression of the heart and cardiac failure. Individuals with a low resistance to infection in recent myocardial injury are particularly at risk. Causes include rheumatic fever, viral or bacterial infections, toxic drugs, trauma, uremia, neoplasms, disorders of connective tissue (lupus erythematosus), and myocardial infarction (MI). Pericarditis can be acute or chronic, fibrinous (constrictive) or exudative (pericardial effusion).

A. Nursing assessment should include a complete history to help determine the presence of the possible causes listed above. The patient may complain of anterior chest pain similar to the pain of myocardial ischemia. Pericardial pain (unlike anginal pain) is aggravated by deep inspiration and changing position. Other symptoms may include a pericardial friction rub (a scratchy, grating, heart sound), shortness of breath from pain or heart failure, and signs of inflammatory processes such as fever and malaise.

B. Diagnostic tests may include laboratory studies, chest films, electrocardiography (ECG), and possibly a pericardial tap. The results of the laboratory studies reflect inflammation. The white blood cell count (WBC) and erythrocyte sedimentation rate (ESR or SED rate) may be elevated. A blood urea nitrogen (BUN) is done to check for uremia, and an antistreptoysin (ASO) titer for rheumatic fever. The ECG will show S-T elevation in all leads. The chest film and echocardiogram may show signs of a pericardial effusion. If a pericardial effusion is present, a pericardial tap is done to perform diagnostic studies to identify a causative organism.

C. Acute pericarditis is characterized by sudden onset and sharp, stabbing pain in the precordial and retrosternal areas with radiation to shoulders, arms, and elbows. Dressler's syndrome (generalized pericarditis) usually occurs within 10 to 14 days post-MI. Nursing care is directed at managing the underlying cause and related signs and symptoms.

D. Patients are placed on bed or chair rest. Positioning in an upright, leaning-forward position alleviates chest pain. Activity may be resumed as pain and pericardial rub abates. Narcotic analgesics to manage pain, and anti-inflammatory drugs, to reduce inflammation, are administered. The patient's response to these methods should be monitored and documented.

E. Dyspnea may occur as a result of splinting related to pericardial pain or as a symptom of constriction. Respiratory rate, rhythm, and breath sounds should be frequently monitored. Oxygen may be ordered.

F. Aspirin, fluids, or sponge bath may help fever.

G. Oral anticoagulants should be discontinued in acute pericarditis because of the potential for effusion and tamponade (p 74). If an anticoagulant must be given, intravenous (IV) heparin is used, which can be reversed with protamine.

H. Frequent monitoring of blood pressure, cardiac rhythm, heart sounds, and neck veins will alert the nurse to potential complications arising from pericardial effusion.

I. A widening pulse pressure, tachyarrhythmias, distant heart sounds, and neck vein distention indicate compression of the heart due to fibrous constriction or pericardial effusion, which may produce effects of heart failure (p 68).

J. If a pericardial effusion accumulates fluid rapidly or accumulates a very large amount of fluid, a cardiac tamponade may occur (p 74). *Tamponade is a medical emergency requiring immediate pericardiocentesis to allow the heart to pump more efficiently.* A pericardial window may be surgically placed to remove recurrent pericardial fluid.

K. Patients recovering from pericarditis will be discharged with instructions regarding medications, activity, and follow-up care.

L. Chronic (constrictive) pericarditis results from a thickening of the pericardium that compresses the heart and reduces cardiac output. Causes include longstanding bacterial and viral infections, tuberculosis (p 120), and incomplete healing of acute pericarditis. Signs and symptoms are those of congestive heart failure. Surgery may be necessary to remove part or all of the pericardium. Postoperative care is similar to that given after cardiothoracic surgery (p 92).

References

Andreoli K, ed. Comprehensive cardiac care. 6th ed. St. Louis: CV Mosby, 1987:121.

Beland IL, Passos JY. Clinical nursing: pathophysiological and psychosocial approaches. 4th ed. New York: Macmillan, 1981:876–878.

Braunwald E, ed. Heart disease: a textbook of cardiovascular medicine. 3rd ed. Philadelphia: WB Saunders, 1988:1487–1492.

Brunner LS, Suddarth DS. Medical-surgical nursing. 6th ed. Philadelphia: JB Lippincott, 1988.

Hamilton HK, ed. Diseases and disorders handbook. 2nd ed. Springhouse, PA: Springhouse Corporation, 1988:561–563.

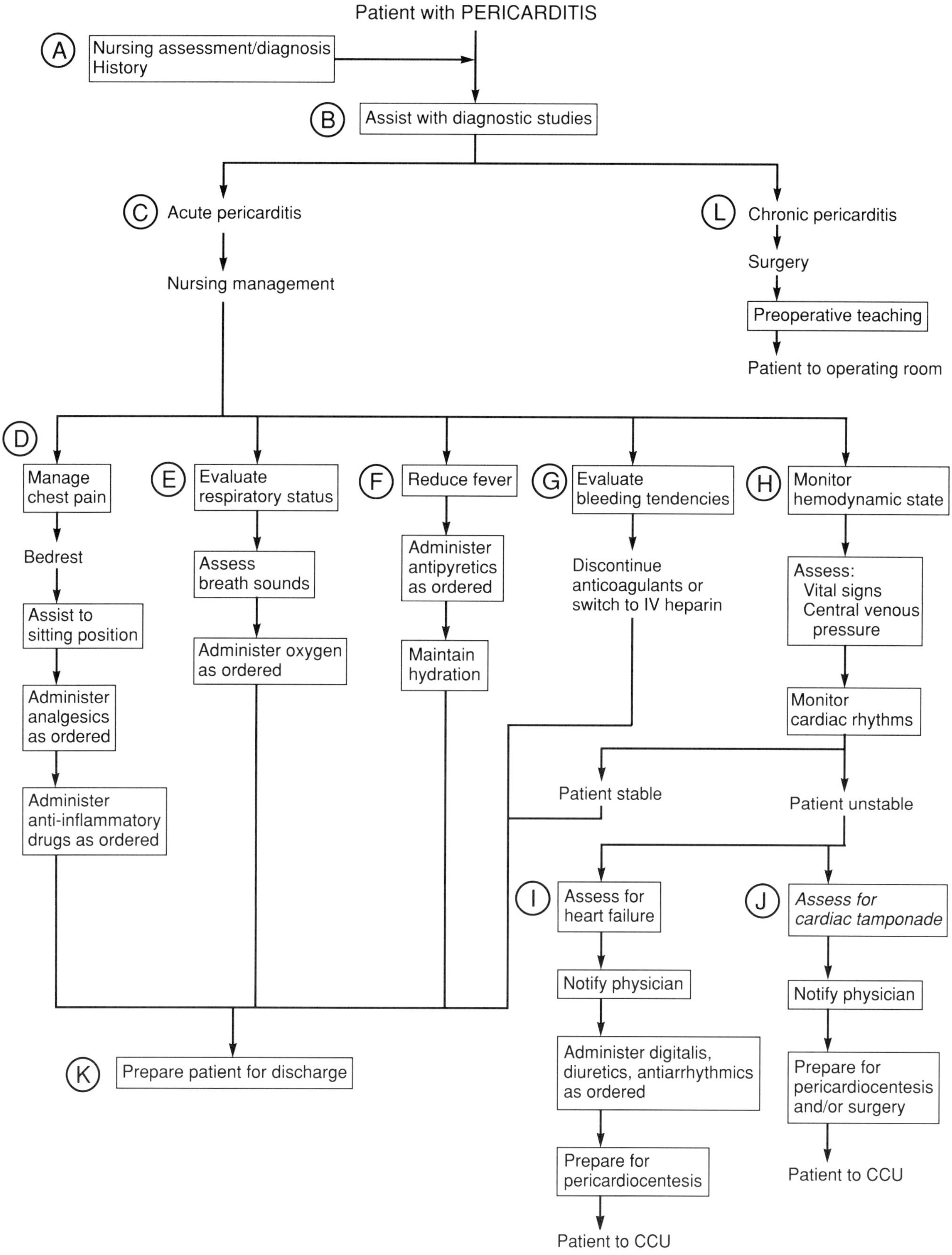
Patient with PERICARDITIS
A
Nursing assessment/diagnosis
History
B
Assist with diagnostic studies
C
Acute pericarditis
Nursing management
L
Chronic pericarditis
Surgery
Preoperative teaching
Patient to operating room
D
Manage chest pain
Bedrest
Assist to sitting position
Administer analgesics as ordered
Administer anti-inflammatory drugs as ordered
E
Evaluate respiratory status
Assess breath sounds
Administer oxygen as ordered
F
Reduce fever
Administer antipyretics as ordered
Maintain hydration
G
Evaluate bleeding tendencies
Discontinue anticoagulants or switch to IV heparin
H
Monitor hemodynamic state
Assess: Vital signs Central venous pressure
Monitor cardiac rhythms
Patient stable
Patient unstable
I
Assess for heart failure
Notify physician
Administer digitalis, diuretics, antiarrhythmics as ordered
Prepare for pericardiocentesis
Patient to CCU
J
Assess for cardiac tamponade
Notify physician
Prepare for pericardiocentesis and/or surgery
Patient to CCU
K
Prepare patient for discharge

ENDOCARDITIS

Laura Luecke

Endocarditis is an infection of the endocardium and/or cardiac valves. The infection is caused by bacterial, fungal, or rickettsial invasion. The valves become crusted with lesions called vegetations, which cause poor valvular function. Valves may become stenosed, causing the heart to work harder to push blood through the chambers. Also, valves may shorten and not close tightly, causing blood to leak or regurgitate backward instead of moving forward. Heart failure from strain and overwork can result (p 72).

A. Patients with hearts already damaged by rheumatic fever or congenital anomalies or patients with artificial valves are predisposed to endocarditis. Infection can be introduced into the blood stream through major cardiac surgery or dental, genitourinary, gynecologic, or gastrointestinal procedures. Drug addicts using contaminated needles are often victims. Endocarditis can be acute or subacute. If untreated, it is usually fatal; with treatment, 70 percent of patients recover.

B. The nursing assessment includes a complete history, noting predisposing factors, e.g., previous heart conditions, recent dental surgery, and intravenous drug abuse. High fever, chills, tachycardia, heart murmurs, and splenomegaly are common symptoms in acute endocarditis. Subacute endocarditis produces more vague symptoms such as moderate fever, malaise, weight loss, and joint pain. Unexplained fever in a patient with a cardiac defect should always be investigated.

C. Laboratory studies show positive blood cultures in 90 percent of patients. The white blood cell count (WBC) and the erythrocyte sedimentation rate (ESR) are elevated. Rheumatoid factor occurs in 50 percent of patients. Echocardiography is performed to check valvular function. The electrocardiogram may show arrhythmias reflective of valvular dysfunction (p 60).

D. Effective antibiotic administration is vital. Usually, parenteral antibiotics are given for 4 to 6 weeks. Administer the antibiotics exactly at prescribed intervals, and rotate intramuscular injection sites to ensure best drug absorption.

E. A long hospitalization is required for antibiotic therapy. As a result, depression, financial worries, or social problems may occur. Referral for psychiatric evaluation and counseling may be necessary.

F. Nursing measures to support the patient include providing a restful environment, adequate hydration, and nutrition.

G. In many cases, embolization of vegetation from valves may occur, causing typical features of occlusion. The nurse should observe the patient for the following manifestations: (1) neurologic—hemiparesis, headache, change in level of consciousness; (2) splenic—upper left abdominal pain radiating to left shoulder; (3) pulmonary—shortness of breath, chest pain, hemoptysis; (4) renal—hematuria, decreased urine output, elevated creatinine and blood urea nitrogen (BUN); (5) peripheral vascular—numbness, tingling, signs of decreased circulation in an extremity; and (6) hematologic—anemia and petechiae. Nursing interventions are tailored to the system affected (see "Stroke," p 20, and "Pulmonary Embolism," p 116).

H. Valvular dysfunction (p 72) may occur, resulting in right or left heart failure (p 68). Nursing responsibilities involve monitoring for cardiac status and development of early symptoms and notifying the physician to initiate appropriate treatment plans.

I. It is important to prepare the patient for discharge. Establish the knowledge level and tailor teaching to the patient's level of understanding. Since endocarditis can recur in vulnerable individuals, be certain that patients understand the need for prophylactic antibiotics when having dental, genitourinary, or gastrointestinal procedures done. Wallet cards with guidelines are available from the American Heart Association. Teach patients to recognize the signs and symptoms of a relapse, e.g., fever, fatigue, and malaise. Stress the importance of seeking medical assistance early before debilitation occurs.

References

Beland IL, Passos JY. Clinical nursing: pathophysiological and psychosocial approaches. 4th ed. New York: Macmillan, 1981:874–876.

Braunwald E, ed. Heart disease: a textbook of cardiovascular medicine. 3rd ed. Philadelphia: WB Saunders, 1988.

Hamilton HK, ed. Diseases and disorders handbook. 2nd ed. Springhouse, PA: Springhouse Corporation, 1988.

Lewis SM, Collier IC. Medical-surgical nursing: assessment and management of clinical problems. New York: McGraw-Hill, 1983.

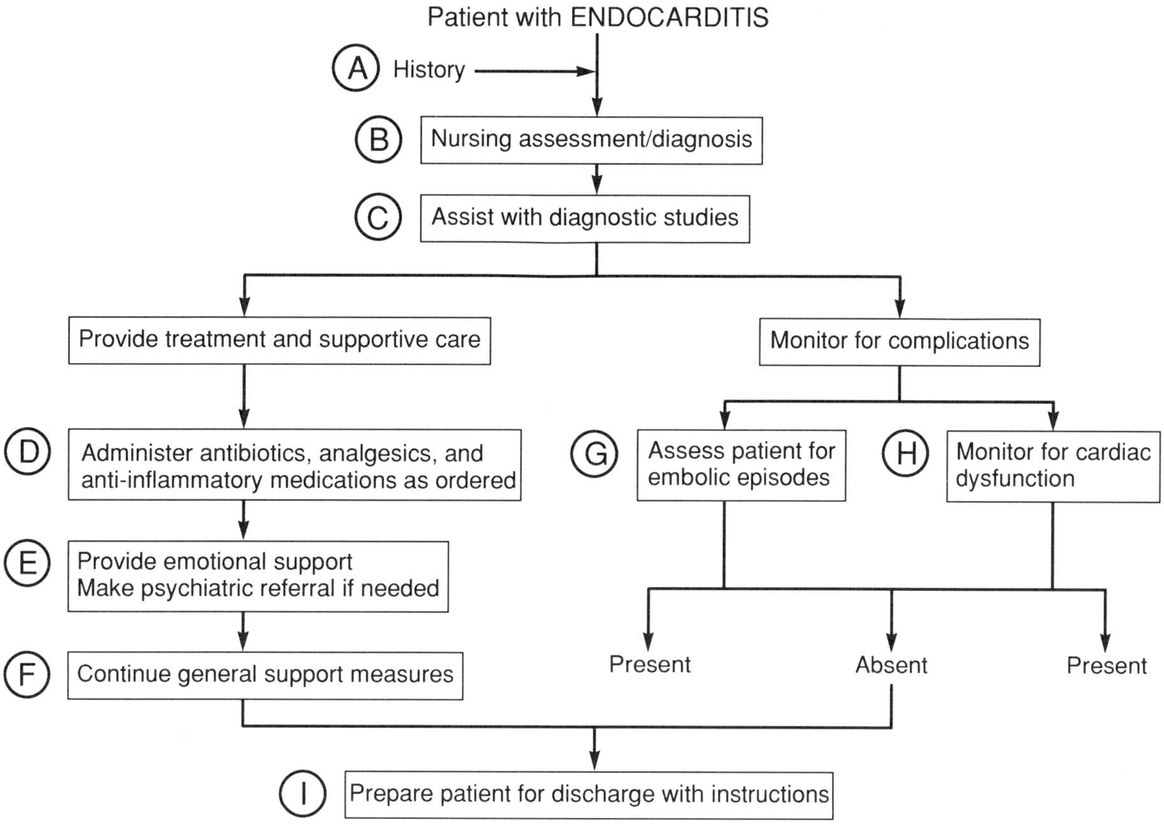
Patient with ENDOCARDITIS
A History
B Nursing assessment/diagnosis
C Assist with diagnostic studies
Provide treatment and supportive care
Monitor for complications
D Administer antibiotics, analgesics, and anti-inflammatory medications as ordered
G Assess patient for embolic episodes
H Monitor for cardiac dysfunction
E Provide emotional support
Make psychiatric referral if needed
F Continue general support measures
Present
Absent
Present
I Prepare patient for discharge with instructions

SYSTEMIC HYPERTENSION

William B. Marshall
Joy Gorzeman

Many standards are set to determine hypertension. The National Heart, Lung and Blood Institute of the National Institutes of Health (NIH) and the World Health Organization (WHO) have established the most widely accepted "norms": a systolic pressure greater than 140 mm Hg and/or a diastolic pressure of greater than 90 mm Hg.

A. One random reading does not constitute hypertension, as there are many factors that can cause a transient rise in either the systolic or diastolic pressures. However, blood pressure elevation on three consecutive occasions indicates hypertension and warrants investigation. Although the cause is often unknown, the nursing history should include questions about lifestyle such as diet (salt and lipid intake), cigarette smoking, exercise, family history, and medications.

B. Primary hypertension is the most common. Patients with primary hypertension do not usually have symptoms, making assessment of anyone with three consecutive elevated blood pressure readings essential. Many patients who are on medical-surgical units for other reasons have primary hypertension.

C. Secondary hypertension is not as common but may be caused by underlying disorders such as endocrine tumors, structural cardiovascular abnormalities, renal disease (p 322), and preeclampsia/eclampsia. Women using oral contraceptives are also at high risk for secondary hypertension. Complaints of headache, palpitations, excessive perspiration, blurred vision, restlessness, or confusion may indicate secondary hypertension.

D. Diagnostic studies include complete blood work, chest film, neurologic tests, and electrocardiography (ECG).

E. Most patients with primary hypertension do not require hospitalization. Weight control; dietary restrictions such as decreasing sodium, coffee, and alcohol; cessation of smoking; need for exercise; and reducing or eliminating stressful situations should be discussed with the patient.

F. If lifestyle changes do not reduce the blood pressure, medical therapy is started. An individualized flexible stepped-care approach is used. Compliance with the medication regimen must be explained and stressed. The medication regimen must be adhered to and monitored in relation to their current disease process.

G. Treatment for patients with secondary hypertension focuses on the underlying cause. Assessment should be ongoing. Vital signs should be checked at least every 2 hours. Daily weights are recorded and fluid intake and output monitored. It is desirable to maintain fluid intake at or below output to avoid increases in intravascular volume; however, patients must also remain adequately hydrated.

H. One of the risks associated with hypertension is hypertensive crisis. Although not a frequent occurrence, this situation is a *medical emergency* and requires an immediate reduction in blood pressure. Hypertensive crisis is manifested by a rapid increase in blood pressure and either grade 3 or 4 retinopathy. Without correction, vital organ damage is imminent. The heart rate increases, pulmonary congestion may occur, and the patient may go into acute renal failure (p 314).

I. Reducing or eliminating negative psychosocial stimuli and providing a quiet, restful environment may help to stabilize or reduce blood pressure. Stimuli such as disputes with family members or staff, loud music, bright lights, and dramatic television shows have been known to trigger a psychosomatic increase in blood pressure. If stabilized, patients may be monitored via telemetry. Unstable patients may require transfer to the ICU for intensive hemodynamic monitoring.

J. Of all nursing interventions, the most important is patient teaching. The presence of hypertension dictates that there must be some lifestyle changes that affect not only the patient but also their significant others. Areas of concentration in the teaching plan must include medication compliance, diet and fluid restrictions, physical fitness, stress avoidance and/or reduction, and follow-up care.

References

Kinney MR, Packa DR, Dunbar SB, eds. AACN's clinical reference for critical-care nursing. 2nd ed. New York: McGraw-Hill, 1988.

Brunner LS, Suddarth DS. The Lippincott manual of nursing practice. 4th ed. Philadelphia: JB Lippincott, 1986.

Luckmann J, Sorensen KC. Medical-surgical nursing: a psychophysiologic approach. 3rd ed. Philadelphia: WB Saunders, 1987.

Muir BL. Pathophysiology: an introduction to the mechanisms of disease. 2nd ed. New York: John Wiley and Sons, 1988.

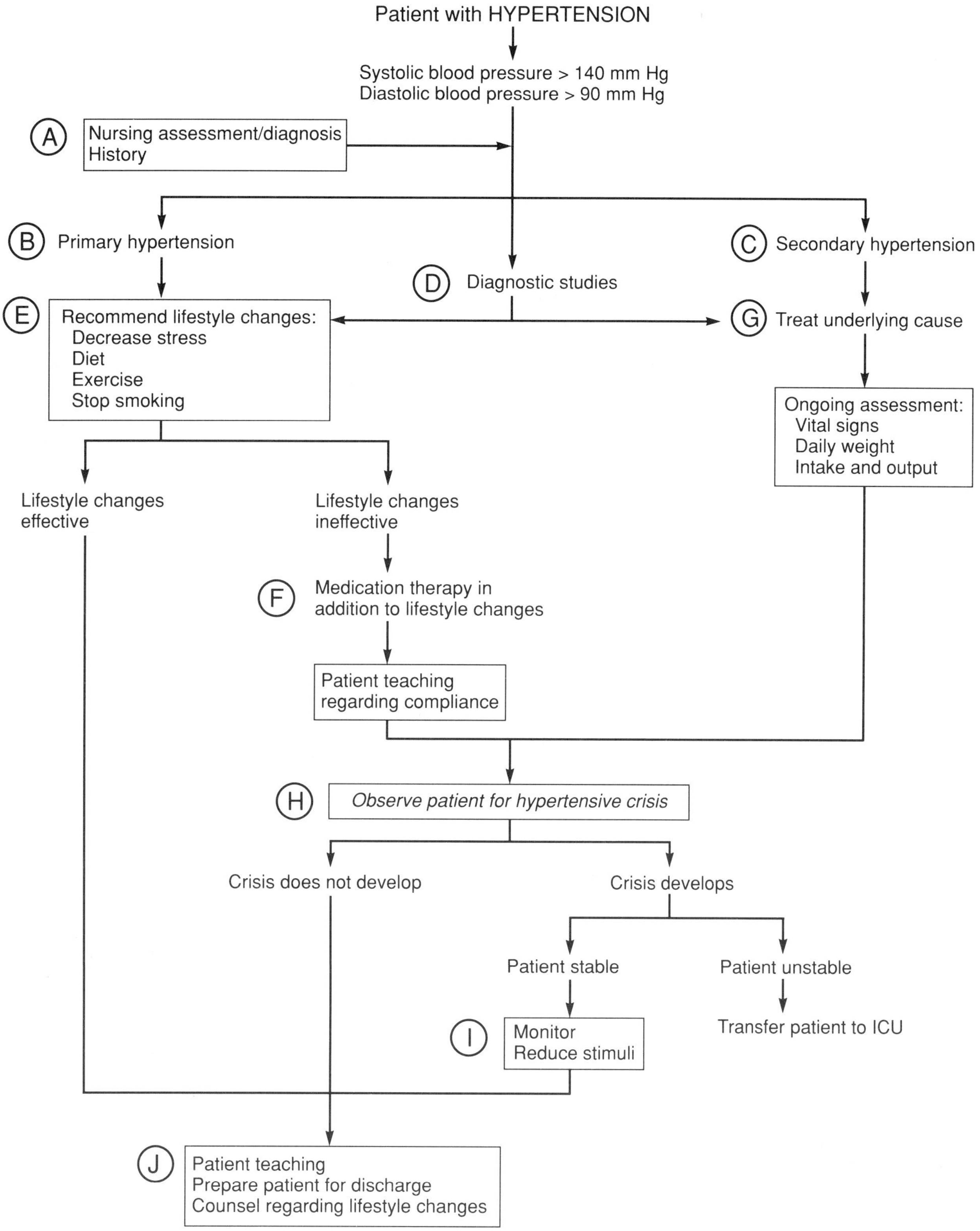

Patient with HYPERTENSION
Systolic blood pressure > 140 mm Hg
Diastolic blood pressure > 90 mm Hg
A
Nursing assessment/diagnosis
History
B
Primary hypertension
C
Secondary hypertension
D
Diagnostic studies
E
Recommend lifestyle changes:
Decrease stress
Diet
Exercise
Stop smoking
G
Treat underlying cause
Ongoing assessment:
Vital signs
Daily weight
Intake and output
Lifestyle changes effective
Lifestyle changes ineffective
F
Medication therapy in addition to lifestyle changes
Patient teaching regarding compliance
H
Observe patient for hypertensive crisis
Crisis does not develop
Crisis develops
Patient stable
Patient unstable
I
Monitor
Reduce stimuli
Transfer patient to ICU
J
Patient teaching
Prepare patient for discharge
Counsel regarding lifestyle changes

CARDIAC CATHETERIZATION

Cindy Drew

Cardiac catheterization is an invasive fluoroscopic test used to determine the status of the heart. It is frequently used to diagnose or assess a cardiac abnormality, especially problems related to coronary artery disease (p 66). This procedure may be done on an outpatient basis in some facilities.

A. The patient undergoing cardiac catheterization may or may not be exhibiting active symptoms of cardiac disease. Cardiac catheterization is used to rule out structural defects (valves, septal defects, ventricular function) and screen candidates for coronary artery surgery (p 92).

B. The nursing assessment is directed toward obtaining baseline physiologic data, evaluating peripheral circulation that may be affected by the test, and assessing the patient's knowledge of the procedure.

C. Evaluation of distal pulses should include palpating and marking the dorsalis pedis and posterior tibial pulses of both extremities (p 88).

D. Have the patient review a cardiac catheterization patient teaching pamphlet. Supplement with additional information, review, and an opportunity to ask questions. Inform patients that they will be awake although sedated during the procedure. Include information about precatheterization preparation, length of procedure, and sensations that may be experienced during the procedure. Make certain that patients adhere to the "NPO after midnight" order. Ensure that a consent form has been signed prior to the procedure.

E. Inquire about a history of allergies. Patients allergic to iodine or shellfish may have a reaction to the contrast dye used during cardiac catheterization.

F. Consult with the physician about continuing medications; cardiac medications may be discontinued.

G. Shave the groin area if required by hospital policy.

H. Establish an intravenous line to provide access for fluids and medications as needed.

I. Obtain a baseline electrocardiogram (ECG) to provide pre- and postprocedure comparison.

J. The postprocedure report from the cardiac catheterization laboratory includes location and appearance of the puncture site and distal circulation, a description of the specific procedures performed and the patient's tolerance, test findings, and medical orders and treatment plan.

K. The patient remains in bed for 6 to 24 hours (depending on hospital procedure). The head of the bed should be flat for the first 6 hours and the involved extremity immobilized. A pressure dressing and sandbag are placed over the puncture site to prevent bleeding. Patients are instructed to avoid activities that increase intra-arterial pressure such as laughing, coughing, and bending the affected leg. The puncture site is checked every 15 minutes for the first hour, every 30 minutes for the next hour, every hour for 4 hours, and every 4 hours for 24 hours postcatheterization. *If acute bleeding occurs, apply direct pressure using gloved hands directly above and below the site, monitor the patient's condition, and notify the physician immediately.*

L. Monitor the distal pulses. A Doppler should be utilized if the pulses are not palpable. *Changes in pulses must be reported immediately.*

M. Monitor the patient's vital signs every 15 minutes for at least the first hour or until stable, then every 4 hours for the next 24 hours. If the patient is not on a cardiac monitor, obtain a 12-lead ECG. *Bradycardia accompanied by hypotension requires immediate intervention.* Place the patient in Trendelenburg's position, administer atropine and fluids per protocol, and notify the physician.

N. If the patient has had angiography, adequate hydration is important to counteract the diuretic effect of the dye.

O. Assess and medicate for incisional pain. Notify the physician if chest pain is present. A stat ECG and serum enzymes should be obtained. Begin oxygen by nasal cannula as ordered. Further treatment with analgesics and nitrates is instituted based on physician's orders or approved protocols. Transfer of the patient to the CCU for stabilization may be indicated.

P. A treatment plan is established in relation to the results of the procedure. Patients may return home with instructions about medications, activity restrictions, and follow-up appointments.

References

Brewin-Wilson D. What you need to know about cardiac catheterization. RN 1984; 47(9):24–30.

Brunner LS, Suddarth DS. Textbook of medical-surgical nursing, 6th ed. Philadelphia: JB Lippincott, 1988.

Vetter PB. Cardiac catheterization. In: Cahill M, ed. Diagnostics. Springhouse, PA: Springhouse Corporation, 1986: 924–932.

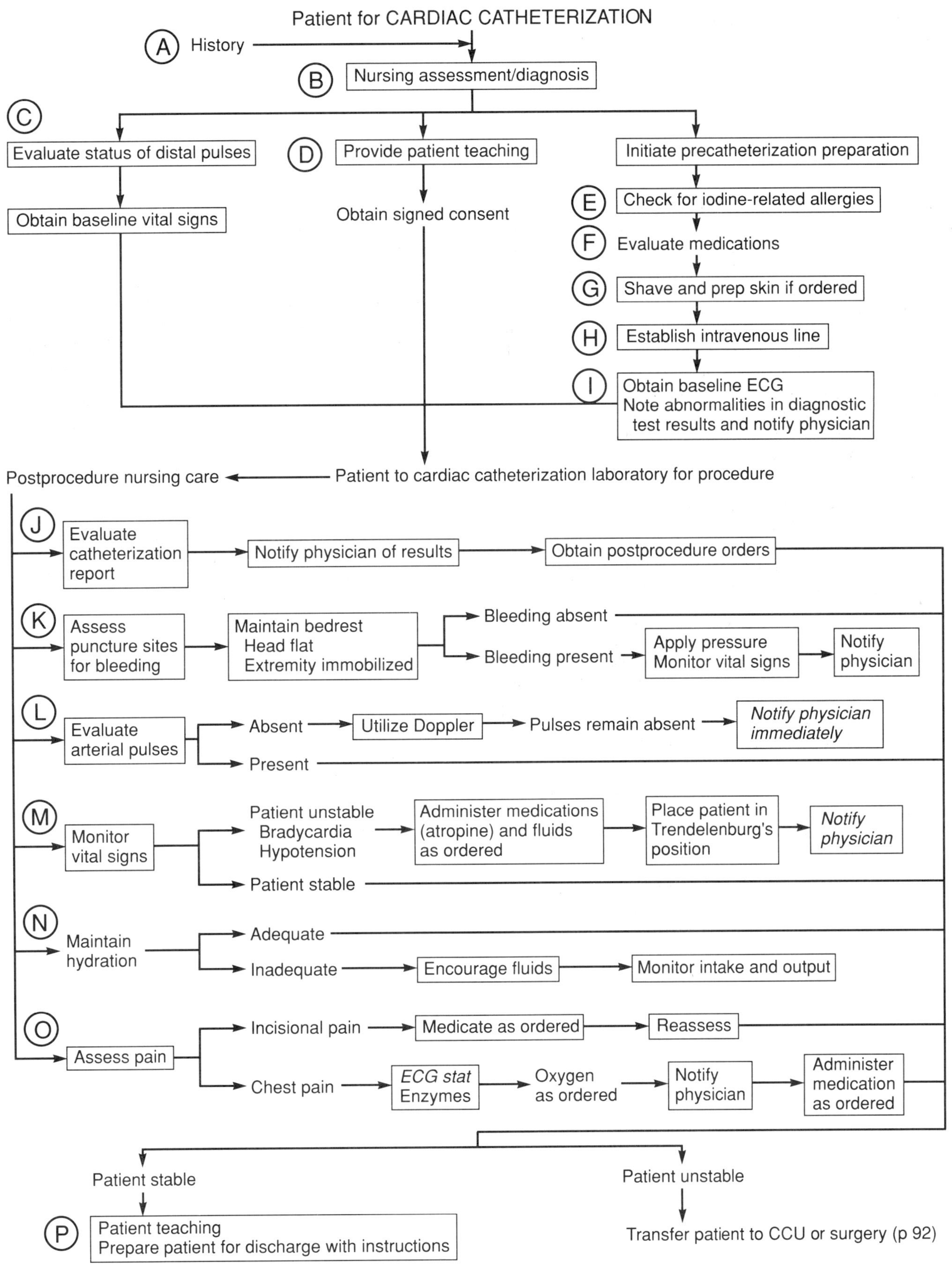
Patient for CARDIAC CATHETERIZATION
A History
B Nursing assessment/diagnosis
C
Evaluate status of distal pulses
Obtain baseline vital signs
D Provide patient teaching
Obtain signed consent
Initiate precatheterization preparation
E Check for iodine-related allergies
F Evaluate medications
G Shave and prep skin if ordered
H Establish intravenous line
I Obtain baseline ECG
Note abnormalities in diagnostic test results and notify physician
Patient to cardiac catheterization laboratory for procedure
Postprocedure nursing care
J Evaluate catheterization report
Notify physician of results
Obtain postprocedure orders
K Assess puncture sites for bleeding
Maintain bedrest
Head flat
Extremity immobilized
Bleeding absent
Bleeding present
Apply pressure
Monitor vital signs
Notify physician
L Evaluate arterial pulses
Absent
Utilize Doppler
Pulses remain absent
Notify physician immediately
Present
M Monitor vital signs
Patient unstable
Bradycardia
Hypotension
Administer medications (atropine) and fluids as ordered
Place patient in Trendelenburg's position
Notify physician
Patient stable
N Maintain hydration
Adequate
Inadequate
Encourage fluids
Monitor intake and output
O Assess pain
Incisional pain
Medicate as ordered
Reassess
Chest pain
ECG stat
Enzymes
Oxygen as ordered
Notify physician
Administer medication as ordered
Patient stable
P Patient teaching
Prepare patient for discharge with instructions
Patient unstable
Transfer patient to CCU or surgery (p 92)

PERMANENT PACEMAKER

Cindy Drew

An artificial pacemaker is utilized to provide electrical stimulation to the heart muscle when the heart's natural pacemaker cells are not initiated or the conduction system is abnormal. Symptomatic bradyarrhythmias (p 56), atrioventricular block (p 58), and tachyarrhythmias (p 64) are also indications for a pacemaker. Most permanent pacemakers are inserted through a transvenous or endocardial approach while the patient is under local anesthesia. The battery-powered pulse generator is placed in a subcutaneous pocket in the chest or abdomen. Every pacemaker includes this pulse generator and the lead or electrode system. Often patients are admitted to the medical-surgical unit with a preexisting or recently inserted pacemaker.

A. The nurse should examine the patient's history to determine the indications for the pacemaker insertion. Refer to the patient's pacemaker identification card for information on the type of pacemaker, programmed rate, date and time of insertion, and personal data.

B. Nursing assessment focuses on maintaining an adequate cardiac output and assessing the patient's knowledge level. A properly functioning pacemaker should have no impact on the treatment regimen for the admitting diagnosis. Any recurrence of problems related to those present before the pacemaker was inserted should be reported to the physician.

C. Patients should be instructed about signs of infection as well as symptoms of pacemaker malfunction. They should be reassured that microwave ovens or radar detectors do not interfere with currently implanted pulse generators.

D. New problems, as well as a drop in pulse rate below the programmed lower rate limit or a pulse rate increase above the programmed upper rate limit, should also be reported to the physician.

E. Consider malfunction of the pacemaker with symptoms such as bradycardia, pallor, shortness of breath, dizziness, prolonged hiccups, syncope, and/or changes in heart rate. *An electrocardiogram (ECG) should be taken and the physician notified.* The ECG will reveal a loss of pacemaker artifact, a change in the amplitude or configuration of the QRS complex, competition, and/or arrhythmias. Emergency treatment (intravenous Isuprel, temporary pacemaker) may need to be instituted to support the patient until the underlying cause is eliminated. Further treatment may require transfer to a coronary care unit.

F. Patients with permanent pacemaker should be instructed to see their physician regularly. Physicians monitor the patients and their pacemakers and may need to reset the pacemaker parameters.

References

Cardiac crises: Nursing now series. Springhouse, PA: Springhouse Corporation, 1984.

Furman S, Hayes DL, Holmes DR. A practice of cardiac pacing. Mount Kisco, NY: Futura, 1986.

Porterfield L. What you need to know about today's pacemakers. RN 1987; 50(3):44–49.

Purcell JA, Burrows SG. A pacemaker primer. Am J Nurs 1985; 85(5):553–568.

Thompson JM, McFarland GK, Hirsch JE, Tucker SM, Bowers AC. Clinical nursing. St. Louis: CV Mosby, 1986.

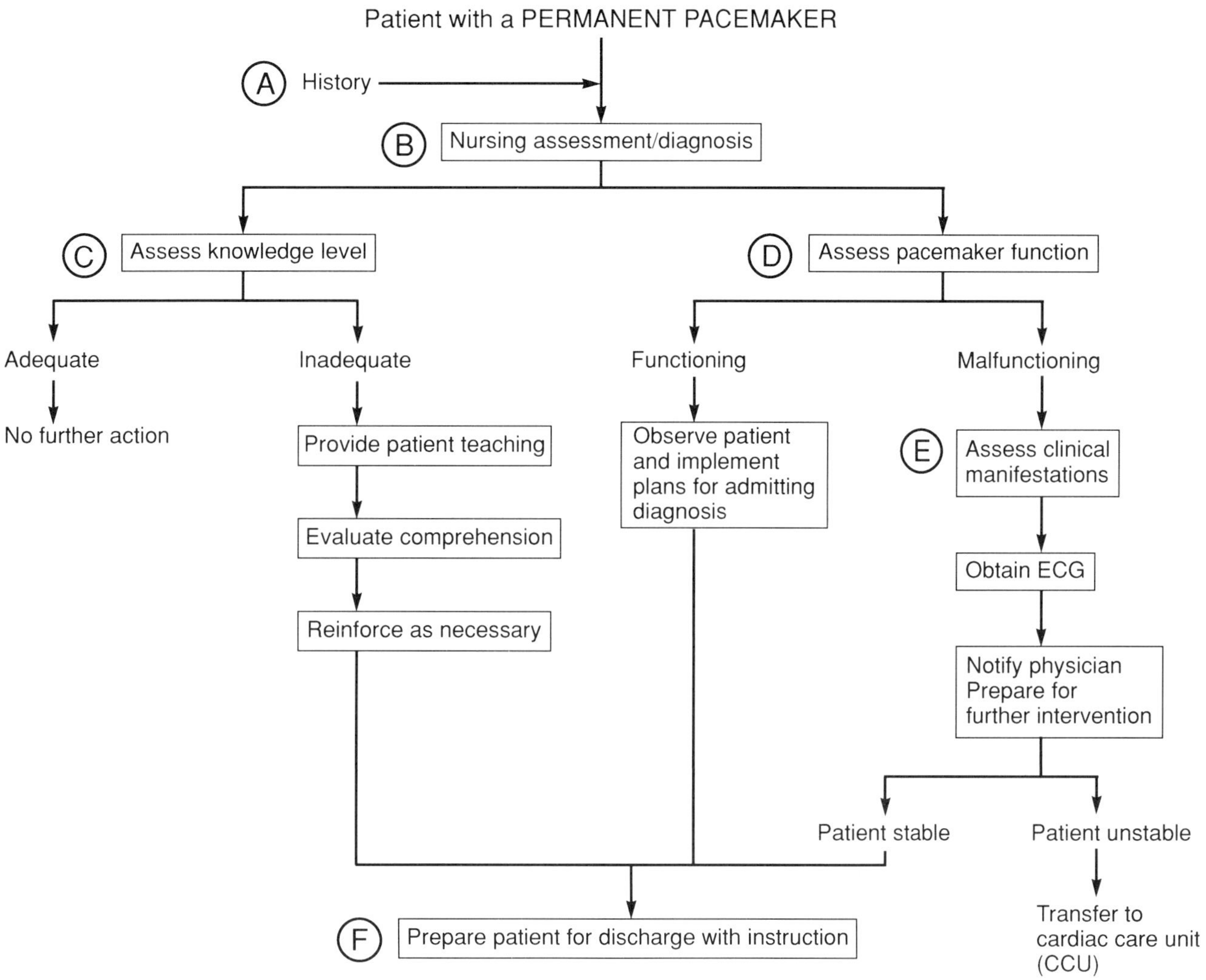
Patient with a PERMANENT PACEMAKER
A
History
B
Nursing assessment/diagnosis
C
Assess knowledge level
D
Assess pacemaker function
Adequate
Inadequate
Functioning
Malfunctioning
No further action
Provide patient teaching
Observe patient and implement plans for admitting diagnosis
E
Assess clinical manifestations
Evaluate comprehension
Obtain ECG
Reinforce as necessary
Notify physician
Prepare for further intervention
Patient stable
Patient unstable
F
Prepare patient for discharge with instruction
Transfer to cardiac care unit (CCU)

VEIN LIGATION

Barbara Kalo

When veins in the lower extremities become dilated, the valves become incompetent and the valve cusps cannot meet, resulting in back-up pressure in the venous system of the legs. The most effective procedure to correct this situation is ligation and stripping of the greater and/or lesser saphenous systems. Because the dilated tortuous veins in the lower extremities may also be unsightly, surgery may be performed for cosmetic purposes. Diagnostic tests to evaluate venous valve competence are done prior to surgery. The most common are the Trendelenburg test, venography, plethysmography, and Doppler ultrasonography.

A. The patient may describe fatigue and an aching discomfort or pain in the lower extremities. Cramping, especially at night, is a frequent symptom. Assessment of edema, pigmentation, and ulceration of the skin is necessary.

B. Preoperative nursing care includes the promotion of comfort, both physically and emotionally. Patient teaching is necessary to provide information about preoperative procedures (p 2) that may be done and postoperative expectations. Physical preparation includes cleansing the legs and lower abdomen with a germicidal soap 3 to 4 days before surgery. It may be necessary to assist the physician in marking the skin to show where incision sites, paths of veins, and dilated tributaries are located.

C. Postoperative nursing care (p 4) is directed toward maintaining an open airway with routine monitoring of level of consciousness and vital signs.

D. Assessment of the circulation to include swelling, color, temperature, and palpable pulses is important. Exercise, movement of legs, and elevating the foot of the bed 30 degrees promotes circulation of the affected extremity.

E. Elastic compression is maintained for approximately 1 week postoperatively from toes to groin. Dressings should be dry, intact, and nonconstricting. Hemorrhage is a possible complication, especially at the groin site. The patient should expect bruising the first week postoperatively. If moderate to large amounts of bleeding are noted or circulation cannot be determined, notify the physician.

F. Medicate the patient for operative pain as needed. Analgesics may help the patient ambulate and move extremities with more ease.

G. Ambulation is begun 24 to 48 hours postoperatively as ordered and is progressive, as tolerated by the patient. Standing still, sitting, and dangling legs at the bedside are contraindicated.

H. If the patient is free of complications, hospital discharge is within 1 week. Patients should be encouraged to wear support hose and elevate their legs periodically. Instructions should also include the avoidance of sitting or standing for long periods of time and the control of excessive weight gain if applicable. The patient should be aware of the existence of patchy numbness that may occur up to 1 year postoperatively.

References

Brunner LS, Suddarth DS. The Lippincott manual of nursing practice. 4th ed. Philadelphia: JB Lippincott, 1986.

Brunner LS, Suddarth DS. Textbook of medical-surgical nursing. 6th ed. Philadelphia: JB Lippincott, 1988.

Krupp MA, Chatton M, Werdegar D, eds. Current medical diagnosis and treatment. Los Altos, CA: Lange, 1985.

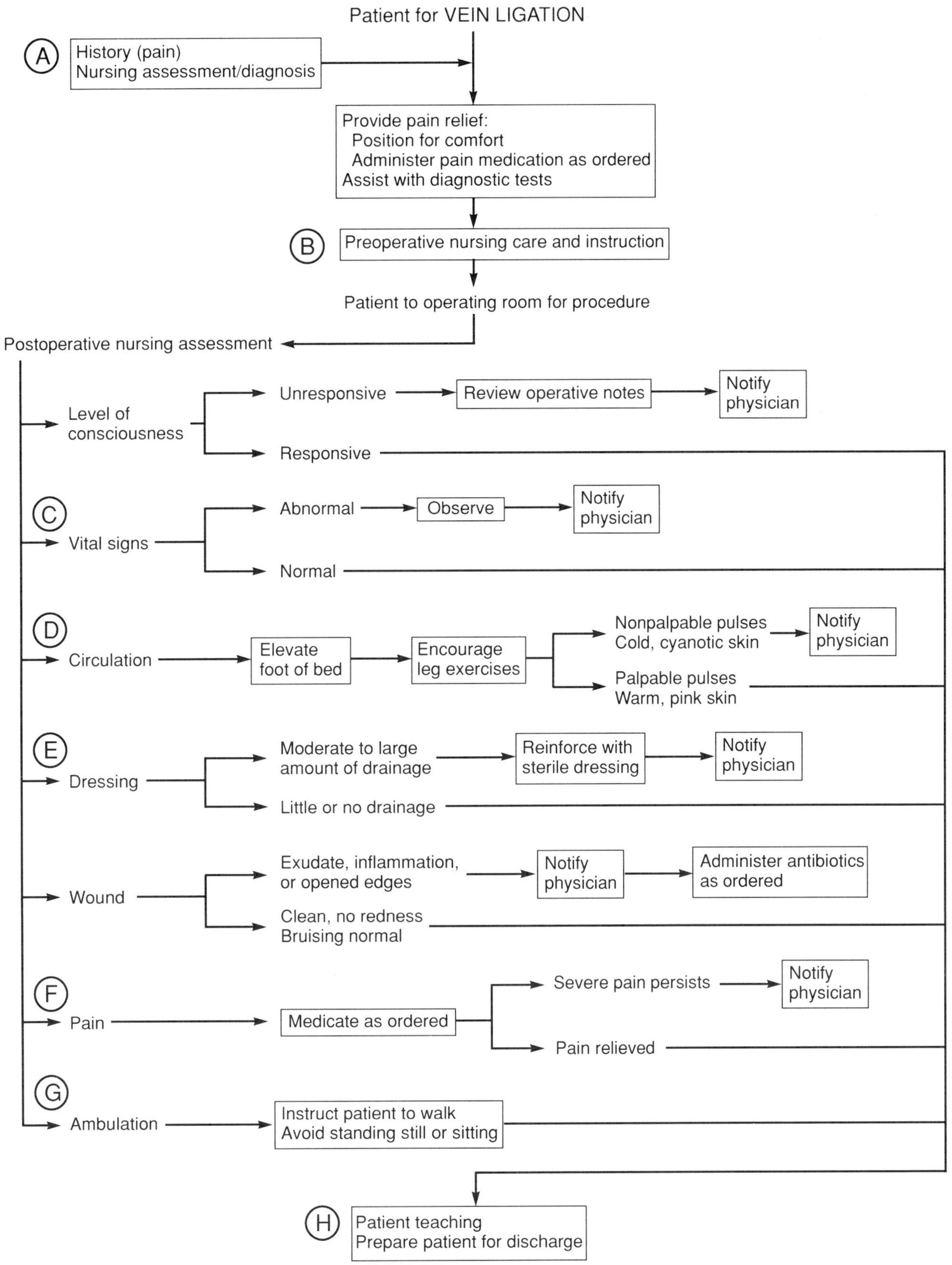
Patient for VEIN LIGATION
A
History (pain)
Nursing assessment/diagnosis
Provide pain relief:
Position for comfort
Administer pain medication as ordered
Assist with diagnostic tests
B
Preoperative nursing care and instruction
Patient to operating room for procedure
Postoperative nursing assessment
Level of consciousness
Unresponsive
Review operative notes
Notify physician
Responsive
C
Vital signs
Abnormal
Observe
Notify physician
Normal
D
Circulation
Elevate foot of bed
Encourage leg exercises
Nonpalpable pulses
Cold, cyanotic skin
Notify physician
Palpable pulses
Warm, pink skin
E
Dressing
Moderate to large amount of drainage
Reinforce with sterile dressing
Notify physician
Little or no drainage
Wound
Exudate, inflammation, or opened edges
Notify physician
Administer antibiotics as ordered
Clean, no redness
Bruising normal
F
Pain
Medicate as ordered
Severe pain persists
Notify physician
Pain relieved
G
Ambulation
Instruct patient to walk
Avoid standing still or sitting
H
Patient teaching
Prepare patient for discharge

FEMORAL-POPLITEAL BYPASS

Joy Gorzeman

Arterial peripheral vascular disease may be acute or chronic and may affect any artery. The arterial lumen is narrowed and/or the endothelial lining is damaged due to atherosclerosis, embolism, thrombosis, trauma, or inflammation. The most common site is the leg.

A. Atherosclerosis is the most common cause of peripheral vascular disease, but the cause of atherosclerosis is not known. However, risk factors that have been associated with atherosclerosis include tobacco use, hypertension, high-cholesterol diets, diabetes, stress, and perhaps most importantly, family history.

B. Diagnostic procedures for peripheral vascular disorders include the Doppler, ankle-arm index (verifies claudication by dividing the ankle systolic pressure by the arm systolic pressure), treadmill exercise to test for intermittent claudication (pain in calf muscles while walking that is relieved by rest), and palpation of peripheral pulses. Other diagnostic procedures are done to identify abnormalities in blood flow resulting from occlusion or narrowing, such as angiography (an invasive procedure in which a dye is injected into the artery) and radiologic studies. Lumbar sympathectomy involves injection of a local anesthetic to improve circulation and to block pain. Patients with peripheral vascular disease should also be worked up for diabetes (p 176) and lipoprotein problems.

C. Classic clinical manifestations of acute peripheral vascular occlusion are pain, loss of sensation, paresthesias, coldness or sensitivity to the cold, pallor, paralysis, and absence of pulse. Quick intervention is essential to save the extremity, since muscle necrosis may start within hours. While preparing the patient for surgery, protect the limb from pressure and trauma, position it level or slightly dependent, and keep it at room temperature.

D. Assessment for chronic occlusive disease includes questions about claudication, rest pain, and numbness and observation of the extremity for blanching, coldness, dusky rubor in dependent positions, presence or absence of pulses, decreased hair growth, thick nails, and shiny skin (trophic changes). Ulceration and gangrenous lesions of the toes may be noted with advanced disease. Other conditions that cause leg pain and need to be ruled out are arthritic disease (p 212), lumbar disk disease (p 46), and muscle cramps.

E. Medical intervention for chronic arterial peripheral vascular disease (arteriosclerosis obliterans) includes vasodilators, anticoagulants and medications that lower serum cholesterol, and/or a nonsurgical procedure that dilates a narrowed artery with a balloon, called percutaneous transluminal angioplasty (PTA).

F. Surgical intervention includes a femoral-popliteal bypass graft for patients who are severely limited because of leg pain or who have ulcers as a result of the poor tissue perfusion. If the saphenous vein is acceptable, it is used for the graft; otherwise, synthetic graft materials are used.

G. If the surgery is not an emergency, preparation should include an explanation of the procedures. Baseline vital signs and location and character of peripheral pulses must be documented. Intravenous lines, a central venous pressure (CVP) line, and a Foley catheter are inserted and prophylactic antibiotics administered. The patient should be free of any infections, especially if a synthetic graft is being used.

H. Postoperatively, monitor blood flow to the extremity. Evaluate peripheral pulses frequently, and rate and record them for consistency in checking (Table 1). *Report changes or cessations of pulses distal to the graft to the physician at once.* Assess color and temperature of skin and movement and sensation of the extremity. Leg position is important and will range from level to slightly elevated, with caution not to constrict blood flow in the popliteal area. Unrelieved edema may result in compartment syndrome and should be reported so a fasciotomy can be done if necessary.

I. Patients will be on bedrest. They should receive heparin intravenously, and antiembolism hose should be applied.

J. Infection is a serious complication in vascular surgeries. Assess the incision and dressing frequently. Report redness, swelling, and drainage.

K. Monitor vital signs and urine output, along with other routine postoperative nursing care (p 4).

L. Patient teaching should include good skin and foot care, a lifestyle that includes rest and exercise, and signs to report that might indicate infection, ulceration, or trauma. Assisting patients with modification of risk factors is an important nursing function.

TABLE 1 Scale for Recording Arterial Pulse Amplitude*

3+	Bounding, hyperkinetic
2+	Normal
1+	Weak, thready, hypokinetic
0	Absent

* Note: Pulses must be evaluated bilaterally in all four extremities for accurate comparison and determination of deficits.

References

Baum PL. Vascular problems. In: Nurse review: a clinical update system. Springhouse, PA: Springhouse Corporation, 1986.

Hincker EA, Malasanos L, eds. The Little Brown manual of medical-surgical nursing. Boston: Little, Brown, 1983.

Phipps WJ, Long BC, Woods NF. Medical-surgical nursing concepts and clinical practice. 3rd ed. St. Louis: CV Mosby, 1987.

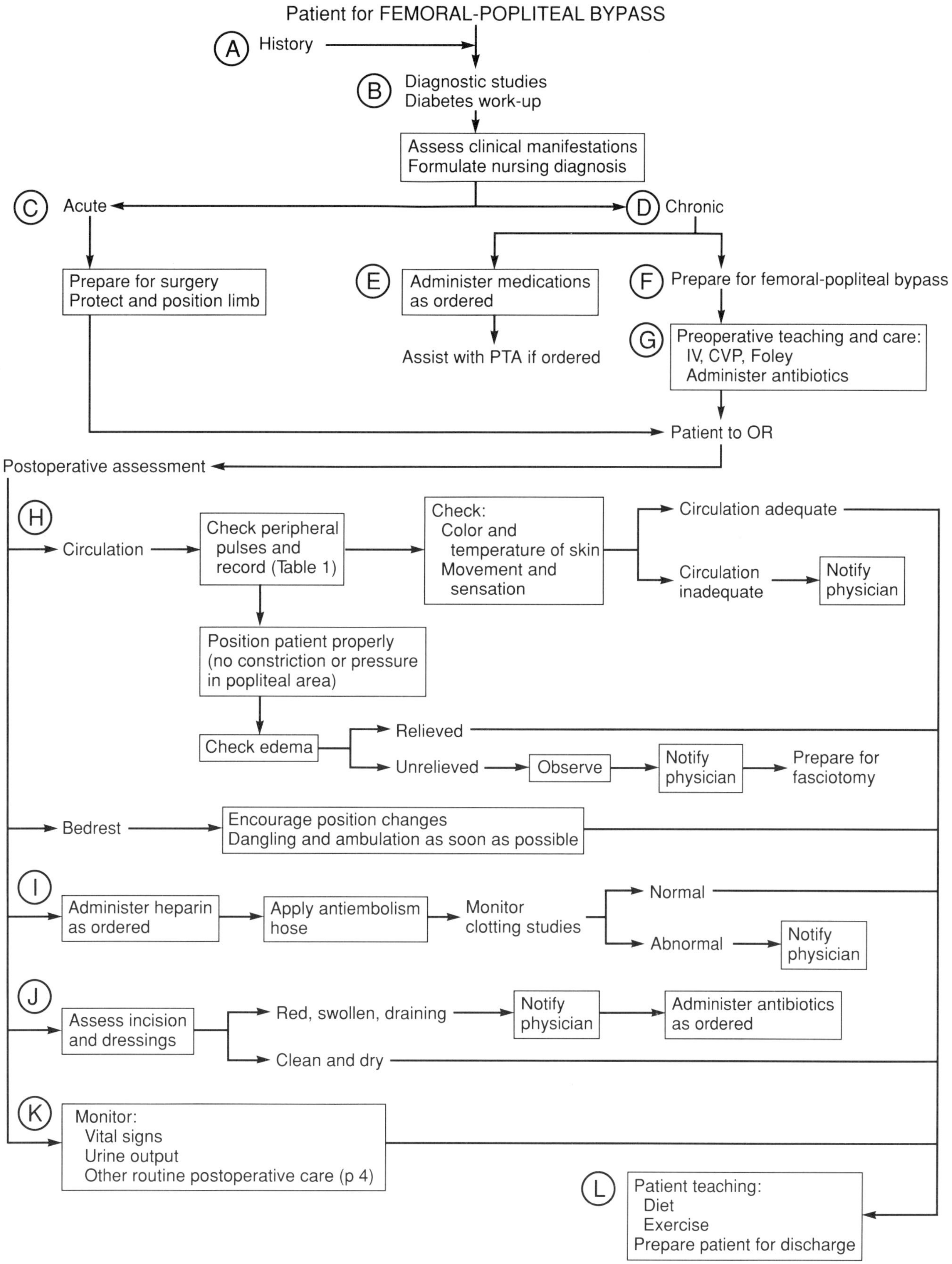

Patient for FEMORAL-POPLITEAL BYPASS
A History
B Diagnostic studies
Diabetes work-up
Assess clinical manifestations
Formulate nursing diagnosis
C Acute
D Chronic
Prepare for surgery
Protect and position limb
E Administer medications as ordered
Assist with PTA if ordered
F Prepare for femoral-popliteal bypass
G Preoperative teaching and care:
IV, CVP, Foley
Administer antibiotics
Patient to OR
Postoperative assessment
H Circulation
Check peripheral pulses and record (Table 1)
Check:
Color and temperature of skin
Movement and sensation
Circulation adequate
Circulation inadequate
Notify physician
Position patient properly (no constriction or pressure in popliteal area)
Check edema
Relieved
Unrelieved
Observe
Notify physician
Prepare for fasciotomy
Bedrest
Encourage position changes
Dangling and ambulation as soon as possible
I Administer heparin as ordered
Apply antiembolism hose
Monitor clotting studies
Normal
Abnormal
Notify physician
J Assess incision and dressings
Red, swollen, draining
Notify physician
Administer antibiotics as ordered
Clean and dry
K Monitor:
Vital signs
Urine output
Other routine postoperative care (p 4)
L Patient teaching:
Diet
Exercise
Prepare patient for discharge

CAROTID ENDARTERECTOMY

Barbara Kalo

Carotid endarterectomy is a surgical procedure done to remove an atherosclerotic plaque from an artery. The most common site of development of the plaque is the region of the carotid bifurcation and the arch of the aorta. Patients who experience transient ischemic attacks (TIAs) have brief episodes of neurologic deficit that pass without apparent residual effects. These are considered a warning signal and are a sign of advanced atherosclerotic disease of the cerebral arterial supply. Carotid endarterectomy is indicated to treat those with TIAs, not those with acute strokes or progressive strokes. It is more of a preventive measure to reduce the frequency of TIA episodes and maintain cerebral blood flow before an infarction occurs.

A. The common signs and symptoms related to cerebral insufficiency are headache, dizziness, blackout spells, memory loss, language dysfunction, and visual defects. There may be numbness and weakness of extremities, absent or diminished carotid pulsations in the neck, and a bruit heard over the carotid artery. Usually no signs of permanent neurologic deficit are present between attacks. These transient periods of neurologic deficit must be differentiated from other causes of cerebral ischemia, such as hematoma or tumor mass (p 38).

B. Preoperative nursing care includes an assessment of the neurologic status, which will be compared to the neurologic assessment postoperatively. Emotional support is necessary to alleviate fears about surgery. Since the majority of patients requiring a carotid endarterectomy are elderly, it is essential that a thorough history and assessment be done (p 412). Other medical problems may be present which must be included in the nursing care of the patient.

C. Postoperative nursing care is directed toward assessment of the neurologic status. The surgery requires temporary clamping of the internal carotid artery, and the blood supply to the brain may be compromised, resulting in a neurologic dysfunction. Any change in the neurologic status (i.e., pupil size or reaction, handgrip, speech, swallowing, mental status) must be reported to the physician (see p 44 for neurologic checklist). Routine procedures such as vital signs and assessment of the surgical site are also done. Patients should be watched for hypotension and bradycardia.

D. The surgical dressing should be dry and intact. A moderate-to-large amount of drainage or a hematoma should be reported to the physician. When dressings are changed, observation of the wound should reveal little or no drainage from the incisional site and no redness or swelling.

E. Medicate the patient for incisional pain as needed. Consider the elderly patient when analgesics are given, since they are more sensitive to central nervous system depressants, and a reduced dose may be required.

F. Assess the bladder for distention. Offer the bedpan or urinal as necessary, and encourage oral fluids when possible to help facilitate the process of voiding.

G. If the patient is free of nausea and vomiting and has a swallowing reflex, clear liquids are offered and a regular diet is resumed as tolerated. Take note of any special diet the patient may have been on preoperatively so that the dietary regimen is maintained.

H. Ambulation may begin on the day of surgery or the first postoperative day. Provide assistance and support as the change to an upright position may cause hypotension. Any support or devices that were needed prior to surgery should be available.

I. If there are no complications, the patient is discharged with specific instructions about dressing changes, wound care, diet, medications, and follow-up care with the physician.

References

Brunner LS, Suddarth DS. The Lippincott manual of nursing practice. 3rd ed. Philadelphia: JB Lippincott, 1982.

Krupp MA, Chatton MJ, Werdegar D, eds. Current medical diagnosis and treatment. Los Altos, CA: Lange, 1985.

Lewis SM, Collier IC. Medical-surgical nursing: assessment and management of clinical problems. New York: McGraw-Hill, 1983.

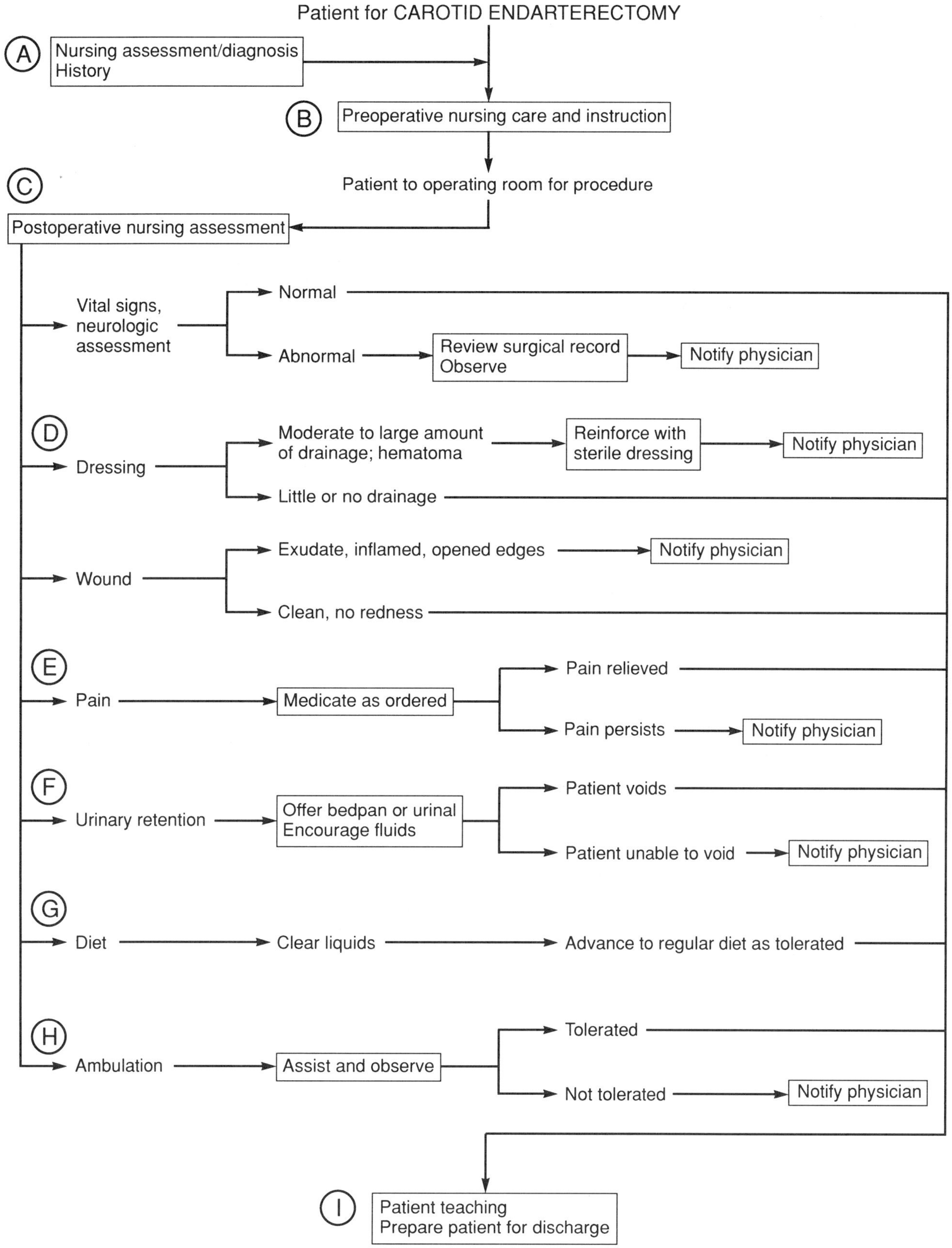
Patient for CAROTID ENDARTERECTOMY
A
Nursing assessment/diagnosis
History
B
Preoperative nursing care and instruction
Patient to operating room for procedure
C
Postoperative nursing assessment
Vital signs, neurologic assessment
Normal
Abnormal
Review surgical record
Observe
Notify physician
D
Dressing
Moderate to large amount of drainage; hematoma
Reinforce with sterile dressing
Notify physician
Little or no drainage
Wound
Exudate, inflamed, opened edges
Notify physician
Clean, no redness
E
Pain
Medicate as ordered
Pain relieved
Pain persists
Notify physician
F
Urinary retention
Offer bedpan or urinal
Encourage fluids
Patient voids
Patient unable to void
Notify physician
G
Diet
Clear liquids
Advance to regular diet as tolerated
H
Ambulation
Assist and observe
Tolerated
Not tolerated
Notify physician
I
Patient teaching
Prepare patient for discharge

CORONARY ARTERY BYPASS

Michele Gann
Linda Weld

Coronary artery bypass graft (CABG) is a surgical procedure that improves blood flow to areas of the myocardium that are in danger because of severely occluded coronary arteries. Vessels used in this procedure may be veins (usually saphenous) or internal mammary arteries. This procedure requires utilization of a cardiopulmonary system to provide oxygenated blood to the body while the heart is in asystole. The patient is anticoagulated while on cardiopulmonary bypass. During the procedure the patient's body temperature is decreased to limit oxygen demand. These patients spend at least 24 hours in an intensive care area after the procedure.

A. Unless the surgery is performed as a result of an acute myocardial infarction, CAB patients usually have a history of chest pain (p 50). Conservative medical management, including nitrates, beta- or calcium-blockers, and/or a percutaneous transluminal angioplasty may have been tried. Prior to the procedure the patient is given a general cardiac workup, which includes electrocardiography, cardiac catheterization (p 82), and a stress test.

B. Preoperative nursing care includes providing emotional support, patient teaching, and physical preparation. Patient teaching should involve the family and include explanations of incisions, chest and mediastinal tubes, endotracheal tubes, Foley catheters, ICU procedures and routines, and coughing and deep breathing exercises. If possible the patient and family should visit the intensive care area. Routine laboratory and radiologic studies are also done. Prior to the procedure the patient should be weighed and a cleansing shower or scrub done.

C. If internal mammary arteries are used for the graft, a pleural chest tube and mediastinal drainage tubes are inserted. All of these tubes should be observed for air leaks, fluctuations, presence of subcutaneous air at the insertion site(s), and type and amount of drainage.

D Assess radial pulses for rate, rhythm, and volume to detect complications such as arrythmias, shock, fever, anxiety, hemorrhage, or hypoxia. Diminished or absent pedal pulses may indicate peripheral emboli. Check the extremity distal to the absent pulse for cyanosis, loss of sensation, and coldness. *Report these findings to the surgeon immediately.*

E. It is possible that the patient may have chest pains from myocardial ischemia after the procedure. The nurse must determine whether the pain the patient is experiencing is incisional or pain from coronary ischemia. The patient must be asked to describe the pain carefully. Any incidents of ischemic pain should be reported to the physician and managed according to agency policy.

F. The patient will progress from dangling on the first postoperative day to full ambulation by the 8th to 10th postoperative day. Vital signs should be taken before and after ambulation. Marked changes in vital signs should be reported to the physician.

G. If there are no complications, the patient is discharged with specific instructions. The incisions should be checked daily for redness or drainage. Instruction for activities of daily living should include diet, medications, exercise, and sexual activities. Follow-up appointments should be made at the time of discharge. Referral to a cardiac rehabilitation program or support group may be indicated.

References

Guzetta CE, Dossey BM. Cardiovascular nursing: bodymind tapestry. St. Louis: CV Mosby, 1984.

Jader GC, Lekander BJ. Open heart surgery: caring for bypass and transplant patients. RN April 1987:40–43.

Kenner CV, Guzzetta CE, Dossey BM. Critical care nursing: body-mind-spirit. 2nd ed. Boston: Little, Brown, 1985.

Lewis SM, Collier IC. Medical surgical nursing: assessment and management of clinical problems. New York: McGraw-Hill, 1983.

Luckmann J, Sorensen KC. Medical-surgical nursing: a psychophysiological approach. 3rd ed. Philadelphia: WB Saunders, 1987.

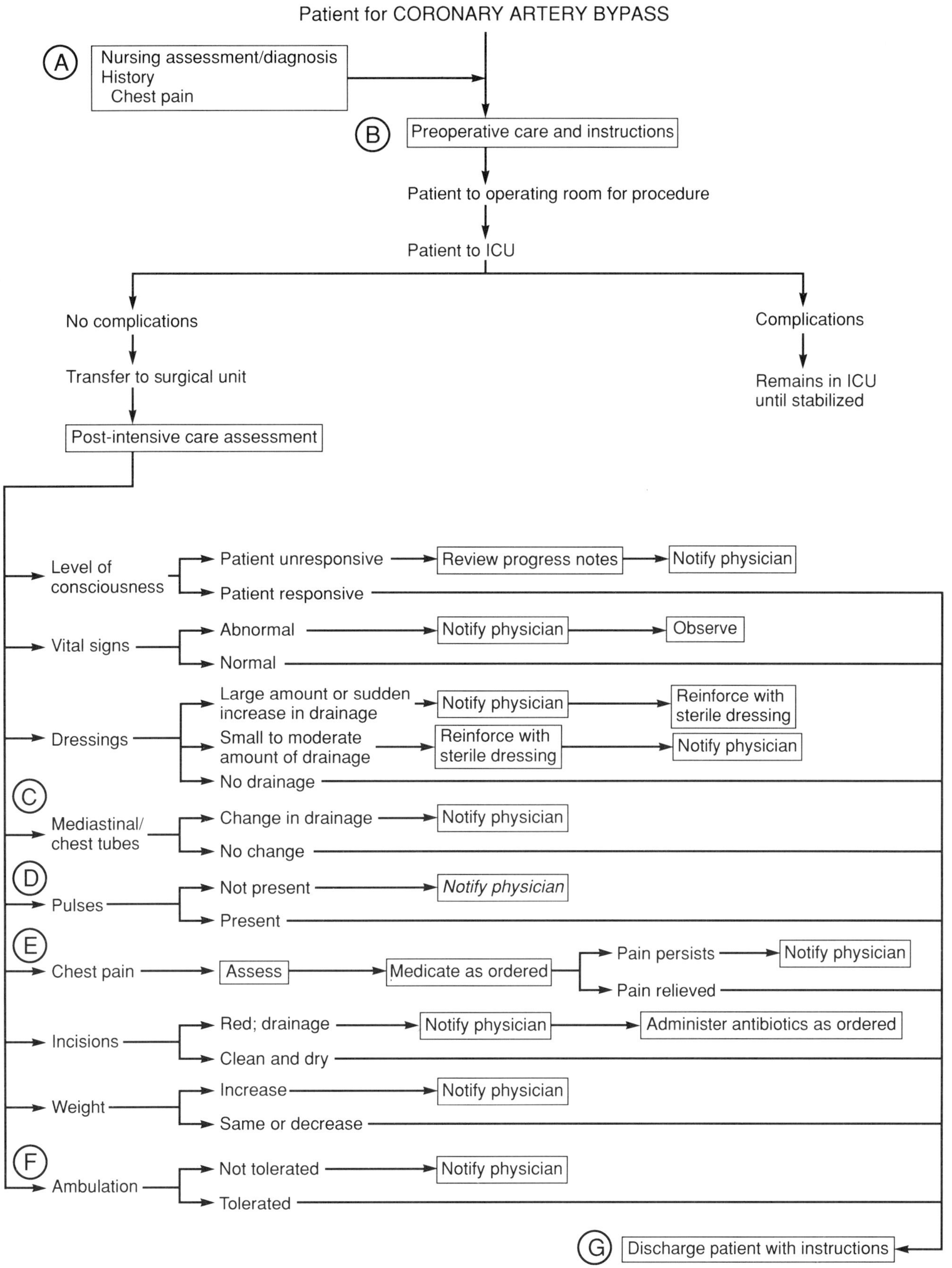

Patient for CORONARY ARTERY BYPASS
A
Nursing assessment/diagnosis
History
Chest pain
B
Preoperative care and instructions
Patient to operating room for procedure
Patient to ICU
No complications
Transfer to surgical unit
Post-intensive care assessment
Complications
Remains in ICU until stabilized
Level of consciousness
Patient unresponsive
Review progress notes
Notify physician
Patient responsive
Vital signs
Abnormal
Notify physician
Observe
Normal
Dressings
Large amount or sudden increase in drainage
Notify physician
Reinforce with sterile dressing
Small to moderate amount of drainage
Reinforce with sterile dressing
Notify physician
No drainage
C
Mediastinal/ chest tubes
Change in drainage
Notify physician
No change
D
Pulses
Not present
Notify physician
Present
E
Chest pain
Assess
Medicate as ordered
Pain persists
Notify physician
Pain relieved
Incisions
Red; drainage
Notify physician
Administer antibiotics as ordered
Clean and dry
Weight
Increase
Notify physician
Same or decrease
F
Ambulation
Not tolerated
Notify physician
Tolerated
G
Discharge patient with instructions

RESPIRATORY SYSTEM

ADULT RESPIRATORY DISTRESS SYNDROME

Robert Steele

Adult respiratory distress syndrome (ARDS) is an acute deterioration of pulmonary function and is manifested by a constellation of symptoms from a variety of causes. Regardless of clinical setting or etiology, the symptoms and management of ARDS are similar. ARDS affects previously normal or healthy lungs as frequently as diseased lungs.

A. Suspicious history and vigilance for predisposing factors may assist the nurse in early identification of symptoms of ARDS. Sepsis, aspiration of gastric contents, and multisystem trauma are the most frequently associated clinical conditions that lead to ARDS. Other conditions include massive transfusions (≥6 units), chest trauma, disseminated intravascular coagulopathy, fat or air embolism, and extracorporeal circulation.

B. Assessment of the patient's airway and cardiopulmonary function is of utmost importance. Abnormal findings include rapid respirations, diminished or absent breath sounds, and use of accessory muscles for respiration. Initially, breath sounds may be clear, but as the syndrome progresses they may be diminished or replaced by rales and rhonchi. Tachycardia with weak pulses, hypotension, reduced urinary output, and diaphoresis are often associated with shock (p 70).

C. The use of sequential blood gas analysis is useful to identify high-risk patients. This method of monitoring blood gases and ventilation has proved to be a reliable means of identifying patients at risk for the development of ARDS.

D. Treatment depends on the severity of the symptoms. Supportive therapy should be initiated as soon as possible or in concert with airway management if symptoms are severe. The sequence of supportive measures is designed for a broad range of patients and does not preclude use of other therapeutic measures specific for coexisting disturbances.

E. Placement of an intravenous catheter and administration of crystalloids at a keep-open rate is indicated. Administration of intravenous fluids may be guided by blood pressure, urine output, and measurement of central filling pressures (CVP).

F. Blood samples should be obtained for complete blood count, serum electrolytes, and clotting studies. Arterial blood gases (ABGs) should be sampled frequently and analyzed for symptoms of respiratory distress.

G. Patients surviving ARDS may have some degree of permanent damage of lung tissues. This damage may result in long-term abnormalities in ABGs and pulmonary function studies. Patients may become short of breath on exertion and are susceptible to more respiratory tract infections. Smoking is contraindicated.

H. Do not withhold oxygen therapy from patients in active respiratory distress. *Notify the physician at once.* Intubation and mechanical ventilation may be indicated. If so, prepare the patient for transfer to the intensive care unit (ICU).

I. If intubation is required, chest roentgenography is useful to confirm placement of the endotracheal tube. In addition, pneumothorax may be diagnosed or ruled out. It is important to note that chest film abnormalities lag behind physiologic changes, so a patient may be in acute distress even though the chest film is essentially normal.

References

Pontoppidan H, Geffin B, Lowenstein E. Acute respiratory failure in the adult. N Engl J Med 1972; 287:690, 743, 799.

Rodgers KM. American Association for Critical Care Nurses. Clinical reference for critical care nursing. New York: McGraw-Hill, 1981:485–497.

Weigelt JA, Snyder WH III, Mitchell RA. Early identification of patients prone to develop adult respiratory distress syndrome. Am J Surg 1981; 142:687–691.

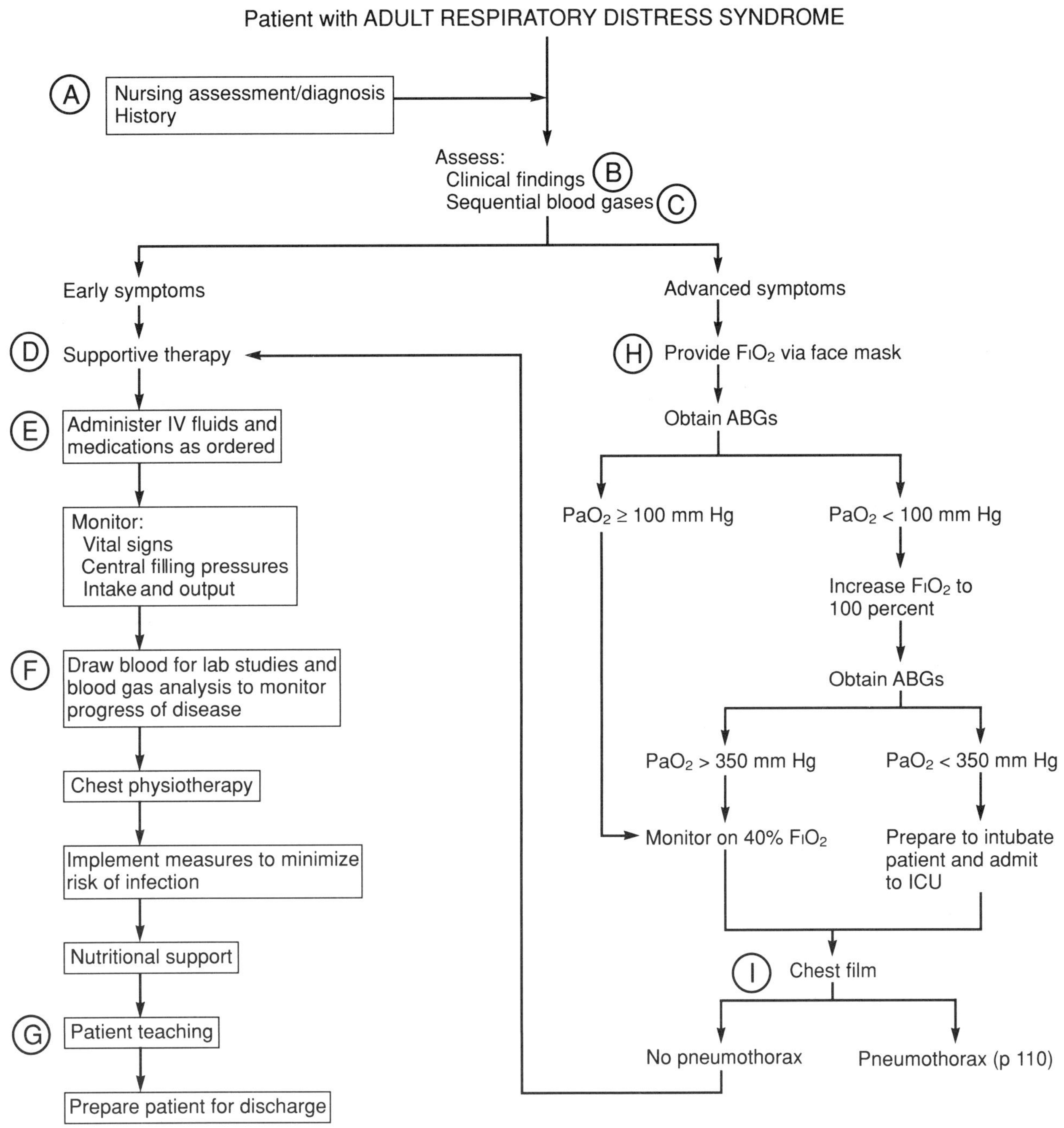

Patient with ADULT RESPIRATORY DISTRESS SYNDROME
A
Nursing assessment/diagnosis
History
Assess:
Clinical findings B
Sequential blood gases C
Early symptoms
D Supportive therapy
E Administer IV fluids and medications as ordered
Monitor:
Vital signs
Central filling pressures
Intake and output
F Draw blood for lab studies and blood gas analysis to monitor progress of disease
Chest physiotherapy
Implement measures to minimize risk of infection
Nutritional support
G Patient teaching
Prepare patient for discharge
Advanced symptoms
H Provide F_IO_2 via face mask
Obtain ABGs
$PaO_2 \geq 100$ mm Hg
$PaO_2 < 100$ mm Hg
Increase F_IO_2 to 100 percent
Obtain ABGs
$PaO_2 > 350$ mm Hg
$PaO_2 < 350$ mm Hg
Monitor on 40% F_IO_2
Prepare to intubate patient and admit to ICU
I Chest film
No pneumothorax
Pneumothorax (p 110)

EMPHYSEMA

David L. Lybarger

Emphysema is one of two types of chronic obstructive pulmonary disease (COPD), type A. It is characterized by permanent abnormal enlargement of the acinus (primary lobule of the lung), with destruction of the alveolar wall. Although other obscure causes of emphysema exist, cigarette smoking and hereditary alpha-1-antitrypsin deficiency are two important causes.

A. Emphysema patients typically present in their 50s, or 60s with progressive, constant dyspnea. Initially, dyspnea only occurs on extreme exertion, but as the condition progresses, it finally occurs even at rest. Cough and sputum production may be absent or mild. The patient with advanced disease may report gradual weight loss to the point of wasting.

B. Nursing assessment of emphysema patients initially includes evaluation of airway clearance, breathing pattern, gas exchange, hydration, and nutrition. Mobility, self-care, self-image, and coping issues should also be evaluated, as well as the degree of support available to the patient in the home environment upon discharge.

C. Diagnostic procedures often include complete blood count (CBC) and arterial blood gas (ABG) determinations, however these are frequently normal until late in the course of the disease. Hypoxemia may be surprisingly mild unless the patient is in obvious respiratory failure. Similarly, pulmonary function tests may be near normal early in the disease.

D. Retained mucopurulent secretions, a major problem in patients with emphysema, is treated by decreasing secretions and by facilitating their removal. Measures that decrease secretions include removing irritants (especially cigarette smoking) and administering steroids as prescribed. Measures that facilitate removal of secretions include encouraging fluid intake within the limits of cardiac reserve, administering bronchodilators, nebulized water, and expectorants as ordered. Utilizing orthopneic and postural drainage positions and providing pulmonary physiotherapy may also enhance gas exchange.

E. Airway infections, detected by sputum culture, are treated with antibiotic therapy guided by sensitivity studies. Ampicillin, erythromycin, tetracycline, and/or trimethoprim-sulfamethoxazole are commonly used.

F. Maintaining nutrition is a formidable problem for emphysemic patients, mainly because of the energy required to prepare, consume, and digest food, but also because of appetite suppression, nausea, and protein depletion caused by drugs such as bronchodilators and steroids. Nursing care includes assisting patients to choose high-protein, high-carbohydrate foods that are easy to chew and swallow, encouraging patients to eat smaller meals more frequently, and administering stool softeners and laxatives as prescribed to relieve constipation.

G. Fiberoptic bronchoscopy may become necessary to remove heavy mucous plug secretions that patients are unable to raise themselves. Nursing care of the patient undergoing bronchoscopy involves keeping the stomach empty (NPO) 8 hours prior to the procedure, administering a preprocedure sedative containing atropine as ordered, removing dental prostheses, carefully observing and positioning the patient during the postanesthesia recovery period, and monitoring for severe complications, especially bronchospasm.

H. If progressive respiratory deterioration ensues, tracheotomy (p 398) may become necessary to permit adequate removal of secretions and/or mechanical ventilation. General nursing care includes providing emotional support through adequate explanation of the procedure and encouraging the patient to share feelings of anxiety; carefully observing for and promptly reporting signs of pneumomediastinum, pneumothorax (p 110), cardiac tamponade (p 28), hemorrhage, or subcutaneous emphysema; suctioning as frequently as necessary; maintaining hygiene of the tracheostomy tube, cannula, and insertion site, and ensuring security of the tracheostomy tube placement.

I. Diuretics and salt restriction may be necessary in the presence of cor pulmonale.

J. Antiarrhythmics such as verapamil are especially helpful in controlling multifocal atrial tachycardia (p 60), commonly seen in emphysemic patients.

K. General supportive care includes assisting the patient to maintain proper body positioning for optimal airway availability; providing hydration to liquify secretions and replace fluids; administering vaporization therapy and postural drainage; monitoring and reporting vital signs, including temperature; assisting with choosing high-protein, high-carbohydrate foods that are easy to chew and swallow; encouraging gradual increase in activities as tolerated to prevent "pulmonary crippling"; problem solving with the patient to determine methods of conserving energy in the performance of activities of daily living (ADL); and assisting the patient in developing coping strategies.

L. Patient and family education should include adaptive breathing and postural drainage techniques; avoidance

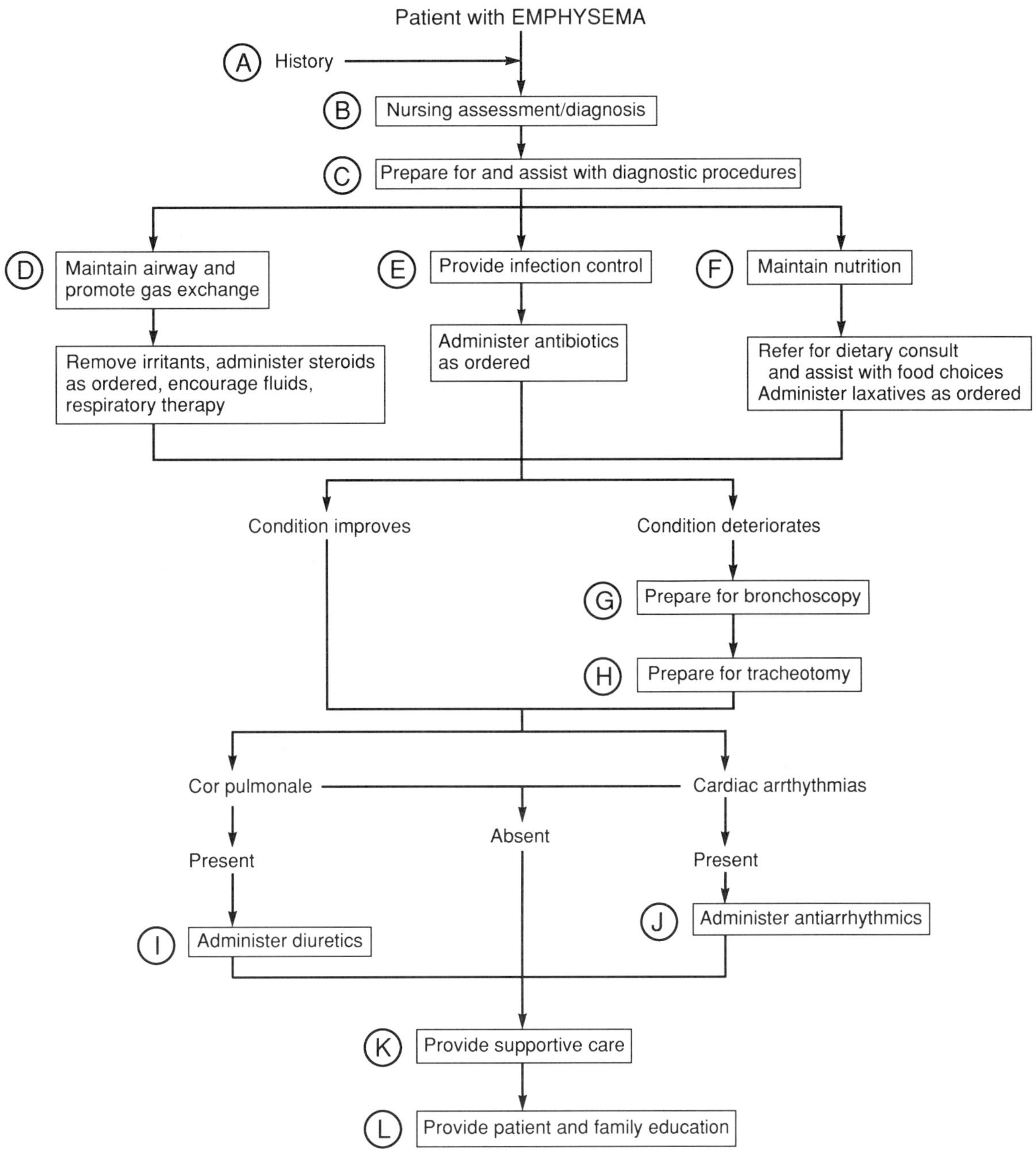

of persons with upper respiratory infections; pneumococcal and influenza vaccines; use, purpose, and importance of medications and compliance; the disease process and signs and symptoms that require medical intervention; importance of consuming up to 4L of fluids per day; avoidance of cigarette smoke and other airborne pollutants; information about the use, care, cleaning, and maintenance of home respiratory care equipment; and information about community support groups and resources.

References

Brunner LS, Suddarth DS, eds. The Lippincott manual of nursing practice. Philadelphia: JB Lippincott 1974:165–168.

Krupp MA, Chatton MJ, Tierney LM, eds. Current medical diagnosis and treatment. Los Altos, CA: Lange, 1986:134–136.

Thompson J. Respiratory system. In: Thompson JM, MacFarland GK, Hirsch JE, Tucker SM, Bowers AC, eds. Clinical nursing. St Louis: CV Mosby, 1986:159–166.

ASTHMA

David L. Lybarger

Bronchial asthma is characterized by narrowing of the large and small airways due to spasm of bronchial smooth muscle, edema and inflammation in the bronchial mucosal wall, and the production of tenacious mucus (Fig. 1). Although the underlying mechanisms responsible for attacks of paroxysmal wheezing are unknown, inherited or acquired imbalance of adrenergic and cholinergic control of airway diameter have been implicated. Bronchial asthma occurs secondarily to a variety of stimuli.

Extrinsic asthma (i.e., asthma precipitated by allergenic exposure and IgE mediated) is seen in 10 to 20 percent of the adult asthmatic population. The symptomatic episodes of 30 to 50 percent of adult asthmatics are triggered by nonallergic factors, and these persons are said to have intrinsic asthma. In many individuals, both allergenic and nonallergenic factors play significant roles.

In bronchial asthma, airway obstruction leads to localized hypoventilation. In an effort to compensate, the patient hyperventilates early in the attack. However, continued airway narrowing and muscle fatigue eventually result in hypoxemia and hypercarbia (respiratory acidosis), and respiratory failure.

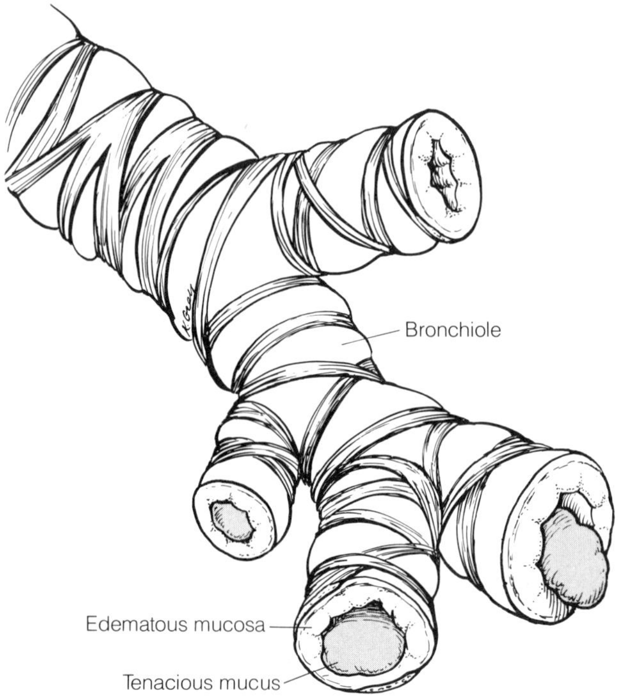

Figure 1 Edematous mucosal wall of bronchiole clogged with tenacious mucus during an asthma attack.

A. Recognition of asthma is frequently based on history. The asthma patient often gives a personal or family history of allergies or of previous episodes of asthma. Careful evaluation of recent stressors is vital. Among the known stressors are infection, exercise, emotional upset, pressure or temperature changes, inhalation of cold air or irritants, and exposure to specific allergens. A careful and complete history of current respiratory-related medications, including evaluation of compliance and time of most recent dose, is essential.

B. Initial nursing assessment includes evaluation of vital signs, breathing pattern and gas exchange, and central nervous system status. Respiratory distress characterized by varying degrees of dyspnea, tachypnea, cough, prolonged expiration, use of accessory muscles, and retractions is common. Chest auscultation usually reveals inspiratory and expiratory wheezing and coarse rhonchi. Tachycardia and cyanosis are commonly present. However, clinical signs of hypoxia such as restlessness, confusion, and combativeness in the absence of wheezes may indicate total small airway obstruction, and can be life threatening. Hydration status and coping ability, self-care and health maintenance abilities, and the degree of support available to the patient in the home environment on discharge are also assessed.

C. Diagnostic tests determine the severity of the attack. Peak expiratory flow rate (PEFR) is measured initially and at intervals during therapy. A PEFR less than 100 L per minute indicates severe airway obstruction. Arterial blood gas (ABG) analysis often shows respiratory alkalosis initially and respiratory acidosis as muscle fatigue and respiratory failure ensue. Sputum examination, chest radiography, electrocardiography (ECG), and theophylline levels are sometimes helpful in ruling out underlying disease, but are seldom diagnostic of asthma itself. Eosinophilia on complete blood count (CBC) supports the diagnosis and indicates an allergic response.

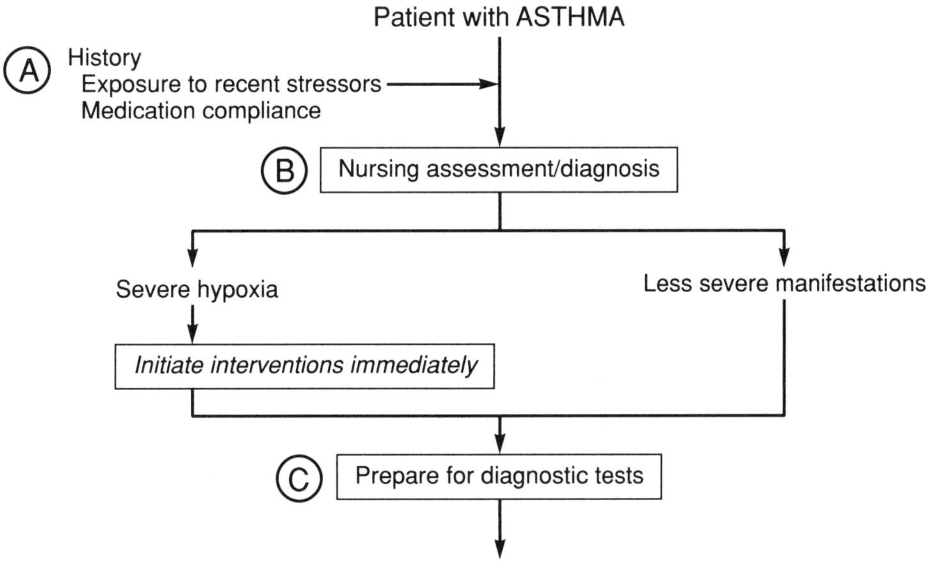

(Cont'd on p 103)

D. Patients with acute, severe asthma should be given supplemental oxygen 3 L per minute per nasal cannula.

E. Epinephrine 0.3 ml (terbutaline 0.25 mg in elderly or cardiac patients) is given subcutaneously. Inhaled sympathomimetic drugs such as isoproterenol, metaproterenol, or isoetharine 0.3 ml in 2.5 ml of normal saline are also used. If the patient fails to respond, intravenous aminophylline is given in doses related to the amount of theophylline already part of the patient's ongoing regimen, usually a maintenance of 0.7 mg per kilogram per hour.

F. If the patient does not respond satisfactorily to parenteral or inhaled bronchodilators, intravenous corticosteroids such as hypocortisone or methylprednisolone are given.

G. Patients subject to infrequent attacks may use bronchodilators such as albuterol, metaproterenol, isoetharine, isoproterenol, terbutaline, or epinephrine by metered-dose inhaler. Long-acting oral theophylline preparations may be used if inhaled bronchodilators alone are unsuccessful. Oral corticosteroids are added when other measures fail to relieve symptoms. Chronic maintenance therapy with oral corticosteroids is seldom necessary, and initial oral therapy may be eliminated or substantially reduced with inhaled corticosteroids such as beclomethasone or triamcinolone.

H. Nursing measures, such as assisting the patient to maintain positioning for optimal gas exchange (sitting straight up leaning forward on an overbed table), instructing the patient in pulmonary hygiene routines, helping the patient to space activities between rest periods, and reducing or eliminating dust factors and other irritants, can also relieve respiratory distress.

I. Anxiety and apprehension resulting from poor oxygen exchange and fear contribute to further exacerbation of hypoxia. The nurse can reduce this anxiety by confident and calm bedside behavior, ensuring a quiet and restful environment, allowing adequate time for the patient to express himself, involving the family in care as appropriate, and encouraging the patient and family to verbalize questions and concerns.

J. Fluid therapy is aimed at liquefying secretions for ease of removal. Within the limits of cardiac reserve, up to 4 L daily of fluids should be provided intravenously and/or orally. Careful monitoring of intake and output is essential, with cautious observation and reporting of symptoms of overhydration and cardiac failure.

K. Patient and family teaching are important prior to discharge.

References

Berkow R, ed. The Merck manual of diagnosis and therapy. 14th ed. Rahway, NJ: Merck, Sharp, & Dohme Laboratories, 1982.

Brunner LS, Suddarth DS, eds. The Lippincott manual of nursing practice. 4th ed. Philadelphia: Lippincott, 1986.

Krupp MA, Chatton MJ, Tierney LM, eds. Current diagnosis and treatment. Los Altos, CA: Lange, 1986.

Thompson JM, MacFarland GK, Hirsch JE, Tucker SM, Bowers AC, eds. Clinical nursing. St. Louis: CV Mosby, 1986.

(Cont'd from p 101)

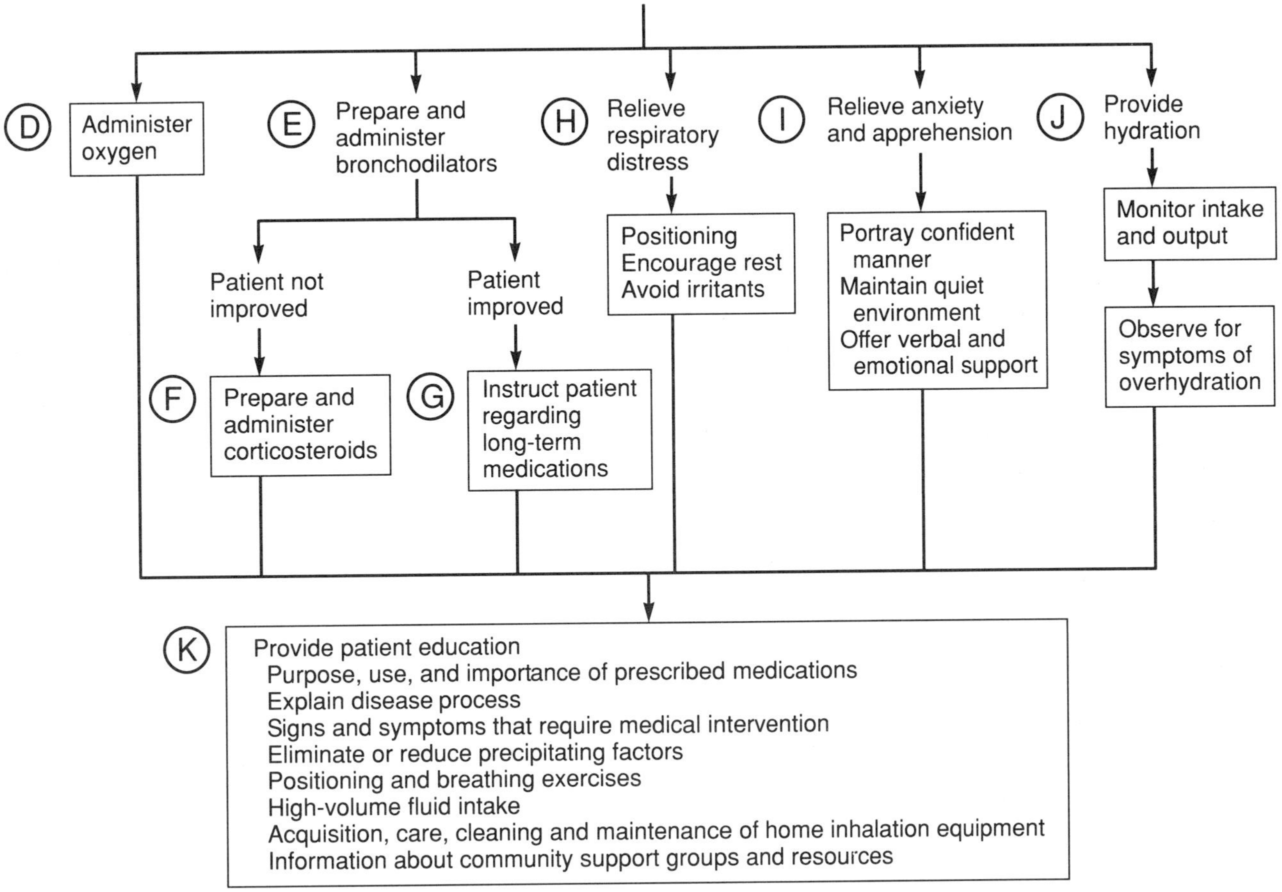

PNEUMONIA

Joy Gorzeman
Nina McIntosh

Pneumonia is an acute infection that causes inflammation of the lung and consolidation of lung tissue (see Fig. 1). It is the most common cause of death from an infectious disease in the United States, especially among the elderly. Legionnaires' disease is an acute form of pneumonia with a patchy pulmonary infiltrate and consolidation, high fever, malaise, headache, nonproductive cough, and a high risk of respiratory failure and death.

A. Symptoms often begin suddenly and include high fever, chills, and cough. The patient may experience "stabbing" chest pain, dyspnea, tachycardia, perspiration, and occasionally gastrointestinal upset. Nursing assessment should include onset and duration of symptoms, self-treatments the patient has used, exposure to persons with infections or to chemical irritants, and a health history. Several conditions predispose to pneumonia, including chronic illness and debility, cancer, thoracic surgery (p 126), and upper respiratory infection. Vital signs should be monitored and a pulmonary examination performed. Respiratory grunting, restricted chest movement, dullness on percussion, and rales all indicate pneumonia.

B. There are several types of pneumonias, caused by different agents. Most pneumonias are caused by an infection and are communicable. Other causes include chemical irritants and aspiration. Early diagnosis and vigorous therapy help to decrease mortality related to pneumonia. *Before* beginning antibiotic therapy, a sterile sputum specimen must be obtained. A Gram stain and culture are done to determine the causative organism. Rusty-color sputum usually indicates bacterial pneumonia. Blood specimens are drawn for culture and white cell count. Blood gases may be measured to assess respiratory status. Chest films are made to check infiltration. In Legionnaires' disease the chest radiograph shows a patchy pattern of pneumonia and small pleural effusions.

C. Overall care for most types of pneumonia is the same. However, it is important that the appropriate medication be ordered, based on the causative agent. Bacterial pneumonias almost always respond to specific antibiotic therapy. Viral pneumonias, however, are not usually treated with antibiotics. Mortality from aspiration pneumonia is high, even with optimal treatment. *The key to overcoming aspiration pneumonia is prevention.*

D. If the pneumonia is bacterial, antibiotics must be administered on schedule to maintain the necessary blood level of medication. Since a penicillin is often the drug of choice, it is important to note any allergies and observe the patient for an allergic reaction.

E. Other facets of care include rest, increased fluid intake (if not contraindicated for other health reasons), coughing and deep breathing (intermittent positive pressure breathing treatments may be ordered), pain relief, ongoing assessment, and observation for complications. Cough may be controlled with codeine if it is nonproductive or causes hypoxemia, but a productive cough should not be suppressed. Universal isolation precautions should be observed to avoid spread of infection.

F. Potential complications include pleurisy and pleural effusion (p 106) atelectasis (p 108), hypoxemia, lung abscess, meningitis (p 32), and pulmonary edema p 114). Complications from Legionnaires' disease include renal failure (p 314), bacteremic shock (p 70) and respiratory failure resulting in death in 15 percent of patients. Physical indications such as high fever, pain, dyspnea, or any unusual behavior or alteration in mental status may be due to cerebral hypoxia and should be reported to the physician immediately.

G. If no complications develop, patient teaching should include advising the patient that fatigue and weakness may linger for several weeks after pneumonia and that adequate rest is important. The patient should continue breathing exercises to expand the lungs. Patients who smoke should be encouraged to stop smoking. It is important to maintain good nutrition to promote resistance to infections.

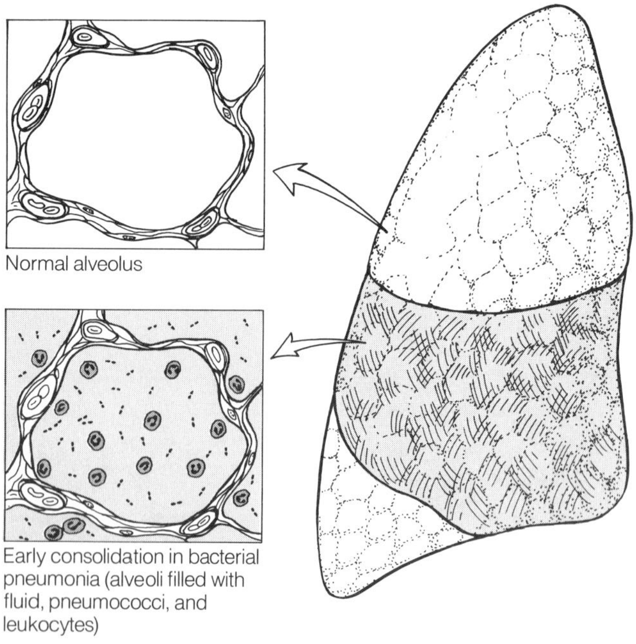

Figure 1 Pneumonia

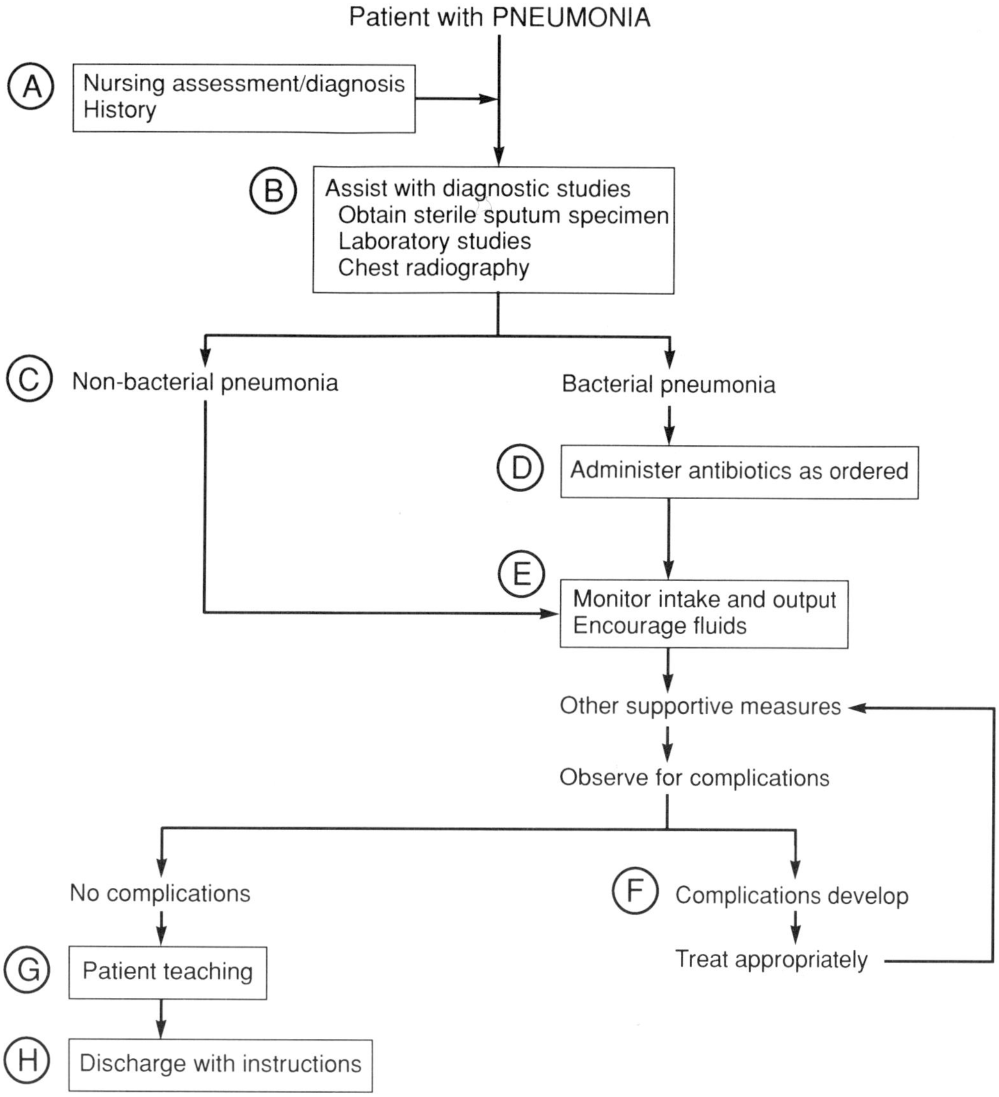

H. The patient must return for a chest film 2 to 4 weeks after discharge; this film should show clear lungs. Individuals at risk (those who are age 55 and older, or have chronic heart or pulmonary disease, diabetes, or metabolic disorders) should discuss with a physician the need for influenza vaccination to prevent infection.

References

Brunner LS, Suddarth DS. The Lippincott manual of nursing practice. 4th ed. Philadelphia: JB Lippincott, 1986.

Luckmann J, Sorensen KC. Medical-surgical nursing: a psychophysiologic approach. 3rd ed. Philadelphia: WB Saunders, 1987.

Phipps WJ, Long BC, Woods NF, eds. Medical-surgical nursing: concepts and clinical practice. 3rd ed. St. Louis: CV Mosby, 1987.

Thompson JM, McFarland GK, Hirsch JE, Tucker SM, Bowers AC. Clinical nursing. St Louis: CV Mosby, 1986.

US Department of Health and Human Services. Recommendations for prevention of HIV transmission in health-care settings. MMWR August 21, 1987; 36 (2S): TU–183.

PLEURISY AND PLEURAL EFFUSION

Mary K. Roberts

Pleurisy is an inflammation of part or all of the visceral and parietal pleura. It usually occurs as a complication of another disease process or traumatic event. Pleural effusion is an excess of fluid in the pleural space.

A. The patient's medical history is important. A history of pulmonary disease or chest trauma could potentiate the development of pleurisy. The patient usually complains of sharp, stabbing pain that increases with inspiration but dissipates when the breath is held. Pain may also radiate to the shoulder or abdomen, with tenderness in the intercostal areas. The nursing assessment should include vital signs, with a focus on respiratory status, noting the rate per minute, pattern, and depth. The patient may also have an increased heart rate and blood pressure secondary to dyspnea. Thoroughly assess the respiratory system. Decreased movement of the chest on the affected side may be observed. Auscultation of breath sounds may reveal decreased breath sounds with a pleural friction rub, caused by the visceral and parietal pleura rubbing together, which may vary from intermittent crackling to a very harsh, grating sound.

B. Administer analgesics to relieve the patient's pain and encourage the patient to take deep breaths and cough. The nurse should know dosage, frequency, and side effects of any analgesics administered in order to prevent overmedication, respiratory depression, and ineffective coughing.

C. The patient should be encouraged to cough frequently and breathe deeply. Teach the patient to splint with a pillow (pressed against affected area) or to lie on the affected side to splint the chest wall; these techniques help to minimize the pain when doing deep breathing and coughing exercises. Applying heat or cold to the areas that are tender may provide symptomatic relief. A restful environment and reassurance should be provided to decrease anxiety and relieve dyspnea.

D. Chest radiography is done to diagnose or rule out pleural effusion and is repeated if symptoms worsen. Radiopaque fluid is seen in dependent regions if pleural effusion has developed.

E. The onset of pleural effusion can be sudden or insidious. Symptoms depend on the underlying pathology. Frequent assessment is essential to identify possible pleural effusion. Assessment should be focused on worsening of symptoms or changes in physical findings since the previous assessment. The most notable sign may be worsening dyspnea. The affected side may have no movement during breathing; absent breath sounds; flat percussion, signifying fluid occupying the space; and a dry cough.

F. Thoracentesis distinguishes different types of pleural effusion, helps pinpoint the underlying disorder, and relieves respiratory distress by removing the space-occupying fluid. Explain that a local anesthetic will be used and that the patient will feel pressure when the needle is inserted. Observe the patient for great discomfort during the procedure and increased difficulty with breathing. Take vital signs to assess for decreased pulse or for hypotension, which may indicate fluid was removed too quickly (hypovolemic shock).

G. A chest film may be performed after thoracentesis to be sure that pneumothorax (p 110) has not developed and to evaluate the effectiveness of the therapy.

H. Arterial blood gases verify the patient's oxygenation status and assist in evaluating the patient's respiratory status and need for supplemental oxygen.

I. If the breath sounds are clear and recovery proceeds without further complications, the patient is discharged with instructions related to activity restrictions and medications ordered.

J. When the underlying cause of pleural effusion is a chronic disease, such as cancer, the effectiveness of thoracentesis is temporary, and the procedure may need to be repeated since fluid will begin to accumulate in the lungs again.

References

Armstrong ME, ed. McGraw-Hill handbook of clinical nursing. New York: McGraw-Hill, 1979.

Brunner LS, Suddarth DS. The Lippincott manual of nursing practice. 4th ed. Philadelphia: JB Lippincott, 1986.

Ford RD, Kangilaski R, eds. Diseases and disorders handbook. Springhouse, PA: Springhouse Corporation, 1988.

Hamilton HK, ed. Diseases. 2nd ed. Springhouse, PA: Springhouse Corporation, 1987:473–475.

Luckmann J, Sorensen KC. Medical-surgical nursing. 3rd ed. Philadelphia: WB Saunders, 1987.

Thompson J, McFarland G, Hirsch J, Tucker S, Bower A. Clinical nursing. St Louis: CV Mosby, 1986.

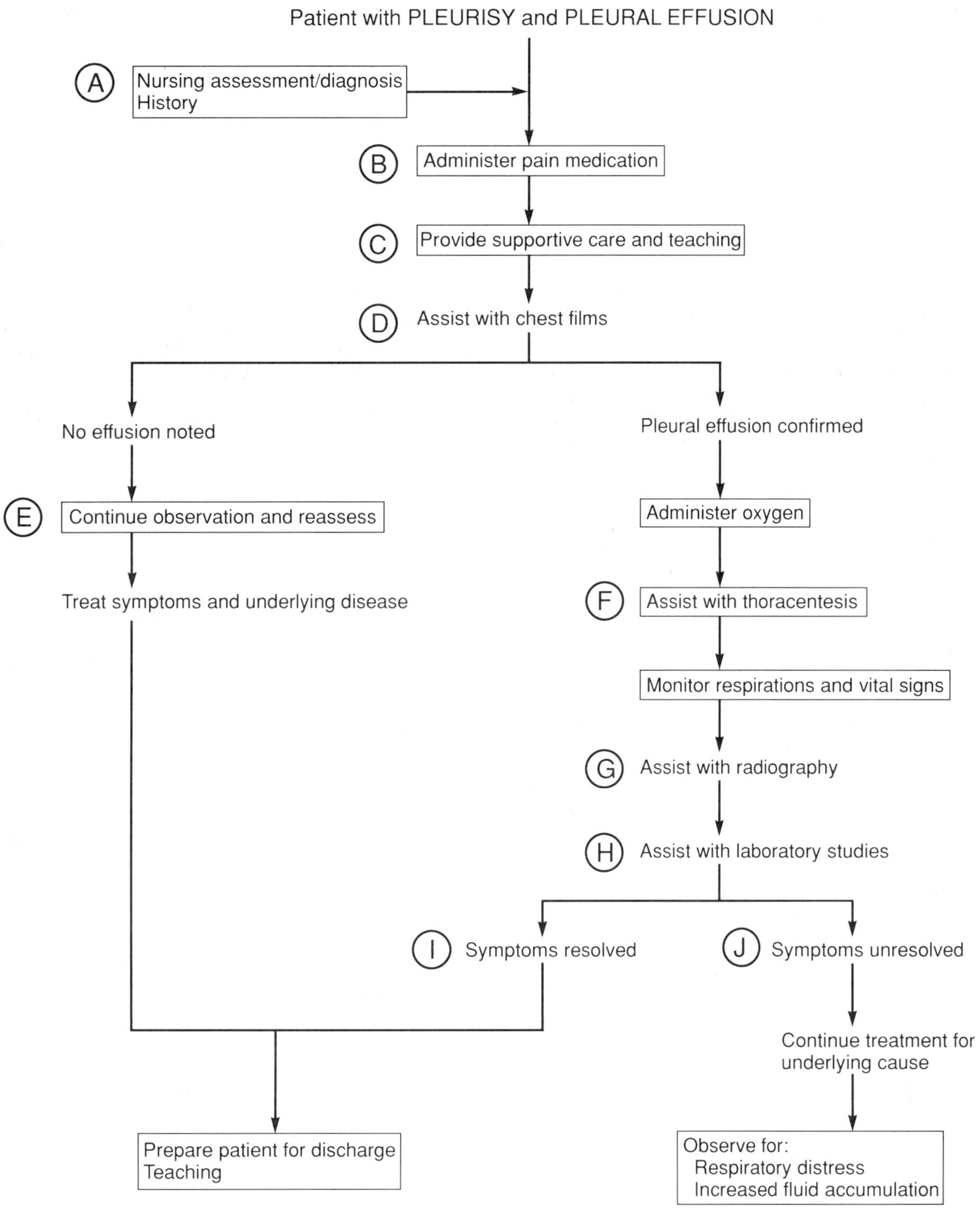
Patient with PLEURISY and PLEURAL EFFUSION
A
Nursing assessment/diagnosis
History
B
Administer pain medication
C
Provide supportive care and teaching
D
Assist with chest films
No effusion noted
E
Continue observation and reassess
Treat symptoms and underlying disease
Pleural effusion confirmed
Administer oxygen
F
Assist with thoracentesis
Monitor respirations and vital signs
G
Assist with radiography
H
Assist with laboratory studies
I
Symptoms resolved
J
Symptoms unresolved
Continue treatment for underlying cause
Prepare patient for discharge
Teaching
Observe for:
Respiratory distress
Increased fluid accumulation

ATELECTASIS

Mary K. Roberts

Atelectasis, or collapsed lung tissue, is not a clinical diagnosis but usually occurs in association with other medical or surgical problems. With atelectasis, there is a loss of area in the lung for gas exchange and the blood passing by these areas remains unoxygenated, thereby producing hypoxia.

A. Patient history is a key factor in identifying patients at risk for atelectasis. Any condition that prohibits full lung expansion or makes deep breathing painful predisposes to atelectasis. Other risk factors include increased respiratory secretions, dry sticky secretions, depression of the respiratory center, and prolonged immobility.

B. Atelectasis may occur suddenly and cause extensive blockages, or it may occur slowly and cause only minor problems. Assessment of vital signs may indicate an increase in temperature, heart rate, blood pressure, and respirations. Auscultation of lung fields reveals decreased breath sounds where the portion of lung is collapsed. Other clinical findings might include dyspnea, anxiety, cyanosis, and diaphoresis.

C. If atelectasis is suspected, draw blood for measurement of arterial blood gases. Expect a decreased PaO_2, indicating that the patient is hypoxemic. Sputum may also be cultured if the patient has a spiking temperature without an identified source of infection. The definitive diagnosis is made by chest radiography.

D. Nursing measures are based on the etiology and the precipitating causes of atelectasis. Etiologies may include chronic obstructive pulmonary disease, bronchiectasis, cystic fibrosis, heavy smoking, and inflammatory disorders (e.g., pneumonia (p 104), pulmonary edema (p 114), inflammatory lung disease, bronchogenic carcinoma). Precipitating factors include external compression of the thorax (obesity or tight dressings around the chest), pain from upper abdominal or thoracic surgical incisions, prolonged immobility from any disease or injury, or central nervous system depression (e.g., drug overdose).

E. If an etiology or precipitating cause cannot be identified, bronchoscopy may be performed to rule out an obstructing neoplasm or foreign body.

F. Patient teaching is crucial to prevent worsening of atelectasis and promote reexpansion of the collapsed lung tissue. Coughing and deep breathing are key components in the treatment. The importance of deep breathing to ventilate the lungs fully, followed by coughing to remove any loosened secretions, needs to be emphasized and clearly demonstrated. The technique of splinting to minimize pain in postoperative patients should also be taught. Evaluate each patient's performance of these techniques and repeat instructions as necessary.

G. Activity further stimulates deep breathing and ventilation of the alveoli and should be encouraged within prescribed limits. Adequate fluid intake further mobilizes secretions and should be encouraged.

H. Respiratory treatments may include incentive spirometry, chest percussion, and postural drainage. Incentive spirometry encourages deep inspiration through a device that presents a visual quantitation of the patient's effort. This provides the patient with a goal and with positive reinforcement to repeat a maximal effort frequently. Chest percussion loosens secretions from the airway walls so that the patient can cough them out easily. It is done by clapping with a cupped hand over areas of the lungs that are being drained, ideally with the patient's head down at a slight angle. Postural drainage requires that the patient assume various positions to facilitate flow of secretions from specific pulmonary lobes and segments.

I. Treatment is the same for the patient who is unable to cooperate, but the nurse takes a more active role in implementation. If the patient cannot be active or produce an effective cough, the nurse should reposition the patient frequently. Bronchodilators may be ordered by the physician to improve mucociliary clearance and dilate the airways. Suctioning to help remove secretions is necessary if the patient does not cough effectively. If antibiotics are ordered, the nurse should know the purpose, correct dosage, frequency, and the side effects.

J. Reassess breath sounds and ventilatory status frequently and note changes. Chest radiography confirms that atelectasis is resolved.

References

Armstrong ME, ed. McGraw-Hill handbook of clinical nursing. New York: McGraw-Hill, 1979.

Ford RD, Kangilaski R, ed. Diseases and disorders handbook. Springhouse, PA: Springhouse Corporation, 1988.

Hamilton HK, ed. Diseases. 2nd ed. Springhouse, PA: Springhouse Corporation, 1987:473–475.

Phipps WJ, Long BC, Woods NF, eds. Medical-surgical nursing: concepts and clinical practice. St. Louis: CV Mosby, 1987.

Shapiro BA, Harrison RA, Trout CA. Clinical application of respiratory care. 2nd ed. Chicago: Year Book, 1979:202–205.

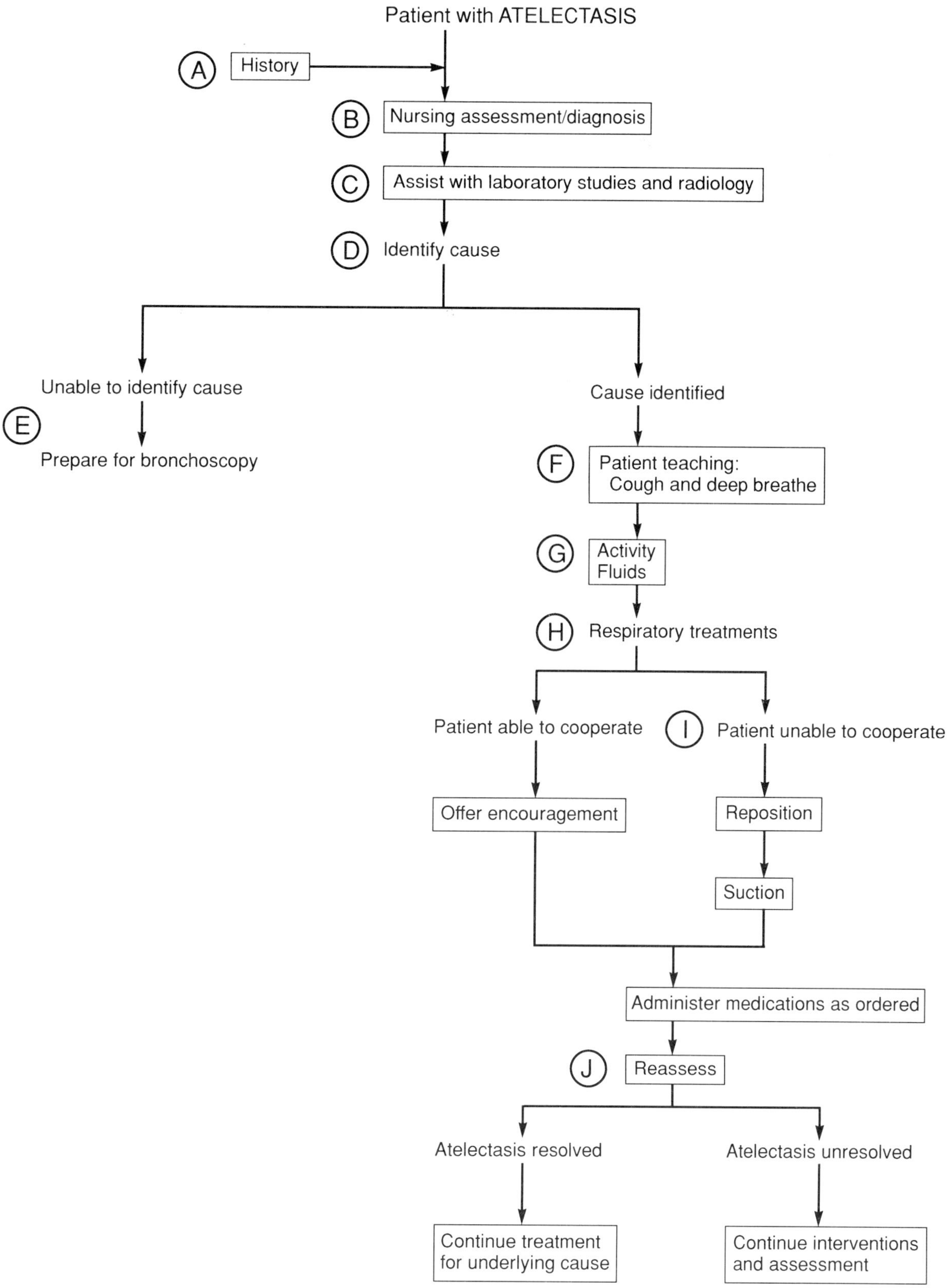
Patient with ATELECTASIS
A
History
B
Nursing assessment/diagnosis
C
Assist with laboratory studies and radiology
D
Identify cause
Unable to identify cause
E
Prepare for bronchoscopy
Cause identified
F
Patient teaching:
Cough and deep breathe
G
Activity
Fluids
H
Respiratory treatments
Patient able to cooperate
I
Patient unable to cooperate
Offer encouragement
Reposition
Suction
Administer medications as ordered
J
Reassess
Atelectasis resolved
Atelectasis unresolved
Continue treatment
for underlying cause
Continue interventions
and assessment

PNEUMOTHORAX AND HEMOTHORAX

Nancy A. Young
Joy Gorzeman

A pneumothorax (Fig. 1) occurs when air escapes from the lung into the pleural cavity, whereas a hemothorax (Fig. 2) results from a collection of blood in the chest due to laceration of the lung or torn intercostal vessels. These insults, whether spontaneous or inflicted, interrupt normal lung function; the severity depends on the amount of bleeding or the cause of air loss. An open pneumothorax involves a hole large enough for air to pass freely in and out of the thoracic cavity with respirations. A tension pneumothorax (Fig. 3), on the other hand, occurs when air is drawn into the pleural space through a lacerated lung or a hole in the chest wall. Since this air cannot escape, pressure continues to accumulate, causing progressive collapse of the lung tissue and possible shifting of the mediastinum (Fig. 4).

A. A thorough history facilitates a definitive diagnosis. Conditions that place individuals at risk for a pneumo- or hemothorax include chest trauma; pneumonia (p 104); degenerative lung diseases such as emphysema (p 98) or bronchitis; airway obstruction; thoracentesis or pericardial tap; central line placement; or positive pressure ventilation. Patients may display symptoms of chest pain on the affected side, dyspnea, confusion and anxiety, or restlessness and fatigue. Clinical indicators reveal changes in chest films, dyspneic breath sounds, asymmetric chest expansion, a decrease in the blood PaO_2, and other signs of respiratory distress such as nasal flaring, cyanosis, or retractions.

B. Even healthy adults can experience a spontaneous closed pneumothorax due to the rupture of pulmonary blebs. The extent of dyspnea depends largely on the extent of lung collapse and the existence of preexisting lung disease.

C. Management of these patients varies from observation for those who remain asymptomatic to needle aspiration (thoracentesis) or chest tube placement.

D. Thoracentesis is the procedure for aspirating fluid or air from the pleural space. Preparation for the procedure includes gathering the equipment, displaying chest films at the bedside, ensuring signed consent, explaining the procedure to the patient, inquiring about the patient's allergy to local anesthetic, and administering sedatives if ordered.

E. During the procedure, the nurse assists the patient with positioning and offers support. The patient should be discouraged from coughing and should be prepared for cold sensations during the preparation and a stinging sensation and pressure while the anesthetic is injected. Document the amount of fluid withdrawn and a description of the fluid (color and viscosity).

F. After the fluid is removed, pressure is applied to the site and a small dressing put in place. The patient is placed on bedrest. Vital signs are checked and recorded every 15 minutes for the first hour. Patients are evaluated periodically for dizziness, tightness in the chest, increased respiration, tachycardia, and signs of hypoxemia, which may indicate pneumothorax.

G. A chest tube is inserted (tube thoracostomy) to evacuate air, blood, or fluid collections. Again, equipment must be gathered, chest film obtained, drainage system assembled, and the procedure explained to the patient.

H. The nurse assists with positioning the patient during the procedure.

I. If water-seal drainage is used, the water should fluctuate in the tube with respiration. Drainage must be assessed for blood or air. Bubbling in the bottle may indicate an air leak. The fluid level should be marked on the outside of the bottle to indicate the amount of fluid loss. A follow-up chest film confirms tube placement and shows any reexpansion of the lung. The tube site should be observed for bleeding, redness, or leakage of air or fluid. The tubing must be kept patent. The nurse can assist in preventing a deterioration in the patient's condition by encouraging turning, coughing, and deep breathing, by suctioning the airway as needed, and by performing chest physiotherapy as ordered by the physician. Pain medication may be administered if needed.

J. A hemothorax may complicate an open pneumothorax that results from a penetrating trauma, particularly when the heart or arteries represent the source of bleeding.

K. Pleural blood should be evacuated and replaced promptly; however, drainage that exceeds 800 to 1,000 ml usually requires an immediate thoracotomy (p 126). This procedure is also indicated for patients who remain in shock after other vigorous resuscitative measures have been implemented.

L. *Tension pneumothorax represents a medical emergency that requires prompt intervention.* It interferes with venous return to the heart, leading to progressive hypoxemia and a falling cardiac output. The patient's physical signs generally change dramatically, to include diminished or absent breath sounds, hyperresonance over the involved area, and a tracheal shift away from the affected side. Immediate chest tube placement is indicated, preceded by needle aspiration for those with severe symptoms.

M. Chest tubes are usually removed in 24 to 72 hours when the lung is reexpanded. An airtight bandage with petroleum gauze is applied to prevent entrance of air.

N. Upon discharge, the patient should understand the importance of keeping follow-up appointments for tests to validate resolution of the pneumothorax and contacting the health care provider if symptoms recur or if new symptoms are experienced.

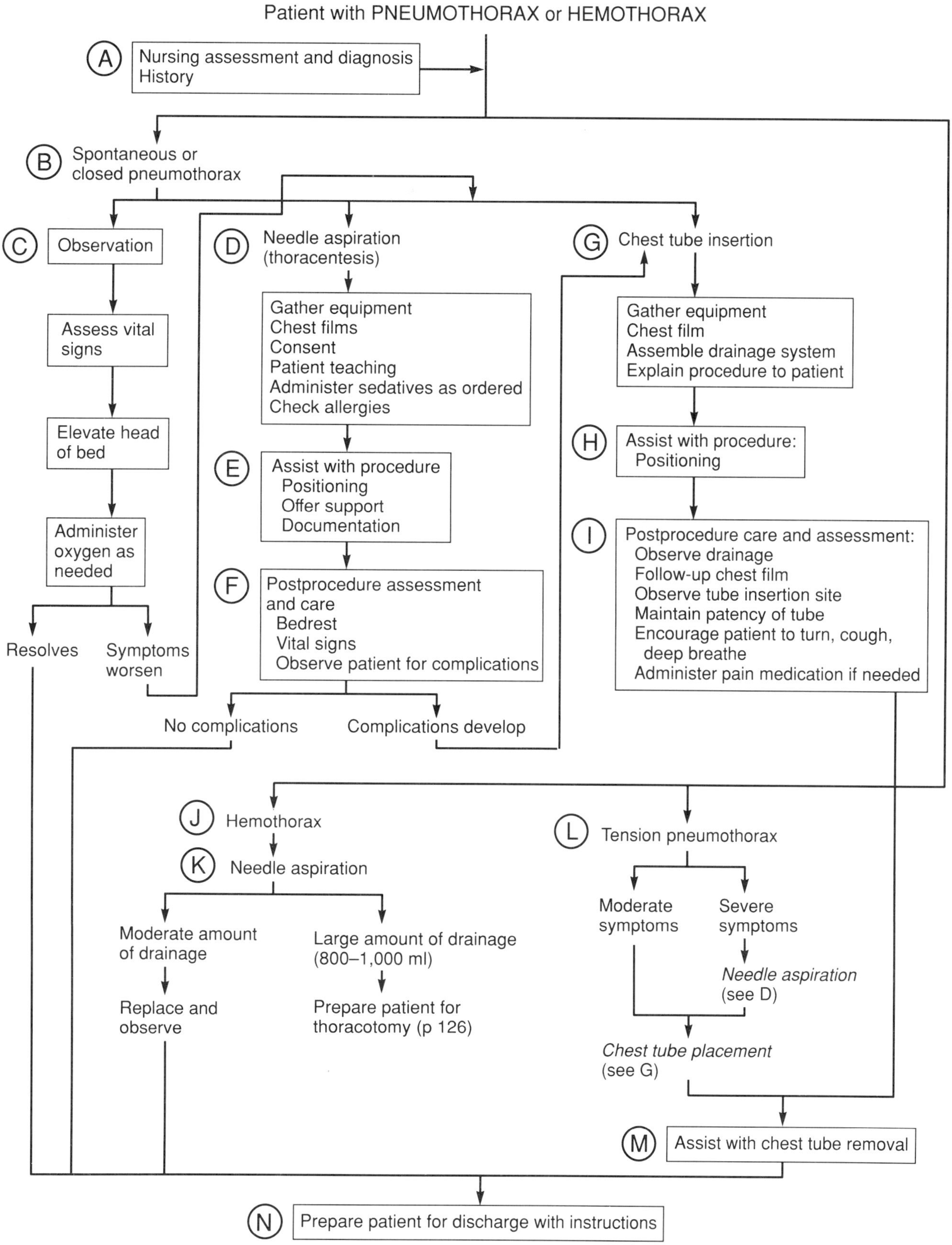
Patient with PNEUMOTHORAX or HEMOTHORAX
A
Nursing assessment and diagnosis
History
B
Spontaneous or closed pneumothorax
C
Observation
Assess vital signs
Elevate head of bed
Administer oxygen as needed
Resolves
Symptoms worsen
D
Needle aspiration (thoracentesis)
Gather equipment
Chest films
Consent
Patient teaching
Administer sedatives as ordered
Check allergies
E
Assist with procedure
Positioning
Offer support
Documentation
F
Postprocedure assessment and care
Bedrest
Vital signs
Observe patient for complications
No complications
Complications develop
G
Chest tube insertion
Gather equipment
Chest film
Assemble drainage system
Explain procedure to patient
H
Assist with procedure:
Positioning
I
Postprocedure care and assessment:
Observe drainage
Follow-up chest film
Observe tube insertion site
Maintain patency of tube
Encourage patient to turn, cough, deep breathe
Administer pain medication if needed
J
Hemothorax
K
Needle aspiration
Moderate amount of drainage
Replace and observe
Large amount of drainage (800–1,000 ml)
Prepare patient for thoracotomy (p 126)
L
Tension pneumothorax
Moderate symptoms
Severe symptoms
Needle aspiration (see D)
Chest tube placement (see G)
M
Assist with chest tube removal
N
Prepare patient for discharge with instructions

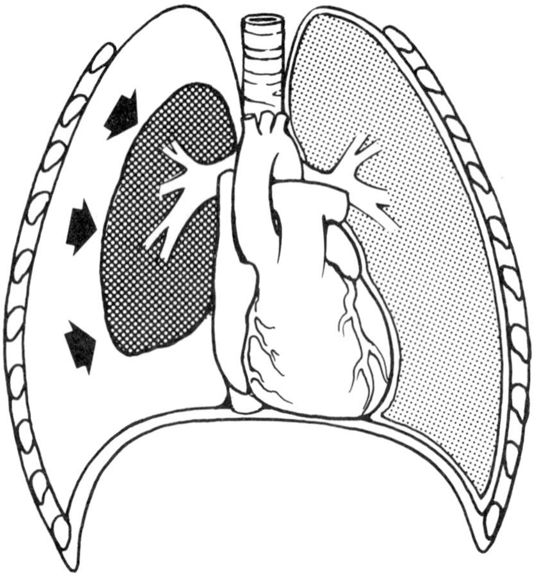

Figure 1 Pneumothorax

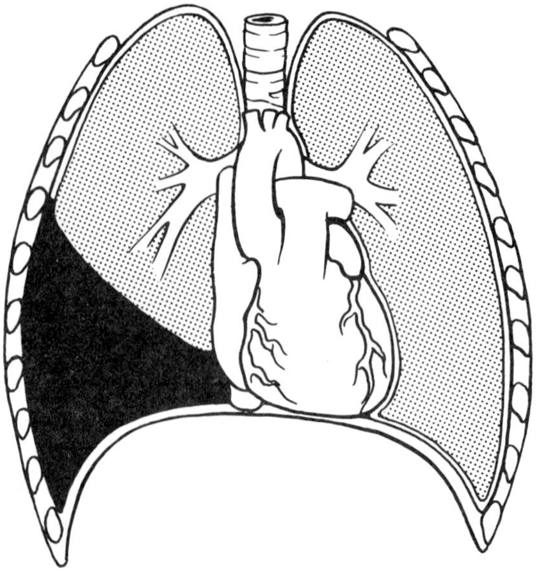

Figure 2 Hemothorax

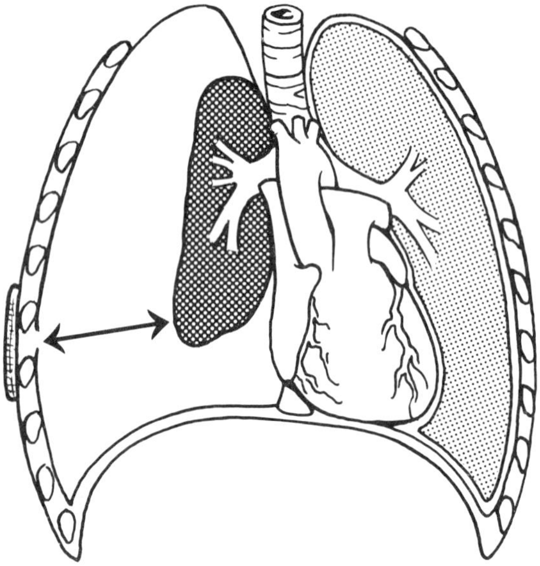

Figure 3 Tension pneumothorax

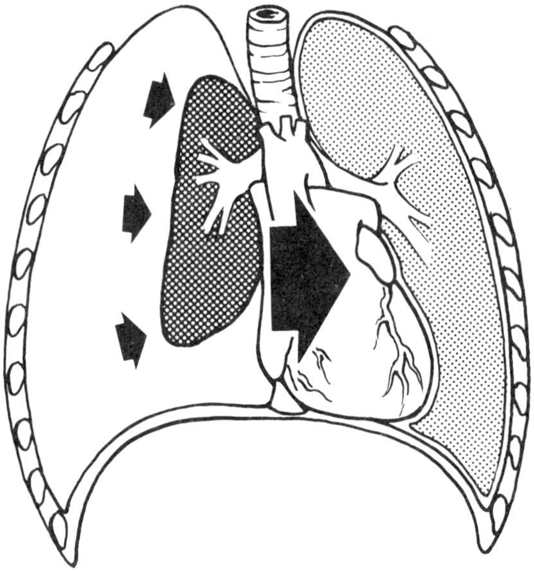

Figure 4 Mediastinal shift

References

Brunner LS, Suddarth DS. Textbook of medical-surgical nursing. Philadelphia: JB Lippincott, 1988.

Holloway NM. Nursing the critically ill adult. Menlo Park, CA: Addison-Wesley, 1988.

May H. Emergency medicine. New York: John Wiley & Sons, 1984.

PULMONARY EDEMA

Carla K. Calloway
Laura Luecke

Pulmonary edema is the accumulation of fluid in the extravascular spaces of the lung. When capillary pressure in the lungs becomes elevated, fluid pours from the blood into the alveoli, bronchi, and bronchioles (Fig. 1). Pulmonary edema may be acute or chronic. Acute pulmonary edema, *a medical emergency,* has an abrupt onset that can rapidly become fatal. The most common cause of pulmonary edema is left ventricular failure. Other causes include infusion of excessive intravenous fluids; narcotic overdose; and decreased serum colloid osmotic pressure as a result of nephrosis, protein-losing enteropathy, extensive burns, hepatic disease, or nutritional deficiency. Impaired lung lymphatic drainage from Hodgkin's disease (p 364), obliterative lymphangitis after radiation, mitral stenosis and left atrial myxoma, which impair left atrial emptying, and pulmonary veno-occlusive disease may also precipitate pulmonary edema.

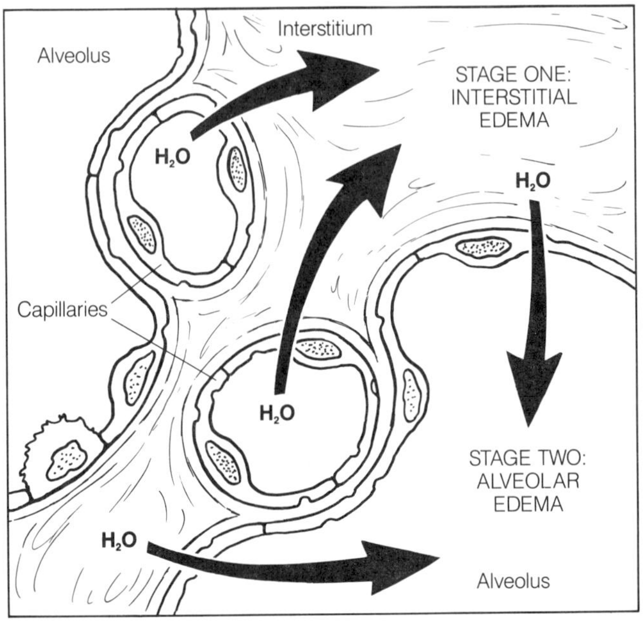

Figure 1 Stages of pulmonary edema.

A. When obtaining the history, attempt to determine the cause and severity of the acute episode. Often, the patient has a history of cardiac disease and may report previous episodes of pulmonary edema. Pulmonary edema is easier to prevent than treat; thus, early identification of symptoms is essential. Dyspnea on exertion, orthopnea, dry hacking cough, a third heart sound (S_3), and paroxysmal nocturnal dyspnea are early indications of pulmonary congestion.

B. Diagnostic tests and procedures assist in determining causative factors, severity, and progression. Obtain a chest film as soon as possible; diffuse haziness, cardiomegaly, and pleural effusion may be seen. Arterial blood gas determinations usually show hypoxia. The patient's P_{CO_2} (partial pressure of carbon dioxide) is variable. Both respiratory acidosis and alkalosis may occur. Other diagnostic studies include electrocardiography (ECG), which may show tachycardia, arrhythmias, hypertrophy, ischemia, and/or infarction; determination of serum electrolytes, creatinine, blood urea nitrogen; urinalysis; and complete blood count.

C. Pulmonary edema often occurs at night after the patient has been lying down. Breathlessness and a feeling of suffocation are early symptoms. Patients with severe pulmonary edema are extremely dyspneic, especially in the supine position, and may also cough up frothy, pink sputum. Wheezes and crackles are heard on auscultation. As the condition worsens, crackles progress from the bases to the apices of the lungs.

D. Oxygen is administered to relieve hypoxia and dyspnea. If significant hypotension does not occur, the patient should be placed in an upright sitting position with legs dangling. This position eases dyspnea and decreases venous return to the heart. Aminophylline is sometimes effective because of its action on bronchial smooth muscle. It reverses bronchospasm induced by hypoxia.

E. Shortness of breath and an impending sense of doom cause patients with acute pulmonary edema to become restless and extremely anxious. Hypoxia may also cause confusion or other signs of altered mental status. Remain with the patient and calmly explain all treatments.

F. Morphine sulfate is frequently used to treat patients with pulmonary edema. In addition to reducing anxiety, morphine causes peripheral venous dilatation, decreasing venous return to the heart. Hypotension caused by the peripheral vasodilatory effect of morphine is quickly remedied by lowering the patient's upper body and elevating the legs. Because morphine is a potent respiratory depressant, ventilation must be closely monitored.

G. In the patient with cardiogenic pulmonary edema, treatment focuses on decreasing the workload of the heart, improving myocardial function, improving gas exchange, and decreasing extravascular fluid. Digoxin or other agents may be given to increase the contractility of the heart and diuretics to decrease circulating volume. Phlebotomy and rotating tourniquets, now rarely ordered treatments, help by decreasing blood volume and pooling volume in the venous periphery.

H. Patients with fulminating pulmonary edema are transferred to the ICU.

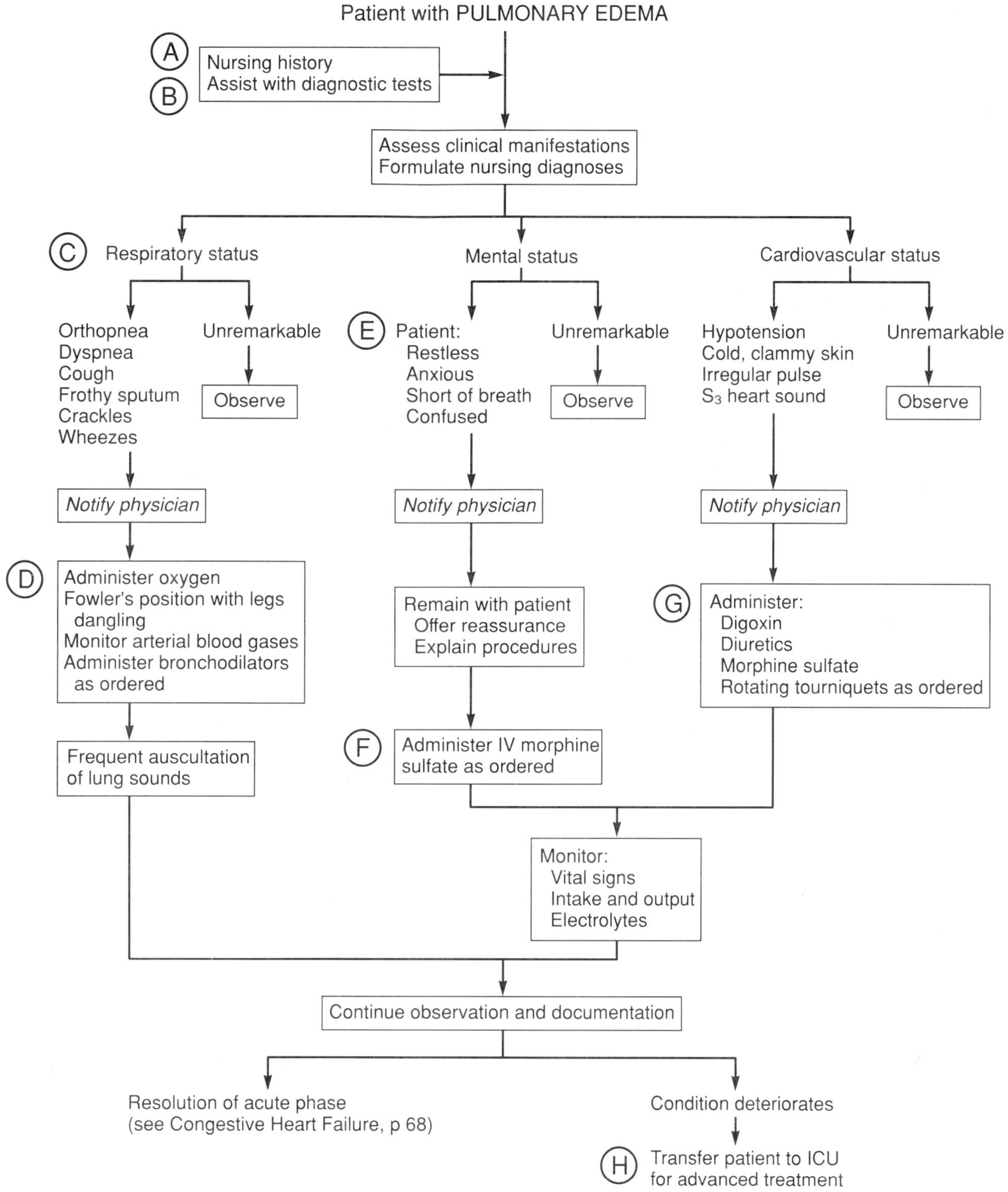

References

Eaton P. Action stat! Pulmonary edema. Nursing 1986; 16:25–26

Hamilton H, ed. Diseases. 2nd ed. Springhouse, PA: Springhouse Corporation, 1987:467–469.

Luckmann J, Sorensen KC. Medical-surgical nursing: a psychophysiologic approach. 2nd ed. Philadelphia: WB Saunders, 1980:810–811.

May HL. Emergency medicine. New York: John Wiley, 1984:84–87, 176.

Mills J, Ho MT, Salber PR, Trunkey DD. Current emergency diagnosis and treatment. 2nd ed. Los Altos, CA: Lange, 1985:55, 57, 59, 489.

PULMONARY EMBOLISM

Kendra Ellis

Pulmonary embolism (PE) is a complete or partial obstruction of one or both branches of the pulmonary artery or its subdivisions. The embolus results in ventilation-perfusion defect because of interruption of the blood flow to that area of the lung. An infarction occurs distal to the site of the PE that can result in sudden death. The embolus is usually a thrombus formed in the legs or pelvic area as a result of venous stasis, venous wall abnormality, and/or clotting abnormalities. Other causes include fat emboli, air emboli, catheter emboli, and septic thrombophlebitis.

A. The majority of patients who experience a PE exhibit classic signs and symptoms, which may be sudden or insidious. The patient is dyspneic and apprehensive and complains of pleuritic chest pain, described as a localized, stabbing sensation that increases with respirations. Substernal pain with apprehension and a sense of impending doom may occur when most of the pulmonary artery is obstructed. *This condition is a medical emergency and demands immediate nursing action.* Patients are tachycardic and tachypneic, with a decrease in blood pressure and engorgement of neck veins. Auscultation of the lung fields may reveal rales, a pleural friction rub, and an S_3 or S_4 heart sound. The patient's current history may include congestive heart failure; recent surgery, especially vascular surgery; impaired peripheral circulation; or trauma. A patient who is on complete bedrest is also at high risk for PE.

B. The diagnosis of PE can be difficult. Fifty percent of the time a chest film shows no abnormalities in a patient with PE; however, the chest film may show diminished vascular markings and increased density in the area of a PE. The only conclusive test is pulmonary angiography. This test is invasive and enables visualization of the pulmonary blood flow. Other tests include perfusion scans, ventilation scans, Doppler ultrasonography, and a fibrinogen uptake study.

C. A PE causes pulmonary hypertension, resulting in increased workload of the right ventricle and, thus decreased blood volume to the left side of the heart. The heart is unable to maintain its cardiac output owing to the decreased volume, with a final result of decreased systemic perfusion. The increased pulmonary vascular resistance causes dilatation of the right ventricle and eventually results in right-sided heart failure. This is evidenced by an increase in central venous pressure, jugular vein distention, and hepatomegaly. Heart sounds heard on auscultation include an accentuated S_2 and a split S_2, indicating resistance at the pulmonic valve. Cardiac complications of a PE include right-sided heart failure, cardiogenic shock, and myocardial ischemia.

D. A patient with a PE is tachypneic and has a nonproductive cough with rales on auscultation of the lung fields. Analysis of the arterial blood gas reveals respiratory alkalosis, caused by hyperventilation, and decreased PaO_2 (partial pressure of arterial oxygen). The embolus causes decreased P_AO_2 (partial pressure of alveolar oxygen) by increasing alveolar dead space—alveoli that are ventilated but not perfused. The lungs then shunt oxygen away from the unperfused area, resulting in hypoxia and vasoconstriction, which can cause an infarction distal to the embolus. Pulmonary infarction occurs in 20 percent of patients with PE. Other pulmonary complications include atelectasis, pulmonary hypertension, and respiratory arrest. When a patient develops sudden pleuritic chest pain, the first line of treatment is oxygen administration supplied with a face mask. If severe hypoxia ensues, intubation with mechanical ventilation may be required.

E. If the patient is unstable or the clot unresolved, surgery is the treatment of choice. A vena cava interruption can be performed to filter out emboli and prevent them from entering the pulmonary arteriole system. An embolectomy, which can be performed in severe cases, involves increased morbidity.

F. The most important preventive method is early and frequent ambulation. Other nursing measures include frequent position changes with range-of-motion exercise, elevation of legs, use of compression hose, and treatment with prophylactic anticoagulants.

G. The goal of treatment is to prevent extension of the clot and to lyse the present clot. This is accomplished with anticoagulants and fibrinolytic drugs. Anticoagulants like heparin and warfarin are used to stabilize the clot, prevent enlargement of the clot, and prevent occurrence of more emboli. Fibrinolytic therapy includes drugs like streptokinase and urokinase. They are used to lyse the clot and prevent pulmonary hypertension. The risk of anticoagulation therapy is hemorrhage.

H. If anticoagulant therapy is effective, the patient is discharged while on the medication. Patient teaching should include instruction to watch for signs of too much anticoagulation, such as bleeding gums and nosebleeds. The patient should be advised against taking any other medication without the physician's approval, especially those with aspirin products, and should avoid prolonged inactivity.

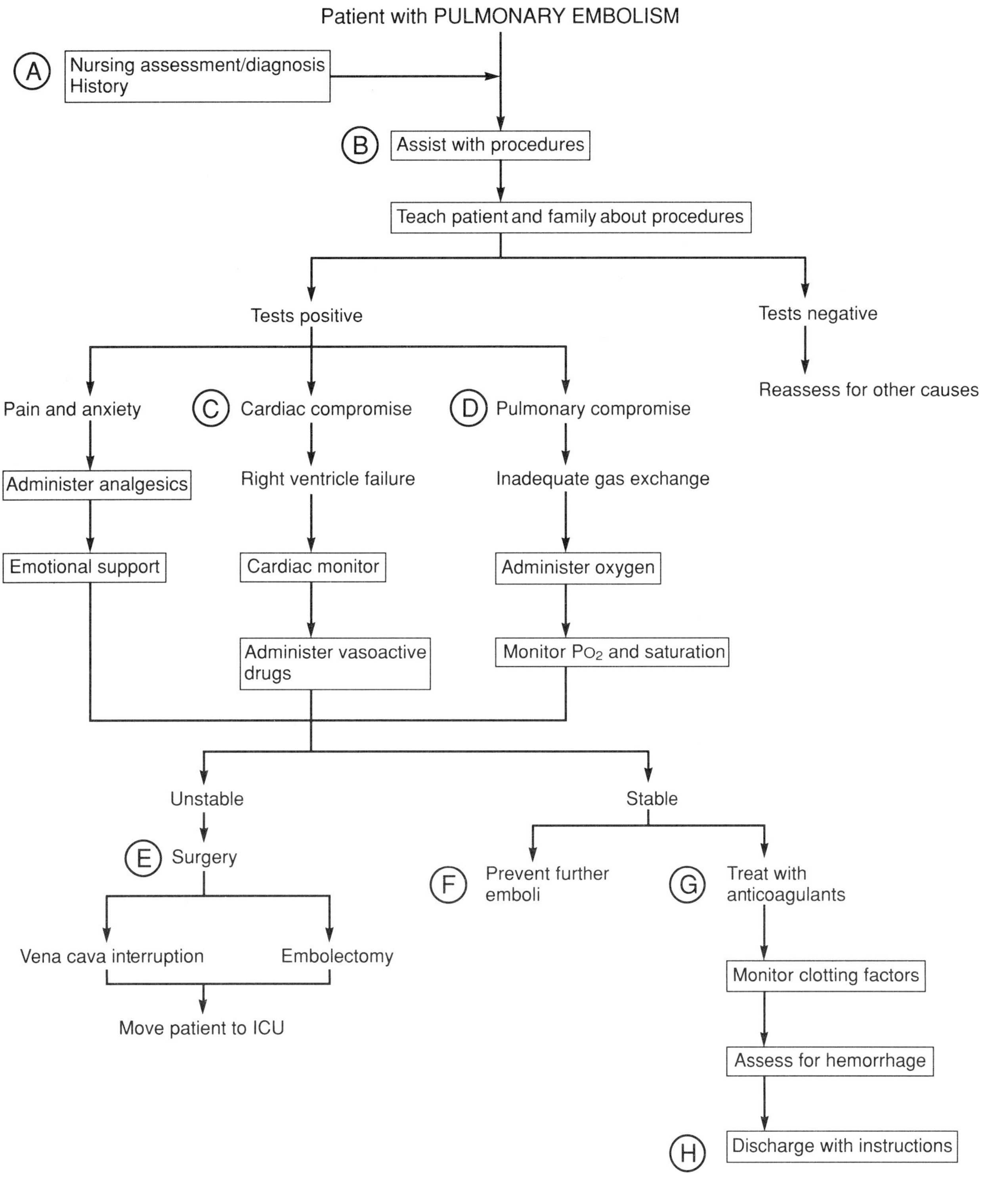

References

Carriere SR, Gulich LG, Schultz KA. Multiple systemic emboli. J Emerg Nurs 1985; 11(3):136–139.

Dossey B, Passons M. Pulmonary embolism: preventing, treating it. Nursing 81, 1981; 14(3):26–33.

Heuy R. Coping with pulmonary embolism. Nursing 81: Nursing Life Booklet. Springhouse, PA: Springhouse Corporation, 1981.

Woodruff M. Pulmonary thromboembolism: risk factors, pathophysiology, and management. Crit Care Nurs, 1984; 4(5):52–63.

INFLUENZA

Nina McIntosh

Influenza is an acute, contagious respiratory disease characterized by sudden onset of headache, fever, and prostration. Hospitalization is not usually required, however influenza reaches epidemic to pandemic proportions and is responsible for thousands of deaths each year, especially among the elderly.

A. Influenza is spread by direct or indirect airborne droplets. The client typically complains of respiratory tract involvement, with symptoms of cough (often productive), sore throat, headache, high fever, chest pain, malaise, apathy, myalgia, anorexia, nausea and vomiting, and prostration. Important factors in making a diagnosis are the patient's history, clinical findings, and knowledge of the current prevalent virus.

B. Influenza is caused by respiratory viruses called influenza types A, B, and C. The virus can sometimes be recovered from nasopharyngeal specimens. In uncomplicated cases, lymphocytopenia and an elevated or normal erythrocyte sedimentation rate may be present.

C. Viral pneumonia (p 104) is one of the main complications of influenza. Persons who have chronic rheumatic heart disease with mitral stenosis are particularly predisposed. Bacterial pneumonia (p 104) most often affects persons with preexisting pulmonary disease, pregnant women, and the elderly. Other groups at risk for developing complications of influenza are infants and patients on immunosuppressive drugs.

D. The primary goals of treatment are supportive measures directed toward symptomatic relief. The patient should be isolated, since influenza is most contagious in the first 3 days and lasts 1 week to 10 days. Encourage frequent intake of fluids to prevent dehydration from the fever and upper respiratory tract secretions. Cough syrup with glycerol guaiacolate may be given for dry hacking coughs. A vaporizer may help reduce irritation to the respiratory mucosa. Aspirin or acetaminophen helps relieve fever and promotes comfort. Encourage bedrest and reduction of physical activity.

E. Advise use of a humidifier in the home; encourage the patient to stop smoking and avoid crowds and exposure to groups; high-risk individuals should be encouraged to have an annual vaccination.

References

Hutchinson R. The common cold primer. Nursing 1979; 9(3):57–61.

Lewis SM, Collier IC. Medical-surgical nursing: assessment and management of clinical problems. New York: McGraw-Hill, 1983.

Rytel MW. Influenza and its complications: recognition and prevention. Hosp Pract 1987; 22:102A–102D.

Thompson JM, McFarland GK, Hirsch JE, Tucker SM, Bowers AC. Clinical nursing. St. Louis: CV Mosby, 1986.

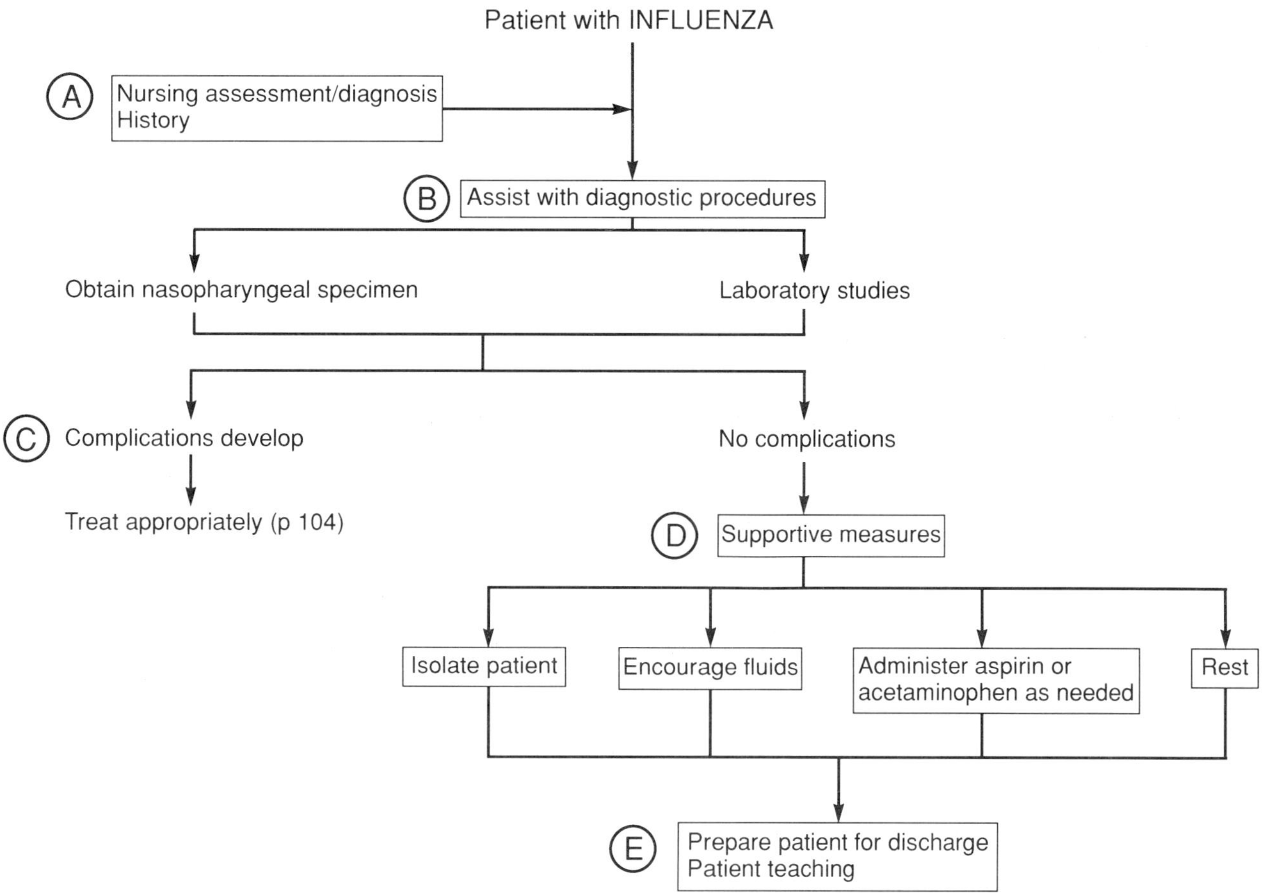
Patient with INFLUENZA
A
Nursing assessment/diagnosis
History
B
Assist with diagnostic procedures
Obtain nasopharyngeal specimen
Laboratory studies
C
Complications develop
Treat appropriately (p 104)
No complications
D
Supportive measures
Isolate patient
Encourage fluids
Administer aspirin or acetaminophen as needed
Rest
E
Prepare patient for discharge
Patient teaching

TUBERCULOSIS

Michele Konnick

Tuberculosis (TB), an infectious communicable disease caused by the tubercle bacillus, is carried on airborne droplets and inhaled by a susceptible person. It is predominantly a pulmonary disease but can also be extrapulmonary, since the bacilli can travel through the lymphatic and blood stream to any other organ of the body. Transmission usually depends on close, frequent, and prolonged exposure to the bacilli. Recent studies have shown a strong comeback of this disease, even though it has been curable since the early 1950s.

A. Prior or current contact with the tubercle bacilli should be determined. The chance of acquiring TB is less with casual contact. Individuals at higher risk for contracting the disease include alcoholics, drug users, prisoners, immunosuppressed patients, and health-care workers.

B. The most common symptoms are cough, blood-streaked sputum, fever, night sweats, weight loss, fatigue, pain, and sometimes swollen glands. Since most of these signs and symptoms can be applied to many other diseases, it is important to obtain a complete patient history. Patients may be placed in respiratory isolation until the diagnosis is confirmed.

C. TB tine tests are only used as a screening tool. The intracutaneous Mantoux test, using five tuberculin units of the antigen PPD (purified protein derivative, 0.1 ml) is the *only* acceptable diagnostic aid to detect TB infections. The test is usually given on the dorsal surface of the forearm. A wheal 6 to 10 mm in diameter must be produced or the test is invalid. Readings for hypersensitivity are done within 48 to 72 hours. An induration 10 mm or greater is considered significant and further testing is done. The tester must also be aware that false-negative reactions can occur because of improper handling of the antigen, not obtaining a "wheal," and such medical conditions as Hodgkin's disease, renal disease, or prolonged usage of steroids.

D. Chest films are suspicious for tuberculosis if any of the following exist: pulmonary infiltrates, lesions, infusions, enlarged hilar lymph nodes, parenchymal infiltrates, or cavitations.

E. The acid-base bacilli culture and smear remains the test of choice for screening the sputum for tuberculosis. Proper collection and handling of the specimen from deep in the lungs (not saliva) is imperative. Several individual specimens obtained at different times on separate mornings are recommended. The smear results are available within 24 to 48 hours, but the culture can take up to 6 weeks. It is not uncommon for the smear to be negative and the culture positive, so if the patient exhibits clinical signs of the disease, proper isolation precautions are taken. Patients may also be screened with the newly developed DNA probe test. Results are available within 2 days with a predictive value of 99 percent.

F. Once the diagnosis is confirmed, patients are placed on therapy. There are six classifications of TB, based on exposure, symptoms, and skin test results (Table 1). The usual treatment is administration of at least two antituberculin drugs for 9 months. Usual drug choices are isoniazid (INH), ethambutol, rifampin, streptomycin, or pyrazinamide.

G. It is important to stress to patients that they must complete the drug regimen. Taking medications intermittently may increase the chances of becoming drug resistant. On drug therapy with negative sputum cultures and smears the patient is no longer infectious; however, noncompliance with medications may make the patient reactive and infectious again. Noncompliance with the treatment regimen is the largest factor in failure to eradicate this disease. The patient must be told of the side effects that may result from the drug therapy.

H. Patients have a 1 percent chance of recurrence after completing treatment. Skin testing is not usually done, since the test result will be significant for some time.

I. Patients with a significant skin test and a negative chest x-ray are placed on prophylactic medications. Patients need to be on one antituberculin drug for 1 year. Usually the drug of choice is INH.

J. Patients must be taught the signs and symptoms of a relapse. Skin testing is usually not done; however, a chest film is made if there has been exposure or if clinical signs of the disease are present.

TABLE 1 Classifications of Tuberculosis

Class	*Characteristics*
0	No contact with TB No Infection Skin test nonsignificant
1	Contact with TB No infection Skin test nonsignificant (Usual classification for health care workers)
2	Contact with disease Infected and significant skin test
3	Active TB
4	Past history of TB Skin test significant or not
5	Diagnosis pending

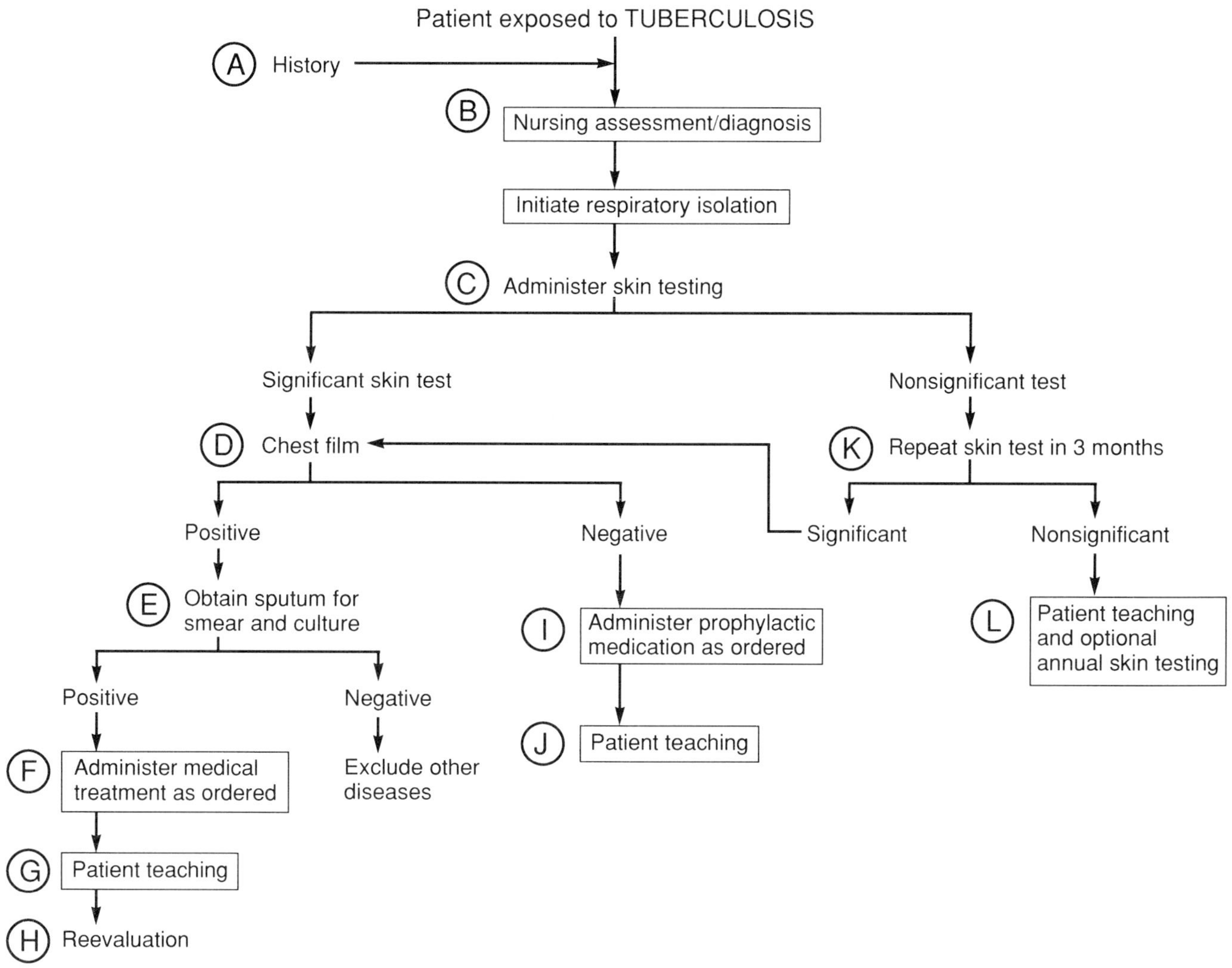

K. If individuals have been exposed to TB and do not have a significant skin test at the time of testing, they are retested within 3 months. It may take as long as 10 to 14 days before the body can produce enough antigens to show up on a skin test. If the second skin test is also nonsignificant, the patient will not acquire TB from that exposure.

L. Annual skin testing is important to continue to rule out contact with tubercle bacilli, especially if the person is a health care-worker and has not converted the skin test to significant. All at-risk individuals should be aware of the signs and symptoms of the disease and seek medical treatment if any of these are present.

References

Coleman DA. TB: the disease that's not dead yet. RN 1984; 47(9):49–57.

Florida State Department of Health and Rehabilitative Services. DNA probe test. Interoffice Memo, February 3, 1988.

Lordia G, Reichman L. Tuberculosis: when not to order roentgenograms. JAMA 1985; 253:1780–1781.

Snider D. BCG vaccinations and TB tests. JAMA 1985; 253:3438–3439.

The tuberculin skin test. Indianapolis: American Lung Association and American Thoracic Society, 1981.

Treatment of tuberculosis and other mycobacterial diseases: control of tuberculosis. Indianapolis: American Lung Association and American Thoracic Society, 1983.

LUNG CANCER

Rosemary Keller

A. A history of repeated exposure to substances that irritate the lungs, such as tobacco smoke, air pollution, and certain metals, fibers, and gases, correlates strongly with lung cancer. Lung cancers are classified according to histologic cell types (Table 1). Prognosis is strongly correlated to cell type.

B. Presenting pulmonary symptoms may include cough, chest pain, hemoptysis, dyspnea, and wheezing. Symptoms of local metastasis may include hoarseness, chest or shoulder and arm pain, dysphagia, or head and neck swelling. Be alert to extrapulmonary systemic manifestations including hypercalcemia (p 188), hyperadrenocorticism, excessive antidiuretic hormone, carcinoid syndrome, hypoglycemia (p 182), erythrocytosis, gynecomastia and myasthenic syndrome (p 18). Staging of lung cancer is based on the TNM system (tumor, node, and metastasis), which includes subsets designated as type I, II, and III. This system facilitates therapeutic decision making and is a prognostic indicator.

C. Diagnosis of lung cancer requires posteroanterior (PA) and lateral chest films and lung tomograms, which indicate the presence of a lesion, a mass in the hilar region, pleural effusion, atelectasis, and erosion of ribs or vertebrae. Cytologic examination of secretions (sputum collection) and/or biopsied tissue (bronchoscopy or percutaneous needle aspiration) reveal cancerous cells. If pleural effusion is present, examination of pleural fluid and a biopsy of pleural tissue confirms the diagnosis. CT scan of the lung, gallium lung scan, transbronchial needle aspiration, and mediastinoscopy are used to evaluate node status. Metastasis can be evaluated through a history and physical examination, routine blood chemistry, and organ radioisotopic scans of liver, bone, and brain. Provide emotional support and information about the required diagnostic procedures.

D. Patients undergoing bronchoscopy, tissue biopsy, or needle aspiration must be monitored for emergencies such as bronchial hemorrhage or pneumothorax (p 110). *If either complication develops, immediate intervention is essential.*

E. The choice of medical treatment for lung cancer is determined by the patient's physiologic status, and classification of the tumor. Surgery, radiation therapy, and chemotherapy (p 408) may be used separately or in combination.

F. A thoracotomy (p 126) involving segmental resection, lobectomy, or pneumonectomy is usually performed for patients with localized tumors with no evidence of metastatic spread whose pulmonary function is adequate.

G. Radiation therapy may be curative for some patients. It may also be used as a palliative treatment to decrease tumor size, control signs and symptoms of metastatic disease, and reduce cough, chest pain, dyspnea, hemoptysis, and bone and liver pain.

H. Before initiation of radiation therapy, provide the patient and family with information about the safety of the treatment and what is involved in the procedure.

I. Localized toxic side effects in normal tissues within the radiation field include esophagitis, pneumonitis and radiation lung fibrosis, anemia (p 342), immunosuppression, and bleeding disorders. Generalized systemic side effects such as fatigue, malaise, headache, nausea, and vomiting frequently occur.

J. Radiation therapy to the chest wall requires assessment of skin integrity for changes ranging from mild erythema to wet desquamation. Nursing instruction includes protecting the skin from irritation as well as avoiding use of soap, lotions, ointments, and powders on the radiated area. Do not remove the ink markings that designate the field for radiation.

K. Integrity of the lining of the esophagus may be altered, causing dysphagia. Patients may need to be placed on a liquid diet, avoiding hot, cold, or spicy foods.

L. Monitoring laboratory blood values for a decrease in red blood cells, white blood cells, and platelets provides information about the degree of bone marrow depression. Weakness and fatigue necessitate assistance with activities of daily living and adequate rest periods.

M. Chemotherapy (p 408) is often used in combination with surgery or radiation as an adjunctive therapy using multiagent protocols.

TABLE 1 Histologic Types of Tumors

Type	*Incidence*	*Site*	*Metastasis*	*Prognosis*
Epidermoid	30%	Bronchial epithelium, bronchial lumen	Less invasive to thorax, regional nodes, pleura, and chest wall	Slow growing Good prognosis
Small cell (oat cell)	25%	Central regions of lung	Early metastasis to liver, adrenals, bones, CNS, and endocrine organs	Rapid growing Poor prognosis
Adenocarcinomas	35%	Peripheral lung	Wide metastasis to uninvolved lung, liver, bone, kidney, CNS	Slow growing If well differentiated, good prognosis If poorly differentiated, poor prognosis
Large cell carcinoma	10%	Peripheral lung	Wide metastasis to mediastinal lymph nodes, pleura, adrenals, CNS, and bone	Poor prognosis

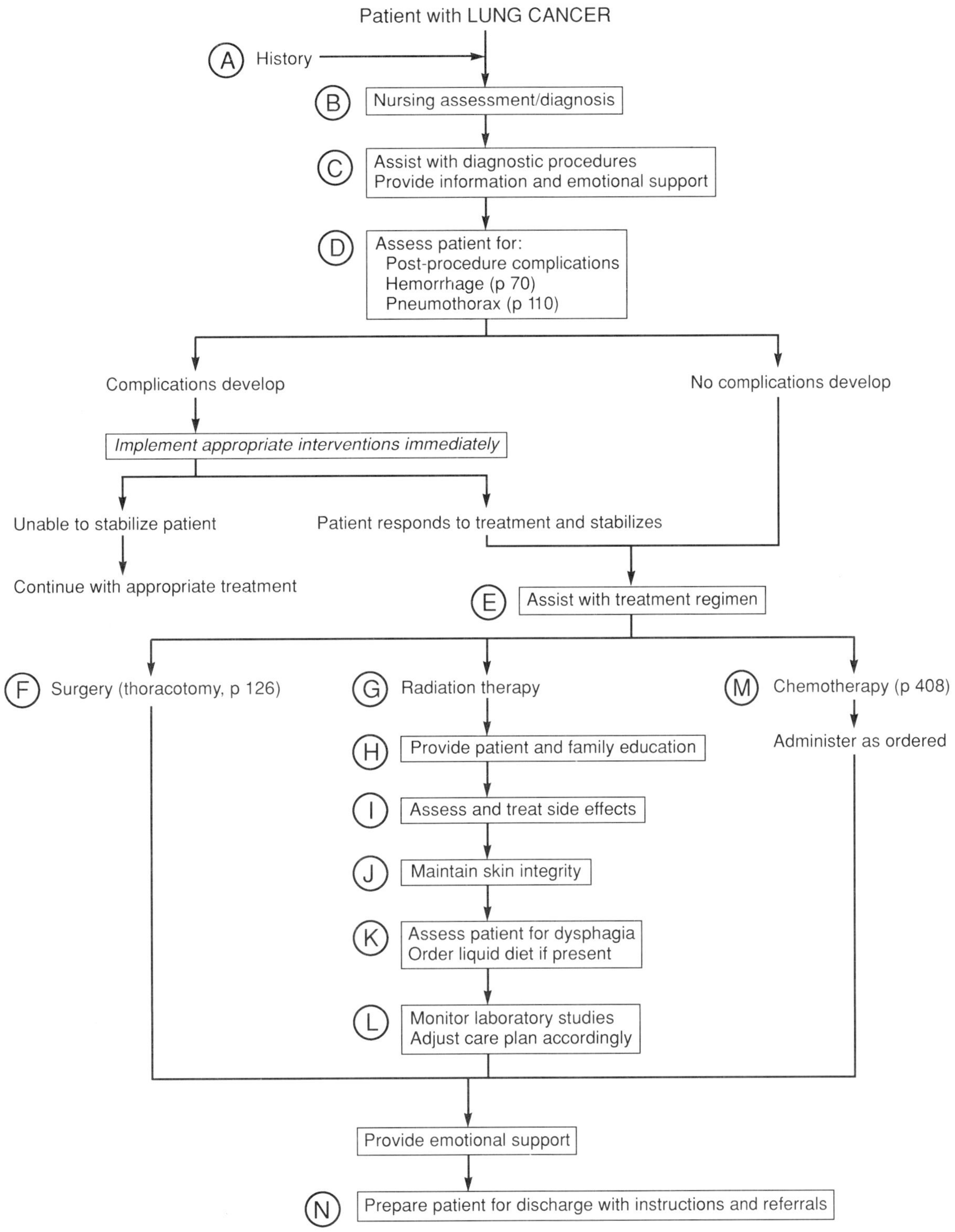

N. Patients and families need emotional support to cope with the treatment and prognosis and to resume as normal a life as possible. Information about the treatment and/or drugs they are receiving, side effects, and measures to reduce the severity of the side effects is required. Assure the patient that side effects will diminish and disappear a few weeks after completion of therapy. Services provided by the American Cancer Society such as the I Can Cope Program and Cancermount Program are of assistance.

References

Greifzu S, Crebase C, Winnick B. Lung cancer: by the time it's detected, it may be too late. RN 1987; 50(3):52–57.

Groenwald SL. Cancer nursing principles and practice. Boston: Jones & Bartlett, 1987.

Rubin P, Bakemeier RS, Kracker SK. Clinical oncology: a multidisciplinary approach. 6th ed. New York: American Cancer Society, 1983.

PULMONARY HYPERTENSION

Michelle Cornish

A. Pulmonary hypertension is an acute condition marked by accumulation of extravascular fluid in the lung tissue and alveoli. It is most commonly caused by congestive heart failure (p 68), but can also be seen in barbiturate and opiate poisoning, renal failure (p 318), near-drowning, and inhalation of irritating gases. Pulmonary hypertension may also occur as the result of rapid administration of whole blood, plasma, and intravenous fluids.

B. Nursing assessment should be as thorough as the condition allows, because this condition may change rapidly. The patient breathes rapidly and shallowly with difficulty, is usually restless, apprehensive, pale or cyanotic, and may cough up frothy, pink-tinged sputum. The peripheral and neck veins may be distended, the blood pressure and heart rate are increased, and the pulse may be full and bounding or weak and thready. There may be edema of the extremities, diffuse rales in the lungs, respiratory acidosis, and diaphoresis.

C. Laboratory studies that should be done include complete blood count (CBC), electrolyte panel, and an arterial blood gas (ABG) measurement. The patient should also have a chest film and electrocardiogram.

D. The symptomatic patient should be placed in high Fowler's position. If possible, allow the feet to dangle over the bedside. This promotes optimal lung expansion, since venous return is decreased by the venous pooling in the legs.

E. An intravenous site should be established to deliver 5 percent dextrose in water (D_5W) at a keep-vein-open (KVO) rate. Care should be taken not to administer more fluids than necessary to further prevent fluid overload. A central venous catheter may be placed to monitor central venous pressure (CVP).

F. Improving oxygenation is a priority. The patient should be placed on high-flow oxygen. Mask is the preferred mode of delivery, but the patient with pulmonary hypertension is usually anxious and may not tolerate the mask. Use caution in delivery of oxygen greater than 24 percent to patients with obstructive disease, since higher concentrations may cause respiratory arrest. Be prepared to suction your patient if secretions compromise the airway. In extreme cases, respiratory status may require intubation. Intermittent positive pressure breathing (IPPB) is an effective means of treatment. It raises pleural pressure, therefore impeding venous return.

G. It is necessary to administer medications to decrease the workload of the heart and to maintain oxygenation. A fast-acting diuretic, such as furosemide, should be given to reduce the circulating and extravascular fluid volumes. Morphine sulfate also acts to decrease cardiac workload by pooling blood peripherally and decreasing venous return. Monitor the patient's respirations and blood pressure carefully, because morphine may depress the respiratory and circulatory systems. A cardiotonic agent, such as digoxin, is usually administered. This increases contractility by slowing the conduction rate and increasing the refractory period of the cardiac cycle. For asthmatic symptoms, bronchodilators are useful to decrease respiratory distress.

H. The patient who does not respond to treatment may be transferred to intensive care for intubation and mechanical ventilation. Additional measures such as rotating tourniquets and phlebectomy may be used to reduce circulating volume.

I. It is of utmost importance to monitor accurate intake and output. Insert a Foley catheter to monitor urinary output after administering medications. Intravenous fluids should be kept at a minimum to avoid increasing circulation blood volume.

J. This condition can provoke anxiety for both the patient and family. Reassuring the patient and significant others and maintaining a calm environment is an important part of the nurse's role.

K. Discharge teaching is ongoing starting with admission. The patient should be instructed to keep follow-up appointments, to adhere to diet and medication regimens, and when to contact medical personnel for advice.

References

Potter D. Assessment. Horsham, PA: Intermed Communications, 1983:310–311.

Potter D. Emergencies. Horsham, PA: Intermed Communications, 1985:199–200.

Sheehy S, Barber J. Emergency nursing: principles and practice. St. Louis: CV Mosby, 1985:451–455.

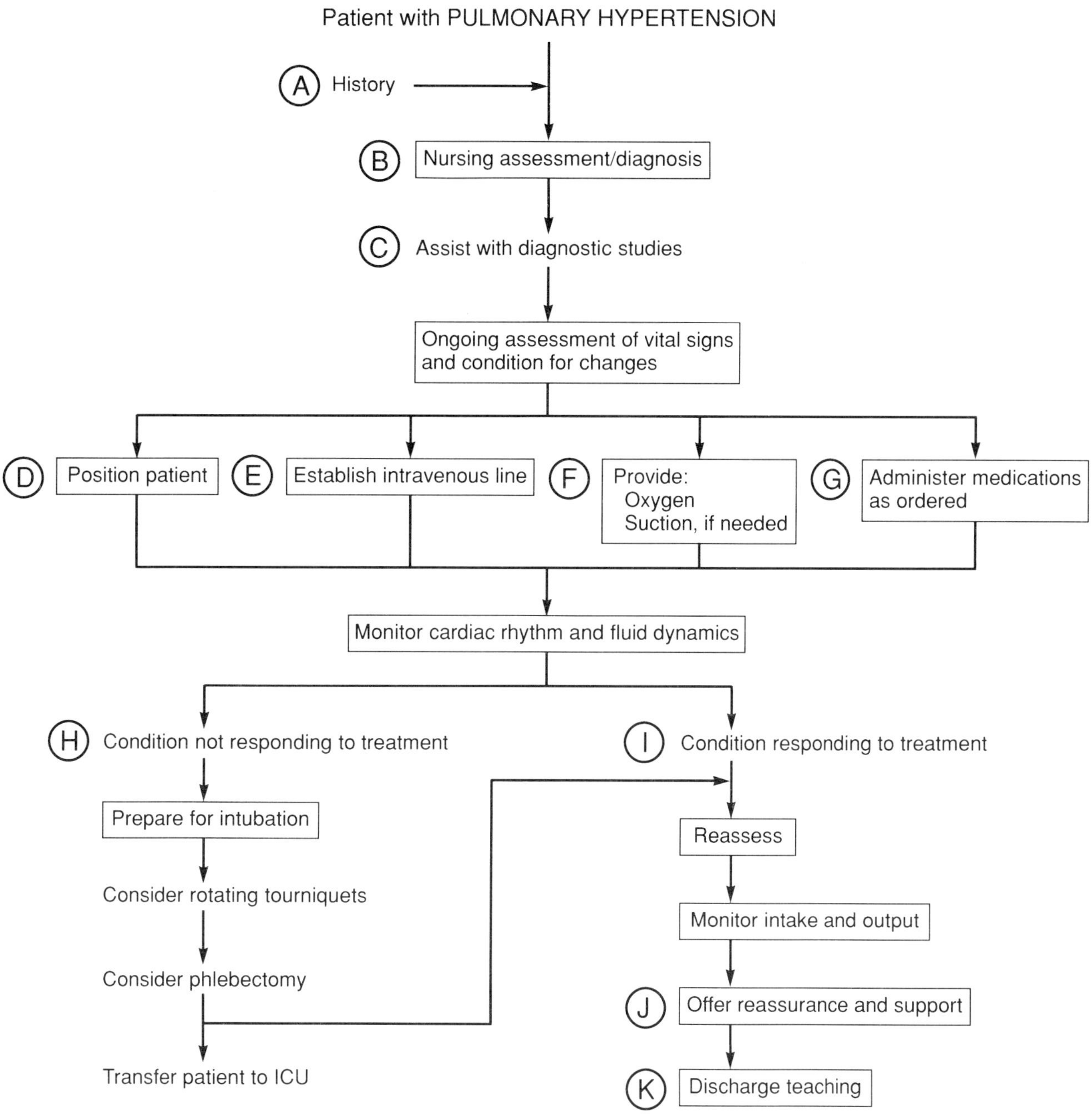
Patient with PULMONARY HYPERTENSION
A History
B Nursing assessment/diagnosis
C Assist with diagnostic studies
Ongoing assessment of vital signs and condition for changes
D Position patient
E Establish intravenous line
F Provide: Oxygen Suction, if needed
G Administer medications as ordered
Monitor cardiac rhythm and fluid dynamics
H Condition not responding to treatment
Prepare for intubation
Consider rotating tourniquets
Consider phlebectomy
Transfer patient to ICU
I Condition responding to treatment
Reassess
Monitor intake and output
J Offer reassurance and support
K Discharge teaching

THORACOTOMY

Michelle Cornish
Joy Gorzeman

Thoracotomy is an incision into the thoracic cavity. During the procedure, the ribs are spread and the pleura is opened. Exploratory thoracotomy is done to perform a biopsy or locate bleeding. Thoracic surgery is most often done to remove portions or all of a lung because of cancer. Lobectomy is the removal of a lobe of the lung; segmental resection, the removal of segments of a lobe; and pneumonectomy, the removal of an entire lung.

A. Patients undergoing chest surgery need routine operative preparation (p 2). Patients who smoke must be advised that it is essential to stop. Many of these patients have a history of pulmonary disease and limited cardiopulmonary reserve, which threatens the postoperative phase.

B. Diagnostic and preoperative studies include pulmonary function tests, chest radiography, electrocardiography and arterial bleed gases (ABGs). Laboratory tests indicated are complete blood count (CBC), prothrombin time, partial thromboplastin time, and electrolyte panel. Blood should be typed and cross-matched, because hypovolemia related to blood loss is a fairly common postoperative complication.

C. Postoperatively, an open airway must be maintained. Frequent suctioning is required because of trauma to the tracheobronchial tree during surgery. Sputum should be colorless; a change in color or consistency may indicate infection.

D. Coughing and deep breathing is essential. Incentive spirometry may also be ordered.

E. ABGs are done to monitor ventilation status. The lungs should be auscultated often. Decreased breath sounds, listlessness, dyspnea, and noisy respiration must be reported because they may indicate atelectasis (p 108). Chest movement should also be observed.

F. Most patients who undergo thoracotomy (except those having a pneumonectomy) have a chest drainage system (chest tubes). Amount and character of drainage should be noted. The amount decreases after the first 12 hours. Color may initially be bloody but should change to serous in about 24 hours.

G. Consistent bloody drainage indicates hemorrhage and should be reported. Blood replacement may be required and surgery may be necessary to stop the bleeding. The tubes must be kept patent. Milking or stripping the tubes should only be done if ordered by the physician. The drainage bottle must be kept below chest level, and covered hemostats should be at the bedside in case a bottle breaks or a tube becomes disconnected.

H. Monitor cardiac output and assess vital signs frequently. Arrhythmias are common in older patients. The physician should be notified if an arrhythmia is noted, and antiarrhythmic intervention should be started immediately.

I. Fluid and electrolyte balance must be maintained. Intake and output must be monitored and recorded. Intravenous fluids are given and oral fluids encouraged when allowed. Hypovolemia and excessive fluid administration must be treated. Report signs of shock (p 70) or pulmonary edema or congestion (p 114).

J. Pain causes the patient to limit chest movement and thereby decreases ventilation. Pain medication (narcotics) should be given in small, frequent doses without depressing the respiratory system. Begin oral analgesics as soon as possible.

K. Positioning is also important in pain control. If condition allows, upright is the best position. Encourage coughing and deep breathing every 1 to 2 hours; helping the patient to support the chest facilitates this process.

L. Observe patients for signs of infection. Fever, purulent drainage on the dressings, redness around the incision, and increased white blood cell count must be monitored and abnormalities reported to the physician.

M. Shoulder stiffness and ankylosis (p 206) may develop on the affected side. Encourage passive and active range of motion and ambulate patients as soon as possible.

N. Discharge teaching includes range of motion exercises to restore function of the affected shoulders and deep-breathing exercises. Advise patients that they will feel weak and tire easily for several weeks and to start activity slowly and build up as tolerance develops. Pain may be relieved by application of heat and/or oral pain medication. Patients should report chest pain, increased shortness of breath, or undue fatigue and be cautioned to avoid respiratory irritants such as smoke or fumes. Follow-up care is important.

References

Brunner LS, Suddarth DS. The Lippincott manual of nursing practice. 4th ed. Philadelphia: JB Lippincott, 1986.

Hamilton H. Procedures. Nurse's reference library. Horsham, PA: Intermed Communications, 1983:502–510.

Luckmann J, Sorensen KC. Medical-surgical nursing: psychophysiologic approach. 3rd ed. Philadelphia: WB Saunders, 1987.

Potter D. Emergencies. Nurse's reference library. Horsham, PA: Intermed Communications, 1985:144–146.

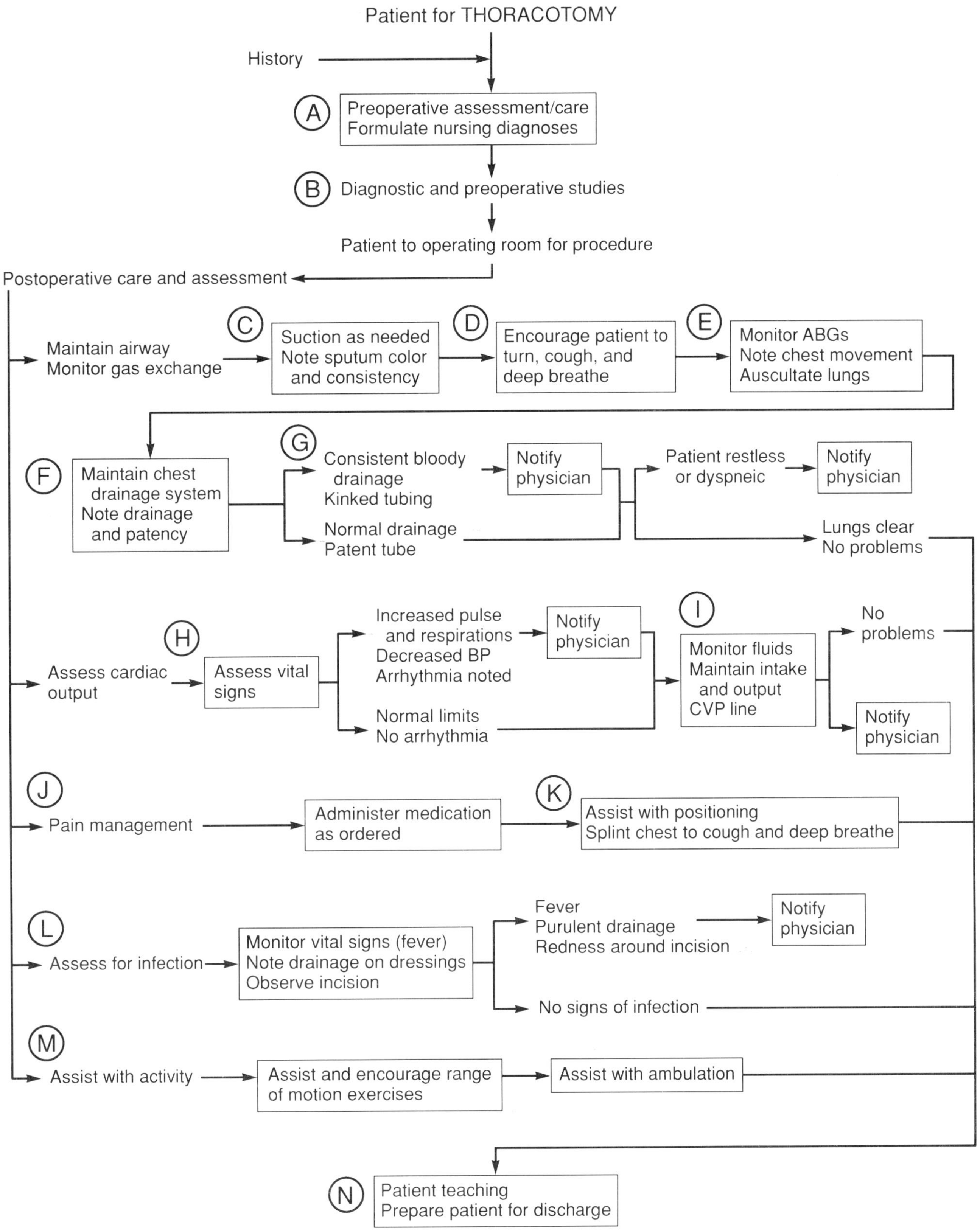
Patient for THORACOTOMY
History
A
Preoperative assessment/care
Formulate nursing diagnoses
B
Diagnostic and preoperative studies
Patient to operating room for procedure
Postoperative care and assessment
Maintain airway
Monitor gas exchange
C
Suction as needed
Note sputum color and consistency
D
Encourage patient to turn, cough, and deep breathe
E
Monitor ABGs
Note chest movement
Auscultate lungs
F
Maintain chest drainage system
Note drainage and patency
G
Consistent bloody drainage
Kinked tubing
Notify physician
Normal drainage
Patent tube
Patient restless or dyspneic
Notify physician
Lungs clear
No problems
H
Assess cardiac output
Assess vital signs
Increased pulse and respirations
Decreased BP
Arrhythmia noted
Notify physician
Normal limits
No arrhythmia
I
Monitor fluids
Maintain intake and output
CVP line
No problems
Notify physician
J
Pain management
Administer medication as ordered
K
Assist with positioning
Splint chest to cough and deep breathe
L
Assess for infection
Monitor vital signs (fever)
Note drainage on dressings
Observe incision
Fever
Purulent drainage
Redness around incision
Notify physician
No signs of infection
M
Assist with activity
Assist and encourage range of motion exercises
Assist with ambulation
N
Patient teaching
Prepare patient for discharge

GASTROINTESTINAL SYSTEM

GASTRIC AND DUODENAL ULCER

Nancy A. Young

Peptic ulcers appear as excavations formed in the mucosal wall of the esophagus, stomach, pylorus, or duodenum. The specific location of the ulcer determines its classification as gastric or duodenal. The erosion sometimes extends as deeply as the muscle layers or into the peritoneum. This erosion results from an increase in concentration or activity of gastric acid or a decrease in the mucosal resistance to these acids. Clinical management depends on the severity of symptoms and the amount and rate of blood loss. Along with gastritis, ulcers are the leading cause of upper gastrointestinal bleeding. Most ulcers respond positively to medical intervention; however, for the 10 to 25 percent of patients who experience uncontrollable rebleeding, surgical intervention is necessary (p 166).

A. A complete history facilitates the diagnosis of peptic ulcer. The patient usually complains of pain and/or burning in the midepigastric area or in the back, which occurs 1 to 3 hours after a meal. Patients may also describe a burning sensation that begins in the stomach or esophagus and moves up to the mouth. The ingestion of food or antacids or vomiting often relieves this pain. Question the patient about food and eating habits, and assess the current level of tension or nervousness and the environmental stressors. Other factors that contribute to ulcer formation include smoking and a family history of ulcer disease.

B. Analysis of hemoglobin and hematocrit in addition to a stool guaiac test for occult blood identifies more specifically the extent and location of the bleeding. Diagnostic procedures such as barium studies or an upper gastrointestinal (GI) endoscopy may also reveal the ulcer.

C. A clinical assessment further aids in the diagnosis of peptic ulcer. In more advanced cases, the patient may experience hematemesis (bright red or coffee ground) or passage of dark tarry stools. The nurse must observe the patient closely for signs of hemorrhage and respond quickly to promote stabilization through control of the bleeding, replacement of blood loss, and identification of the source of bleeding. The patient may require transfusions of whole blood or plasma and nasogastric intubation to classify the type of blood and to perform iced lavage. An indwelling urinary catheter monitors output, and taking frequent vital signs alerts the nurse to any change in status.

D. Tachycardia, hypotension, cool skin, faintness, or mental confusion may also indicate anemia (p 340) and further support the possibility of GI bleeding. On physical examination the patient may exhibit abdominal tenderness, distention, or absence of bowel sounds. If severe, these symptoms may indicate a perforation of the ulcer.

E. The use of medication and antacids that neutralize and inhibit gastric acid secretion plays a prominent role in pain management for the ulcer patient. In addition, the nurse should encourage other pain relief measures such as avoidance of ulcerogenic over-the-counter medications, avoidance of foods and beverages that exacerbate stomach irritation, planning of meals and snacks at regular intervals, and eating small pieces of food very slowly. Severe abdominal pain accompanied by distention and vomiting (or a nasogastric [NG] tube residual aspiration in excess of 200 to 400 ml) can indicate perforation or pyloric obstruction. *The physician should be notified immediately of these symptoms.*

F. Patients may be concerned about the development of complications. They should be encouraged to verbalize concerns, and all treatments should be thoroughly explained to prevent unnecessary worrying.

G. Often, patients who develop ulcers have a type A personality. The importance of rest and the need for a less stressful environment and lifestyle should be discussed. Counseling and/or sedatives may promote relaxation.

H. To promote complete healing of the ulcer and to minimize the possibility of recurrent attacks, the nurse must offer a discharge teaching plan that meets the patient's individual needs and knowledge deficits. The patient should understand the medication schedule and diet regimen, which includes avoidance of cigarettes, caffeine, colas, alcohol, and highly seasoned or fried foods. Help the patient to identify and reduce the stressors in the environment and plan activities to allow for adequate rest and energy conservation. Relaxation methods include meditation, distraction, imagery, and development of successful coping methods. Finally, the need for follow-up medical appointments should be emphasized. Instruct the patient to resume taking antacids if symptoms recur in the future. The patient must understand the symptoms of potential complications and the importance of seeking prompt treatment should they occur.

References

Brunner LS, Suddarth DS. Textbook of medical-surgical nursing. 6th ed. Philadelphia: JB Lippincott, 1988.

Feickert DM. Gastric surgery: your crucial pre- and postop role. RN 1987; 50(1):24–33.

Gitrick G. Handbook of gastrointestinal emergencies. 2nd ed. New York: Medical Examination Publishing Company, 1987.

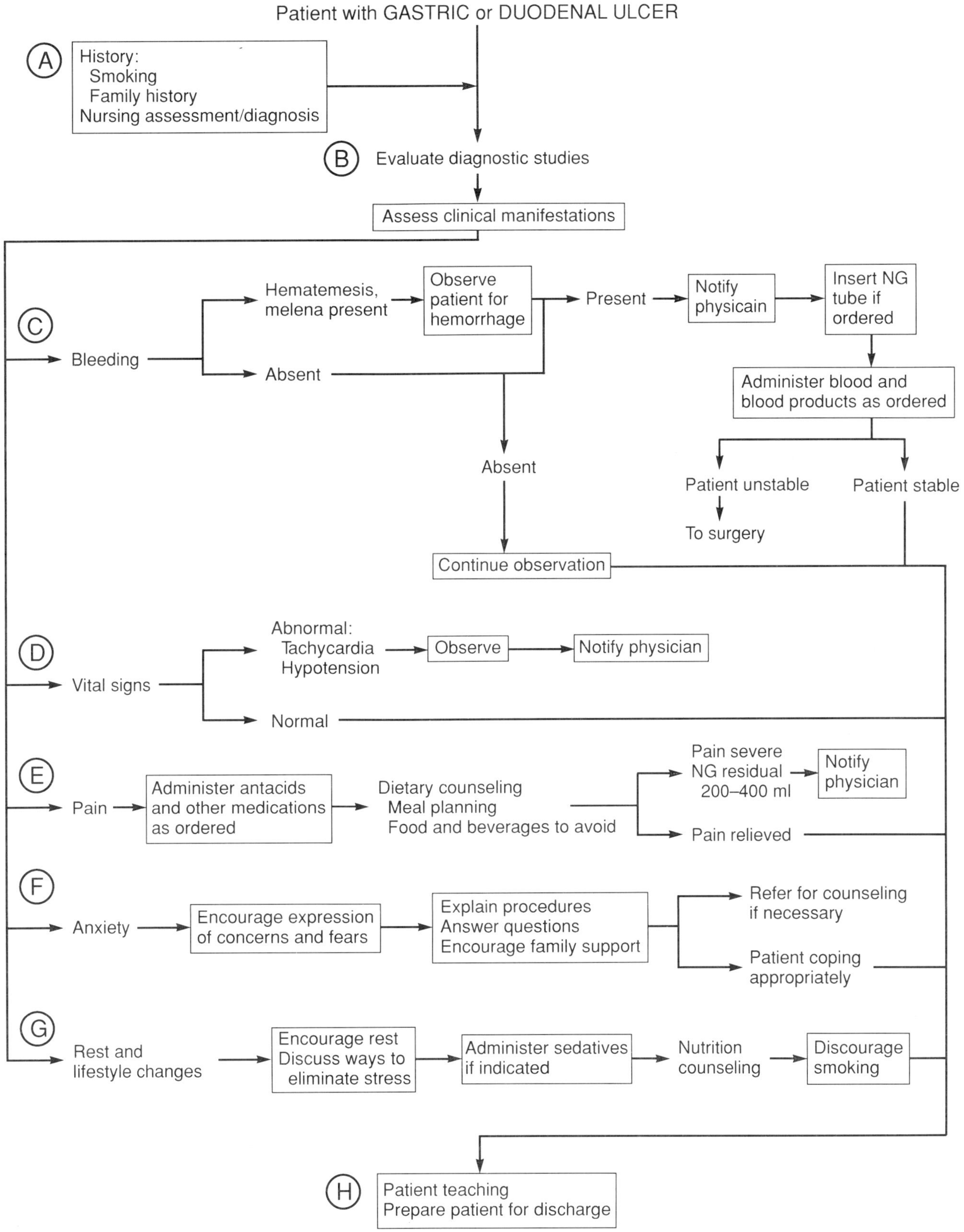
Patient with GASTRIC or DUODENAL ULCER
A
History:
Smoking
Family history
Nursing assessment/diagnosis
B
Evaluate diagnostic studies
Assess clinical manifestations
C
Bleeding
Hematemesis, melena present
Observe patient for hemorrhage
Present
Notify physicain
Insert NG tube if ordered
Administer blood and blood products as ordered
Patient unstable
To surgery
Patient stable
Absent
Absent
Continue observation
D
Vital signs
Abnormal:
Tachycardia
Hypotension
Observe
Notify physician
Normal
E
Pain
Administer antacids and other medications as ordered
Dietary counseling
Meal planning
Food and beverages to avoid
Pain severe
NG residual 200–400 ml
Notify physician
Pain relieved
F
Anxiety
Encourage expression of concerns and fears
Explain procedures
Answer questions
Encourage family support
Refer for counseling if necessary
Patient coping appropriately
G
Rest and lifestyle changes
Encourage rest
Discuss ways to eliminate stress
Administer sedatives if indicated
Nutrition counseling
Discourage smoking
H
Patient teaching
Prepare patient for discharge

VOLVULUS

Mary K. Roberts

Volvulus is a twisting of the intestine on its mesentery that results in compression of blood vessels, which can lead to ischemia and infarction, if unrelieved (Fig. 1). This condition most often occurs in children and the elderly (p 412). It commonly occurs in the sigmoid area of the bowel in the adult; other common sites include the stomach and cecum.

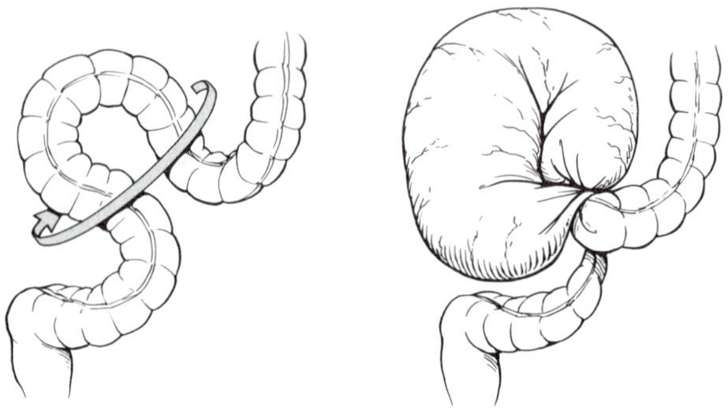

Figure 1 Sigmoid volvulus.

A. The patient presents with a complaint of sudden onset of severe abdominal pain with vomiting. Inspection of the abdomen may reveal markedly rapid abdominal distention with a palpable mass. Bowel sounds are markedly increased upon auscultation. The patient should be assessed for signs and symptoms of dehydration, since fluids and electrolytes are lost because the obstruction prevents reabsorption in the bowel. Profound fluid loss can result in hypovolemic shock (p 70). There may be a history of similar transient attacks in which there was spontaneous reduction of volvulus.

B. Diagnosis is made with characteristic findings of the partial or complete obstruction on radiographic tests. The special tests include abdominal films, which may be normal in the patient with midgut volvulus, but show abnormal air-fluid levels in the patient with either sigmoid or cecum volvulus; upper gastrointestinal series of films, which assists in the diagnosis of midgut volvulus, because barium does not pass by the obstruction; a barium enema, which fills the colon distal to the section of cecum in the patient with cecal volvulus and takes on an ''ace of spades'' configuration in the patient with sigmoid volvulus.

C. If the severity of the symptoms of a patient with a sigmoid volvulus does not require emergent surgery, a proctoscopy is done to check for infarction of the bowel.

D. For the patient with an infarcted bowel, the surgery of choice is resection with anastomosis (p 168). If the bowel is gangrenous or the patient is an at-risk candidate for surgery, a temporary colostomy or ileostomy may be performed, deferring anastomosis to a later time.

E. Nonsurgical reduction may be attempted in a patient with cecal or sigmoid volvulus. A colonoscopy is performed to untwist and decompress the bowel for the patient with cecal volvulus. A soft rectal tube passed through a sigmoidoscope may successfully deflate the bowel of the sigmoid volvulus patient. Success is indicated by the expulsion of gas and immediate relief of abdominal pain. Other treatment measures may include insertion of a gastrointestinal (GI) tube to decompress the bowel by removing fluid and fecal material above the obstruction. Document the color, odor, and amount of fluid removed. Comfort measures such as oral care, gargles, and lozenges are indicated. Use of an antibiotic mouthwash is recommended to prevent colonic bacterial growth. The tube is gradually removed as continuity of the GI tract is reestablished. Attention to the skin integrity of the nares is important, with frequent cleansing and lubrication.

F. Discharge planning includes recognition of the symptoms of recurrent volvulus, dietary and personal practices to promote elimination, and follow-up care.

G. Detorsion or untwisting of the bowel is the surgical procedure used when attempts to decompress the bowel per rectum are unsuccessful. This surgical procedure is also used to treat midgut volvulus.

References

Armstrong ME, ed. McGraw-Hill handbook of clinical nursing. New York: McGraw-Hill, 1979.

Billings DM, Stokes LG. Medical-surgical nursing: common health problems of adults and children across the lifespan. 2nd ed. St. Louis: CV Mosby, 1987.

Ford RD, Kangilaski R, eds. Diseases and disorders handbook. Springhouse, PA: Springhouse Corporation, 1988.

Hamilton HK, ed. Diseases. 2nd ed. Springhouse, PA: Springhouse Corporation, 1987.

Schrock TR. Large intestine. In: Dunphy HE, Way LW, eds. Current surgical diagnosis and treatment. 5th ed. Los Altos, CA: Lange, 1981:572–610.

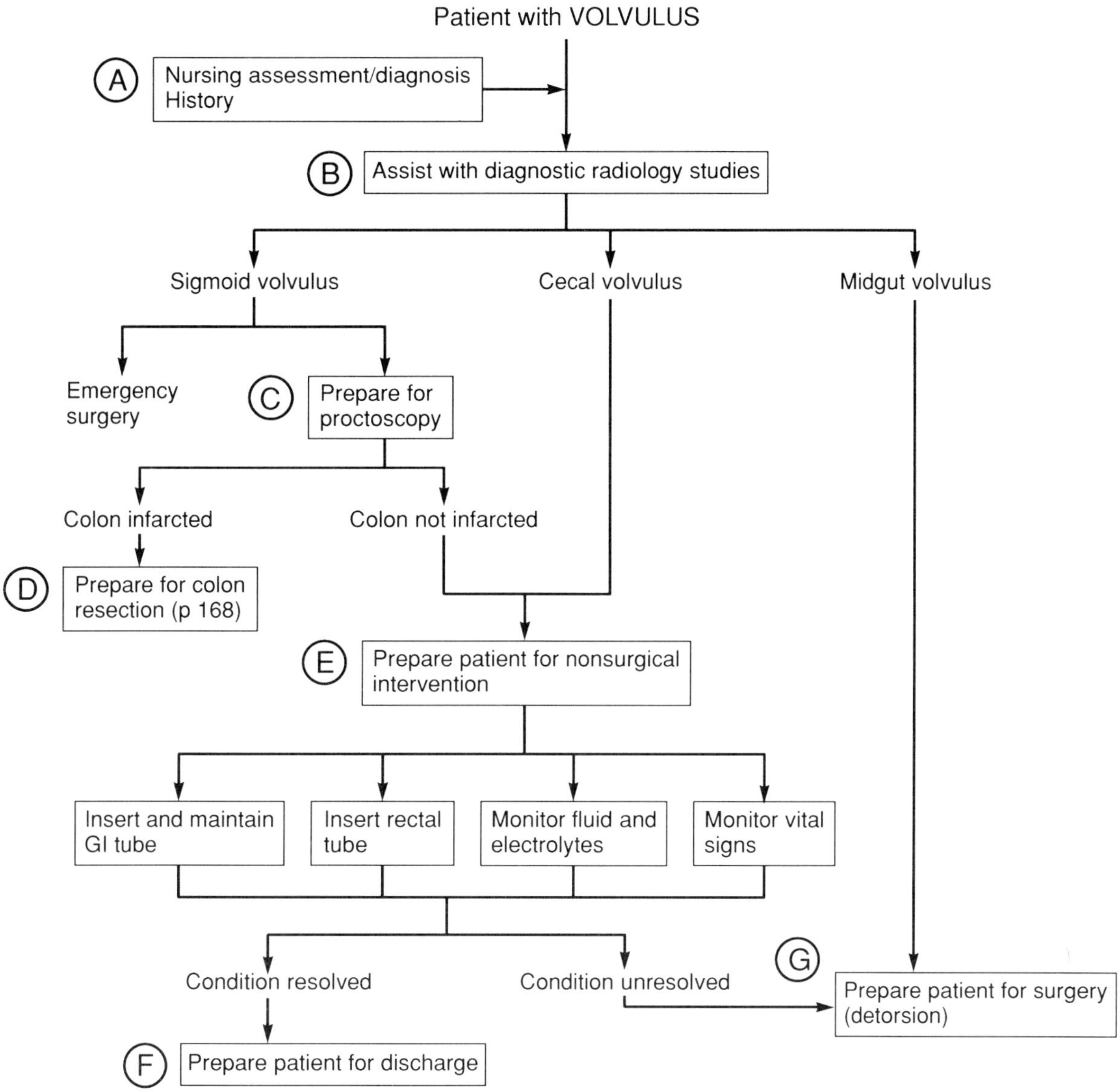
Patient with VOLVULUS
A
Nursing assessment/diagnosis
History
B
Assist with diagnostic radiology studies
Sigmoid volvulus
Cecal volvulus
Midgut volvulus
Emergency surgery
C
Prepare for proctoscopy
Colon infarcted
Colon not infarcted
D
Prepare for colon resection (p 168)
E
Prepare patient for nonsurgical intervention
Insert and maintain GI tube
Insert rectal tube
Monitor fluid and electrolytes
Monitor vital signs
Condition resolved
Condition unresolved
G
Prepare patient for surgery (detorsion)
F
Prepare patient for discharge

INTESTINAL ISCHEMIA

Mary K. Roberts

The celiac, superior mesenteric, and inferior mesenteric arteries with collateral connections comprise the blood supply to the gastrointestinal tract. Intrinsic vascular disease, systemic illness, pharmacologic agents, and surgical procedures can contribute to lesions that occlude the arteries and decrease blood flow to the intestine, producing ischemia.

A. The history is important in differentiating acute occlusive ischemia, chronic occlusive ischemia, and nonocclusive ischemia. With acute occlusive disease, the patient complains of severe, gripping abdominal pain, often poorly localized. Nausea, vomiting, diarrhea, and constipation are symptoms that occur variably. The primary complaint with chronic occlusive disease is postprandial epigastric pain that characteristically appears 15 to 30 minutes after the beginning of a meal and lasts for 1 hour or more. These patients usually present with a significant weight loss because of reluctance to eat. A suspected diagnosis of nonocclusive ischemia can be made on the basis of the patient's medical history. A history of other acute diseases, such as a cardiac arrhythmia or sepsis, can lead to nonocclusive ischemia because of low perfusion pressure and flow. These patients usually have acute abdominal pain.

B. Blood should be drawn and sent to the laboratory for a complete blood count and liver enzyme studies. Leukocytosis, reflected in an elevated white blood cell count, is usually present with intestinal ischemia, and an elevated serum amylase may also be present. Barium studies reveal "thumbprinting" and disordered motility. The most definitive procedure for accurate diagnosis is arteriography. This procedure also documents the absence of vascular occlusion, which categorizes the ischemia as a nonocclusive intestinal ischemia.

C. Nursing assessment begins with vital signs to check for signs of hypovolemia and immediate need for intravenous (IV) fluid resuscitation. An increased temperature may indicate infection that can develop into peritonitis (p 138). A thorough gastrointestinal assessment includes auscultation of bowel sounds and palpation for abdominal tenderness and distention. Stool and gastric contents are checked for the presence of blood.

D. Acute occlusive disease requires continued, careful nursing monitoring. Stabilization of the patient is a priority before laparotomy. Surgical options are related to the extent of injury to the bowel (p 168).

E. Chronic occlusive ischemia of the celiac and/or mesenteric arteries is caused by atherosclerosis or external compression by ligamentous bands. Stabilization of fluid and electrolyte balance guides clinical management. Surgery for atherosclerotic lesions with viable bowel involves revascularization by either endarterectomy or graft replacement.

F. Assessing the patient for signs of hypovolemia is crucial with acute occlusive ischemia. The patient incurs fluid losses through vomiting and diarrhea as well as through a large amount of fluid loss to the peritoneal cavity and the intestinal lumen.

G. The principal effect of a major vascular occlusion is hemorrhagic necrosis of the mucosa, which accounts for blood loss and also contributes to potential hypovolemia. Fluid losses should be replaced with IV fluids and blood products, the type of replacement and amount determined by close monitoring of vital signs, central venous pressure measurements, urine output, and hematocrit values.

H. The patient is at risk for electrolyte imbalances because of fluid loss and the resulting hypovolemic state. The risk of electrolyte imbalance is greater if the level of occlusion is very high in the small bowel. Electrolytes that should be assessed immediately and monitored frequently during the hypovolemic phase and stabilization of the patient for surgery are potassium, sodium, and chloride, which might be low.

I. Visceral ischemia may be due to the compression of the celiac artery by the median arcuate ligament. Thin women 25 to 50 years of age are most commonly affected.

J. Surgery involves an abdominal incision with a simple division of the median arcurate ligament. This relieves the compression of the celiac artery in 50 percent of cases. Postoperative care is similar to that for laparotomy or other bowel surgery (p 168). Continued ischemia may require further surgery for vascular reconstruction.

K. Patients with no complications after ligament revision are discharged 3 to 5 days after surgery, with instruction about medication, incision care, diet, resumption of normal activities, and follow-up care.

L. When nonocclusive intestinal ischemia is diagnosed, treatment involves 24-hour IV vasodilator therapy. An arterial line is usually placed during arteriography for direct infusion to the superior mesenteric artery. The patient is sent to the ICU for further therapy and fluid replacement. Surgery is usually required after vasodilator therapy to exclude other disease that may simulate intestinal ischemia and to resect the infarcted bowel.

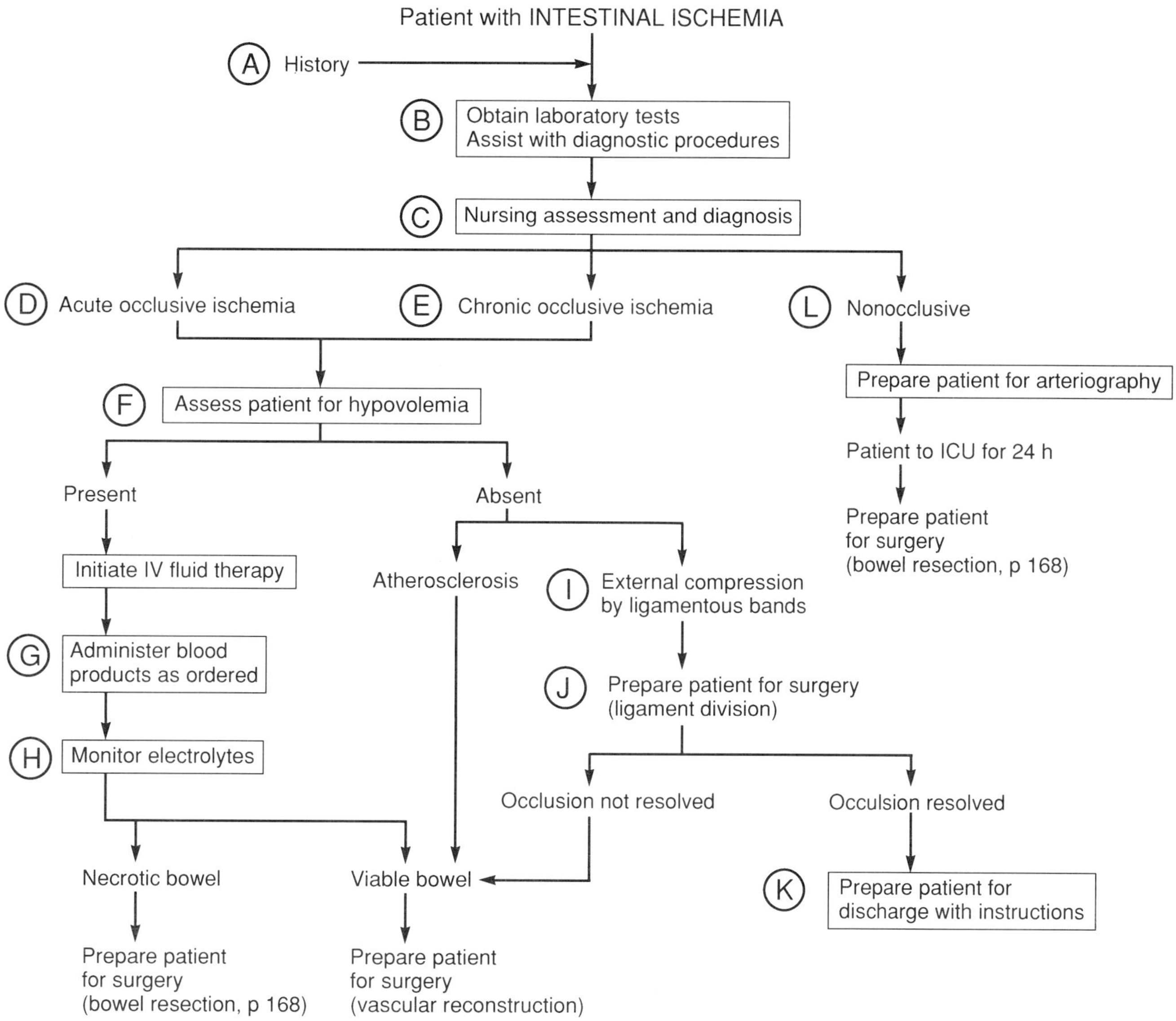

References

McConnell EA. Meeting the challenge of intestinal obstruction nursing. Nursing 87, 1987; 17(7):34–41.

Shrock TR. Small intestine. In: Dunphy JE, Way LW, eds. Current surgical diagnosis and treatment. 5th ed. Los Altos, CA: Lange, 1981:547–571.

Silen W. Acute intestinal obstruction. In: Isselbacher KJ, Adams RD, Braunwald E, Petersdorf RG, Wilson JD, eds. Harrison's principles of internal medicine. 9th ed. New York: McGraw-Hill, 1980:1437–1439.

Wylie EJ, Effeney DJ, Ehrenfeld WK, Moore WS. Arteries. In: Dunphy JE, Way LW, eds. Current surgical diagnosis and treatment. 5th ed. Los Altos, CA: Lange, 1981:657–660.

DIVERTICULOSIS

Mary K. Roberts

Bulging pouch-like herniations in the gastrointestinal (GI) wall that push the mucosal lining through the surrounding muscle are called diverticula and cause diverticular disease or diverticulosis. They may develop at any point in the GI system from the proximal end of the pharynx to the anus. Congenital weakness and bowel distention are common causes of this disease. Diverticula also develop because of the normal slowing of the GI tract in later maturity.

A. Diverticulosis is more prevalent in men over age 40. The history should include diet and bowel habits. The patient with diverticulosis usually has a diet that consists primarily of highly refined foods; the lack of dietary roughage leads to a history of constipation. The presenting symptom is usually recurrent left lower-quadrant abdominal pain, which is relieved by passage of flatus or defecation.

B. Diverticulosis can progress to diverticulitis when the diverticula become inflamed, which may cause potentially fatal obstruction, infection, or hemorrhage. A complete nursing assessment, including vital signs, needs to be done with particular attention to the GI system.

C. The symptoms are considered mild if the patient history confirms constipation related to diet and left lower-quadrant pain relieved by flatus while vital signs are within normal limits.

D. Explain diverticula and how they form to the patient with mild symptoms. Patient teaching should focus on dietary and bowel habits and exercise. The importance of dietary roughage (foods high in undigestible fiber), and the harmful effects of constipation need to be emphasized. When constipation is a problem, advise the patient to take stool softeners or bulk-forming laxatives. Stress that bulk-forming laxatives must be taken with large amounts of water to prevent their sticking in and obstructing the esophagus.

E. A low-grade fever is present in the patient with moderate symptoms. This patient may also exhibit some tenderness in the left lower quadrant on palpation and complain of mild nausea.

F. A patient previously diagnosed with diverticulosis may exhibit symptoms classified as severe. The left lower-quadrant pain may be intensified and constipation may be chronic. Bowel sounds may be diminished and the abdomen tender, with the possibility of a mass in the left lower quadrant. Elevated temperature, increased pulse, and decreased blood pressure suggest an inflammatory process of the diverticula. Carefully observe the patient's bowel patterns, noting frequency, color, and consistency of all stools.

G. A patient with moderate or severe symptoms must undergo confirming diagnostic studies for diverticulosis and assessment for progression to diverticulitis. A barium enema confirms diverticulosis of the lower bowel; an upper GI series confirms or rules out diverticulosis of the esophagus and upper bowel. Abdominal films are helpful to check for perforation of the diverticula, which show up as free air. Blood studies may reveal an elevated white blood cell count, which combined with fever suggests an inflammatory process.

H. The patient without complications should remain on bedrest with continued monitoring of vital signs, intake and output, and careful observation of stools.

I. Mild to massive bleeding may occur in patients with diverticulosis. This is assessed by the stool examination and by hemoglobin and hematocrit counts.

J. Inflammation of the diverticula (diverticulitis) is a complication and needs further medical treatment with intravenous antibiotics.

K. Controlling infection and preventing constipation is the goal of medical therapy. Treatment may also include meperidine to control pain and relax smooth muscle, a broad-spectrum antibiotic, stool softeners, and an antispasmodic to control muscle spasms. Be aware of the purpose, correct dosage, frequency, and side effects of all drugs administered.

L. If hemorrhage does not resolve spontaneously, further medical therapy may include vasopressin administered through an intravenous line placed directly into the bleeding vessel. Catheter placement is done via arteriography, and the patient is moved to the ICU for infusion and treatment of hemorrhagic shock (p 70).

M. Further complications may include perforation, abscess, peritonitis (p 138), and bowel obstruction. The nurse must continually assess the GI system, noting bowel sounds, abdominal tenderness, abdominal softness or rigidity, and character of pain; monitor fluid intake and output; and continue careful observation of stools. Vital signs must be closely watched, since they may signal developing complications.

N. If the inflammatory process does not resolve with medical therapy or further complications develop, surgical intervention (colon resection [p 168] to remove the involved segments of the colon) is necessary.

References

Billings DM, Stokes LG. Medical-surgical nursing: common health problems of adults and children across the lifespan. 2nd ed. St. Louis: CV Mosby, 1987:927–928.

Ford RD, Kangilaski R, eds. Diseases and disorders handbook. Springhouse, PA: Springhouse Corporation, 1988.

Greenberger NJ. Gastrointestinal disorders. 3rd ed. Chicago: Year Book, 1986.

Hamilton HK, ed. Diseases. 2nd ed. Springhouse, PA: Springhouse Corporation, 1987.

Phipps WJ, Long BC, Woods NF, eds. Medical-surgical nursing. St. Louis: CV Mosby, 1987:1289–1290.

Schroeder SA, Krupp MA, Tierney LM, eds. Current medical diagnosis and treatment. Norwalk, CT: Appleton & Lange, 1988:389–390.

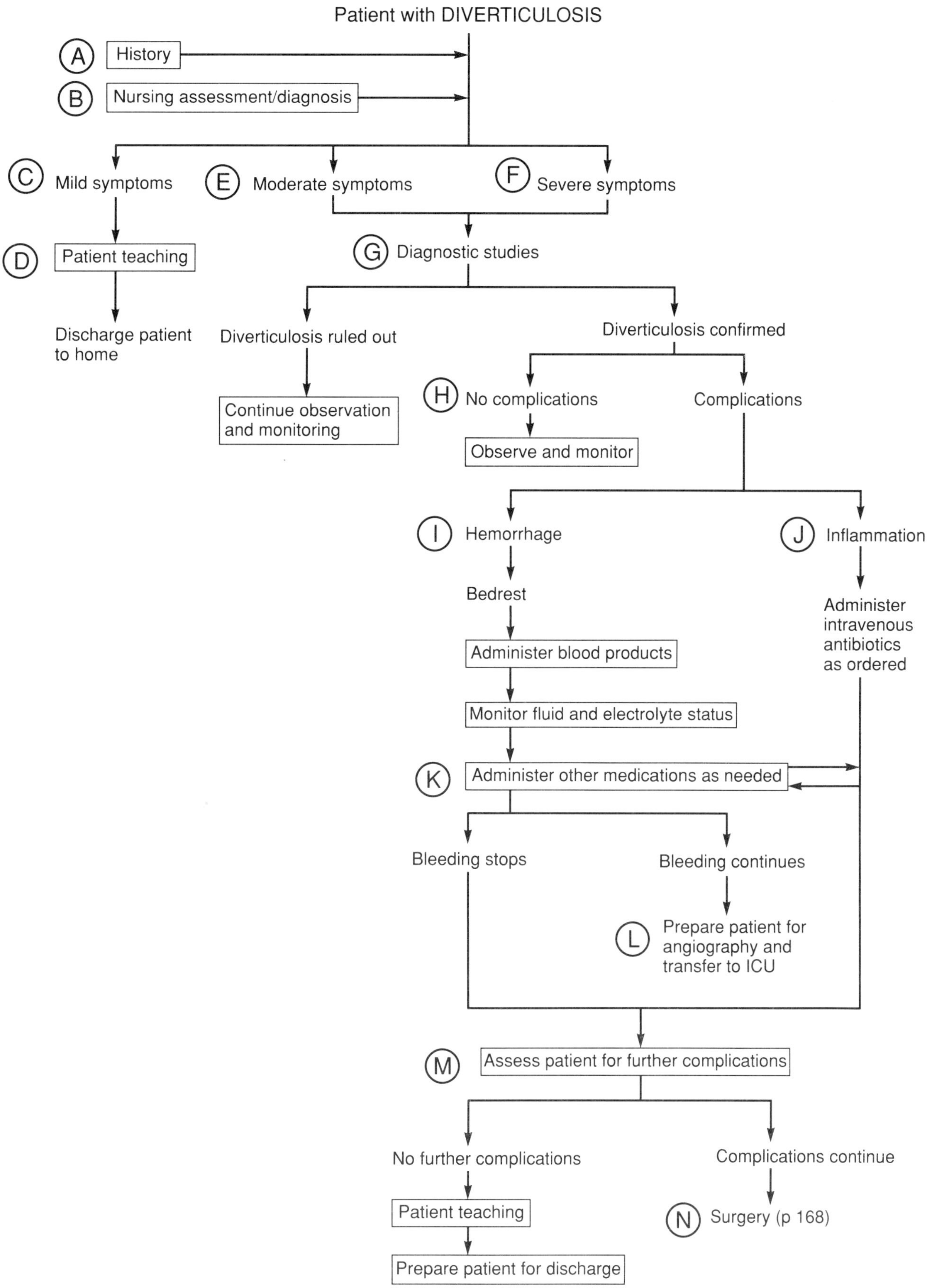
Patient with DIVERTICULOSIS
A History
B Nursing assessment/diagnosis
C Mild symptoms
E Moderate symptoms
F Severe symptoms
D Patient teaching
Discharge patient to home
G Diagnostic studies
Diverticulosis ruled out
Continue observation and monitoring
Diverticulosis confirmed
H No complications
Observe and monitor
Complications
I Hemorrhage
Bedrest
Administer blood products
Monitor fluid and electrolyte status
K Administer other medications as needed
J Inflammation
Administer intravenous antibiotics as ordered
Bleeding stops
Bleeding continues
L Prepare patient for angiography and transfer to ICU
M Assess patient for further complications
No further complications
Patient teaching
Prepare patient for discharge
Complications continue
N Surgery (p 168)

PERITONITIS

Joy Gorzeman

Peritonitis is inflammation of the peritoneum, the semipermeable membrane covering the organs in the abdominal cavity.

A. Primary peritonitis is usually seen in children with urinary tract infections. Secondary peritonitis is more commonly seen in acutely ill medical-surgical patients. It results from contamination of the peritoneum and is caused by invasion of bacterial or chemical irritants through trauma, inflammation, or neoplastic disease. The site of inflammation secretes a plasma-like fluid. If the source of contamination is not sealed, edema and paralytic ileus may result. Extra blood is shunted to the site, peristalsis decreases, and oxygen requirement is increased. Peritonitis is a common complication of many acute disease processes that involve rupture or perforation of digestive organs, such as ruptured appendix (p 164), perforated ulcer, gangrenous cholecystitis, and gunshot wounds.

B. Clinical manifestations are related to the location and extent of the inflammation. Pain may be diffuse at first and become more localized. Abdominal muscles become rigid. Patients try to lie very still and usually draw up their legs. Anorexia, nausea, and vomiting are often present. Other assessment factors include increased temperature and pulse and decreased bowel sounds.

C. Confirmative diagnostic findings include leukocytosis and free air in the diaphragm, which may be seen on radiologic examination. Primary peritonitis may be indicated in urinalysis or peritoneal aspirate.

D. If peritonitis is localized, treatment is targeted at the cause, usually through surgery. If it is generalized, surgery is not done until distention and fluid and electrolyte problems are under control.

E. The best intervention for peritonitis is prevention. Early signs and symptoms should be reported. Strict aseptic technique must be maintained with any surgical procedure. Early diagnosis and treatment are important to prevent severe shock, septicemia, or major organ failure.

F. Ongoing assessment includes frequent monitoring of vital signs and central venous pressure (CVP), hourly urine output, and laboratory studies, such as blood gases and electrolytes.

G. Patients are made NPO, and intravenous fluids are maintained. Meticulous oral hygiene is a must. Intake and output should be monitored and recorded. Antibiotics must be administered as ordered. Placing the patient in Fowler's position helps facilitate drainage. Nasogastric suction is implemented and patency of the tube must be assured.

H. The degree of pain is assessed and documented.

I. The patient should be offered reassurance because peritonitis is a serious, possibly fatal complication. Mortality is influenced by age, type of contamination, and tissue perfusion.

J. After acute symptoms are resolved, surgery may be performed if necessary. Discharge teaching includes wound care, information about medications, and follow-up care.

References

Brunner LS, Suddarth DS. The Lippincott manual of nursing practice. 4th ed. Philadelphia: JB Lippincott, 1986.

Deters GE. Managing complications after abdominal surgery. RN, 1987; 50(3):27–32.

Luckmann J, Sorensen KC. Medical-surgical nursing: a psychophysiologic approach. 3rd ed. Philadelphia: WB Saunders, 1987.

Thompson JM, McFarland GK, Hirsch JE, Tucker SM, Bowers AC. Clinical nursing. St. Louis: CV Mosby, 1986.

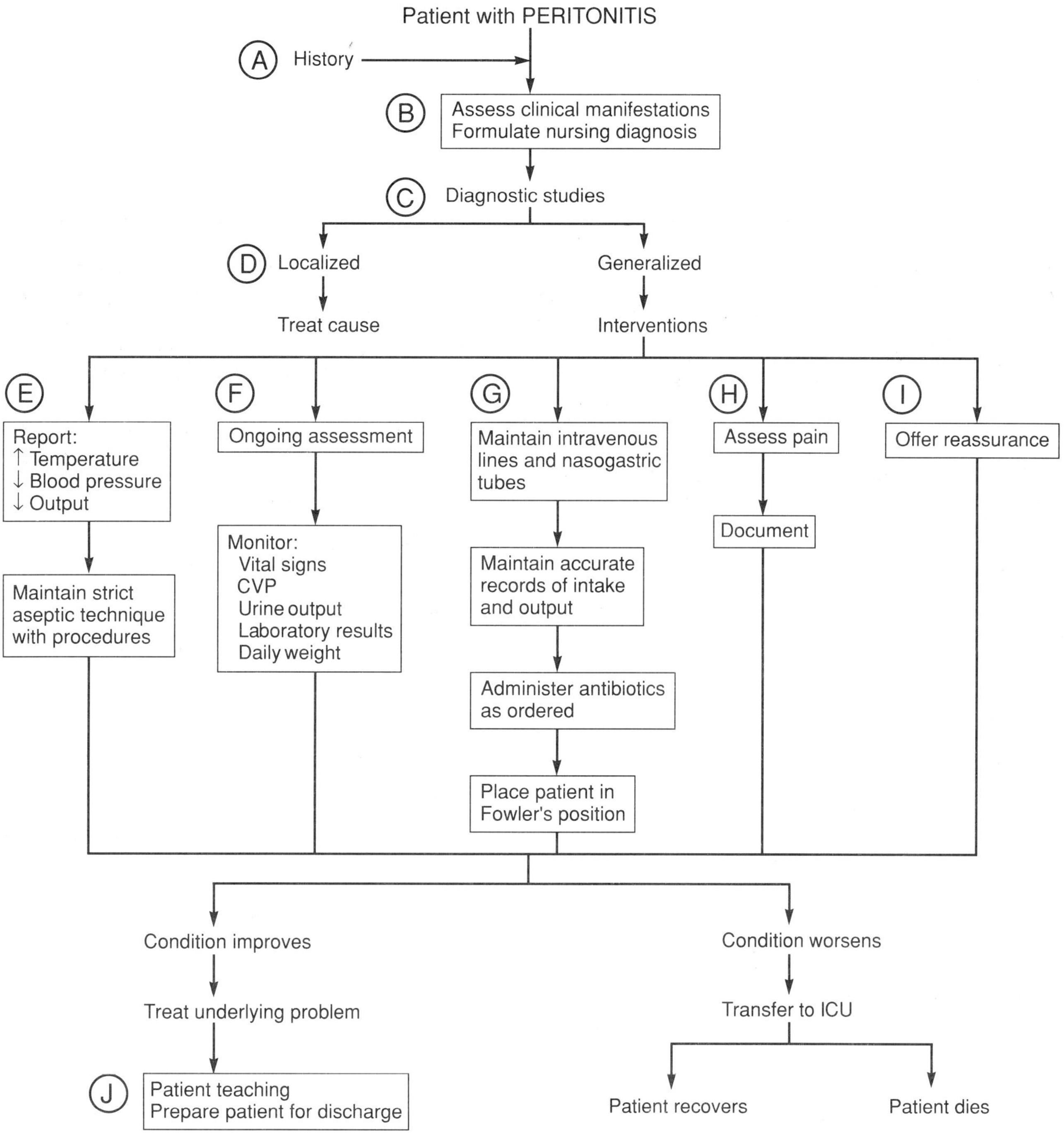
Patient with PERITONITIS
A
History
B
Assess clinical manifestations
Formulate nursing diagnosis
C
Diagnostic studies
D
Localized
Generalized
Treat cause
Interventions
E
Report:
↑ Temperature
↓ Blood pressure
↓ Output
Maintain strict aseptic technique with procedures
F
Ongoing assessment
Monitor:
Vital signs
CVP
Urine output
Laboratory results
Daily weight
G
Maintain intravenous lines and nasogastric tubes
Maintain accurate records of intake and output
Administer antibiotics as ordered
Place patient in Fowler's position
H
Assess pain
Document
I
Offer reassurance
Condition improves
Treat underlying problem
J
Patient teaching
Prepare patient for discharge
Condition worsens
Transfer to ICU
Patient recovers
Patient dies

CROHN'S DISEASE

Gail Shores

Crohn's disease, or regional enteritis, falls into a group of diseases known as inflammatory bowel disease (IBD). IBD denotes all diseases causing inflammation of the small and/or large intestine. Crohn's disease most commonly occurs before 40 years of age, with a peak incidence in the 20s. It occurs equally among men and women, is more common in the Jewish population, and has definite familial tendencies. Although the cause is unknown, a prominent theory suggests that autoimmune factors may play a role, since Crohn's disease is often associated with arthritis (p 212), skin rash, and thyroid (pp 184–187) disease. There is a psychological component, and stress and emotional upset can cause a relapse or return of symptoms. The lower ileum is most frequently affected, although the colon and other parts of the gastrointestinal (GI) tract may be affected. Inflammation frequently involves all three layers of the bowel wall. Granulomas, or groups of inflammatory cells, are also characteristic. The intestinal walls can become thick and rigid, with the formation of fibrous tissue causing narrowing of the lumen and eventual obstruction.

A. Symptoms of Crohn's disease include right lower-quadrant abdominal pain, stools alternating between diarrhea and constipation, low-grade fever, anorexia, nausea and vomiting, and weight loss. These symptoms may appear abruptly or insidiously and are characterized by exacerbations and remissions. Perianal fissures or fistulas are common, resulting from diarrhea. Complications can arise from hemorrhage, stricture, or perforation. The incidence of cancer is increased in these patients. Other systemic complications include arthritis, iritis, uveitis, skin lesions, and disease of the liver, kidney, and gallbladder. Regional enteritis causes symptoms similar to appendicitis (p 164); thus, appropriate assessment and diagnosis are important.

B. Diagnostic studies include complete blood count with differential, electrolytes, sedimentation rate, albumin, and liver function tests. Stool samples are collected and examined to rule out bacterial infection or parasites. A chest film and flat plate of the abdomen are also done. The results of these tests reflect the extent and severity of the inflammatory reaction.

C. Sigmoidoscopy is done to check for mucosal inflammation and to test the friability of the rectal lining. Suspicious lesions can be biopsied. After a rigid 48-hour prep involving dietary restrictions and cleansing of the colon, colonoscopy (direct visualization of the lining of the entire colon using a fiberoptic scope) and/or barium enema study (radiologic evaluation) is done to determine the extent of involvement and to distinguish Crohn's disease from ulcerative colitis (p 142). In the former a "cobblestone" appearance (coarse irregularities in the mucosal surface) is characteristic, as are pseudopolyps, edema, and strictures. Biopsies reveal granulomas in 30 to 50 percent of the specimens taken from involved areas of the mucosal lining. A barium enema frequently reveals small rectal ulcerations or irregular nodules, and irregular thickening, which lead to areas of stricture.

D. Treatment is aimed at reducing inflammation and relieving symptoms caused by involvement of other areas of the body.

E. Antispasmodic and antidiarrheal agents may be ordered to relieve abdominal cramps and diarrhea. Antibiotics may be given to prevent infection. Symptoms may be aggravated by high stress levels. Psychotherapy and/or antianxiety medications or sedation are frequently employed. Prednisone may be given, initially in high doses, and decreasing as symptoms permit. Sulfasalazine (Azulfidine) is also given to reduce inflammation. 6-Mercaptopurine has been effective in 65 percent of the cases treated.

F. Cortisone enemas may be ordered to reduce the mucosal inflammation locally.

G. These patients usually require dietary counseling about a low residue, low fiber, low fat diet that is high in calories, protein, carbohydrates, and vitamins (especially vitamin K).

H. If the patient is extremely malnourished, hyperalimentation may be administered. This also allows for complete rest of the intestine.

I. Surgery may be required to relieve obstructed areas, repair perforations, or when medical therapy fails (p 168). In children, because the disease may retard normal growth and development, surgery may be utilized more frequently, in addition to medications and hyperalimentation. Recurrence of the disease is possible even after surgery.

J. Prior to discharge, patients are instructed regarding diet, medications, and lifestyle. These patients may also have concerns about frequent malodorous stools. Referral to support groups for encouragement and coping strategies assist these individuals to return to a satisfying and productive life. Patients should be instructed to contact their physician at the first sign of IBD recurrence.

References

Brunner LS, Suddarth D. The Lippincott manual of nursing practice. 4th ed. Philadelphia: JB Lippincott, 1987.

Knapp AB. Gastroenterology. Baltimore: Williams & Wilkins, 1985.

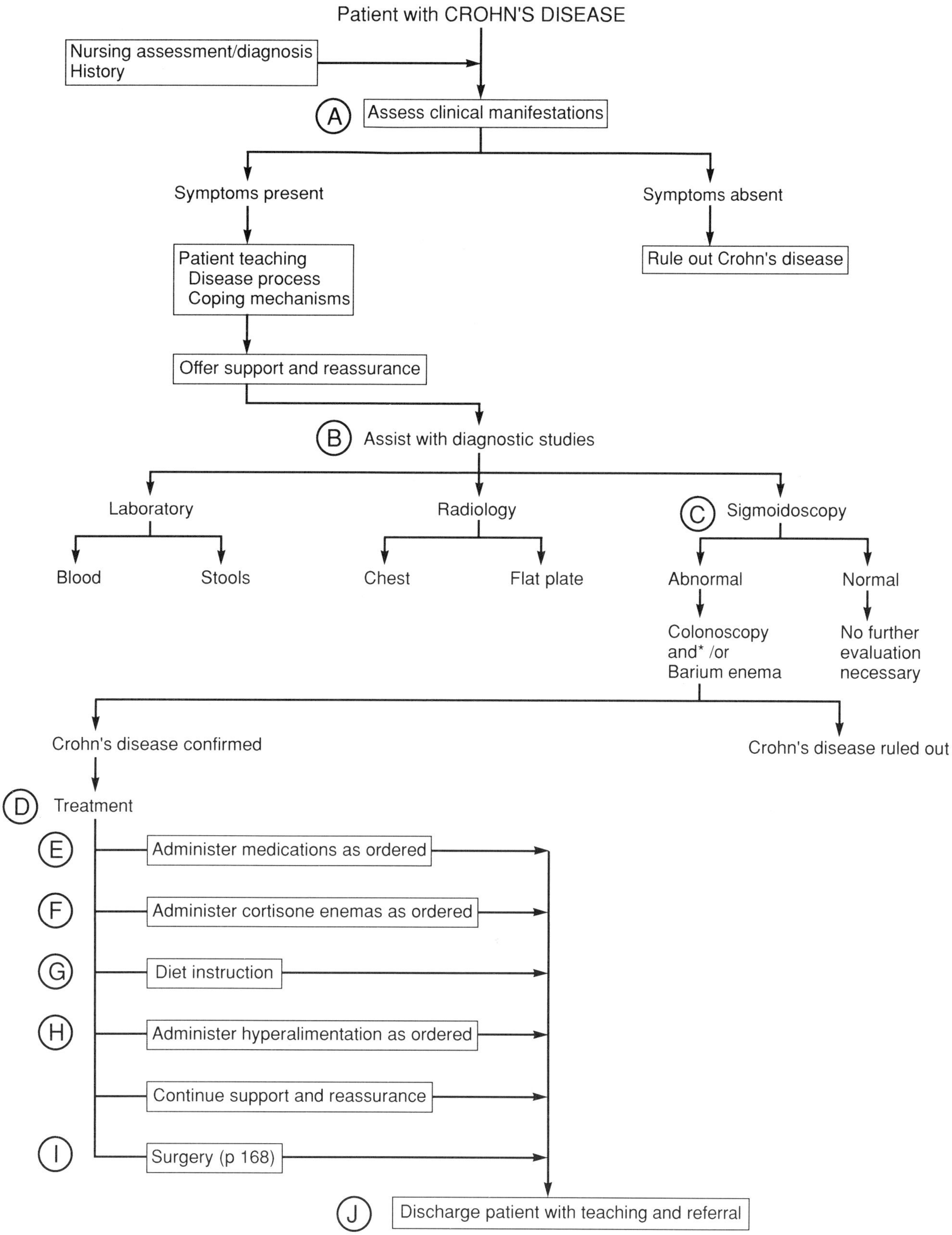

* If both colonoscopy and barium enema are to be done, schedule barium enema last.

Luckmann J, Sorensen KC. Medical-surgical nursing: a psychophysiologic approach. 3rd ed. Philadelphia: WB Saunders, 1987.

Sugawa C, Schumau B. Primer of gastrointestinal fiberoptic endoscopy. Boston: Little, Brown, 1981.

ULCERATIVE COLITIS

Gail Shores

Ulcerative colitis is one of a group of diseases known as chronic inflammatory bowel disease (IBD). IBD denotes any disease causing inflammation of the small and/or large intestine. Ulcerative colitis generally involves the large intestine (colon), and the inflammation and ulcerations are limited to the inner lining, unlike Crohn's disease (p 140), which often extends through all the layers of the intestinal wall and involves the small intestine as well. In severe cases of ulcerative colitis, the bowel wall may become very thin and the mucosa worn through with inflammation, causing dilation and eventual perforation.

A. Ulcerative colitis is more common than Crohn's disease (p 140), and the incidence peaks between the ages of 15 and 35 years, being equally prevalent among males and females. A strong familial tendency has been observed, which suggests either a genetic or an environmental cause, but as yet no definite cause has been identified. As with Crohn's disease, an autoimmune cause has been considered because of the extraintestinal symptoms such as arthritis, pericholangitis, liver involvement, and thyroid problems, which are often also seen in patients with ulcerative colitis. Psychological features need to be noted, since the initial presentation of the disease frequently occurs after a period of emotional stress, and recurrent episodes or exacerbations can be traced to emotional upsets.

B. The major symptoms of ulcerative colitis are bloody diarrhea and abdominal pain, frequently with associated fever and weight loss. In mild cases the patient may have one or two loose stools and no other symptoms. In severe cases there can be frequent liquid stools with blood and pus, severe cramping, and the patient may have anemia, dehydration, and anorexia.

C. The diagnostic work-up is essentially the same as for Crohn's disease. The following laboratory tests are done: complete blood count (CBC) with differential, electrolytes, erythrocyte sedimentation rate (ESR), and albumin and liver function tests. Radiography of the chest and abdomen is also performed. The results of these tests indicate the severity of the body's overall reaction to the inflammation in the colon. Sigmoidoscopy is done to check involvement of the rectal-sigmoid area. Any suspicious areas can be biopsied, and stool samples collected for examination to rule out parasites or bacterial infection.

D. After a rigid 48-hour preparation involving dietary restrictions and cleansing of the colon, one of two additional diagnostic tests is done: (1) colonoscopy, which involves direct visualization of the lining of the entire colon using a fiberoptic scope; or (2) a barium enema study, which is a radiologic evaluation of the colon following the insertion of barium. Upon direct visualization it is generally noted that in ulcerative colitis the rectum is almost always involved and the areas of involvement along the colon are continuous, without the "rectal sparing" and "skip areas" of uninvolved colon often seen in Crohn's disease. The colon radiograph often has a straight, "pipe-stem" appearance, and the normal haustra (pouchline markings) are absent.

E. Treatment is often difficult, but the goal is to reduce the inflammation and relieve the symptoms in the colon and other areas of the body that may be involved. Psychotherapy and sedation are often utilized to reduce stress.

F. Dietary management to eliminate irritating foods is helpful. Antidiarrheal and anticholinergic medications may be utilized in some cases. Vitamin and iron supplements are recommended for some patients to combat deficiencies and/or anemic conditions.

G. In patients with severe ulcerative colitis, hospitalization may be required. In these cases transfusions may be needed to treat anemia (p 340), and hyperalimentation may be required in order to allow the colon to rest. Corticosteroids or ACTH may be used, as well as azulfidine, to decrease inflammation.

H. Surgery may be required to relieve obstruction or repair perforation (p 168).

I. These patients need a good deal of nursing intervention in order to provide necessary teaching and support, and to assist in goal-setting and implementation of new habits and lifestyle changes.

References

Braunwald E, Isselbacher K, Petersdorf F, Wilson J, Martin J, Fauci A, eds. Harrison's principles of internal medicine. 11th ed. New York: McGraw-Hill, 1987.

Cello JP. Gastrointestinal disease: pathophysiology, diagnosis, management. 3rd ed. Philadelphia: WB Saunders, 1983.

Knapp AB. Gastroenterology. Baltimore: Williams & Wilkins, 1985.

Sugawa C, Schuman B. Primer of gastrointestinal fiberoptic endoscopy. Boston: Little, Brown, 1981.

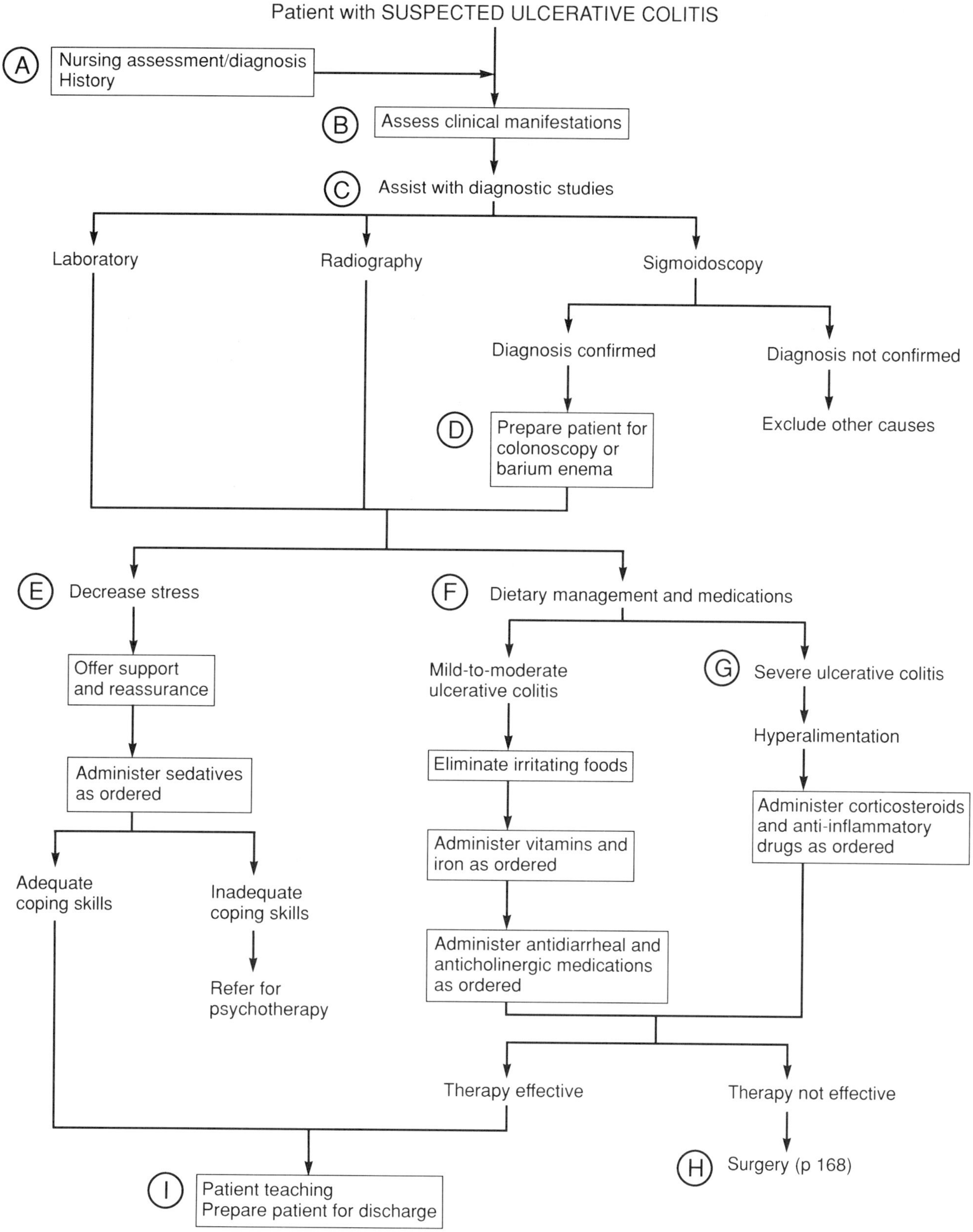
Patient with SUSPECTED ULCERATIVE COLITIS
A
Nursing assessment/diagnosis
History
B
Assess clinical manifestations
C
Assist with diagnostic studies
Laboratory
Radiography
Sigmoidoscopy
Diagnosis confirmed
Diagnosis not confirmed
D
Prepare patient for colonoscopy or barium enema
Exclude other causes
E
Decrease stress
F
Dietary management and medications
Offer support and reassurance
Mild-to-moderate ulcerative colitis
G
Severe ulcerative colitis
Hyperalimentation
Eliminate irritating foods
Administer sedatives as ordered
Administer corticosteroids and anti-inflammatory drugs as ordered
Administer vitamins and iron as ordered
Adequate coping skills
Inadequate coping skills
Administer antidiarrheal and anticholinergic medications as ordered
Refer for psychotherapy
Therapy effective
Therapy not effective
H
Surgery (p 168)
I
Patient teaching
Prepare patient for discharge

HEMORRHOIDS

Cecile A. Lengacher

Hemorrhoids are a condition of varicose veins or dilated internal or external veins in the rectal area and anus. The flow of blood through the hemorrhoidal venous plexus is impaired and causes dilatation and congestion of vessels of the rectum and anus. If the veins are above the internal sphincter, they are internal hemorrhoids; if they are outside the external sphincter, they are called external hemorrhoids. Causes of hemorrhoids can be linked to pregnancy, chronic liver disease, chronic constipation, straining on defecation, not taking time for defecation, obesity, constant sitting or standing, heavy lifting, heredity, and lack of exercise.

A. Diagnosis and treatment is based on the diagnostic test findings. A digital examination can confirm whether hemorrhoids are present: proctoscopy or anoscopy can identify internal hemorrhoids, and a radiography-barium enema can identify hemorrhoids and rule out carcinoma and inflammatory disease. This is of particular concern to patients over 40 years of age. A complete blood count (CBC) may reveal a decreased hemoglobin and hematocrit. Iron deficiency anemia (p 340) may develop if bleeding continues over a prolonged period.

B. Patients with external hemorrhoids have the clinical manifestations of anal pain with defecation, and pain without defecation if the hemorrhoids are inflamed or thrombosed. Other symptoms include protrusion of hemorrhoids, rectal bleeding, bleeding during defecation, anal prudish, and symptoms of incomplete defecation.

C. Medical treatment is determined by the extent of the problem. A conservative treatment plan includes diet therapy (high-fiber, low-roughage) and increased fluid intake. Patient teaching also addresses weight loss, exercise, and avoidance of constipation and straining on defecation.

D. Relief of anal pain may be obtained with the use of analgesics, stool softeners, sitz baths, hydrocortisone cream, antipruritics, and laxatives. The patient may be instructed to replace prolapsed hemorrhoids manually. However, they may later become irreducible. Privacy during defecation should be provided for, and sitz baths with perineal care after defecation should occur.

E. Patients with hemorrhoids should be encouraged to maintain proper evacuation at home with a program of routine exercise, proper diet, increased fluids, and weight control.

F. Alternative procedures such as surgery (p 172) may be indicated when symptoms are not relieved and/or the hemorrhoids are no longer reducible.

References

Brunner LS, Suddarth DS. Textbook of medical-surgical nursing. 4th ed. Philadelphia: JB Lippincott, 1988.

Boyd M, Tower B. Medical-surgical nursing: a study and learning tool. Springhouse, PA: Springhouse Corporation, 1988.

Sorensen K, Luckmann J. Basic nursing: psychophysiologic approach. 2nd ed. Philadelphia: WB Saunders, 1986.

Thompson JM, McFarland GK, Hirsch JE, Tucker SM, Bowers AC. Clinical nursing. St. Louis: CV Mosby, 1986.

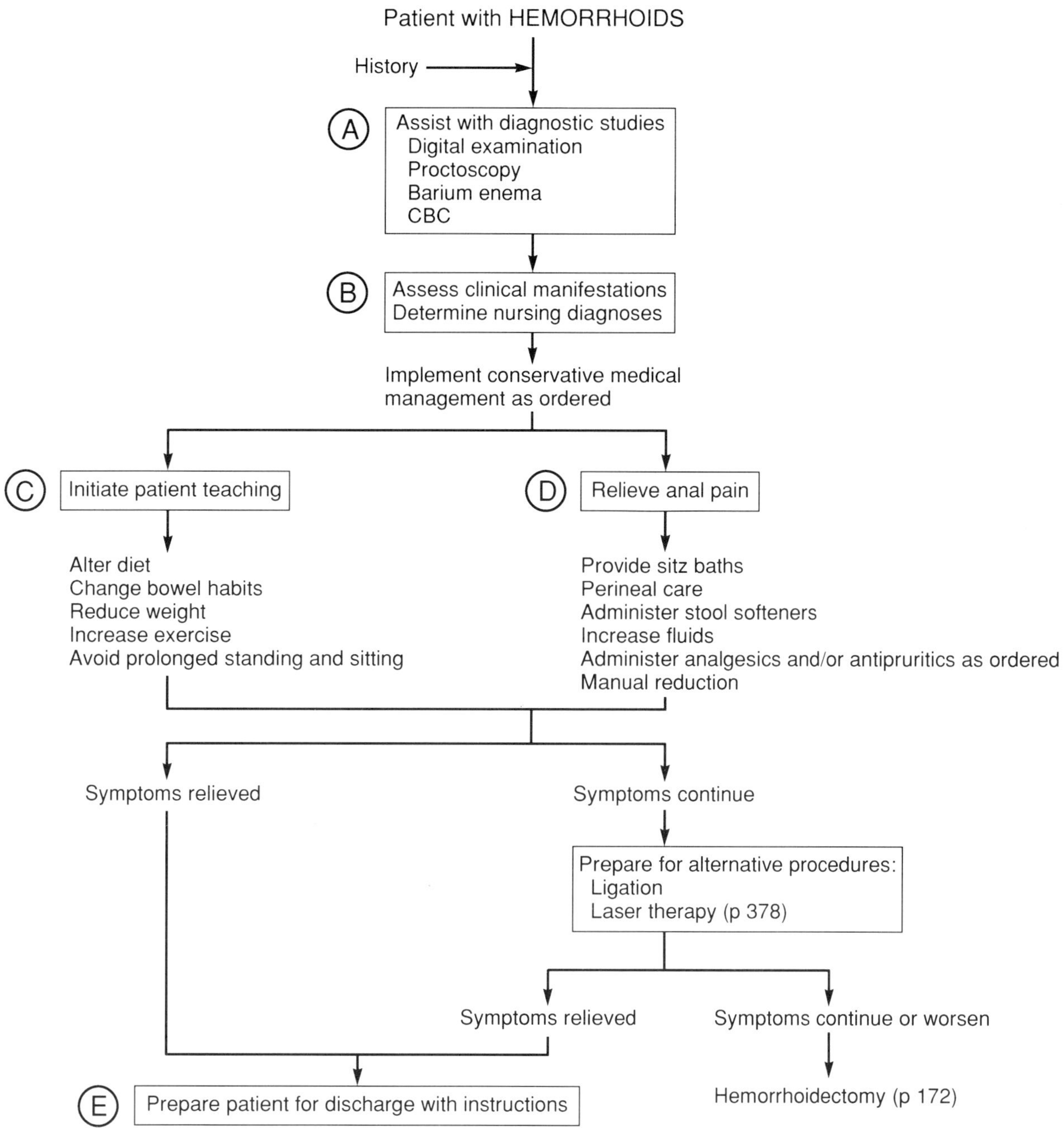
Patient with HEMORRHOIDS
History
A
Assist with diagnostic studies
Digital examination
Proctoscopy
Barium enema
CBC
B
Assess clinical manifestations
Determine nursing diagnoses
Implement conservative medical management as ordered
C
Initiate patient teaching
Alter diet
Change bowel habits
Reduce weight
Increase exercise
Avoid prolonged standing and sitting
D
Relieve anal pain
Provide sitz baths
Perineal care
Administer stool softeners
Increase fluids
Administer analgesics and/or antipruritics as ordered
Manual reduction
Symptoms relieved
Symptoms continue
Prepare for alternative procedures:
Ligation
Laser therapy (p 378)
Symptoms relieved
Symptoms continue or worsen
Hemorrhoidectomy (p 172)
E
Prepare patient for discharge with instructions

HEPATIC CIRRHOSIS

Barbara Kalo

Hepatic cirrhosis is a chronic disease of the liver. Diffuse inflammation and fibrosis of the liver results in loss of liver function and obstructs the flow of portal venous blood through the liver, resulting in portal hypertension. Ascites occurs as a manifestation of portal hypertension. With profound liver failure, the damaged liver cells fail to detoxify and convert ammonia into urea. This increase of ammonia in the blood causes brain dysfunction and damage, resulting in hepatic coma. The major causes of cirrhosis are excessive consumption of alcohol (p 402) and chronic viral hepatitis (p 150). Men between the ages of 40 and 60 are most commonly affected.

A. The patient presents with anorexia, weight loss, edema, weakness, and fatigue. There may be jaundice, fever, change in bowel habits, esophageal varices, and ascites. Changes in neurologic status such as level of consciousness, concentration, memory, and asterixis may indicate the progression of liver damage.

B. Explanation of laboratory studies and diagnostic tests alleviates patient fears. If jaundice is present, the serum bilirubin is elevated. Serum glutamic oxaloacetic transaminase (SGOT) is elevated if alcoholic cirrhosis is present. A complete blood count shows anemia, leukopenia, and thrombocytopenia. Diagnostic procedures may include liver biopsy (p 158), paracentesis (p 158), esophagoscopy, ultrasonography, angiography, percutaneous transhepatic portography, and electroencephalography.

C. Medications that may be given to patients with cirrhosis of the liver include diuretics such as Aldactone, Diuril, and Lasix; neomycin sulfate, to decrease the bacterial flora so the formation of ammonia is decreased; and lactulose, which decreases the pH of the colon from 7.0 to 5.0 (the acidic environment discourages bacterial growth and traps the ammonia so it is eliminated in the feces).

D. Management is directed toward removal or treatment of the causative factors and preventing additional liver damage. Supportive nursing care and observation of the symptoms are necessary to determine the course of the liver disease. Evaluate vital signs and neurologic status as ordered, and notify the physician when they are abnormal. Changes in the mental status may indicate the onset of hepatic coma.

E. Provide small frequent feedings that are high in calories, carbohydrates, and protein and low in fat and sodium. If the patient cannot tolerate food by mouth, tube feedings and/or hyperalimentation may be indicated. Vitamin supplements (A, D, and E), folic acid, and iron may be prescribed. A dietary referral may be indicated.

F. Measure weight daily to assess weight gain where anorexia and weight loss are symptoms. If ascites is present, measurement of abdominal girth is necessary to determine the progression of ascites and its response to treatment. Monitoring and documenting intake and output are important at any stage of liver disease.

G. Poor nutritional status, fatigue, and immobility may lead to skin breakdown. Frequent turning and positioning and keeping the patient's skin clean and dry are important aspects of care.

H. Plan care to allow for rest between treatments, procedures, and visitors. Position the patient for maximum respiratory function with minimum effort. Oxygen may be given to reduce the effort of breathing.

I. If coagulopathy causes bleeding, the patient must be monitored closely and immediate intervention instituted. Techniques to protect the patient include padded siderails, avoiding sharp objects, and using small-gauge needles for injection. Hemorrhage from ruptured esophageal varices may also occur in patients with advanced liver disease and is life-threatening. Signs and symptoms include melena, hematemesis, hypotension, tachycardia, and cool, clammy skin. Immediate intervention is required, e.g., iced saline lavage, balloon tamponade, vasopressors, and injection sclerotherapy. Transfer the patient to the ICU for stabilization. Surgery may be indicated to reduce portal hypertension (portal-system shunt) or ligate the varices.

J. Treatment may be a slow process. Discharge instructions include measures to prevent further damage to the liver, such as abstinence from alcohol and drugs, and a dietary regimen specific to salt and protein intake, vitamin supplements, and fluid restriction. Weight gain, edema, bleeding, fever, or increased abdominal girth should be reported. As the disease progresses and coma occurs, provide support and teaching to the family.

References

Brunner LS, Suddarth DS. The Lippincott manual of nursing practice. 4th ed. Philadelphia: JB Lippincott, 1986.

Brunner LS, Suddarth DS. Textbook of medical-surgical nursing. 6th ed. Philadelphia: JB Lippincott, 1988:873–886.

Lewis SM, Collier IC. Medical-surgical nursing: assessment and management of clinical problems. New York: McGraw-Hill, 1983.

Thompson JM, McFarland GK, Hirsch JE, Tucker SM, Bowers AC. Clinical nursing. St. Louis: CV Mosby, 1986.

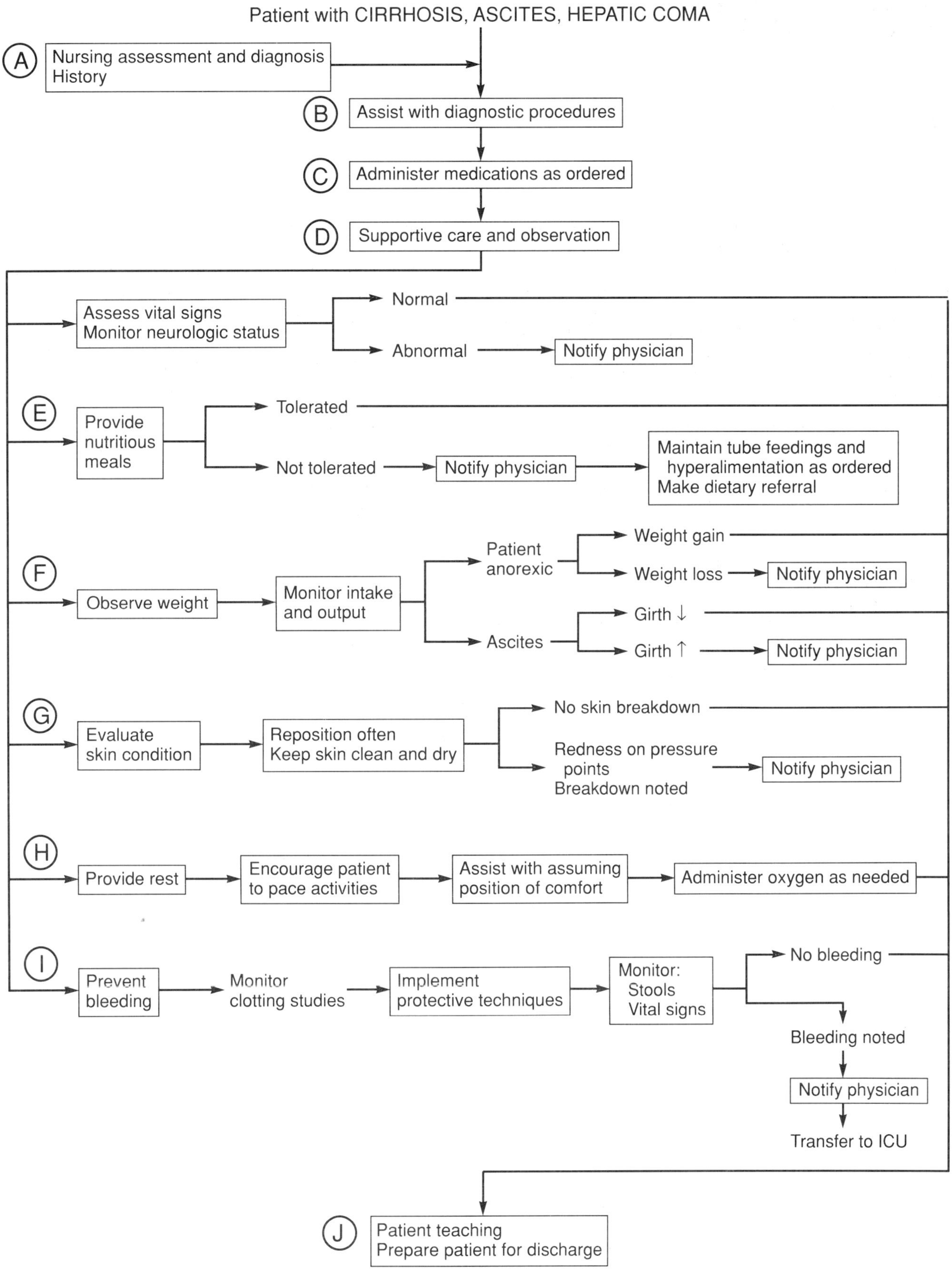

Patient with CIRRHOSIS, ASCITES, HEPATIC COMA
A
Nursing assessment and diagnosis
History
B
Assist with diagnostic procedures
C
Administer medications as ordered
D
Supportive care and observation
Assess vital signs
Monitor neurologic status
Normal
Abnormal
Notify physician
E
Provide nutritious meals
Tolerated
Not tolerated
Notify physician
Maintain tube feedings and hyperalimentation as ordered
Make dietary referral
F
Observe weight
Monitor intake and output
Patient anorexic
Weight gain
Weight loss
Notify physician
Ascites
Girth ↓
Girth ↑
Notify physician
G
Evaluate skin condition
Reposition often
Keep skin clean and dry
No skin breakdown
Redness on pressure points
Breakdown noted
Notify physician
H
Provide rest
Encourage patient to pace activities
Assist with assuming position of comfort
Administer oxygen as needed
I
Prevent bleeding
Monitor clotting studies
Implement protective techniques
Monitor:
Stools
Vital signs
No bleeding
Bleeding noted
Notify physician
Transfer to ICU
J
Patient teaching
Prepare patient for discharge

PANCREATITIS

Barbara Kalo

The pancreas facilitates digestion through the secretion of enzymes into the proximal duodenum. Pancreatitis is inflammation of the pancreas and can be brought about by several factors, primarily alcoholism (p 402) and biliary tract diseases. Trauma, viral infections, or the digestion of the pancreas by one of the enzymes it produces may also cause pancreatitis, which may be acute or chronic. The severity of the disease varies with the degree of destruction of the pancreas.

A. The nursing assessment reveals abdominal pain, which may be epigastric or in the left upper quadrant. Nausea, vomiting, and fever may be present. In a more advanced form of pancreatitis, restlessness, hallucinations, coarse tremors, or shock may be noted.

B. Explain the diagnostic procedures to the patient to help alleviate fears. The serum amylase level is elevated in acute pancreatitis, but often is not elevated in chronic pancreatitis. Arteriography and radiography allow visualization of the pancreas and assessment of its structure and function. Serum and urine tests are also done. An amylase-creatinine clearance ratio (ACCR) gives the best indication of pancreatic disease. A ratio greater than 6 percent indicates pancreatitis. Fecal fat determination helps assess fat digestion. Abnormally low lipase levels may lead to fat maldigestion and malabsorption.

C. Nursing care is primarily supportive—focusing on relieving symptoms, assessment, and observation. Provide relief from pain as necessary. Opiates cause spasms of the sphincter of Oddi, which compounds the obstruction, so meperidine (Demerol) is usually ordered.

D. Observation of vital signs is important to assess the severity of fever, hypotension, and tachycardia that may be present. Vital signs may also identify impending shock (p 70) caused by hemorrhage or toxemia from activated pancreatic enzymes. Monitoring arterial blood gases (ABGs) enables detection of early signs of respiratory failure.

E. Antiemetics may be ordered for nausea or vomiting. A nasogastric (NG) tube may be inserted and connected to suction to remove hydrochloric acid from the stomach. Patients are given nothing by mouth to reduce enzyme stimulation. Intravenous fluids are maintained, and blood may be ordered. Intake and output should be recorded. Diet is resumed slowly as nausea and vomiting subside. A bland, low-fat diet in six small daily feedings may be ordered for chronic pancreatitis.

F. If the patient is free of complications, discharge with specific instructions about diet, rest, and medication. Patients with acute pancreatitis are at risk of infection, so they should be instructed to avoid high-risk situations. These patients also frequently develop diabetes (p 176) and should be aware of reportable symptoms such as thirst, weight loss, and increased urination.

References

Brunner LS, Suddarth DS. The Lippincott manual of nursing practice. 4th ed. Philadelphia: JB Lippincott, 1986.

Brunner LS, Suddarth DS. Textbook of medical-surgical nursing. 6th ed. Philadelphia: JB Lippincott, 1988.

Lewis SM, Collier IC. Medical-surgical nursing: assessment and management of clinical problems. New York: McGraw-Hill, 1983.

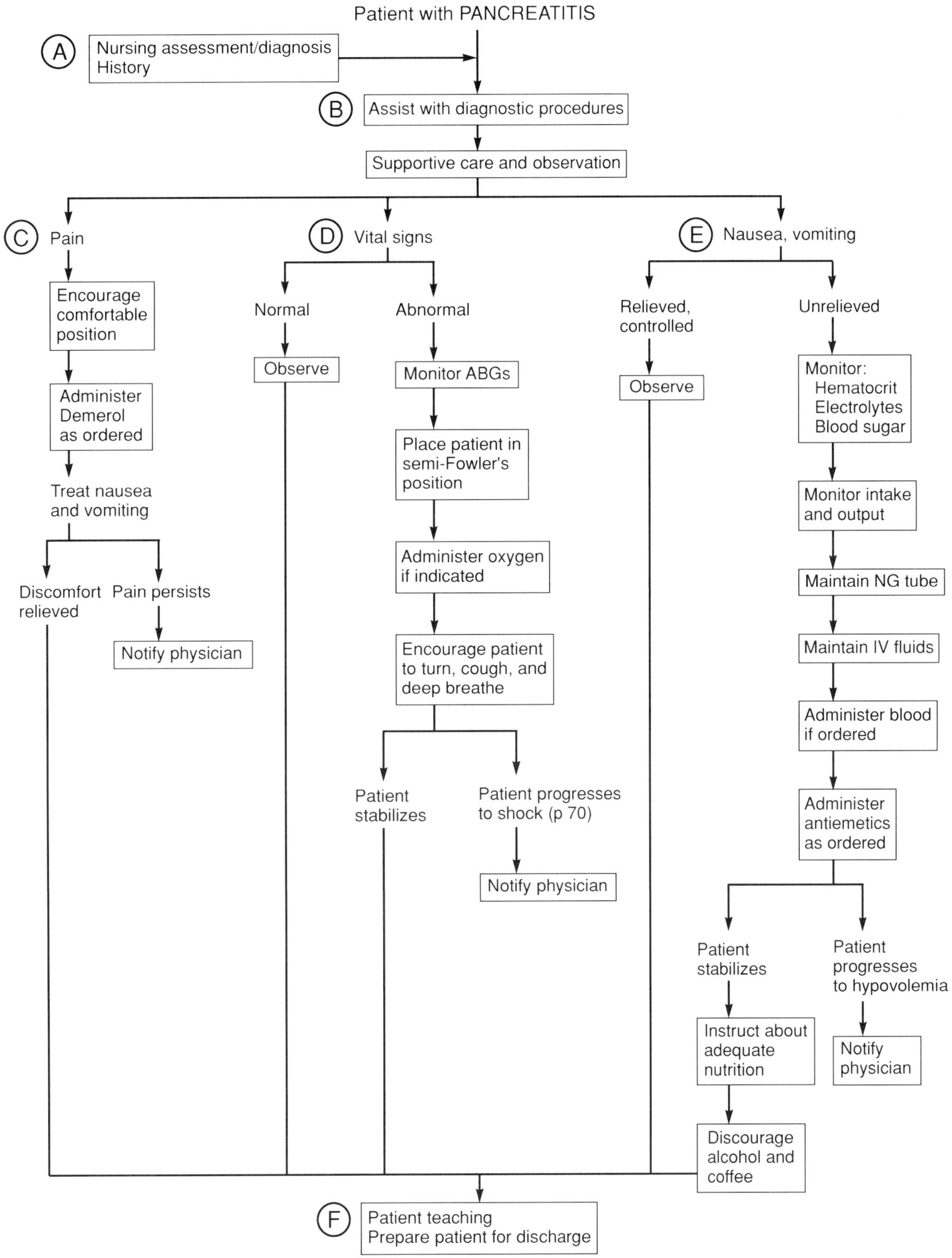
Patient with PANCREATITIS
A
Nursing assessment/diagnosis
History
B
Assist with diagnostic procedures
Supportive care and observation
C
Pain
Encourage comfortable position
Administer Demerol as ordered
Treat nausea and vomiting
Discomfort relieved
Pain persists
Notify physician
D
Vital signs
Normal
Observe
Abnormal
Monitor ABGs
Place patient in semi-Fowler's position
Administer oxygen if indicated
Encourage patient to turn, cough, and deep breathe
Patient stabilizes
Patient progresses to shock (p 70)
Notify physician
E
Nausea, vomiting
Relieved, controlled
Observe
Unrelieved
Monitor:
Hematocrit
Electrolytes
Blood sugar
Monitor intake and output
Maintain NG tube
Maintain IV fluids
Administer blood if ordered
Administer antiemetics as ordered
Patient stabilizes
Instruct about adequate nutrition
Discourage alcohol and coffee
Patient progresses to hypovolemia
Notify physician
F
Patient teaching
Prepare patient for discharge

VIRAL HEPATITIS

Joy Gorzeman

Hepatitis is an inflammation of the liver that results in a disturbance of bilirubin excretion. There are three forms of hepatitis, each caused by a different virus: hepatitis A or infectious hepatitis; hepatitis B or serum hepatitis; and Non-A, Non-B hepatitis, which is most often seen after blood transfusions. Hepatitis A and B are most common. Hepatitis may also occur as a secondary infection to other illness such as cytomegalovirus (p 360), herpes simplex, rubella, and Epstein-Barr syndrome (p 358).

A. Hepatitis A is primarily transmitted through the oral-fecal route via contaminated food, water, or shellfish and is often associated with poor sanitation. Hepatitis B is transmitted through saliva, blood, and semen. Health-care workers, homosexuals, morticians, and parenteral drug abusers are at higher risk for contracting hepatitis B.

B. Immune serum globulin should be administered within 72 hours to individuals who have been exposed to hepatitis A. Hepatitis B vaccine may be given to individuals who are identified as being at high risk of exposure to hepatitis B.

C. An increased SGPT and/or the presence of IgM (immunoglobulin M) indicates hepatitis A; hepatitis B is diagnosed on the basis of the presence of HBsAg (the hepatitis B antigen). The bilirubin is also usually elevated. The absence of any of these laboratory findings indicates non-A, non-B hepatitis or some other viral infection.

D. Clinical manifestations reflect liver cell damage and are similar for any form of viral hepatitis. Although patients with hepatitis A are highly contagious early in the disease, they may not experience symptoms until jaundice appears a couple of weeks later. Preicteric symptoms that may occur include headache, fatigue, anorexia, and fever. Hepatitis B patients may develop rashes and complain of arthralgia. During the icteric phase, patients may manifest dark urine, jaundiced sclera, and liver enlargement with tenderness. Non-A, non-B symptoms are similar to those of hepatitis B.

E. Treatment for any form of hepatitis is primarily directed at relief of symptoms and providing support.

F. Universal precautions must be implemented. Patients and families need instructions regarding personal hygiene and transmission of the disease. Special attention should be given to enteric precautions with hepatitis A and to body fluids and blood with hepatitis B.

G. Recovery is long and slow. Activities must be restricted as patients need a great deal of rest. Although hepatitis is not usually a severe or fatal disease, the length of the illness requires emotional support, and diversional activities should be planned as the patient begins to feel better.

H. Maintaining nutrition is frequently a challenge because of the anorexia and the body's diseased state. Fluids should be encouraged. Meals should be balanced and incorporate the patient's food preferences whenever possible. Low-fat and high-carbohydrate foods are advised. Alcohol must be avoided because of the toxicity to the liver.

I. Liver function is monitored, and the nurse must observe the patient for complications. Jaundice may cause pruritus. Skin integrity must be assessed. Antipruritic medications may be ordered. The enlarged liver may cause discomfort. Pain should be assessed and recorded. If pain occurs suddenly or becomes severe, notify the physician.

J. Chronic, persistent hepatitis and fatal hepatitis, although rare, are more common from hepatitis B. Development of confusion, asterixis, or bleeding should be reported and observed.

K. Preparation for discharge should include instructions regarding activity level, diet, and disease transmission. The patient and family should be advised about personal hygiene and precautions such as handwashing, not sharing personal items such as razors, and avoiding preparation of food by the patient. Patients must be reminded to avoid alcohol and nonprescribed drugs, especially aspirin and sedatives. The importance of follow-up visits and laboratory studies must be stressed. Patients should avoid sexual activity until tests are clear.

References

Brunner LS, Suddarth DS. The Lippincott manual of nursing practice. 4th ed. Philadelphia: JB Lippincott, 1986.

Luckmann J, Sorensen KC. Medical-surgical nursing: a psychophysiologic approach 3rd ed. Philadelphia: WB Saunders, 1987.

Thompson JM, McFarland GK, Hirsch JE, Tucker SM, Bowers AC. Clinical nursing. St. Louis: CV Mosby, 1986.

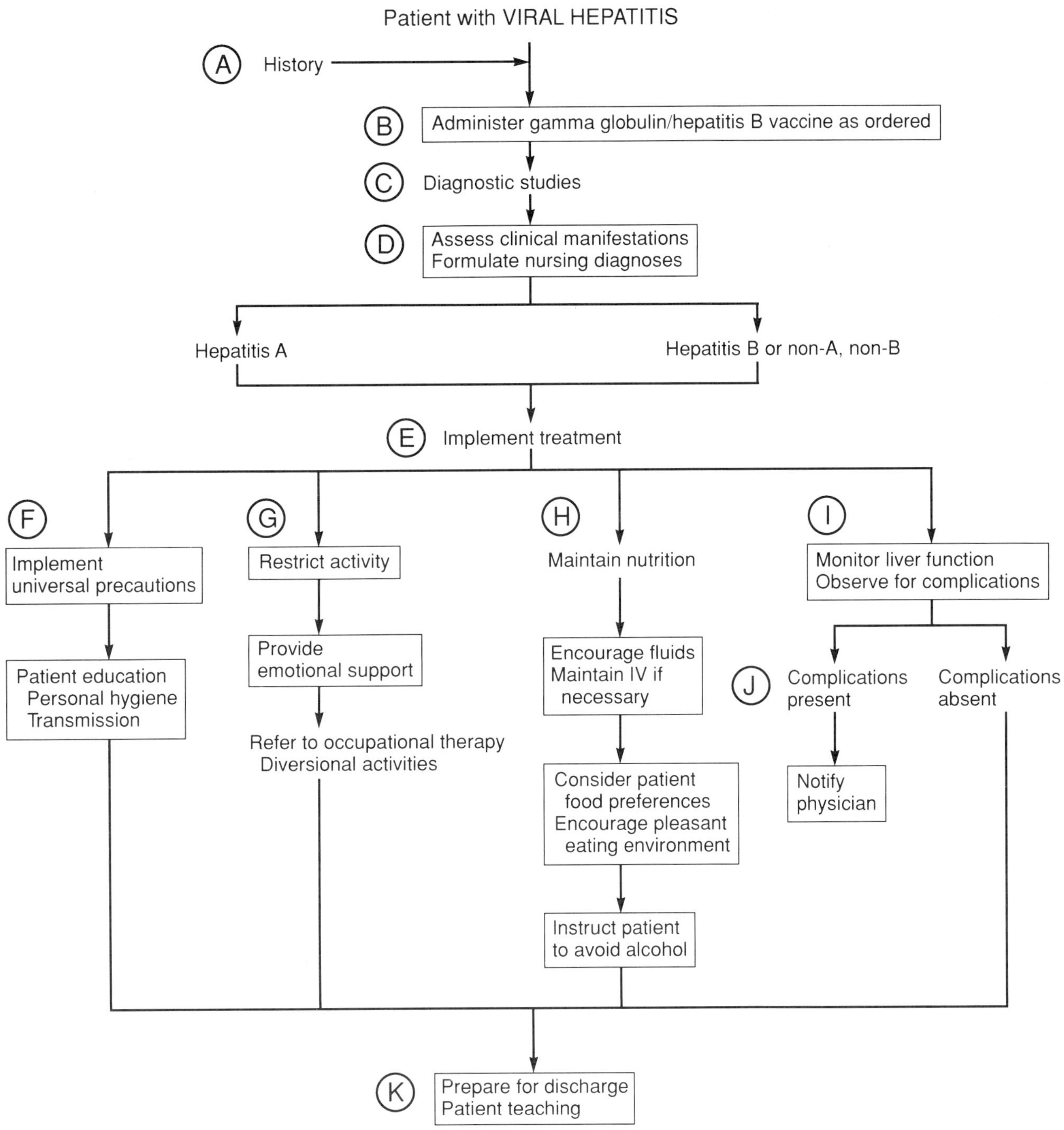
Patient with VIRAL HEPATITIS
A History
B Administer gamma globulin/hepatitis B vaccine as ordered
C Diagnostic studies
D Assess clinical manifestations
Formulate nursing diagnoses
Hepatitis A
Hepatitis B or non-A, non-B
E Implement treatment
F Implement universal precautions
Patient education
Personal hygiene
Transmission
G Restrict activity
Provide emotional support
Refer to occupational therapy
Diversional activities
H Maintain nutrition
Encourage fluids
Maintain IV if necessary
Consider patient food preferences
Encourage pleasant eating environment
Instruct patient to avoid alcohol
I Monitor liver function
Observe for complications
J Complications present
Complications absent
Notify physician
K Prepare for discharge
Patient teaching

ESOPHAGEAL AND STOMACH CANCER

Joy Gorzeman

Esophageal cancers usually occur in people over age 50, more often in men and in blacks. Primary adenocarcinoma of the esophagus is rare; however, metastasis from other cancers, such as breast cancer, may affect the esophagus. At least half of esophageal cancers occur at the esophagogastric junction and arise from the stomach. Stomach cancers are most common in males of middle age and usually occur in the lower half of the stomach. The incidence of stomach cancer has decreased in recent years.

A. Esophageal cancer may be related to the use of alcohol and tobacco, ingestion of hot foods and drinks, and environmental carcinogens. Stomach cancer has been associated with eating smoked fish and with ulcers (p 130). Genetic factors are also believed to play a role in stomach cancer.

B. Clinical manifestations of esophageal and stomach cancer do not usually appear until late in the disease process. Patients with esophageal cancer may notice difficulty swallowing, which may progress to pain with swallowing, and results in anorexia, weight loss, weakness, and anemia. Pain in the chest and respiratory difficulty may indicate metastasis. Other late symptoms may be foul breath and regurgitation. Patients with stomach cancer may feel full after minimal intake and experience a distaste for meat. Persistent indigestion or midepigastric pain should be investigated. Often, patients complain of ulcer-like symptoms and the lesion is later found to be malignant. Vomiting, especially coffee-ground material, is another late symptom.

C. Diagnostic studies for any of these clinical manifestations include a barium swallow to identify sources of gastrointestinal bleeding and to outline the tumor. Chest films, bronchoscopy, endoscopy, and liver function tests may be done to assess for metastasis. If stomach tumor is suspected, hematocrit is checked for anemia from blood loss, and stools are checked for occult blood.

D. Since symptoms rarely occur early in the disease, prognosis is often poor and treatment is basically palliative. Providing a way to eat may be the goal rather than removal of the tumor. Surgical procedures depend on the type and location of the lesion. Gastric pull-up or resection may be done for esophageal tumors. If necessary, a gastrostomy is done to relieve obstruction and allow for nutrition. Another method of nutritional assistance may be insertion of a Celestin tube to facilitate swallowing. Subtotal or total gastrectomy may be done for patients with stomach tumors (p 166).

E. Combinations of radiation and chemotherapy (p 408) are used postoperatively, although radiation has not proved effective for stomach tumors.

F. Patients need the opportunity to discuss their feelings and concerns about their illness and its grim prognosis.

G. In addition to routine postoperative and postprocedural care, special emphasis must be given to nutritional support and the promotion of physical comfort.

H. Patient teaching must include rationale for treatment, caring for tubes that are in place, elevating the head of the bed, and not lying down after eating in order to prevent aspiration or regurgitation. Referral to available support groups should be made, and arrangements for home care must be confirmed. Potential side effects of radiation or chemotherapy and a schedule of treatment and follow-up must be explained.

References

Brunner LS, Suddarth DS. The Lippincott manual of nursing practice. 4th ed. Philadelphia: JB Lippincott, 1986.

Luckmann J, Sorensen KC. Medical-surgical nursing: a psychophysioplogic approach. 3rd ed. Philadelphia: WB Saunders, 1987.

Thompson JM, McFarland GK, Hirsch JE, Tucker SM, Bowers AC. Clinical nursing. St. Louis: CV Mosby, 1986.

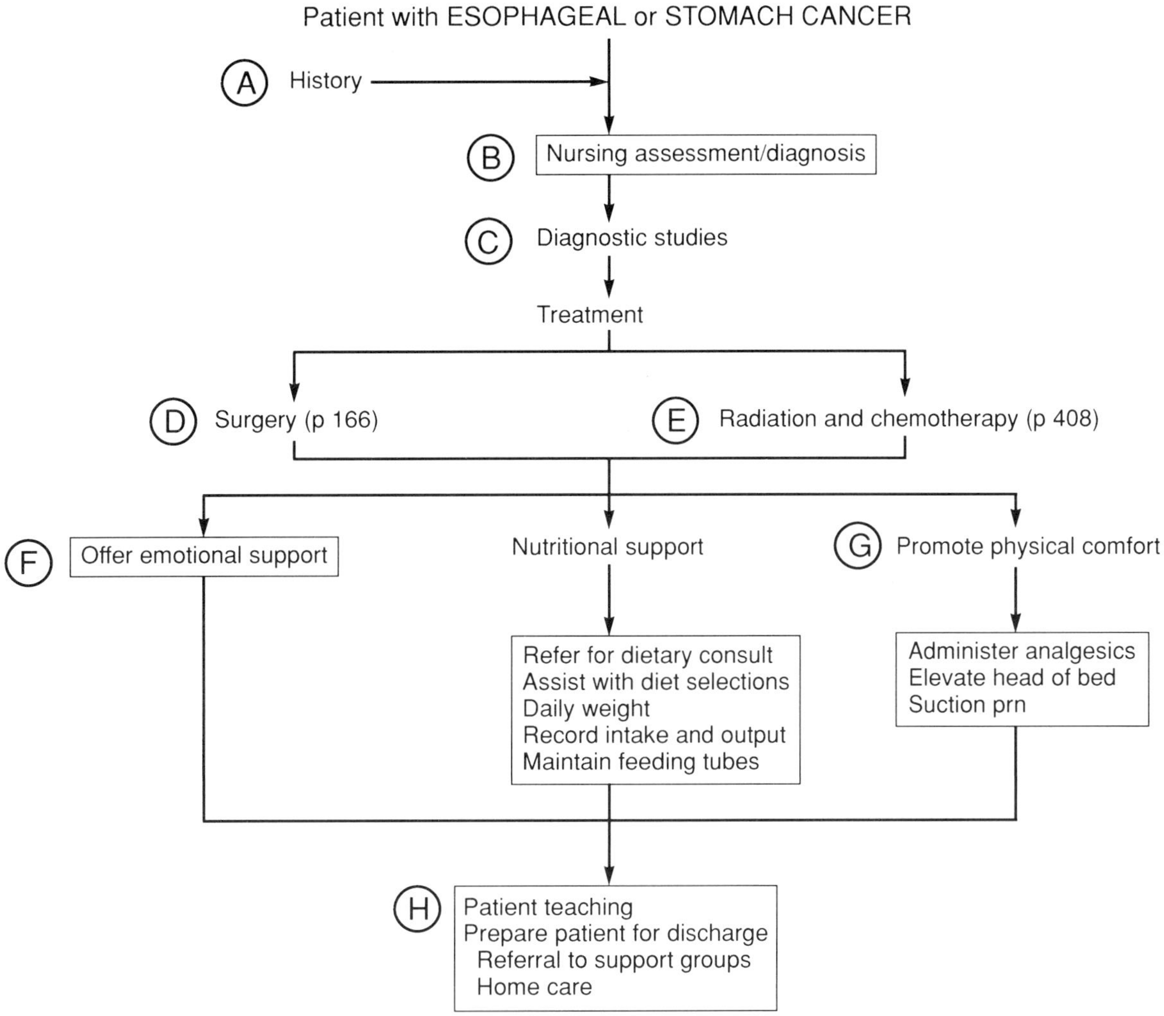
Patient with ESOPHAGEAL or STOMACH CANCER
A History
B Nursing assessment/diagnosis
C Diagnostic studies
Treatment
D Surgery (p 166)
E Radiation and chemotherapy (p 408)
F Offer emotional support
Nutritional support
G Promote physical comfort
Refer for dietary consult
Assist with diet selections
Daily weight
Record intake and output
Maintain feeding tubes
Administer analgesics
Elevate head of bed
Suction prn
H Patient teaching
Prepare patient for discharge
Referral to support groups
Home care

PANCREATIC CANCER

Carol Bowdoin
Barbara Greaux

Cancer of the pancreas is a disease primarily affecting males 60 to 70 years of age who often have a history of alcoholism (p 402), cigarette smoking, excessive caffeine and fat intake, and exposure to chemicals. The cancer may arise in the head, tail, or body of the pancreas. The insulin-secreting (beta) cells may or may not be affected. Metastasis occurs first in the regional lymph nodes and liver; spread may be to the lungs, intestines, adrenals, and bone. Prognosis is extremely poor, with death usually occurring within 1 year of the appearance of symptoms.

A. Initial symptoms are often vague, with complaints developing 4 to 9 months prior to diagnosis, thereby reducing cure rate. Symptoms present as a triad of weight loss, abdominal pain, and jaundice. The patient may complain of bloating and nonspecific dull to severe pain in the back or epigastic area after eating, which may be worse at night when lying down. Patients may say that relief is obtained by drawing up the legs or walking in a bent position.

B. The patient may present with right or left upper quadrant pain, clay-colored stools, dark urine, jaundice, and itching. Pain in the right upper quadrant suggests a tumor of the head of the pancreas; left upper quadrant pain suggests involvement of the body or tail of the pancreas. Anorexia with resulting malnutrition may occur because the patient is afraid of precipitating episodes of pain. Patients are often anxious and have a "Sense of impending doom" or premonition of serious illness. Trousseau's sign or migratory thrombophlebitis may also be detected.

C. Diagnostic studies include serum bilirubin, alkaline phosphatase, serum aspartate aminotransferase (AST), and prothrombin time. The carcinoembryonic antigen (CEA) level is elevated in 90 percent of these patients. A titer of 20 mg/ml is associated with metastasis. Radiologic procedures such as upper gastrointestinal series, gallbladder series, and fiberoptic examination (endoscopic retrograde cholangiopancreatography—ERCP) of the duodenum and pancreatic ducts may be beneficial. Computed tomography (CT), ultrasonography, angiography, and fine-needle biopsy are effective tools to ascertain a differential diagnosis, eliminating unnecessary surgery.

D. Surgical intervention is the primary treatment for a resectable tumor. Five-year survival is about 25 percent. The tumor is removed unless it has invaded adjacent vital structures. The Whipple procedure removes the head and/or neck of the pancreas, adjacent stomach, distal portion of the common duct and duodenum. Severe malnutrition results. Cholecystojejunostomy or gastrojejunostomy is done to relieve obstruction when the Whipple procedure cannot be done. Distal pancreatectomy and splenectomy are indicated in cancer of the body and tail of the pancreas. Total pancreatectomy involves removal of the common bile duct, stomach, duodenum, pancreas, and spleen resulting in severe, brittle diabetes (p 176).

E. Preoperative nursing care is similar to that for the patient preparing for major surgery (p 2). The patient may require nutritional building prior to surgery with a bland, low-fat diet. Hyperalimentation may be indicated for the severely malnourished patient. Vitamin K may be administered for prothrombin deficiencies.

F. Postoperative nursing care is similar to that for patients receiving gastrointestinal surgery, e.g., cholecystectomy (p 160) and gastrectomy (p 166). Conditions such as malnutrition or diabetes that result from a specific surgical procedure are managed symptomatically. Pancreatic enzymes (Pancrease or Viokase) are administered with meals. Nursing care focuses on relief of pain, stimulation of appetite, and psychological support.

G. Complications such as hemorrhage, vascular collapse, or hepatorenal failure may necessitate transfer to the ICU because of the multiple intravenous and arterial lines needed to monitor fluid and blood replacement.

H. The immediate and long-term outcomes of treatment are uncertain, which requires the nurse to be especially sensitive to the apprehension of both patient and family. The family may experience anticipatory grief. Referral to the psychiatric liaison nurse may help them to cope with the stresses of this illness and its prognosis.

I. Palliative treatment involves radiation therapy and chemotherapy (p 408). A Hickman catheter may be inserted to provide access for medications and nutrition.

J. Families should be referred to a local hospice organization for assistance with pain management in the terminal phase of the illness.

References

Brunner LS, Suddarth DS. The Lippincott manual of nursing practice. 3rd ed. Philadelphia: JB Lippincott, 1982:466–467.

Brunner LS, Suddarth DS. Medical-surgical nursing. 6th ed. Philadelphia: JB Lippincott, 1988:982–983.

Bullock BL, Rosenthal PP. Pathophysiology: adaptations and alterations in function. 2nd ed. Boston: Scott, Foresman/Little, Brown College Division, 1988:554–555.

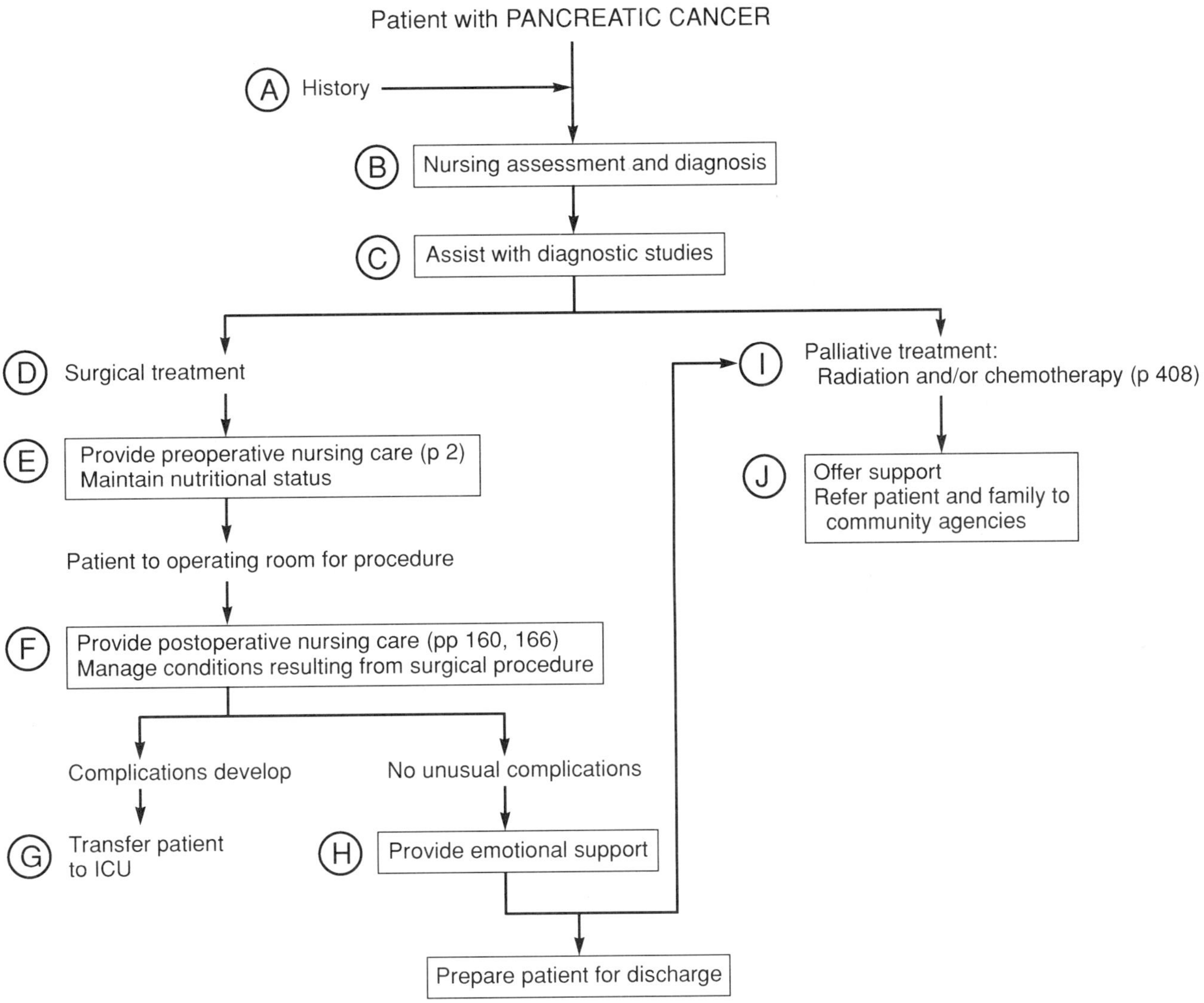

Jones DA, Dunbar CF, Jirovec MM. Medical-surgical nursing: a conceptual approach. 2nd ed. New York: McGraw-Hill, 1982:684–685.

Thompson JM, McFarland GK, Hirsch JE, Tucker SM, Bowers AC. Clinical nursing. St. Louis: CV Mosby, 1986:1435–1436.

CANCER OF THE LIVER

Barbara Greaux

Cancer of the liver is usually metastatic in origin. Primary tumors are related to a history of cirrhosis (p 146) or chronic liver disease (type B viral hepatitis, p 150). A rare form of tumor is associated with exposure to polyvinyl chloride. Symptoms arise as the liver is unable to function normally. The clinical course is marked by rapid deterioration, resulting in death after several months. The disease usually develops insidiously with vague, nonspecific symptoms and occurs predominately in men.

A. Patients present with complaints of recent weight loss, extreme weakness, anorexia, and a continual ache in the epigastric and back areas. Rapid liver enlargement, jaundice, ascites, and other signs of liver failure such as bruising, may indicate a terminal state.

B. A complete nursing care plan is made after gathering data and doing a thorough physical assessment. Care focuses on comfort, nutrition, preventing injury, and emotional support.

C. Explain and prepare patient for procedures and treatment protocols. A signed, witnessed, and dated consent must precede each procedure. Intake is restricted prior to initiating a new protocol. Allay patient and significant others' concerns, obtain vital signs, monitor intravenous infusion, observe biopsy or surgical sites and dressings, and evaluate medications or anesthesia used. Fluids, nutrition, and activity levels may be resumed after the procedure, unless contraindicated. A position of comfort and rest should be provided.

D. Medical treatment may pursue a palliative or surgical direction based on the findings from diagnostic tests to rule out other disease processes: radiographic tests such as ultrasonography, CT scan, a liver biopsy (p 158), magnetic resonance imaging (MRI), arteriography, and radioactive scintigraphy. Laboratory studies reveal an elevated CEA level (malignancy), elevated serum enzyme and ammonia levels (liver failure), and abnormal blood count (anemia). Prothrombin time, partial thromboplastin time, and platelet levels are altered if bleeding tendencies exist.

E. Liver lobectomy may effect a cure, depending on the health of the patient and the extent of the disease. A liver transplant may also be considered. The patient requires constant monitoring in the ICU for the first 2 days postoperatively, due to extensive blood loss and possible cardiopulmonary or metabolic complications.

F. Treatment is geared toward symptom control and palliation. Radiation is used to reduce tumor size and increase comfort and mobility. Chemotherapy (p 408) can be delivered by continuous infusion via an implantable pump to the liver, through the hepatic artery. Percutaneous biliary or transhepatic drainage can be used to reestablish biliary drainage if obstruction is present.

G. Treatment of pain is symptomatic and palliative. Brompton's mixture can be given orally and titrated to suit the individual patient's needs. Intravenous morphine can be given with the dosage controlled on demand by the patient. Spiritual and psychological distress and grieving can be assessed by the experienced nurse or referred to a minister, psychiatric liaison nurse, or grief counselor.

H. Weight loss with marked cachexia is treated by lipid therapy and hyperalimentation. Observe the central line closely to prevent complications (e.g., infection, bleeding, erosion). Potential hyperglycemia (p 176) is avoided with frequent glucoscan monitoring and insulin coverage. If diarrhea becomes a problem, adjust hyperalimentation to prevent excoriation and breakdown of skin. Offer frequent, small feedings and adequate hydration on a regular schedule. Maintain an accurate intake and output record. Record daily morning weights.

I. Debilitation occurs with loss of strength and muscle wasting as hepatomegaly increases. Radiation therapy and chemotherapy may be contributing factors. Activities should be planned to conserve strength and provide rest between treatments. Referral to physical therapy for exercises to increase muscle tone and maintain joint mobility is indicated. A Balkan bedframe may be helpful.

J. Anemia may result from bleeding (p 340) or bone marrow suppression related to radiation or chemotherapy. Assess for fatigue, petechiae, purpura, bruising, epistaxis, and melena. Bedrest, oxygen therapy, vitamin and iron dietary supplements, and blood transfusions may be indicated. Measures to protect the patient from injury should be taken.

K. Jaundice may cause pruritus. Administration of antihistamines, trimming nails, or wearing cotton gloves may decrease scratching. Avoid soaps and alcohol-based lotions. Starch baths may soothe itching.

L. Measure abdominal girth at least daily. Ascites may be reduced with diuretics and sodium restriction. Paracentesis (p 158) is reserved for severe cases.

M. Hepatic encephalopathy may herald the terminal phase. Changes in level of consciousness and mentation, or confusion are common. Care is directed to providing for patient safety and supporting family.

N. Assist the patient and significant others to verbalize feelings, fears, and concerns related to changes in the patient's appearance, role, and lifestyle. Assess coping mechanisms and make appropriate referrals.

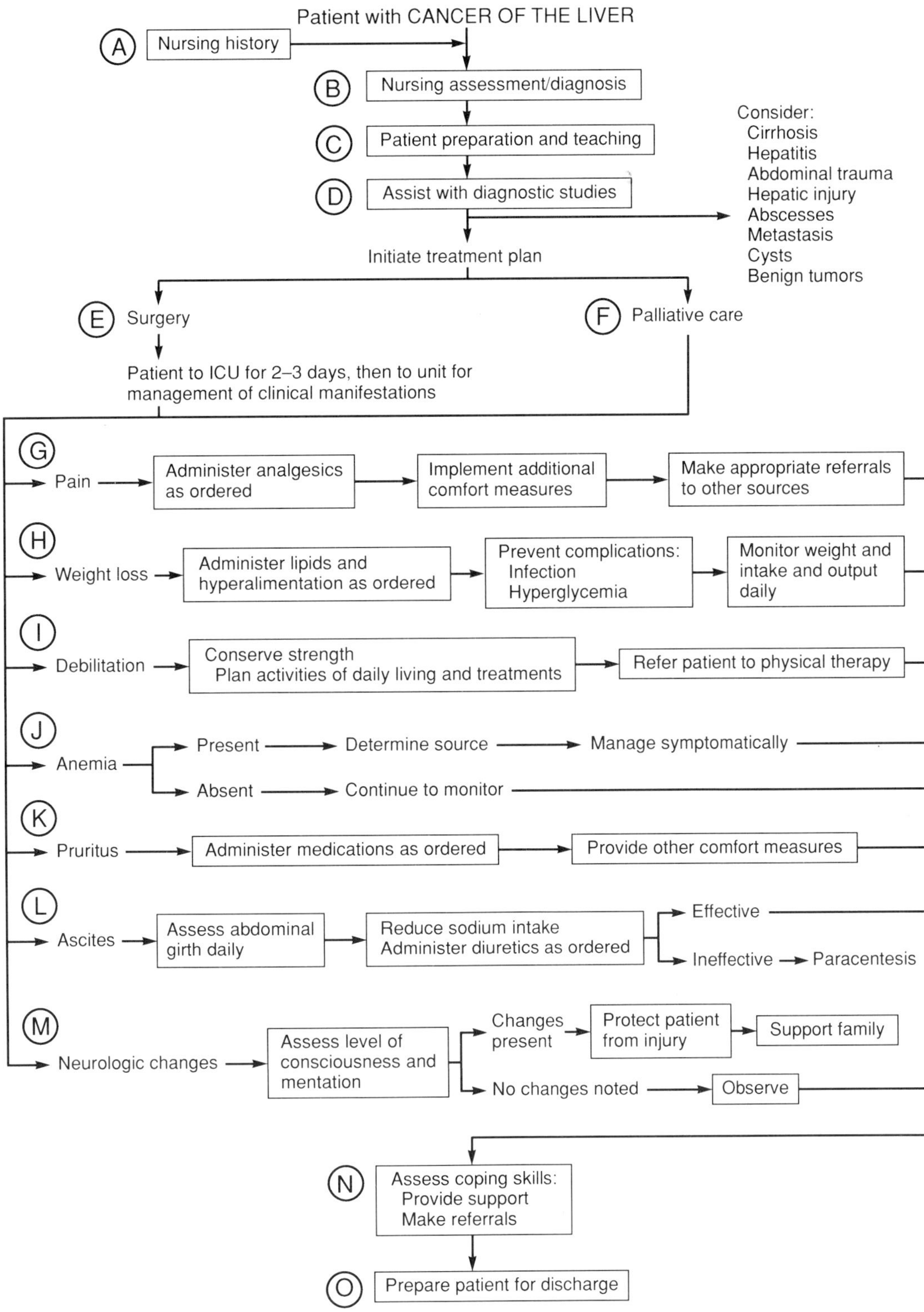

O. Discharge plans include instructions for physical care, outpatient therapy, and coordination with home health. Hospice or other community resources can be utilized for support during the transition to home care.

References

Bullock BL. Alterations in Hepatobiliary Function. In: Bullock BL, Rosendahl PP., eds. Pathophysiology: adaptations and alterations in function. 2nd ed. Glenview, IL: Scott, Foresman, 1988:613–614.

Doenges M, Townsend MC, Moorhouse MF. Psychiatric care plans: guidelines for client care. Philadelphia: FA Davis, 1989:255–270.

Jones DA, Dunbar CF, Jirovic MM. Disturbances in Hepatic Function. In: Jones DA, Dunbar CF, Jirovic MM, eds. Medical-surgical nursing: a conceptual approach. 2nd ed. New York: McGraw-Hill, 1982:741–742.

PARACENTESIS AND LIVER BIOPSY

Carol Bowdoin
Barbara Greaux

Paracentesis and liver biopsy are diagnostic procedures performed by a physician to obtain samples of ascitic fluid and liver tissue for examination. Paracentesis may be used to treat massive ascites resistant to other methods of treatment and to diagnose intra-abdominal bleeding following trauma. Procedures can be done in the hospital room or in a special procedures room.

A. These procedures are indicated in the diagnosis and treatment of hepatic cirrhosis (p 146), liver cancer (p 156), or abdominal trauma. A thorough nursing history and assessment assist the nurse to prepare the patient adequately and plan for the procedure. Paracentesis may precipitate hepatic coma in patients with chronic liver disease.

B. Patient teaching includes the purpose and steps of the procedure to allay anxiety and to promote cooperation. Instruct the patient that a stinging sensation will be felt when the local anesthetic is injected, and some pressure may be felt when the trocar or needle is introduced. Provide reassurance that close monitoring will be done during and after the procedure. Ensure that the patient understands, and obtain a signed consent.

C. Preparation for the paracentesis includes instructing the patient to void just before the procedure and obtaining baseline vital signs, weight, and abdominal girth. Position the patient in a sitting position, and remind him or her to be as still as possible during the procedure. A heparin lock or intravenous line may be established as a precaution. Set up the paracentesis tray, using sterile technique. Monitor the patient for signs of hypovolemia throughout the procedure. Be prepared to assist the physician in collecting peritoneal fluid samples. If a large amount of fluid is to be removed, connect a three-way stopcock for slow removal. Hypovolemic shock (p 70) may result if more than 1,500 cc is removed at one time. Document all pertinent data such as location of site, amount and characteristics of fluid removed, and reaction to procedure.

D. After the needle is removed, a sterile pressure dressing is applied to the site, and the patient is assisted to a comfortable position. The patient's vital signs and dressing are checked frequently per protocol to detect possible complications such as peritoneal fluid leakage, shock, perforation of abdominal organs, and wound infection. Any change in vital signs, increase in abdominal girth, or scrotal edema should be reported immediately.

E. Liver biopsy requires a baseline evaluation of clotting mechanisms. Ensure that a prothrombin time and blood type with cross-match have been done and blood is on hand. Reinforce previous teaching, and restrict intake 4 to 8 hours prior to the procedure. Inform the patient that a brief sharp pain in the right shoulder may be felt as the needle passes through the phrenic nerve. Place the patient flat with the right arm under the head. Disinfect skin per policy, and prepare the biopsy tray per agency procedure using sterile technique. After the site is selected and local anesthetic is introduced, instruct the patient to take several deep breaths, exhale, and then hold breath. The needle is inserted, tissue aspirated and needle removed in 5 to 10 seconds, after which the patient may resume normal breathing.

F. Immediately assist the patient to turn onto the right side with pillow support to lower the rib cage. The patient remains in this position for several hours. Bedrest for 24 hours is advisable. Assess vital signs every 15 minutes for the first hour. Tachycardia and hypotension may indicate hemorrhage (p 340) and must be reported immediately. Diffuse abdominal pain, abdominal rigidity, nausea and vomiting, and fever may indicate bile peritonitis (p 138). Observe the patient for symptoms of pneumothorax (p 110).

G. Analgesics may be administered for discomfort at the procedure site. Barring any complications, a normal diet may be resumed. Treatment and evaluation based on test results will continue.

References

Brunner LS, Suddarth DS. Lippincott manual of nursing practice. 3rd ed. Philadelphia: J.B. Lippincott, 1982:448–449, 455–457.

Smeltzer, SC. Assessment & management of patients with hepatic & biliary diseases. In Brunner LS, Suddarth DS. Medical-surgical nursing. 6th ed. Philadelphia: JB Lippincott, 1988:860–861, 865–867.

Ford RD, ed. Diagnostic tests handbook. Springhouse, PA: Springhouse Corporation, 1987: 295–299, 454–455.

Vigeant S, Okun P. Abdominal paracentesis. In: Hamilton, HK ed. dir. Diagnosis. 2nd ed. Springhouse, PA: Springhouse Corporation, 1986:527–529.

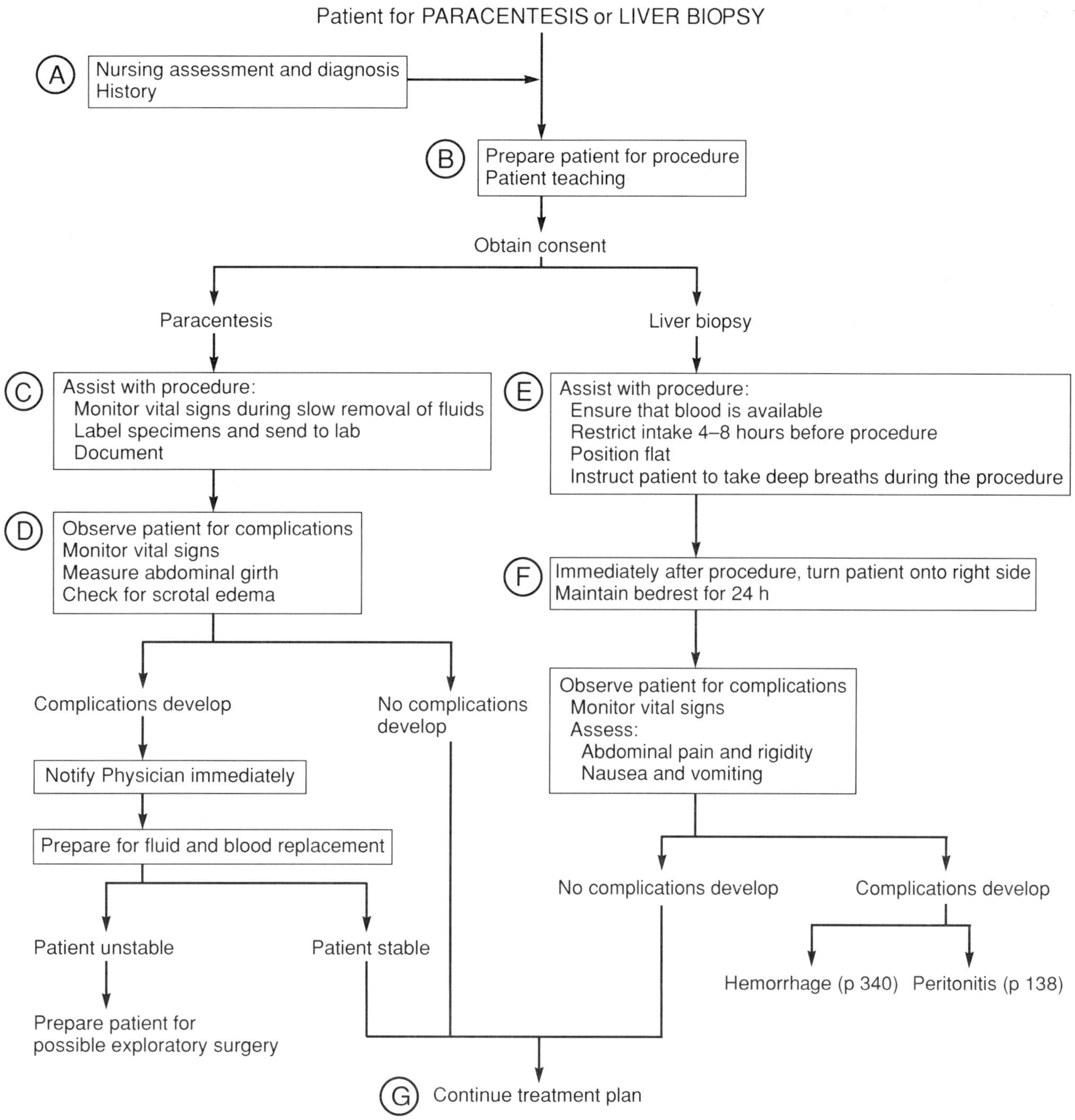
Patient for PARACENTESIS or LIVER BIOPSY
A
Nursing assessment and diagnosis
History
B
Prepare patient for procedure
Patient teaching
Obtain consent
Paracentesis
Liver biopsy
C
Assist with procedure:
Monitor vital signs during slow removal of fluids
Label specimens and send to lab
Document
E
Assist with procedure:
Ensure that blood is available
Restrict intake 4–8 hours before procedure
Position flat
Instruct patient to take deep breaths during the procedure
D
Observe patient for complications
Monitor vital signs
Measure abdominal girth
Check for scrotal edema
F
Immediately after procedure, turn patient onto right side
Maintain bedrest for 24 h
Complications develop
No complications develop
Observe patient for complications
Monitor vital signs
Assess:
Abdominal pain and rigidity
Nausea and vomiting
Notify Physician immediately
Prepare for fluid and blood replacement
No complications develop
Complications develop
Patient unstable
Patient stable
Hemorrhage (p 340)
Peritonitis (p 138)
Prepare patient for
possible exploratory surgery
G
Continue treatment plan

CHOLECYSTECTOMY

Barbara Kalo

Cholecystectomy, the most common surgery in acute or chronic cholecystitis, is the removal of the gallbladder after ligation of the cystic duct. Cholecystitis is inflammation of the gallbladder usually caused by the presence of stones. A calculus becomes impacted in the cystic duct and inflammation develops behind the obstruction. In the absence of stones, cholecystitis is caused by bacteria in the gallbladder. This disease occurs more frequently in women who are over 40 years of age, multiparous, and overweight.

A. The primary symptoms are moderate to severe pain and tenderness in the right hypochondrium and epigastrium with frequent radiation to the infrascapular area. Nausea, vomiting, jaundice, fever, and leukocytosis may occur. Chronic cholecystitis is episodic, usually with colicky pain and associated with nausea and vomiting. An acute attack is usually precipitated by a large or fatty meal with sudden, severe pain. Severe vomiting and weight loss are reported. Right upper quadrant tenderness with muscle guarding and rebound pain is noted. Use the basic steps in evaluating gastrointestinal functions, such as inspection, palpation, auscultation, and percussion. Jaundice usually indicates choledocholithiasis, which involves stones in the common bile duct.

B. Pain is relieved with narcotic analgesics, such as Demerol and anticholinergics to relax smooth muscle and decrease ductal tone. Antiemetics and a nasogastric tube may be utilized to relieve nausea and vomiting.

C. Laboratory tests and radiography are done to determine a differential diagnosis of perforated peptic ulcer (p 130) or acute pancreatitis (p 148). Serum laboratory results show an increase in the white blood cell (WBC) count, transaminase, alkaline phosphatase, and amylase. A HIDA (technetium-labeled iminodiacetic acid, ^{99m}TcHIDA) scan shows an obstructed cystic duct and is reliable if the bilirubin is under 5 mg/dl. Explain the tests and prepare the patient for them.

D. Preoperative nursing care includes promoting comfort and relieving pain, nausea, and vomiting. Care of the nasogastric tube, if used, and explanation for the tube are necessary. Patient teaching should include expectations of surgery and the postoperative period. Provide emotional support to alleviate fear of the surgery.

E. Postoperative nursing care is directed toward adequate ventilation and preventing postoperative infection. Routine procedures such as vital signs and assessment are done (p 4), plus fluid replacement with intravenous fluids.

F. The surgical dressing used to protect the incision from contamination and physical stress should be kept dry to prevent irritation to the skin. The drainage may be moderate to heavy with serosanguineous bile-tinged drainage. A Penrose drain inserted into a stab wound near the incision allows for drainage of the fluid away from the incision site. The patient may have a T-tube to maintain an open common bile duct. The T-tube drains by gravity into a closed system (drainage bag). It is important to allow enough tubing to permit the patient to move in bed. Nursing care includes measuring and noting the character and color of drainage.

G. A nasogastric tube connected to low suction provides relief from vomiting, reduces abdominal distention, and eliminates gastric juices that stimulate cholecystokinin and increases peristalsis. The tube is irrigated as ordered to maintain patency and is taped securely but comfortably to the patient's nose, allowing enough tubing to permit patient movement. Oral and nasal care are essential for any patient with a nasogastric tube.

H. Medicate the patient for incisional pain with narcotics as needed. Encourage the patient to splint the incisional area when coughing or sneezing to protect the site and lessen pain.

I. Fluids and food are withheld while the nasogastric tube is in place. When peristalsis resumes and the nasogastric tube is removed, clear liquids are resumed and the diet is advanced as tolerated. A low-fat diet may be maintained for 2 to 3 months; fatty foods are then added as tolerated.

J. Ambulation may begin on the day of surgery or the first postoperative day. Provide assistance and support, and encourage the patient to stand up straight to prevent shortening of the abdominal muscles.

K. If there are no complications, the patient is discharged with specific instructions about diet, dressing changes, wound care, and follow-up care with the physician.

References

Brunner LS, Suddarth DS. Textbook of medical-surgical nursing. 6th ed. Philadelphia: JB Lippincott, 1988.

Cahill M, ed. Diagnostics. Springhouse, PA: Springhouse Corporation, 1986:793–794.

Jermier BJ, Treloar DM. Bringing your patient through gallbladder surgery. RN 1986; 49(11):318–325.

Kearns PC. Exercises to ease pain after abdominal surgery. RN 1986; 49(7):45–48.

Munn NE. Diagnosis: acute abdomen. Nursing 1988; 18(9):34–41.

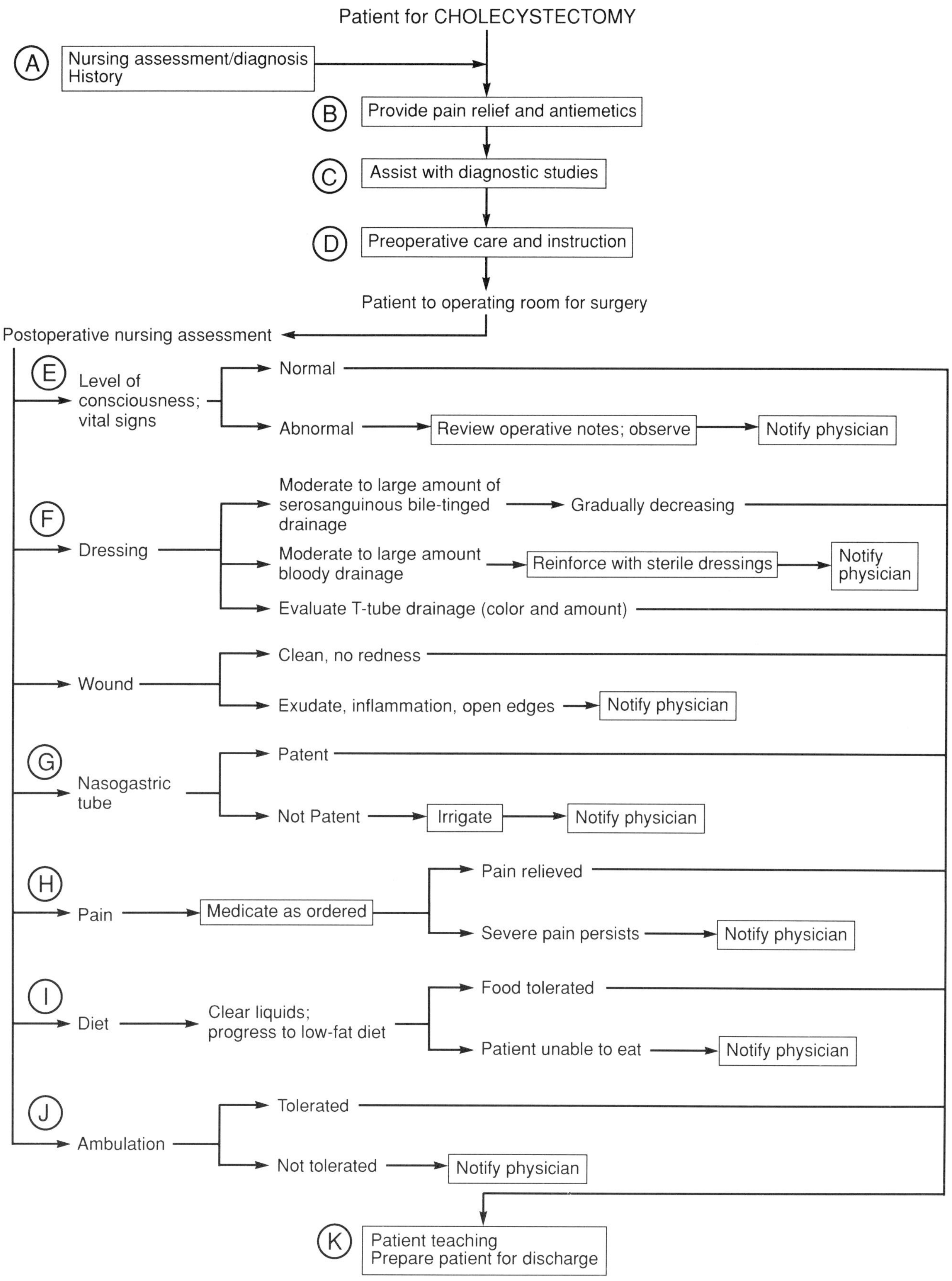
Patient for CHOLECYSTECTOMY
A
Nursing assessment/diagnosis
History
B
Provide pain relief and antiemetics
C
Assist with diagnostic studies
D
Preoperative care and instruction
Patient to operating room for surgery
Postoperative nursing assessment
E
Level of consciousness; vital signs
Normal
Abnormal
Review operative notes; observe
Notify physician
F
Dressing
Moderate to large amount of serosanguinous bile-tinged drainage
Gradually decreasing
Moderate to large amount bloody drainage
Reinforce with sterile dressings
Notify physician
Evaluate T-tube drainage (color and amount)
Wound
Clean, no redness
Exudate, inflammation, open edges
Notify physician
G
Nasogastric tube
Patent
Not Patent
Irrigate
Notify physician
H
Pain
Medicate as ordered
Pain relieved
Severe pain persists
Notify physician
I
Diet
Clear liquids; progress to low-fat diet
Food tolerated
Patient unable to eat
Notify physician
J
Ambulation
Tolerated
Not tolerated
Notify physician
K
Patient teaching
Prepare patient for discharge

HERNIA AND HERNIORRHAPHY

Barbara Kalo

Hernia is defined as a protrusion of an organ or tissue through the wall of the affected cavity, and herniation can occur in any part of the body. Generally, herniation occurs as a protrusion of the abdominal viscus through the wall of the abdominal cavity at various sites. A weakness of the abdominal wall may be congenital or acquired. This condition is more common in men. Herniorrhaphy is the surgical repair that is usually required to prevent strangulation of the hernia. There are five types of abdominal hernias: inguinal (Fig.1), umbilical, ventral or incisional, hiatal, and femoral.

A. Patients may complain of a lump, and a bulge or protrusion is observed as the patient changes position, strains, coughs, laughs, or cries. On examination, a weakened area is palpable at the site of the hernia. If strangulation occurs, the patient experiences abdominal distention, severe pain, and nausea and vomiting. This condition requires *emergency surgery*. The only cure for hernias is surgery to repair the weakened area.

B. Preoperative nursing care includes physical preparation and emotional support to alleviate fears about the procedure (p 2). Patient teaching should include expectations of surgery and the postoperative period. The preparation and teaching may vary depending on what kind of herniorrhaphy the patient is having. The surgery is postponed if the patient has an upper respiratory infection, because sneezing and coughing may break sutures postoperatively.

C. Postoperative nursing care is directed toward the prevention of infection at the operative site. Routine procedures such as checking of vital signs and assessment of level of consciousness are done (p 4).

D. The surgical dressing should be dry and intact. If a moderate to large amount of drainage is noted, it should be reinforced and reported to the physician.

E. When dressings are changed, observation of the wound should reveal little or no drainage from the incisional site and no signs of infection. If the scrotal area is edematous, ice bags may be applied.

F. Medicate the patient for incisional pain as needed. Depending on the complexity of the herniorrhaphy, the medication may range from oral analgesics to narcotic injections. Encourage the patient to splint the incision when coughing or sneezing to protect the incision site and lessen the pain.

G. Urinary retention may be a problem after herniorrhaphy. Assess the bladder for distention. Offer the bedpan or urinal as necessary and encourage oral intake of fluids to facilitate voiding.

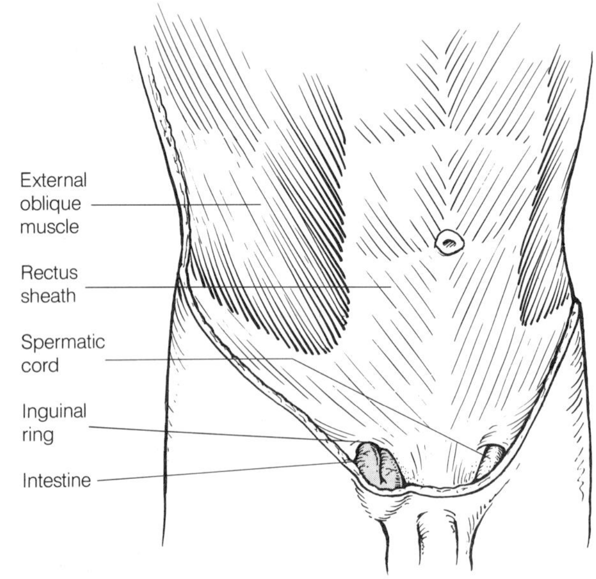

Figure 1 Incarcerated inguinal hernia

H. The patient is offered clear liquids when free of nausea and vomiting; regular diet is resumed as tolerated.

I. Ambulation is usually begun on the day of surgery. Provide assistance and support when needed. Encourage the patient to stand up straight and ambulate without stooping to prevent shortening of the abdominal muscles.

J. If there are no complications, the patient is discharged with specific instructions about dressing changes, wound care, and follow-up care with the physician. Instruct the patient not to lift heavy objects and to avoid strenuous activity and driving for 3 to 6 weeks. Contact sports should be avoided for 12 weeks. Patients should be reassured that sexual function is not affected by this surgery.

References

Brunner LS, Suddarth DS. The Lippincott manual of nursing practice. 3rd ed. Philadelphia: JB Lippincott, 1982.

Brunner LS, Suddarth DS. Textbook of medical-surgical nursing. 6th ed. Philadelphia: JB Lippincott, 1988.

Kearns PC. Exercises to ease pain after abdominal surgery. RN, 1986; 49(7):45–48.

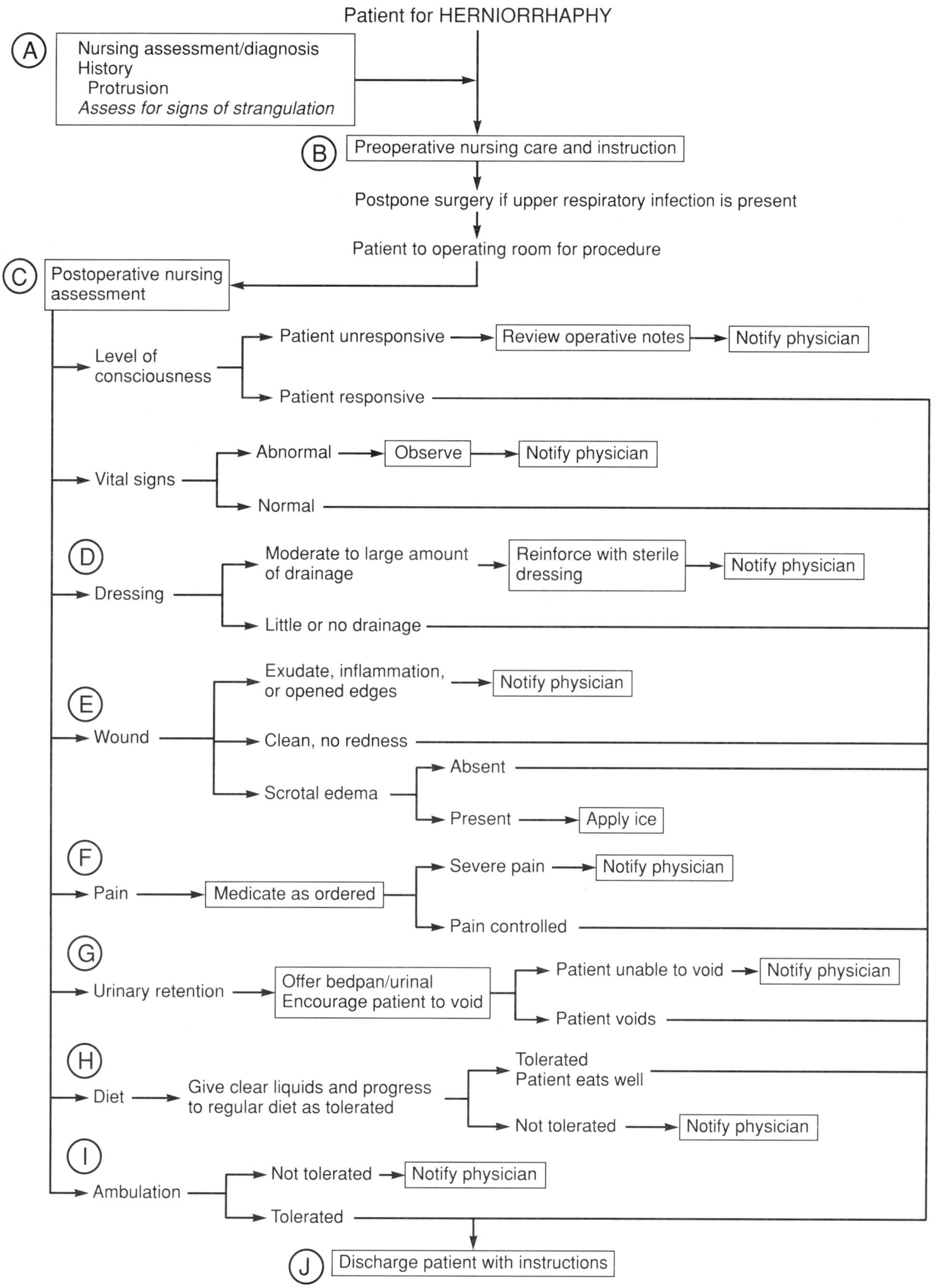
Patient for HERNIORRHAPHY
A
Nursing assessment/diagnosis
History
Protrusion
Assess for signs of strangulation
B
Preoperative nursing care and instruction
Postpone surgery if upper respiratory infection is present
Patient to operating room for procedure
C
Postoperative nursing assessment
Level of consciousness
Patient unresponsive
Review operative notes
Notify physician
Patient responsive
Vital signs
Abnormal
Observe
Notify physician
Normal
D
Dressing
Moderate to large amount of drainage
Reinforce with sterile dressing
Notify physician
Little or no drainage
E
Wound
Exudate, inflammation, or opened edges
Notify physician
Clean, no redness
Scrotal edema
Absent
Present
Apply ice
F
Pain
Medicate as ordered
Severe pain
Notify physician
Pain controlled
G
Urinary retention
Offer bedpan/urinal
Encourage patient to void
Patient unable to void
Notify physician
Patient voids
H
Diet
Give clear liquids and progress to regular diet as tolerated
Tolerated
Patient eats well
Not tolerated
Notify physician
I
Ambulation
Not tolerated
Notify physician
Tolerated
J
Discharge patient with instructions

APPENDICITIS AND APPENDECTOMY

Barbara Kalo

Appendectomy is a surgical procedure done to remove an inflamed appendix. The appendix can become obstructed with a fecalith (fecal concretion), foreign body, neoplasm, or inflammation. The obstruction of the appendiceal lumen is followed by an infection, and surgical intervention is indicated.

A. The patient describes the pain as progressively severe abdominal pain, which becomes localized in the right lower quadrant (McBurney's point) after 6 to 12 hours. On examination, rebound tenderness is noted, and the pain is aggravated by walking or coughing. Nausea, vomiting, and anorexia may also be noted. Many patients present with a low-grade fever and tachycardia.

B. Monitoring and assessing the location and severity of the pain is important to the diagnosis of appendicitis. The patient is placed in Fowler's position, and an ice bag may be ordered for comfort. Narcotics are usually not given to relieve the pain, but tranquilizing agents are not contraindicated. Laboratory findings show a leukocyte count that exceeds 10,000 per cubic millimeter and a shift to the left (more than 75 percent neutrophils) may occur. Abdominal radiography visualizes a radiopaque shadow consistent with fecalith in the appendix.

C. If perforation has occurred and generalized peritonitis has developed, conservative treatment is initiated prior to surgical intervention, to include intravenous fluids, antibiotic therapy, and drainage.

D. Preoperative nursing care (p 2) includes close observation of signs and symptoms to help make a definitive diagnosis. The patient is placed on bedrest and receives nothing by mouth. Along with the physical preparation, comfort measures, and patient teaching, emotional support is necessary to help alleviate fears regarding surgery. Expectations after surgery should also be included.

E. Postoperative nursing care is directed toward maintaining an open airway, with routine monitoring of level of consciousness and vital signs (p 4).

F. The surgical dressing should be dry and intact. If a moderate to large amount of drainage is noted, the dressing should be reinforced and the physician notified. When dressings are changed, observation of the wound should reveal little or no drainage from the incisional site and no signs of infection.

G. Medicate the patient for incisional pain as needed. Splinting the abdomen when the patient coughs or sneezes should be encouraged to help alleviate incisional pain and facilitate coughing and deep breathing.

H. If patient is free of nausea and vomiting, clear liquids are offered and the diet gradually expanded as peristalsis and gastrointestinal function return. Intravenous fluids are administered as needed.

I. Assess the bladder for distention. Offer the bedpan as necessary, and encourage oral fluids when possible to help facilitate voiding.

J. Ambulation is usually begun the day of surgery. Provide assistance and support when needed. Encourage the patient to stand up straight, without bending forward, to facilitate strengthening of abdominal muscles.

K. The patient who is free of complications is discharged from the hospital within a week. In some instances, the patient may go home the same day. Discharge instructions should include dressing and/or wound care. Normal activity may be resumed 2 to 3 weeks after surgery.

References

Brunner LS, Suddarth DS. The Lippincott manual of nursing practice. 4th ed. Philadelphia: JB Lippincott, 1986.

Brunner LS, Suddarth DS. Textbook of medical-surgical nursing. 6th ed. Philadelphia: JB Lippincott, 1988.

Krupp MA, Chatton MJ, Werdegar D, eds. Current medical diagnosis and treatment. Los Altos, CA: Lange, 1985.

Thompson JM, McFarland GK, Hirsch JE, Tucker SM, Bowers AC. Clinical nursing. St. Louis: CV Mosby, 1986.

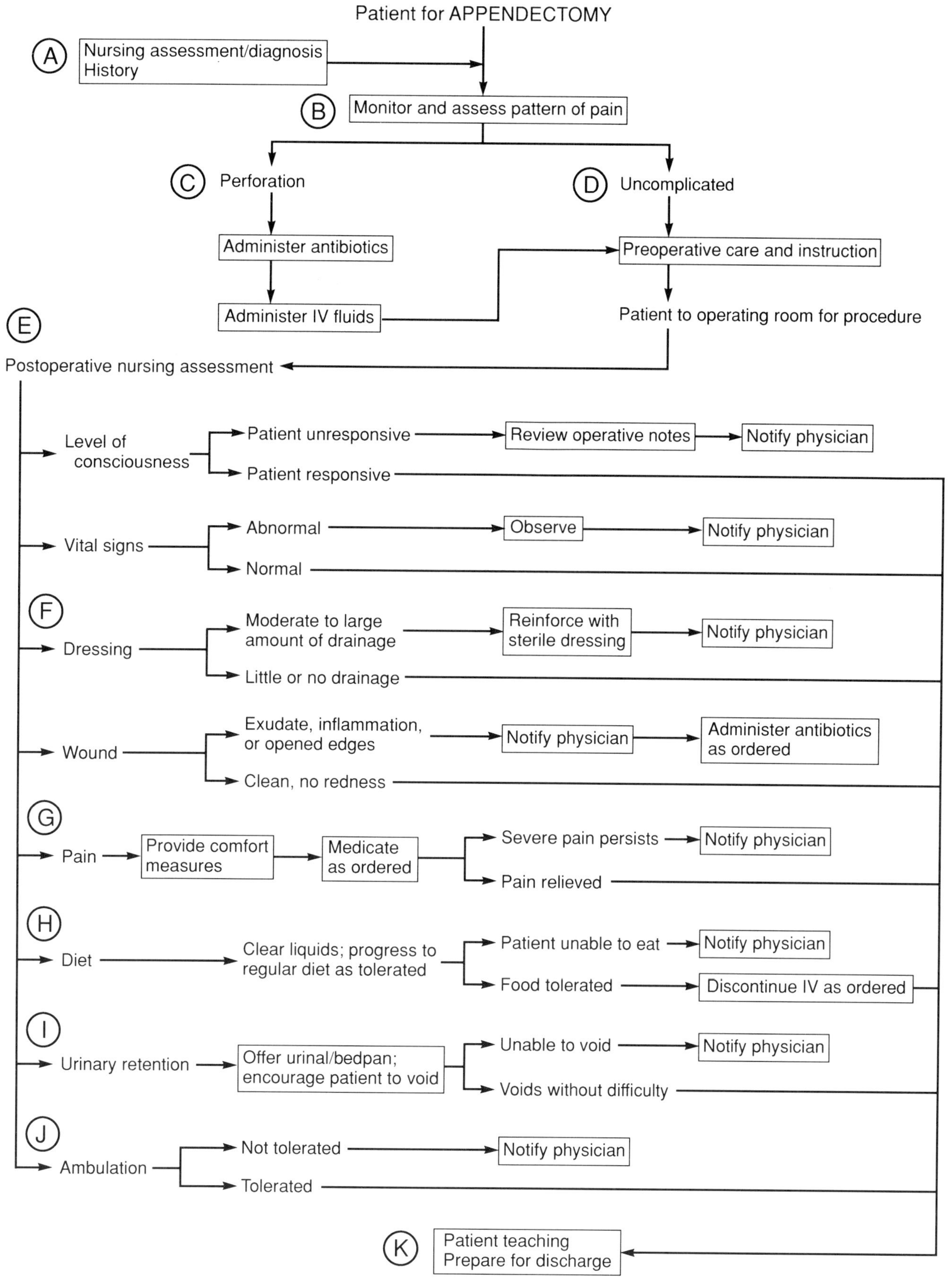

Patient for APPENDECTOMY
A
Nursing assessment/diagnosis
History
B
Monitor and assess pattern of pain
C
Perforation
D
Uncomplicated
Administer antibiotics
Administer IV fluids
Preoperative care and instruction
Patient to operating room for procedure
E
Postoperative nursing assessment
Level of consciousness
Patient unresponsive
Review operative notes
Notify physician
Patient responsive
Vital signs
Abnormal
Observe
Notify physician
Normal
F
Dressing
Moderate to large amount of drainage
Reinforce with sterile dressing
Notify physician
Little or no drainage
Wound
Exudate, inflammation, or opened edges
Notify physician
Administer antibiotics as ordered
Clean, no redness
G
Pain
Provide comfort measures
Medicate as ordered
Severe pain persists
Notify physician
Pain relieved
H
Diet
Clear liquids; progress to regular diet as tolerated
Patient unable to eat
Notify physician
Food tolerated
Discontinue IV as ordered
I
Urinary retention
Offer urinal/bedpan; encourage patient to void
Unable to void
Notify physician
Voids without difficulty
J
Ambulation
Not tolerated
Notify physician
Tolerated
K
Patient teaching
Prepare for discharge

GASTRECTOMY

Barbara Kalo

Gastrectomy is a surgical procedure performed to relieve hemorrhage, perforating ulcer, pyloric stenosis, or obstruction. The stomach may be removed partially or totally. Partial gastrectomy involves removal of the distal one-third to one-half of the stomach. The duodenum is anastomosed to the remaining stomach. Hemigastrectomy involves removal of the first part of the duodenum, pylorus, and up to half of the stomach; the duodenal stump is closed, and the jejunum is anastomosed to the remaining stomach. Total gastrectomy is removal of the entire stomach, a resection of the lower esophagus and anastomosis of the esophagus to the jejunum. Vagotomy (i.e., severing of the vagus nerve), which may be necessary in some of the surgeries, causes a reduction in gastric mobility.

A. A thorough objective and subjective assessment is important. The patient usually presents with abdominal pain. It is necessary to identify the character of the pain and when it occurs. Besides pain, the patient may have vomiting, bleeding, and occult blood in the stool. Projectile vomiting may indicate an obstruction. During the assessment and history taking, stressful factors in the patient's life may be identified; these may be important contributors to the original problem. If perforation of an ulcer (p 130) has occurred, the patient presents with vomiting, diffuse abdominal pain, diminished bowel sounds, board-like abdomen with diffuse distention, tachycardia, and shallow respirations. The head of the bed should be elevated to localize gastric content.

B. Once a definite diagnosis has been made, analgesics may be given for abdominal pain. A nasogastric (NG) tube may be placed to control bleeding by irrigating the stomach with cool saline until clear. The NG tube is later connected to suction.

C. A gastrectomy may be indicated as an immediate procedure in the presence of hemorrhaging. Preparation for surgery, which includes promoting comfort, relieving pain, and explaining procedures and diagnostic tests, may need to be done quickly. Patient teaching should include expectations of surgery and the postoperative period (p 4). Emotional support is necessary to alleviate fears about the seriousness of the underlying problem and the surgery.

D. Postoperative nursing care is directed toward adequate ventilation, preventing postoperative infection, and assessing gastric aspirant. Care of the NG tube and explanation for the tube are necessary. Routine procedures such as vital signs and assessment are done, plus fluid replacement with intravenous fluids.

E. The surgical dressing used to protect the incision from contamination and physical stress should be kept dry and intact. If a moderate to large amount of drainage is noted, the dressing should be reinforced and reported to the physician. When dressings are changed, little or no drainage should be noted from the incision site and there should be no signs of infection.

F. Postoperatively, the NG tube is not irrigated unless ordered. The purpose of the tube is to drain the stomach contents to promote healing, reduce stress on the suture line, and prevent secretions from infiltrating the site of anastomosis. The tube should be taped firmly but comfortably to the patient's nose, allowing enough tubing so as not to pull on the nose when the patient moves. Good oral and nasal care is essential for any patient with an NG tube. Observe the gastric aspirant for color and odor. The color is bright red initially and gradually darkens within the first 24 hours after surgery. Within 36 to 48 hours, the color changes to yellow-green. A fecal odor may indicate a reflux of the contents of the large intestine into the operative area. If the NG tube is not patent or the color or odor is not normal, notify the physician.

G. Medicate with narcotics as needed for pain. Encourage the patient to splint the incisional area when coughing or sneezing to protect the incisional site and lessen the pain.

H. Intake of food and fluids is held until gastric and intestinal motility returns and the internal incision is healed. The diet begins with clear liquids and progresses to a bland diet with six small feedings daily. Encourage the patient to avoid taking fluids with meals, to eat foods low in simple carbohydrates, high in protein, and moderately high in fat, and to rest after meals to help avoid the dumping syndrome.

I. Ambulation may begin the first day postoperatively. Provide assistance and support when needed. Encourage the patient to stand up straight and ambulate without stooping to prevent shortening of the abdominal muscles.

J. If there are no complications, the patient is discharged with instructions about dressing changes, wound care, and follow-up care with the physician. Specific dietary instructions, rest after eating, and avoidance of known stressors are necessary.

References

Brunner LS, Suddarth DS. Textbook of medical-surgical nursing. 6th ed. Philadelphia: JB Lippincott, 1988.

Kearns PC. Exercises to ease pain after abdominal surgery. RN 1986; 49(7):45–48.

Munn NE. Diagnosis: acute abdomen. Nursing 1988; 18(9):34–41.

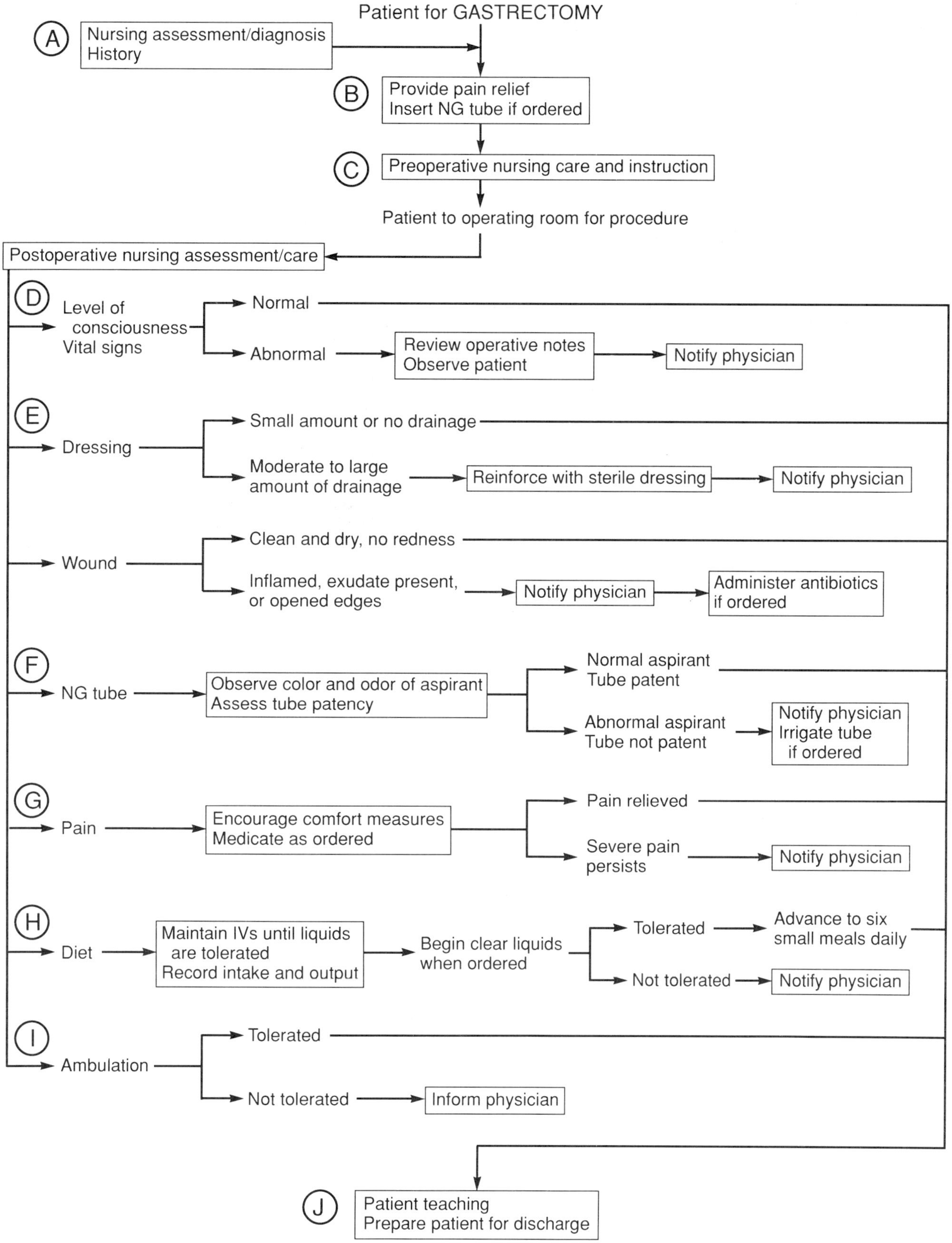
Patient for GASTRECTOMY
A
Nursing assessment/diagnosis
History
B
Provide pain relief
Insert NG tube if ordered
C
Preoperative nursing care and instruction
Patient to operating room for procedure
Postoperative nursing assessment/care
D
Level of consciousness
Vital signs
Normal
Abnormal
Review operative notes
Observe patient
Notify physician
E
Dressing
Small amount or no drainage
Moderate to large amount of drainage
Reinforce with sterile dressing
Notify physician
Wound
Clean and dry, no redness
Inflamed, exudate present, or opened edges
Notify physician
Administer antibiotics if ordered
F
NG tube
Observe color and odor of aspirant
Assess tube patency
Normal aspirant
Tube patent
Abnormal aspirant
Tube not patent
Notify physician
Irrigate tube if ordered
G
Pain
Encourage comfort measures
Medicate as ordered
Pain relieved
Severe pain persists
Notify physician
H
Diet
Maintain IVs until liquids are tolerated
Record intake and output
Begin clear liquids when ordered
Tolerated
Advance to six small meals daily
Not tolerated
Notify physician
I
Ambulation
Tolerated
Not tolerated
Inform physician
J
Patient teaching
Prepare patient for discharge

COLOSTOMY AND ILEOSTOMY

Joy Gorzeman

A colostomy is a surgical procedure that bypasses or removes a segment of diseased or injured colon and brings an open end or loop of colon through an opening in the abdominal surface (stoma) for purposes of elimination. An ileostomy brings the ileum through the abdominal wall after the entire colon and rectum are removed (Fig 1).

A. Colostomy or ileostomy is done to treat obstructions, inflammatory conditions (pp 140, 142), and cancer of the colon. Cancer of the colon and rectum accounts for the second highest death rate from cancer. It is slightly more common in men than in women and is seen more often in persons over 50 years of age. Chronic ulcerative colitis, diverticulosis (p 136), and diets low in fiber have been related to the development of colon cancer. The survival rate for colon cancer with treatment is 40 to 50 percent.

B. Blood in the stool should always be examined. Occult blood is revealed by hematesting fecal samples (guaiac). Bleeding may result in anemia over time that is manifested in a low hemoglobin (p 340). Anemia may cause the patient to feel tired and weak. Patients may note constipation alternating with diarrhea, lower abdominal cramping, and distention, which may result in anorexia and weight loss. These symptoms may indicate an obstruction. Rectal masses are often detected during digital examination, making regular physical examinations a must, especially in people over 40 years of age.

C. Unless the surgery is emergent, preoperative care includes a bowel preparation. Enemas and a low-residue or liquid diet help decrease fecal contents. Lack of a bowel preparation, as in emergencies, increases the risk of infection and peritonitis (p 138) postoperatively. Preoperative preparation also includes the administration of antibiotics, and blood transfusions if indicated. Teaching about the postoperative course is extremely important. Measures to prevent complications (coughing, deep breathing, and leg exercises) are reviewed. Patients need to know about having a nasogastric (NG) tube after surgery. These patients need support and may have many questions. Visits from the enterostomal therapist and a member of the Ostomy Association who has had similar surgery may help allay the patient's anxiety.

D. Pre- and postoperative care depend on the reason for surgery and the location of the resection. Occasionally colostomy is done as a temporary measure. Surgery for colon cancer is always permanent.

E. Postoperative vital signs, level of consciousness, and routine assessment (p 4) are done.

F. The NG tube is connected to suction, and drainage must be observed, measured, and recorded. The return of peristalsis is indicated by passing of flatus, return of bowel sounds, or discharge from the stoma. A rectal tube inserted for about 20 minutes may provide some relief for abdominal cramps and distention. Oral fluids are started when peristalsis returns, and the diet is increased gradually.

G. Check dressings, drains, and/or Hemovacs often. An abdominoperineal resection involves a deep rectal incision that requires frequent dressing changes. A colostomy/ileostomy bag is placed over the stoma to prevent wound contamination. Monitor drainage for character, odor, and amount. Report a red or swollen wound or drainage that is odoriferous or purulent. Cultures are taken and antibiotics administered as ordered. Isolation may be required to reduce the spread of infection.

H. Bowel elimination may be regulated in patients with a colostomy. Stools are usually normal. In patients with sigmoid colostomies, irrigation may encourage a regular elimination pattern. The patient with an ileostomy has almost constant drainage of liquid stools, requiring continuous wearing of an ileostomy appliance. Ileostomies are not irrigated.

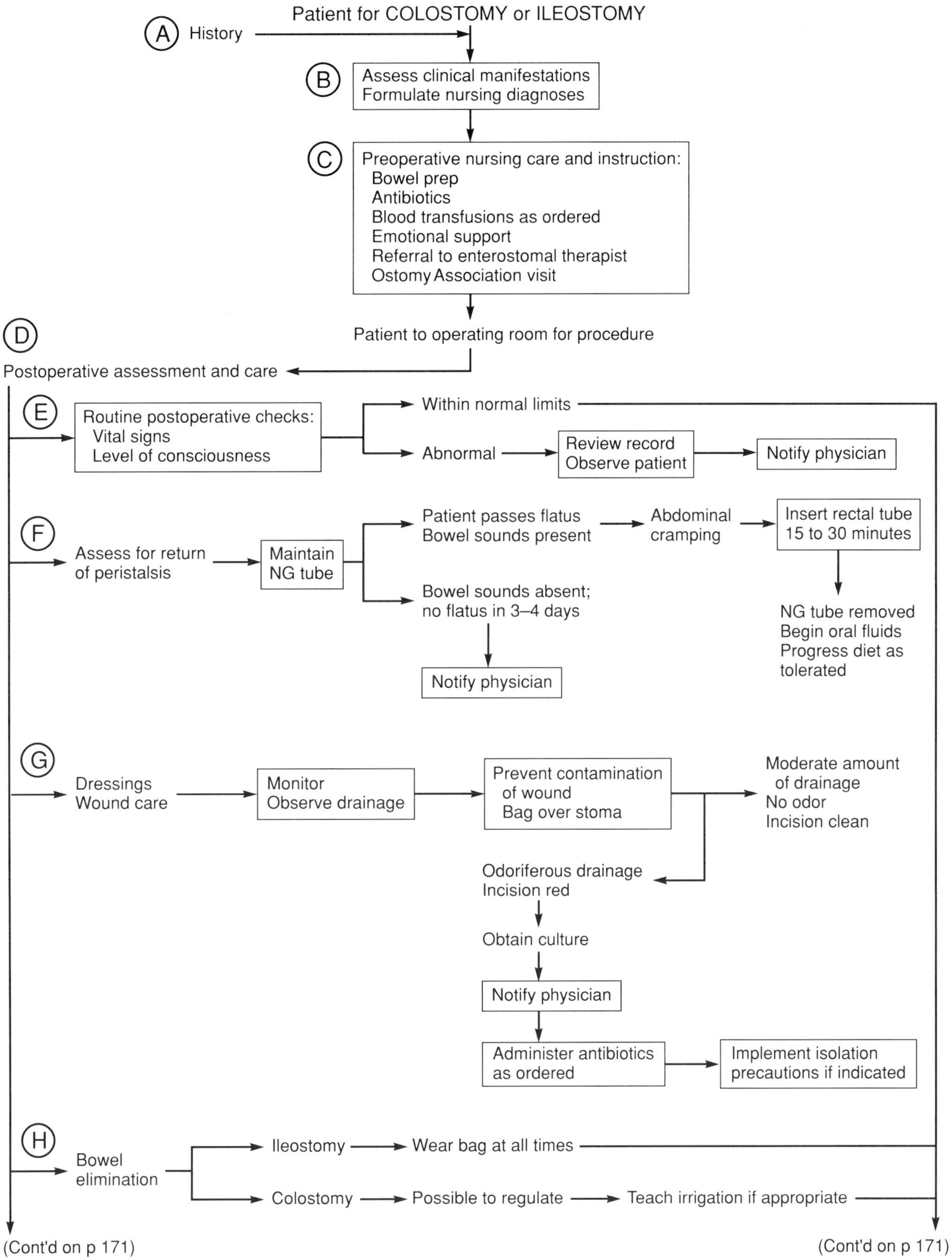
Patient for COLOSTOMY or ILEOSTOMY
A History
B Assess clinical manifestations
Formulate nursing diagnoses
C Preoperative nursing care and instruction:
Bowel prep
Antibiotics
Blood transfusions as ordered
Emotional support
Referral to enterostomal therapist
Ostomy Association visit
Patient to operating room for procedure
D Postoperative assessment and care
E Routine postoperative checks:
Vital signs
Level of consciousness
Within normal limits
Abnormal
Review record
Observe patient
Notify physician
F Assess for return of peristalsis
Maintain NG tube
Patient passes flatus
Bowel sounds present
Abdominal cramping
Insert rectal tube 15 to 30 minutes
NG tube removed
Begin oral fluids
Progress diet as tolerated
Bowel sounds absent; no flatus in 3–4 days
Notify physician
G Dressings
Wound care
Monitor
Observe drainage
Prevent contamination of wound
Bag over stoma
Moderate amount of drainage
No odor
Incision clean
Odoriferous drainage
Incision red
Obtain culture
Notify physician
Administer antibiotics as ordered
Implement isolation precautions if indicated
H Bowel elimination
Ileostomy
Wear bag at all times
Colostomy
Possible to regulate
Teach irrigation if appropriate
(Cont'd on p 171)
(Cont'd on p 171)

I. The constant loss of fluids puts the patient with an ileostomy at risk for fluid and electrolyte imbalance. Weight, intake and output, and serum electrolytes are monitored and recorded.

J. Skin integrity is especially important in the patient with a stoma. Prevention of skin breakdown is much easier than treatment. Change a leaking bag immediately. An enterostomal therapist can assist with choosing the appropriate pouch, changing the pouch, skin care, and patient instruction.

K. Complications of ileostomies include food blockage and intestinal obstruction. Observe for and investigate abdominal distention, nausea, vomiting, and lack of output. A hot shower or assuming the knee-chest position may relieve the blockage; however, symptoms that persist for 3 to 4 hours should be reported.

L. Diet is an important part of the postoperative care of "ostomy" patients. Gas-producing foods such as cabbage, beans, and beer and odor-producing foods such as garlic, fish, and eggs are avoided to reduce self-consciousness or embarrassment.

M. Adjustment to a colostomy or ileostomy requires time and support. Patients and family need to be allowed to grieve and express their feelings. A positive, realistic approach is helpful. Encourage patients to resume a normal, active life. Some men suffer impaired sexual function and potency; often this is temporary. Radical surgery such as abdominoperineal resection results in sexual disability, and a penile implant (p 304) may be considered. Women with ostomies can have successful pregnancies with careful medical supervision. Unwillingness to participate in self-care and social isolation indicate ineffective coping, and referral for counseling is suggested.

N. Patient teaching includes bowel training and stoma and skin care. Patients and families must learn to change the pouch and perform other stoma care. Ileostomy patients are instructed not to take laxatives, because the increased fluid loss could cause a fluid and electrolyte imbalance. Enteric-coated or time-release capsules should not be taken, as they are not absorbed. Review the signs and symptoms of obstruction.

O. A visiting nurse may be needed to ensure patient capability for self-care and adequate supplies. Referral to the Ostomy Association may be helpful.

References

Brunner LS, Suddarth DS. The Lippincott manual of nursing practice. 4th ed. Philadelphia: JB Lippincott, 1986.

Casedonte LB. The patient with a fistula, a colostomy, and an ileal conduit. RN 1984; 47(9):42–47.

Doering KJ, LaMountain P. Flow charts to facilitate caring for ostomy patients—recuperative care: pt. III. Nursing 1984; 14(11):54–57.

Luckmann J, Sorensen KC. Medical-surgical nursing: a psychophysiologic approach. 3rd ed. Philadelphia: WB Saunders, 1987.

Thompson JM, McFarland GK, Hirsch JE, Tucker SM, Bowers AC. Clinical nursing. St. Louis: CV Mosby, 1986.

Volk SH, Christich GD, Green SH. Against all odds. Nursing 1987; 17(8):53–55.

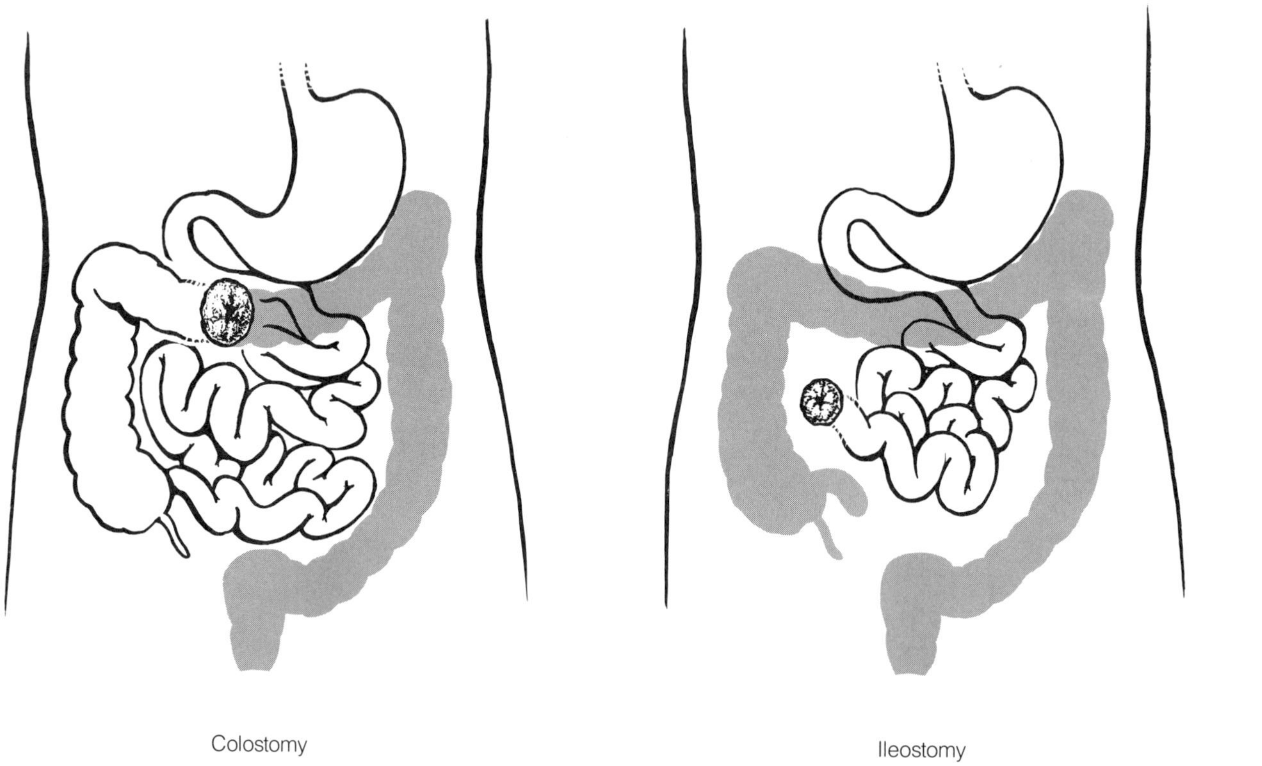

Figure 1 Colostomy and ileostomy. Shaded area indicates resected intestine.

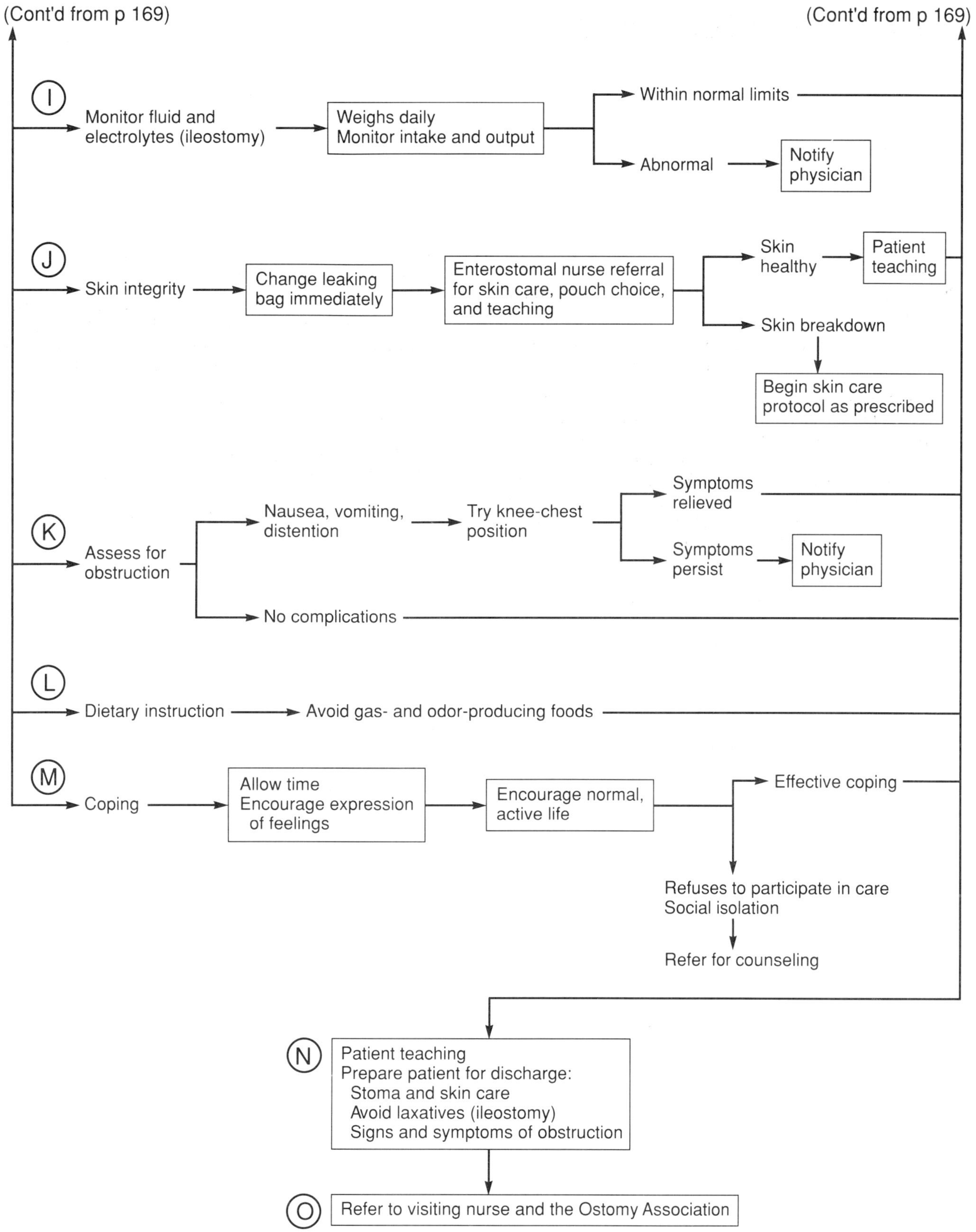
(Cont'd from p 169)
(Cont'd from p 169)
I
Monitor fluid and electrolytes (ileostomy)
Weighs daily
Monitor intake and output
Within normal limits
Abnormal
Notify physician
J
Skin integrity
Change leaking bag immediately
Enterostomal nurse referral for skin care, pouch choice, and teaching
Skin healthy
Patient teaching
Skin breakdown
Begin skin care protocol as prescribed
K
Assess for obstruction
Nausea, vomiting, distention
Try knee-chest position
Symptoms relieved
Symptoms persist
Notify physician
No complications
L
Dietary instruction
Avoid gas- and odor-producing foods
M
Coping
Allow time
Encourage expression of feelings
Encourage normal, active life
Effective coping
Refuses to participate in care
Social isolation
Refer for counseling
N
Patient teaching
Prepare patient for discharge:
Stoma and skin care
Avoid laxatives (ileostomy)
Signs and symptoms of obstruction
O
Refer to visiting nurse and the Ostomy Association

HEMORRHOIDECTOMY

Cecile A. Lengacher
Carol Bowdoin

Hemorrhoidectomy is the surgical removal of hemorrhoids (p 144) because of chronic pain, prolonged bleeding, intolerable itching, or unrelieved discomfort due to thrombosed or prolapsed hemorrhoids.

A. A complete history, physical examination, and diagnostic work-up are done upon admission as required.

B. Preoperative nursing care includes conservative management of discomfort in addition to traditional preparatory measures, e.g., patient teaching and bowel preparation (p 2). The nurse should particularly be concerned with allaying the patient's anxiety about surgery in the genitorectal area. It is important to ensure personal hygiene and respect the patient's privacy during examinations and treatments.

C. Postoperatively the nursing assessment is directed toward preventing complications while promoting comfort and wound healing.

D. Changes in neurologic function, vital signs, and urinary output may be secondary to effects of anesthesia (p 4).

E. Surgical dressings should be routinely inspected. Increased amounts of bright red drainage and changes in vital signs may indicate hemorrhage. The physician must be notified, dressings reinforced, and a STAT hemoglobin and hematocrit obtained. The nurse should be prepared for the administration of blood products and a possible return of the patient to surgery. In uncomplicated cases, the rectal packing is removed several days postoperatively.

F. Pain management (p 406) is a priority during the postoperative period. Analgesics should be administered prior to defecation. Stool softeners, sitz baths, and use of an air ring reduce discomfort to the rectal area.

G. Early ambulation facilitates a return of bowel and bladder function.

H. Prior to discharge, instruct the patient about perianal hygiene to reduce the possibility of infection, diet, and use of medications. Activity is gradually increased. Regular follow-up care is necessary to prevent recurrence.

References

Boyd M, Tower B. Medical-surgical nursing: a study and learning tool. Springhouse, PA: Springhouse Corporation, 1988.

Brunner LS, Suddarth DS. The Lippincott manual of nursing practice. 3rd ed. Philadelphia: JB Lippincott, 1986.

Lewis SM, Collier IC. Medical-surgical nursing: assessment and management of clinical problems. New York: McGraw-Hill, 1983.

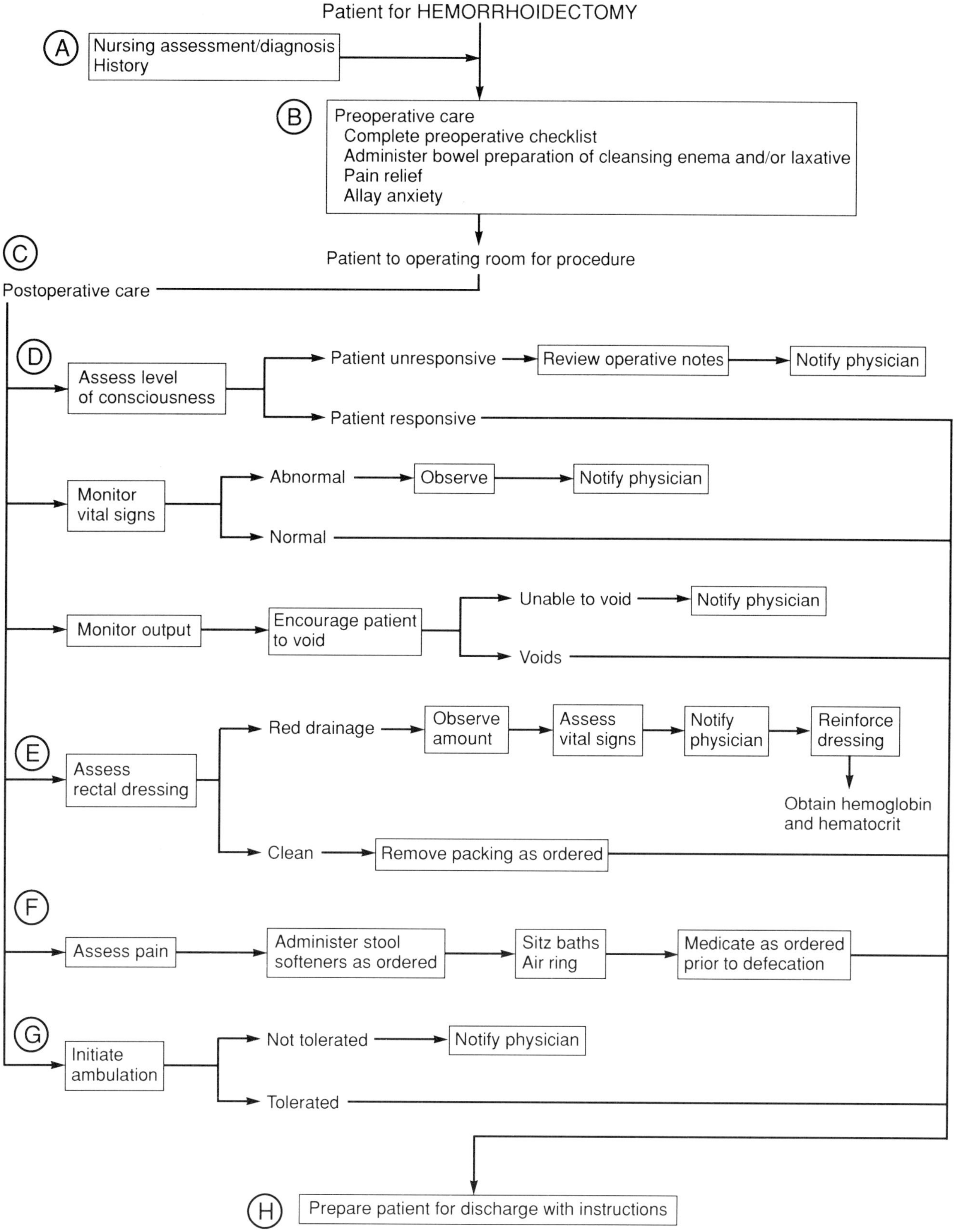
Patient for HEMORRHOIDECTOMY
A
Nursing assessment/diagnosis
History
B
Preoperative care
Complete preoperative checklist
Administer bowel preparation of cleansing enema and/or laxative
Pain relief
Allay anxiety
Patient to operating room for procedure
C
Postoperative care
D
Assess level of consciousness
Patient unresponsive
Review operative notes
Notify physician
Patient responsive
Monitor vital signs
Abnormal
Observe
Notify physician
Normal
Monitor output
Encourage patient to void
Unable to void
Notify physician
Voids
E
Assess rectal dressing
Red drainage
Observe amount
Assess vital signs
Notify physician
Reinforce dressing
Obtain hemoglobin and hematocrit
Clean
Remove packing as ordered
F
Assess pain
Administer stool softeners as ordered
Sitz baths
Air ring
Medicate as ordered prior to defecation
G
Initiate ambulation
Not tolerated
Notify physician
Tolerated
H
Prepare patient for discharge with instructions

ENDOCRINE AND METABOLIC SYSTEMS

Diabetes Mellitus
Diabetes Insipidus
Diabetic Ketoacidosis
Hyperinsulinemia (Hypoglycemia)
Hyperthyroidism
Hypothyroidism
Hypercalcemia
Hypocalcemia
Hyperkalemia
Hypokalemia

ENDOCRINE SURGERY

Thyroidectomy

DIABETES MELLITUS

Jean Oswald Konrady

Diabetes mellitus causes elevated blood sugar with a tendency toward vascular complications. In 1979, the following classification system was adopted by the American, British, Australian, and European Diabetes Associations: Type I—insulin-dependent diabetes mellitus (IDDM); Type II—non-insulin dependent diabetes mellitus (NIDDM); Impaired glucose tolerance (IGT); Gestational diabetes mellitus (GDM); and Diabetes mellitus associated with other conditions or syndromes.

Diabetes afflicts 5 percent of Americans. It occurs more frequently after age 40. It is the third leading cause of death by disease and the major cause of new blindness in the United States today. Although diabetes doubles the incidence of heart attack and stroke, kidney disease accounts for 50 percent of the deaths in insulin-dependent diabetics.

A. The symptoms of diabetes vary with type. Eighty percent of patients with Type II (NIDDM) have no symptoms. However, symptoms may be associated with complications of diabetes, for example, extremity numbness or burning and tingling of the feet, worsening at night, might indicate the presence of diabetic neuropathy, which may be present at diagnosis. Patients may complain of rashes, genital yeast infections, tiredness, or vision problems. The Type I IDDM patient experiences more pronounced symptoms such as polyuria, polydipsia, polyphagia, rapid weight loss, and progressive fatigue. As the condition worsens, the patient experiences nausea, vomiting, and acetone odor to the breath. Dehydration, shock, and coma result if treatment is not instituted. Patients with IGT and GDM usually experience no symptoms.

B. Patient education is the foundation for all nursing management. Diabetes education is started at the time of diagnosis and is a lifelong process. Emphasis should be on self-reliance and establishing a knowledge base to facilitate daily problem-solving. Assess the patient's physical, emotional, and experiential readiness to learn.

C. The complex treatment regimen of insulin therapy, self-monitoring of blood glucose, and meal planning leaves room for error and noncompliance. One study of diabetic patients taking insulin found that 50 percent were administering incorrect dosages. Taking extra time for demonstration and return demonstration when teaching insulin administration and self-monitoring of blood glucose is the best insurance against patient error (Table 1).

D. The patient not taking insulin relies on diet, exercise, and/or oral antidiabetic medication to control the diabetes. Weight control is usually the behavior change that needs to be emphasized. In addition to the importance of meal planning, benefits of exercise should also be stressed. Explain the influence of exercise on blood sugar, and review the components of an individual exercise plan. Explain oral medications so that patients know the name of the drug, the correct dosage, when to take the medication, how the medication works, and possible side effects.

E. All diabetes patients, whether or not they take insulin, need education. Discuss the importance of good hygiene and susceptibility to infection. The impact of diabetes on lifestyle and the necessity for health management are also important aspects of discharge planning. Patients must be aware of conditions such as illness, stress, increased or decreased exercise, and dietary changes that increase the likelihood of complications. Short-term complications include diabetic

TABLE 1 Survival Skills for Diabetic Patients

Insulin administration
Inject air into the insulin bottle
Check for and remove air bubbles
Draw up correct dose
Pinch skin correctly
Insert needle at the proper angle
Rotate injection sites
Proper procedure for mixing insulin if appropriate
Self-monitoring of blood glucose
Appropriate sites for obtaining blood samples
Apply blood to reagent strip correctly
Time reagent strip accurately
Utilize specific meter correctly and record results
Meal planning
Meal distribution
Decreased use of concentrated sweets
Calorie level
Reading labels
Effect of alcohol on blood sugar
Dining out
Importance of fiber in the diet
Hypoglycemia and hyperglycemia
Causes
Signs and symptoms
Treatment and prevention
Sick day rules
Monitor blood sugar frequently
Monitor urine ketones
Report nausea and vomiting
Meal substitutions
Adjustment of insulin in relation to blood sugar
Relationship of food, exercise, and insulin
Somogyi effect
Adjustment of medication or insulin relative to exercise
Adjustment of medication or exercise relative to food intake
Urine ketone testing
Significance of ketones in urine
When to perform tests
Types of tests available
Correct timing of tests

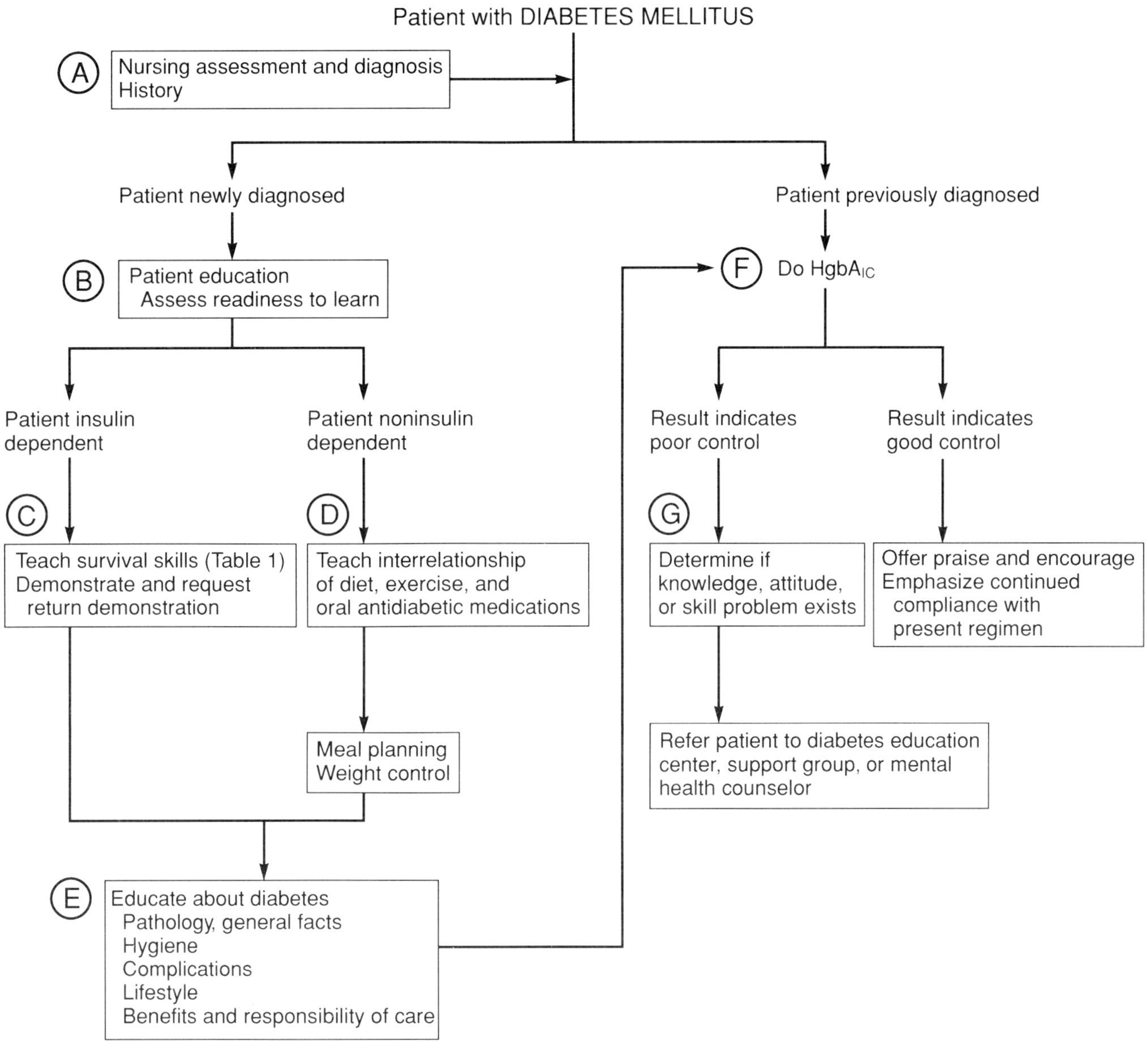

ketoacidosis (p 180), hypoglycemia (p 182), and nonketotic hyperosmolar coma. Common long-term complications of diabetes mellitus are nephropathy, neuropathy, retinopathy, and cardiovascular difficulties with associated foot problems. Patients should be aware of symptoms of these complications and how to avoid them.

F. The effectiveness of diet, exercise, and oral antidiabetic medication or insulin can be assessed with a glycosylated hemoglobin (HgbA$_{1C}$). HgbA$_{1C}$ is hemoglobin with glucose attached to it. If a high sugar concentration is in the blood, it is reflected by the amount of glucose attached to the red blood cells. The red blood cell lives for 2 to 3 months, so this test is a reliable assessment of blood glucose control for the previous 2 to 3 months.

G. When the HgbA$_{1C}$ indicates poor control, it must be determined if a knowledge, attitude, or skill problem exists. The patient's attitude about health is very important. Diabetes care is a day-to-day challenge, and patients are constantly exposed to temptations to deviate from the diabetes management program. Making appropriate referral to diabetes education centers, support groups, or mental health counselors may be useful.

References

Franz M, Krosnick A, Maschak-Carey BJ, Parker T, Wheeler F. Goals of diabetes education. Alexandria, VA: American Diabetes Association, 1986.

Guidelines for diabetes care. Alexandria, VA: American Diabetes Association/American Association of Diabetes Educators, 1981.

Nath C. Lessons in living with type II diabetes mellitus. Nursing 88 1988;18(8):44–49.

The physician's guide to type II diabetes (NIDDM): diagnosis and treatment. Alexandria, VA: American Diabetes Association, 1984.

The physician's guide to type I diabetes (IDDM): diagnosis and treatment. Alexandria, VA: American Diabetes Association, 1987.

DIABETES INSIPIDUS

Jean Oswald Konrady

Diabetes insipidus (DI) is a disorder of water metabolism, defined as a urine output greater than 250 ml per hour. It can affect either sex and occurs at any age. DI may be central (neurogenic or pituitary) or nephrogenic in origin. Antidiuretic hormone (ADH or vasopressin) is synthesized in the hypothalamus. The posterior pituitary stores and releases ADH in response to changes in osmolality, blood volume, or blood pressure. ADH acts on the kidneys to enhance the absorption of water from the collecting tubules into the medullary interstitium, thereby conserving water and concentrating urine.

A. Central DI is related to a decrease or total lack of ADH production and may be caused by head trauma, neurosurgery, or infections such as meningitis (p 32). At least half of the cases are idiopathic. Nephrogenic DI is related to the kidney's failure to respond to ADH. It may be seen in association with chronic renal disease (p 318), electrolyte disturbances, or with certain medications that may affect ADH production in some individuals. Nephrogenic DI may also be inherited by boys as an autosomal dominant trait, but this is rare.

B. Primary symptoms of DI include polyuria (which may have an insidious onset, or if it is related to an injury, the onset may be sudden) and polydipsia, which may be intense. Patients may drink 4 to 10 L of fluid daily. Cold water is usually preferred.

C. The urine of a patient with DI is very dilute, has a low specific gravity (1.000 to 1.005), and contains no abnormal substances, such as sugar or protein. A fluid deprivation test confirms the diagnosis of DI. Oral intake is held for 6 to 8 hours, until the urine osmolality of three consecutive urine specimens (obtained at 15-minute to hourly intervals) varies by less than 30 mOsm/kg. Then 5 to 10 U of aqueous vasopressin (mammalian ADH) are injected subcutaneously. The urine osmolality is measured 1 hour later. Even after fluids have been withheld, patients with DI pass urine that is hypotonic in relation to their serum. If the cause is nephrogenic, the administration of ADH subcutaneously will cause no change in urine osmolality. If the cause is neurogenic, the urine osmolality will increase by at least 50 percent with administration of vasopressin.

D. Complete and permanent loss of the ability to secrete ADH occurs with the destruction of the supraoptic nuclei of nerve tracts above the level of the median eminence (located in the medulla oblongata) and results in a permanent disturbance of water metabolism. Lesions lower on the pituitary stalk result in a partial decrease in ADH production and are usually transitory. When medications are the cause of the disturbance, their discontinuation resolves the condition.

E. Intake and output are monitored and recorded; however, fluids should be available and not withheld.

F. Serum electrolytes (especially serum sodium), urine specific gravity, and osmolality are gauges of the patient's condition.

G. Patients should be weighed daily before breakfast and after dinner in the same amount of clothing and on the same scale. A fluid increase or decrease of 1 L is a weight change of 1 kg. Signs of hypovolemia are tachycardia, dry mucous membranes, extreme thirst, decreased skin turgor, weight loss, sunken eyeballs, constipation, and lethargy. Signs of water intoxication are periorbital, pedal, digital, or sacral edema.

H. Since the patient may not want to eat because he is drinking so much fluid, a nutritional assessment is recommended. The patient is asked to keep a food diary and calorie count.

I. Treatment with medications depends on the severity of the condition. Chlorpropamide, carbamazepine, and/or clofibrate may be used for mild polyuria due to neurogenic DI. Aqueous vasopressin, vasopressin tannate in oil, pituitrin, intravenous or intranasal desmopressin (DDAVP), or lypressin intranasal spray may be used for moderate-to-severe polyuria caused by neurogenic DI. Hydrochlorothiazide and indomethacin are used for nephrogenic DI. The medications must be administered on time because diuresis begins when the effects of the drug diminish. Vasopressin tannate must be shaken vigorously and the vial warmed before administration because the active component settles at the bottom of the vial.

J. The patient and family are usually relieved to know the condition can be treated. DI in children and teens requires special consideration. Bedwetting and frequent urination and thirst may be sources of embarrassment. Patient and family teaching includes medication administration; side effects and signs that the medication is not working properly; how to check urine specific gravity; allowing fluids as desired; weighing daily; and the importance of periodic laboratory work and continued, regular check-ups.

References

Brunner LS, Suddarth DS. Textbook of medical-surgical nursing. Philadelphia: JB Lippincott, 1988.

Germon K. Fluid and electrolyte problems associated with diabetes insipidus and syndrome of inappropriate antidiuretic hormone. Nurs Clin North Am 1987; 22:785–796.

Stewarts M. When the patient has the "other" diabetes. RN 1985; 48(5):54–58.

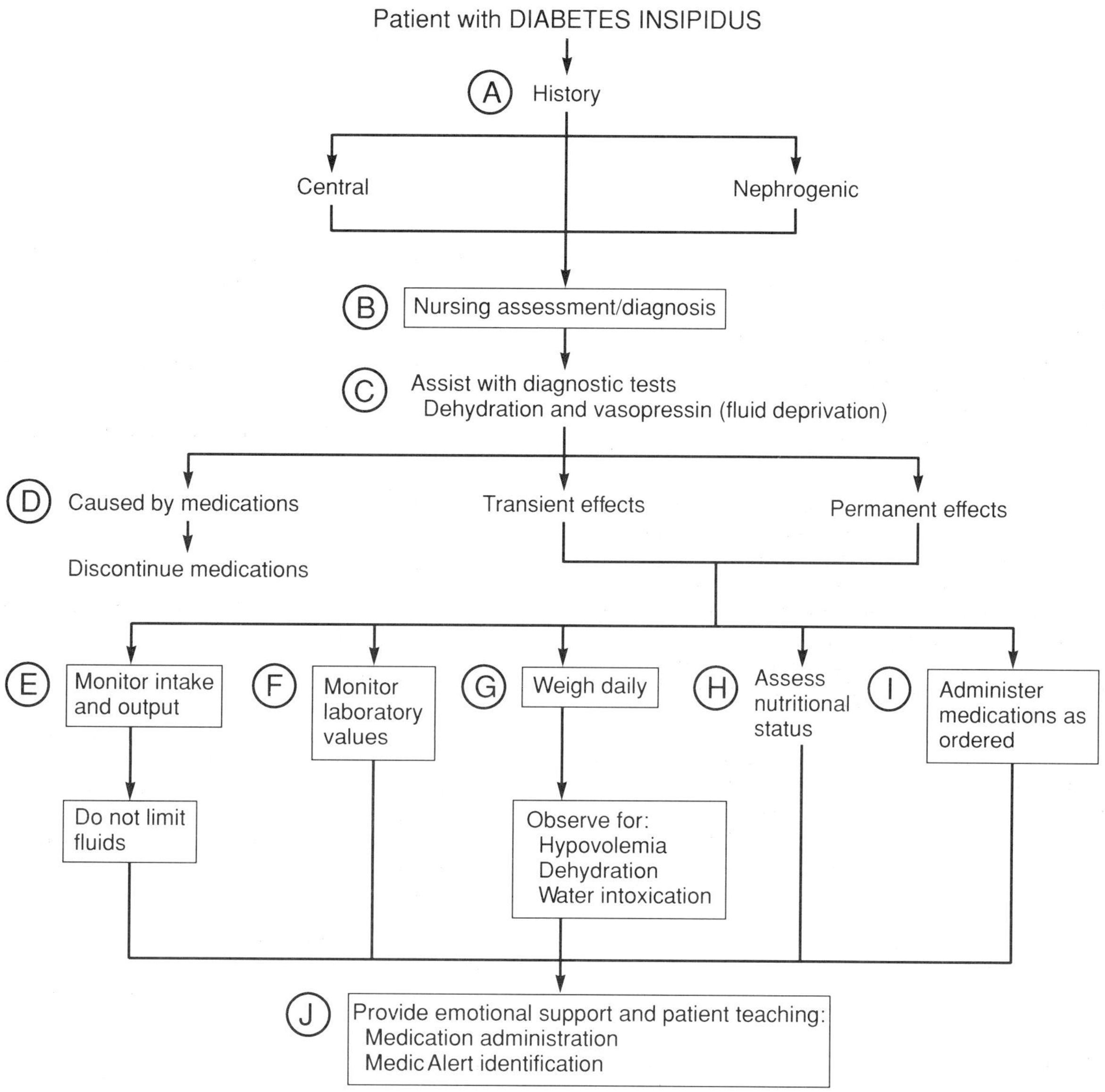
Patient with DIABETES INSIPIDUS
A History
Central
Nephrogenic
B Nursing assessment/diagnosis
C Assist with diagnostic tests
Dehydration and vasopressin (fluid deprivation)
D Caused by medications
Discontinue medications
Transient effects
Permanent effects
E Monitor intake and output
Do not limit fluids
F Monitor laboratory values
G Weigh daily
Observe for:
Hypovolemia
Dehydration
Water intoxication
H Assess nutritional status
I Administer medications as ordered
J Provide emotional support and patient teaching:
Medication administration
Medic Alert identification

DIABETIC KETOACIDOSIS

Jean Oswald Konrady

Diabetic ketoacidosis (DKA) is an acute metabolic disorder that results primarily from a sustained lack of insulin. Carbohydrate, protein, and fat metabolism are affected. The body cannot effectively use glucose, and fat is metabolized instead of carbohydrate. Ketones are produced from the fatty acids oxidized by the liver. Metabolic acidosis results, with lowering of serum bicarbonate level, P_{CO_2}, and pH. The clinical picture includes hyperglycemia, water and electrolyte loss, and acidemia.

A. The most common causes of DKA are infections of the skin, respiratory system, and urinary tract, which affect the amount of insulin needed. Previously undiagnosed cases account for 25 percent of DKA episodes. Less common causes include lack of patient education about DKA and its causes, failure to follow sick-day rules (p 176, Table 1), and failure to change insulin doses for stress, trauma, illness, pregnancy, or rapid growth of children with diabetes.

B. Early manifestations of DKA include symptoms such as nausea, vomiting, abdominal pain, fatigue, and drowsiness, which may cause newly diagnosed patients to think they have the "flu." Later symptoms may include hypotension, semiconsciousness, acetone breath, soft eyeballs, flushed face, dry skin, dry lips and tongue, subnormal temperature, pleural rub, coffee ground vomitus, gastric distention, tender and rigid abdomen, and cold extremities.

C. Blood and urine samples should be obtained immediately. The serum glucose level is usually greater than 300 mg/dl. Blood and urine are positive for ketones. Potassium levels may be high, normal, or low. Serum bicarbonate and blood pH are decreased. Serum lipids, hematocrit, blood urea nitrogen (BUN), and white blood cell count may be increased. Peaked T-waves may indicate a hyperkalemic state (p 196).

D. Fluid replacement depends on the patient's condition. The deficit may range from 6 to 10 L. Intravenous (IV) isotonic or hypotonic saline is started immediately, initially at a rapid rate, to expand blood volume, stabilize blood pressure, and promote urine flow.

E. The method of choice for insulin administration is to give low doses of regular insulin subcutaneously (SQ), intramuscularly, or by intermittent or continuous IV, with IV administration generally preferred. One of the following insulin regimens may be prescribed. Specific hospital protocol should be followed.

High Dosage

1. 50 U insulin IV push followed by 50 to 60 U per hour IV drip
2. 50 to 200 U insulin IV push and repeat IV bolus injections of 25 to 100 U every 1 to 2 hours
3. 100 U insulin (½ IV and ½ SQ) repeated every 2 to 4 hours

Low Dosage

1. 5 to 10 U insulin IV push followed by 2 to 4 U per hour IV
2. 5 U intramuscularly every 1 hour

F. Hourly monitoring of blood glucose, serum electrolytes (signs of hyperkalemia and/or hypoglycemia [p 182]), urine ketones, pH, BUN, and vital signs, is essential. Level of consciousness, hydration status, intake and output, and electrocardiogram should also be assessed every hour. Changes in the patient's status are easily detected by the use of flow sheets.

G. Evaluate patient knowledge, attitude, and skills to determine the cause of a DKA episode. Determine if reeducation is necessary, and refer the patient to diabetes education classes. Review fingerstick blood glucose monitoring, insulin administration, diet and meal planning, signs and symptoms of hyperglycemia, sick-day rules, and when to call the physician.

References

Brunner LS, Suddarth DS. Textbook of medical-surgical nursing. Philadelphia: JB Lippincott, 1984.

Davidson M. Diabetes mellitus: diagnosis and treatment. New York: Churchill Livingstone, 1986:225–265.

Johanson B, Dungca C, Hoffmeister D, Wells S. Standards for critical care. St. Louis: CV Mosby, 1985.

McCarty J. The continuum of diabetic coma. Am J Nurs 1985; 85(8):878–880.

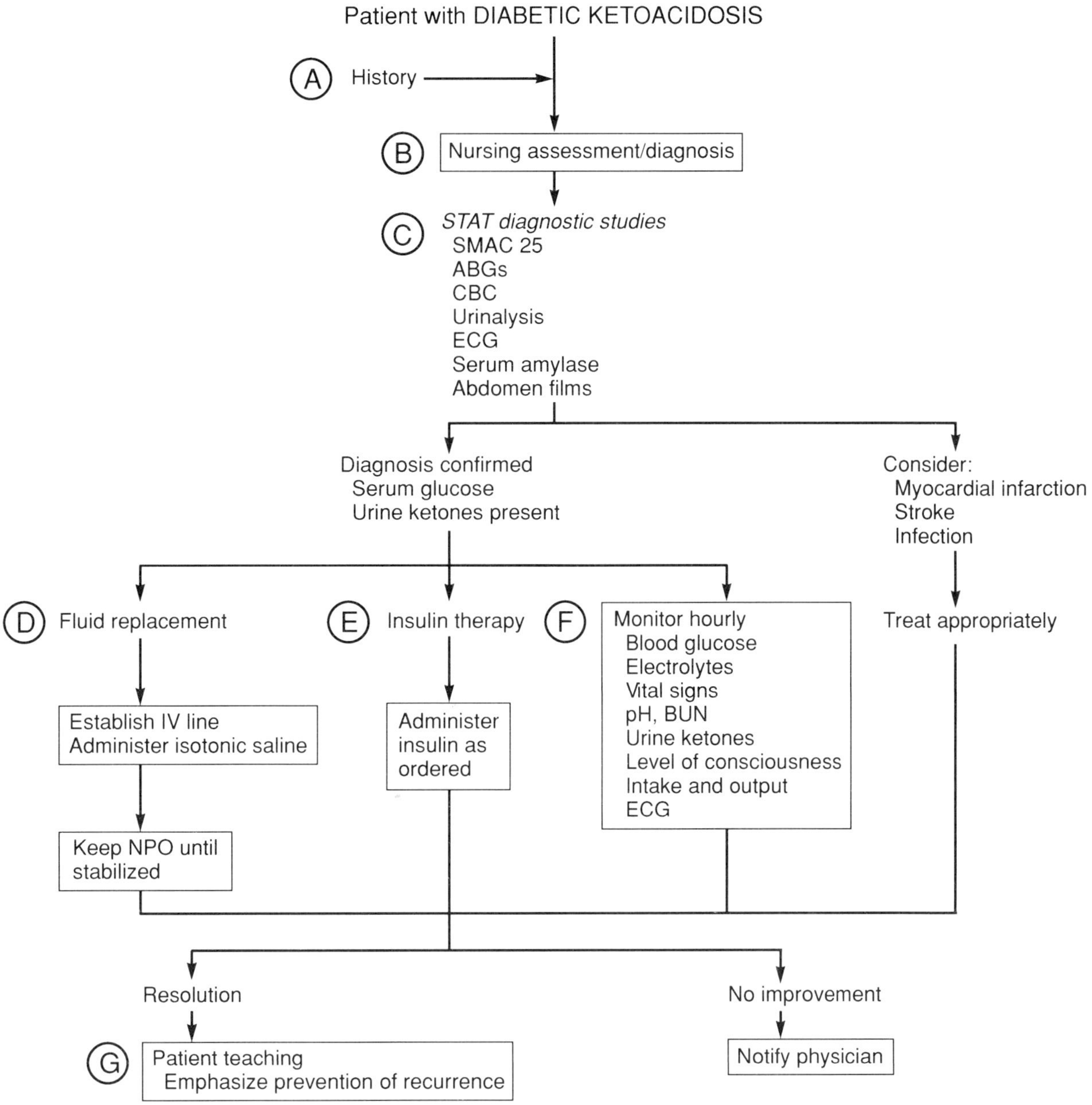
Patient with DIABETIC KETOACIDOSIS
A
History
B
Nursing assessment/diagnosis
C
STAT diagnostic studies
SMAC 25
ABGs
CBC
Urinalysis
ECG
Serum amylase
Abdomen films
Diagnosis confirmed
Serum glucose
Urine ketones present
Consider:
Myocardial infarction
Stroke
Infection
D
Fluid replacement
E
Insulin therapy
F
Monitor hourly
Blood glucose
Electrolytes
Vital signs
pH, BUN
Urine ketones
Level of consciousness
Intake and output
ECG
Treat appropriately
Establish IV line
Administer isotonic saline
Administer insulin as ordered
Keep NPO until stabilized
Resolution
No improvement
G
Patient teaching
Emphasize prevention of recurrence
Notify physician

HYPERINSULINEMIA (HYPOGLYCEMIA)

Jean Oswald Konrady

Hypoglycemia is an abnormally low blood glucose level (less than 50 mg/dl). Any well-controlled diabetic who takes insulin experiences hypoglycemic reactions. Usually symptoms occur around meal times, when blood sugars are naturally decreased prior to feeding. However, an insulin reaction may occur at any time.

A. Common causes of hypoglycemia include excessive doses of insulin or antidiabetic oral medication, especially the peaking of insulin; unusual physical activity without adjustment of food or insulin; skipping, delaying, or not eating a full meal without changing insulin dose; unpredictable absorption of insulin from the injection site; and ingestion of alcohol without food. Determination of blood glucose should be done at the onset of symptoms, preferably by reflectance photometer. Symptoms may vary considerably in different patients and in the same patient at different times.

B. If the blood glucose level falls rapidly, the body responds by secreting adrenalin, glucagon, cortisone, and growth hormone. Adrenalin is the hormone responsible for the early warning signs of hypoglycemia such as diaphoresis, hunger, tachycardia, fatigue, irritability, nervousness, and trembling. If the blood sugar level falls slowly, the brain eventually suffers from glucose deprivation, and symptoms of cerebral hypoglycemia follow. These symptoms include headache, stupor, combativeness, amnesia, confusion, incoordination, double vision, slurred speech, convulsions, and coma.

C. When the first warning signs appear, if the patient is able to swallow and the blood sugar level is less than 80 mg/dl, orange juice, apple juice, a soft drink containing sugar, LifeSavers, or commercially prepared sugar such as dextrosols or glucose tablets (commercially prepared sucrose) should be taken. The equivalent of at least one fruit exchange (15 g of simple carbohydrate or 60 calories, i.e., one glass of juice, soft drink) is given. *If the symptoms persist the treatment should be repeated.* If the next meal is more than 1 hour away, one meat and one starch exchange (half a sandwich) is given.

D. If the patient is unable to swallow and the blood sugar level is less than 80 mg/dl, glucagon or 50 ml of 50 percent glucose in water may be given. Glucagon is a hormone secreted by the alpha cells of the pancreas. It causes glycogenolysis in the liver (if hepatic glycogen stores are not depleted). It is available by prescription in 1-mg vials and given in the same manner as insulin. The onset of action is 10 to 20 minutes. The patient should be given 15 g of simple carbohydrate (one glass of juice) as soon as possible after awakening.

E. Any patient taking insulin should know the warning signs of hypoglycemia and have a source of simple, fast-acting carbohydrate readily available. Personal medical identification should be worn by all patients taking insulin or oral antidiabetic medications. Tell the patient to exercise when the blood sugar level is highest, 1 to 2 hours after a meal. Patients should be taught to adjust insulin or food for exercise. Family members and close friends should be taught the symptoms and treatment of hypoglycemia. The meal plan should be followed carefully; all meals and prescribed snacks should be eaten at the correct times.

F. If the blood glucose level is greater than 80 mg/dl, the patient should be observed and the blood sugar measured again in 5 to 10 minutes. At that time, appropriate treatment must be initiated if the result is below 80 mg/dl. Consider stress–anxiety reaction or hyperventilation if the symptoms persist and the blood sugar level remains 80 or above.

References

Brunner LS, Suddarth DS. Textbook of medical-surgical nursing. Philadelphia: JB Lippincott, 1984:903.

Cassmeyer VL. Preventing, recognizing and treating diabetic shock. Nursing Life 1987, 7(1):33–40.

Davidson M. Diabetes mellitus, diagnosis and treatment. New York: Churchill Livingstone, 1986:516.

Lumley W. Controlling hypoglycemia and hyperglycemia. Nursing 1988; 18(10):34–41.

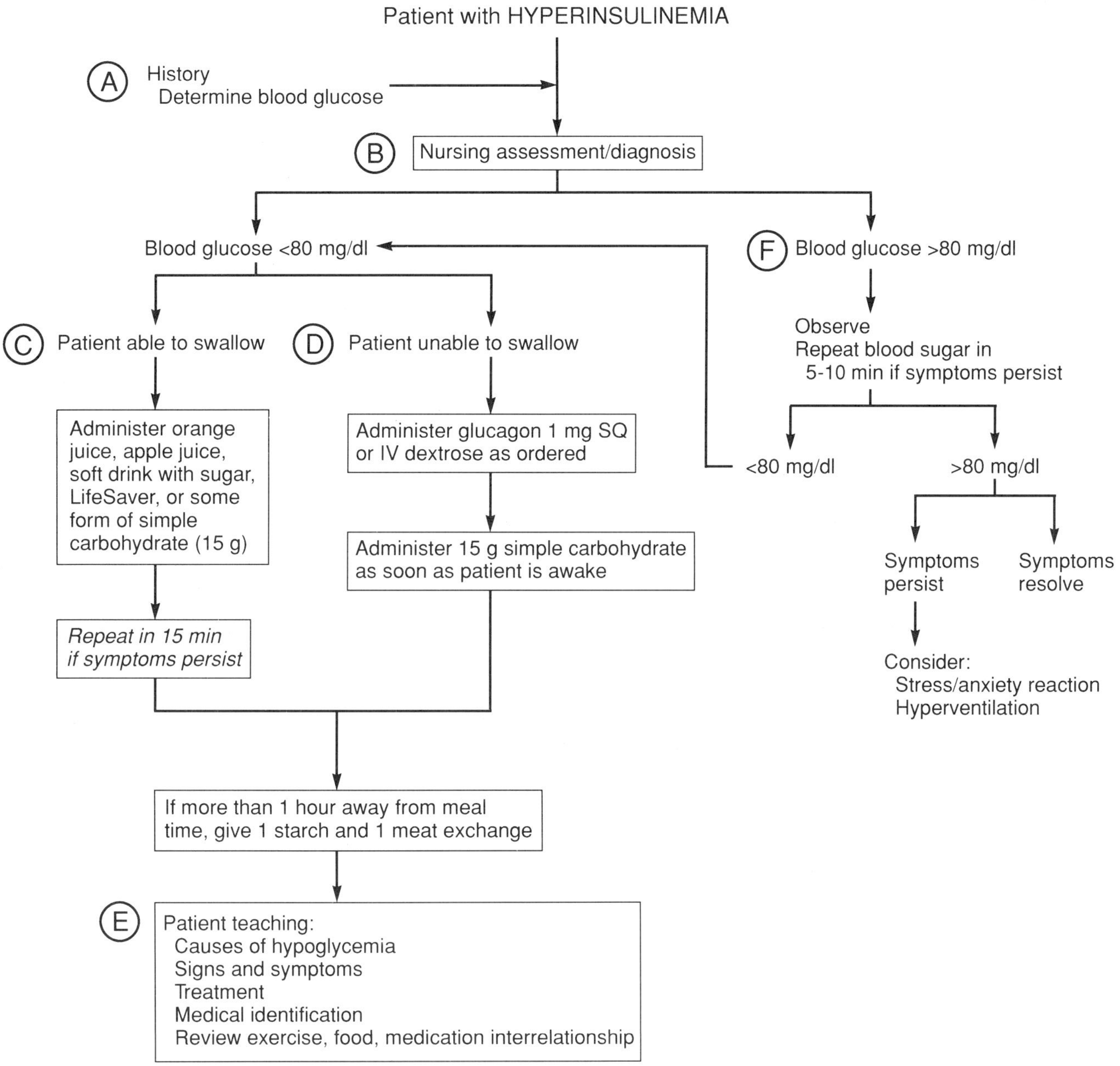
Patient with HYPERINSULINEMIA
A History
Determine blood glucose
B Nursing assessment/diagnosis
Blood glucose <80 mg/dl
F Blood glucose >80 mg/dl
C Patient able to swallow
D Patient unable to swallow
Observe
Repeat blood sugar in 5-10 min if symptoms persist
Administer orange juice, apple juice, soft drink with sugar, LifeSaver, or some form of simple carbohydrate (15 g)
Administer glucagon 1 mg SQ or IV dextrose as ordered
<80 mg/dl
>80 mg/dl
Administer 15 g simple carbohydrate as soon as patient is awake
Symptoms persist
Symptoms resolve
Repeat in 15 min if symptoms persist
Consider:
Stress/anxiety reaction
Hyperventilation
If more than 1 hour away from meal time, give 1 starch and 1 meat exchange
E Patient teaching:
Causes of hypoglycemia
Signs and symptoms
Treatment
Medical identification
Review exercise, food, medication interrelationship

HYPERTHYROIDISM

Gail Shores

Hyperthyroidism is a condition in which there is an excess output of thyroid hormones. The etiology is unknown, but it is thought to be caused by abnormal stimulation of the thyroid gland by circulating immunoglobulins; hence it is one of the little understood autoimmune illnesses. It affects women five times more frequently than men, generally occurs in the 30s or 40s age group, and is more likely to appear after an emotional shock, stress, pregnancy, or infection.

A. Patients often present with a history of nervousness, restlessness, irritability, weakness, fatigue, heat intolerance, fine tremors, weight loss despite a ravenous appetite, menstrual irregularities, impotence, and/or changes in bowel habits to either constipation or diarrhea.

B. Physical findings may include resting tachycardia (heart rate 90 to 160 beats per minute), fine tremor of the hands or tongue, hyperreflexia, warm moist skin, and atrial fibrillation. The thyroid gland is frequently enlarged, soft, and pulsates, causing a palpable "thrill" and a bruit heard over the thyroid arteries. Many patients develop exophthalmos, a condition in which edema develops in the tissue behind the eyes, causing them to protrude and giving the patient a startled or "bug-eyed" expression. Emotional changes are common and may range from mild exhilaration to delirium and exhaustion, progressing to severe depression. These patients may initially present on an inpatient psychiatric unit, because they often feel as if they are "going crazy." Support and encouragement are major nursing interventions during this phase. This includes teaching the patient methods for coping with this disease process.

C. When hyperthyroidism is suspected because of a patient's history and presenting symptoms, a panel of thyroid function testing is done (including T_4, T_3 by radioimmune assay [RIA], and thyroid stimulating hormone [TSH] blood levels). Frequently one or more of these values is elevated. A radioactive iodine uptake measures the rate of iodine uptake by the thyroid gland. Patients with hyperthyroidism accumulate a high proportion of ^{131}I (in some cases up to 90 percent) administered in the testing procedure.

D. There is no curative therapy; however, a reduction in thyroid hyperactivity can provide symptomatic relief and thus remove the cause of the resulting complications. Persons with uncontrolled hyperthyroidism, especially Graves' disease, are susceptible to the medical emergencies of thyroid crisis or storm. The crisis is precipitated by stress, e.g., infection or trauma, and occurs abruptly. The cause of thyroid crisis is unknown. Signs and symptoms are caused by increased metabolism. Fever is always present. Sinus or ectopic tachypnea may lead to cardiac failure. The patient is extremely restless and exhibits tremors. Psychosis, delirium, or coma may occur. Treatment consists of large doses of propylthiouracil along with a saturated solution of potassium iodide (SSKI). Other drugs may also be given to inhibit the release of thyroid hormones. Supportive therapy includes fluids, control of fever, and treatment of cardiac failure. Nursing care involves monitoring cardiac output, providing complete care and comfort, and elimination of all stressors.

E. Administration of antithyroid drugs, such as PTU (propylthiouracil) or Tapazole interferes with the synthesis of thyroid hormones, and other drugs such as Inderal (propranolol) help to control many other manifestations of the disease. Patients should be taught the importance of taking medications at regularly spaced intervals to maintain necessary blood levels. Fever, sore throat, or skin eruptions should be reported to the physician, because these symptoms may indicate drug toxicity. Toxicity may be verified through blood counts showing leukopenia. These individuals may need to discontinue medication.

F. Radioactive iodine therapy (^{131}I) can decrease thyroid activity. A single dose is usually effective within 3 weeks, and thyroid function returns to normal within a couple of months. The medication may be taken at home unless unusually large doses are prescribed. Precautions should include flushing the toilet several times after use and sleeping alone for several nights. Patients need extra reassurance that radioactivity is quickly dissipated. This method of treatment is not used for pregnant women because of the potential effect on the fetus.

G. A thyroidectomy (p 202) is performed if medication and/or radioactive therapy is ineffective.

H. Depending on the form of treatment, the patient is discharged with instructions regarding the treatment and medication regimen and need for medical follow-up.

References

Braunwald E, Isselbachek K, Petersdorf F, et al, eds. Harrison's principles of internal medicine. 11th ed. New York: McGraw-Hill, 1987.

Cassmeyer VL. Interventions for persons with problems of the endocrine system. In: Phipps WJ, Long BC, Woods NF, eds. Medical-surgical nursing: concepts & clinical practice. St. Louis: CV Mosby, 1987:558–564.

Mulvihill ML. Human diseases: a systemic approach. 2nd ed. Norwalk, CT: Appleton & Lange, 1987.

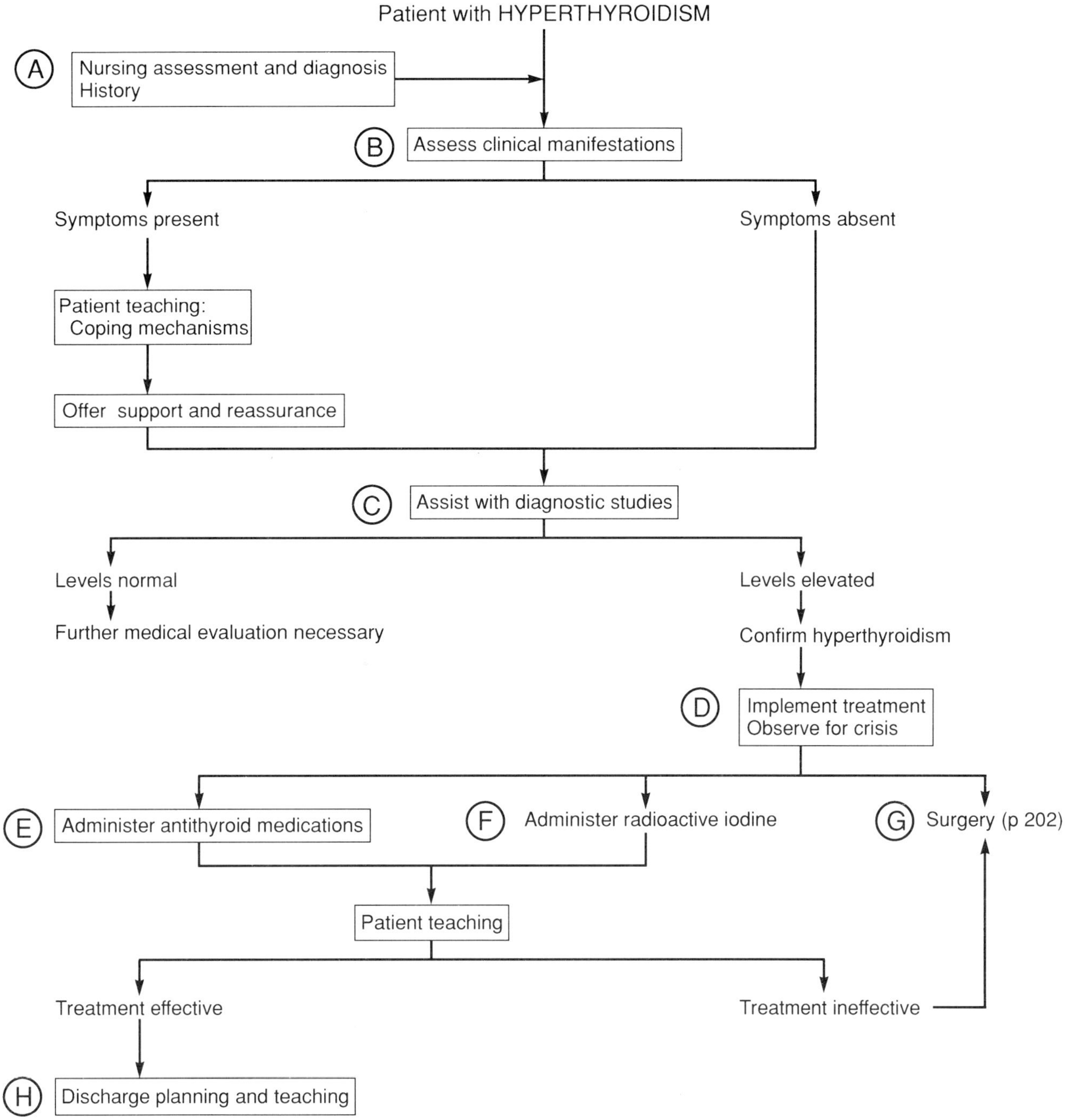

Patient with HYPERTHYROIDISM
A
Nursing assessment and diagnosis
History
B
Assess clinical manifestations
Symptoms present
Symptoms absent
Patient teaching:
Coping mechanisms
Offer support and reassurance
C
Assist with diagnostic studies
Levels normal
Further medical evaluation necessary
Levels elevated
Confirm hyperthyroidism
D
Implement treatment
Observe for crisis
E
Administer antithyroid medications
F
Administer radioactive iodine
G
Surgery (p 202)
Patient teaching
Treatment effective
Treatment ineffective
H
Discharge planning and teaching

HYPOTHYROIDISM

Gail Shores

Hypothyroidism, sometimes called myxedema, is underactivity of the thyroid gland. The gland produces only small amounts of thyroid hormone (thyroxine—thyroid stimulating hormone, or TSH), and all chemical processes in the body slow down. Hypothyroidism affects women five times more frequently than men and occurs most often between the ages of 30 and 60 years.

A. Hypothyroidism has several causes, but it also can occur for no apparent reason. Treatment for hyperthyroidism (p 184) may cause the previously overactive gland to become underactive (e.g., owing to surgical removal of a large portion of the thyroid gland or damage from radiation). A more unusual cause is a lack of TSH, caused by a disorder of the pituitary gland (hypopituitarism—the anterior lobe of the pituitary gland is underactive and does not produce sufficient hormone). Hypothyroidism may also occur in Hashimoto's disease, a disorder in which an inflammatory thyroid condition (probably caused by an autoimmune reaction) destroys the body's thyroid gland. Rarely, a baby is born with either a defective thyroid or no gland at all. If this condition is not detected and treated, it can lead to cretinism or irreversible mental retardation and dwarfism.

B. Symptoms of hypothyroidism may develop slowly over months or years. Patients complain of fatigue, frequent aches and pains, and thus move more slowly. They tend to sleep 14 to 16 hours a day, have slow reflexes, a thick tongue, slurred speech, and a slow heart rate. This leads to slowed circulation, which can cause edema, constipation, and generalized weight gain. There is a sensitivity to cold, and the hair becomes thin, dry, and dull. The skin becomes dry and scaly and thickens, giving the face a bloated appearance. Edema may cause a deeper, hoarse quality to the voice; loss of auditory acuity; and numbness and tingling sensations in the wrist and hands. Women frequently experience heavier menstrual periods, and both men and women experience a loss of libido.

C. Hypothyroidism can be fatal if myxedema coma develops. Although rare, *this is a medical emergency.* The patient becomes cold, lethargic, and drowsy, lapsing into an unconscious state and death, if untreated.

D. Diagnosis can be made easily by thyroid function studies. The serum T_3 (triiodothyronine) and T_4 (thyroxine) levels are generally subnormal, while the serum TSH or thyrotropin levels are elevated. A radioactive iodine uptake (RAI) test may also be done to measure the rate of iodine uptake by the thyroid gland. The patient is given a tracer dose of ^{131}I, and a count is made over the thyroid, using a scintillation counter. Patients with hypothyroidism exhibit a very low uptake of iodine.

E. The goal of treatment is to restore the thyroid hormone in the tissues to a level high enough to relieve the symptoms of hypothyroidism and low enough to prevent symptoms of hyperthyroidism (p 184). Synthetic levothyroxine (Synthroid) is the preferred medication for supplementing the body's own production of thyroid hormone. The dosage is based on the patient's normal or suppressed serum TSH concentration. Dosage usually varies from 0.1 mg to 0.2 mg daily. Desiccated thyroid is also used occasionally, but it has been known to cause an elevated serum T_3 level and resultant symptoms of hyperthyroidism. If replacement therapy is sufficient, a normal metabolic state is restored, and the patient feels much better in a short time.

F. Patient teaching includes methods to help the patient cope with the physical and emotional effects of the disease process. Referrals to the psychiatric liaison nurse may be appropriate. The nurse should provide emotional support and reassurance during treatment.

G. During discharge teaching, it must be stressed that a daily regimen of supplemental thyroid medication is necessary for the remainder of the patient's life to prevent recurrence of the symptoms. Blood tests should be done at the annual physical assessment to be certain the precise dosage is being given.

References

Braunwald E, Isselbachek K, Petersdorf F, et al, eds. Harrison's principles of internal medicine. 11th ed. New York: McGraw-Hill, 1987.

Hamilton HK, Rose MB. Professional guide to diseases. Springhouse, PA: Intermed Communications, 1982.

Mulvihill ML. Human diseases: a systemic approach. 2nd ed. Norwalk CT: Appleton & Lange, 1987.

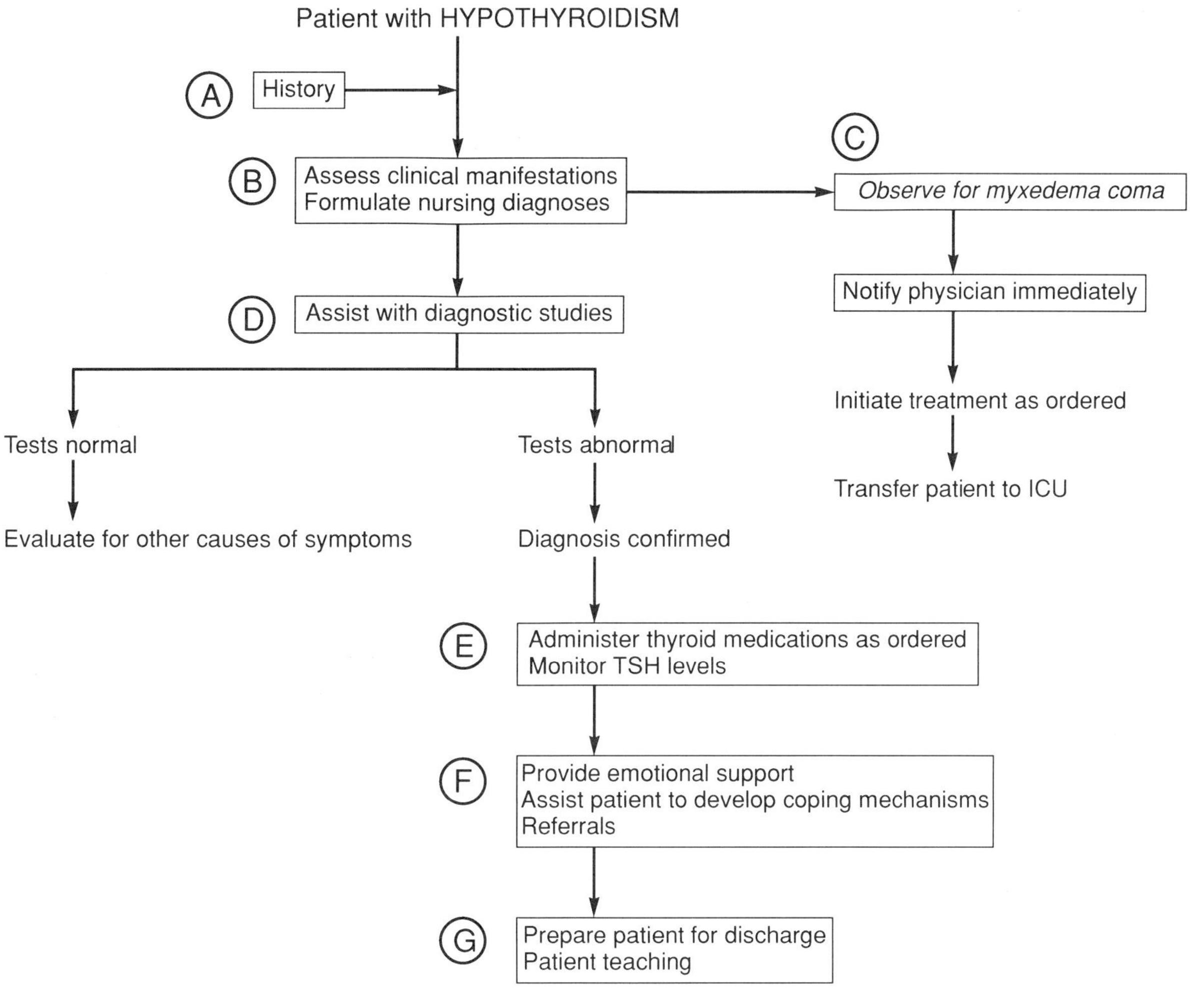
Patient with HYPOTHYROIDISM
A
History
B
Assess clinical manifestations
Formulate nursing diagnoses
C
Observe for myxedema coma
Notify physician immediately
Initiate treatment as ordered
Transfer patient to ICU
D
Assist with diagnostic studies
Tests normal
Evaluate for other causes of symptoms
Tests abnormal
Diagnosis confirmed
E
Administer thyroid medications as ordered
Monitor TSH levels
F
Provide emotional support
Assist patient to develop coping mechanisms
Referrals
G
Prepare patient for discharge
Patient teaching

HYPERCALCEMIA

Marsha Cloak

Hypercalcemia is a metabolic condition characterized by an elevation in serum calcium levels above 10.5 mg/dl. When hypercalcemia is detected, a diagnosis of the underlying disease process must be made. In 90 percent of patients with hypercalcemia, the cause is either primary hyperparathyroidism or a neoplastic disease. Malignancies most commonly associated with hypercalcemia are carcinomas of the breast, lung (p 122), prostate (p 294), pancreas, kidneys, or bladder (p 298), multiple myeloma (p 362), and lymphoma. A thorough history is important to assess symptoms, drug intake, and diet.

A. Clinical manifestations of hypercalcemia and their degree of severity are determined by the serum calcium level. When the calcium level is above 12.0 mg/dl, symptoms are usually present. Clinical manifestations of hypercalcemia can be categorized by systems (Table 1). Nursing care is planned to assess each system continually while maintaining function. Emotional and physical support are especially important to prevent long-term debilitation.

B. To diagnose hypercalcemia, more than one serum calcium level must be taken. Hypercalcemia can be established when at least three levels are increased above the normal range. Hypercalcemia in a person who is asymptomatic is most often caused by hyperparathyroidism; however, a differential diagnosis must be made. Immunoassay for parathyroid hormone (iPTH) should be done to determine if the underlying cause is primary hyperparathyroidism. If the serum iPTH is normal, a work-up is done to identify a neoplastic disease. Other studies that can be done to determine if the hypercalcemia is parathyroid- or nonparathyroid-related include serum phosphate, magnesium, potassium, chloride, alkaline phosphatase, hematocrit, and erythrocyte sedimentation rate. Urinary studies include cyclic adenosine monophosphate (AMP) excretion levels and measurement of 24-hour urine calcium levels. To determine the severity of hypercalcemia, the serum albumin must also be evaluated. If the serum albumin level is low, the severity of the hypercalcemia is greater than that indicated by the serum calcium level. For every gram per deciliter reduction in the serum albumin, the measured total serum calcium should be adjusted upward by 0.8 mg/dl. This recalculation of the serum calcium gives a more accurate reflection of the degree of hypercalcemia.

TABLE 1 Clinical Manifestations of Hypercalcemia by System

System	*Symptoms*
Neuromuscular system	Fatigue Muscle weakness Muscle atrophy
Central nervous system	Impaired concentration Loss of memory Somnolence Confusion Lethargy Stupor Coma
Renal system	Polyuria Nocturia Renal tubular defects Decreased ability to concentrate Nephrolithiasis Nephrocalcinosis
Cardiovascular system	Hypertension Electrocardiographic changes (shortened Q-T interval) (Fig. 1) Arrhythmias Digitalis toxicity
Gastrointestinal system	Anorexia Nausea and vomiting Constipation Pancreatitis Peptic ulcer

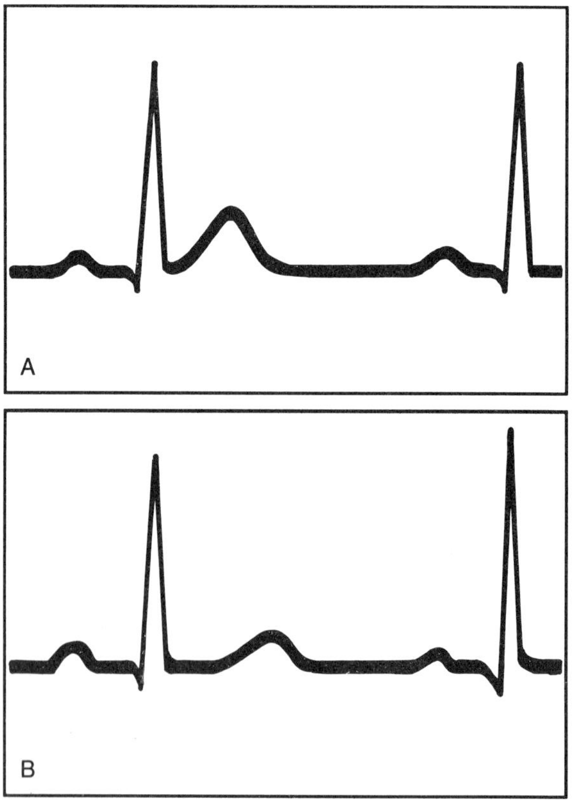

Figure 1 *A.* Electrocardiographic changes in hypercalcemia (short Q-T segment). *B.* Normal serum calcium.

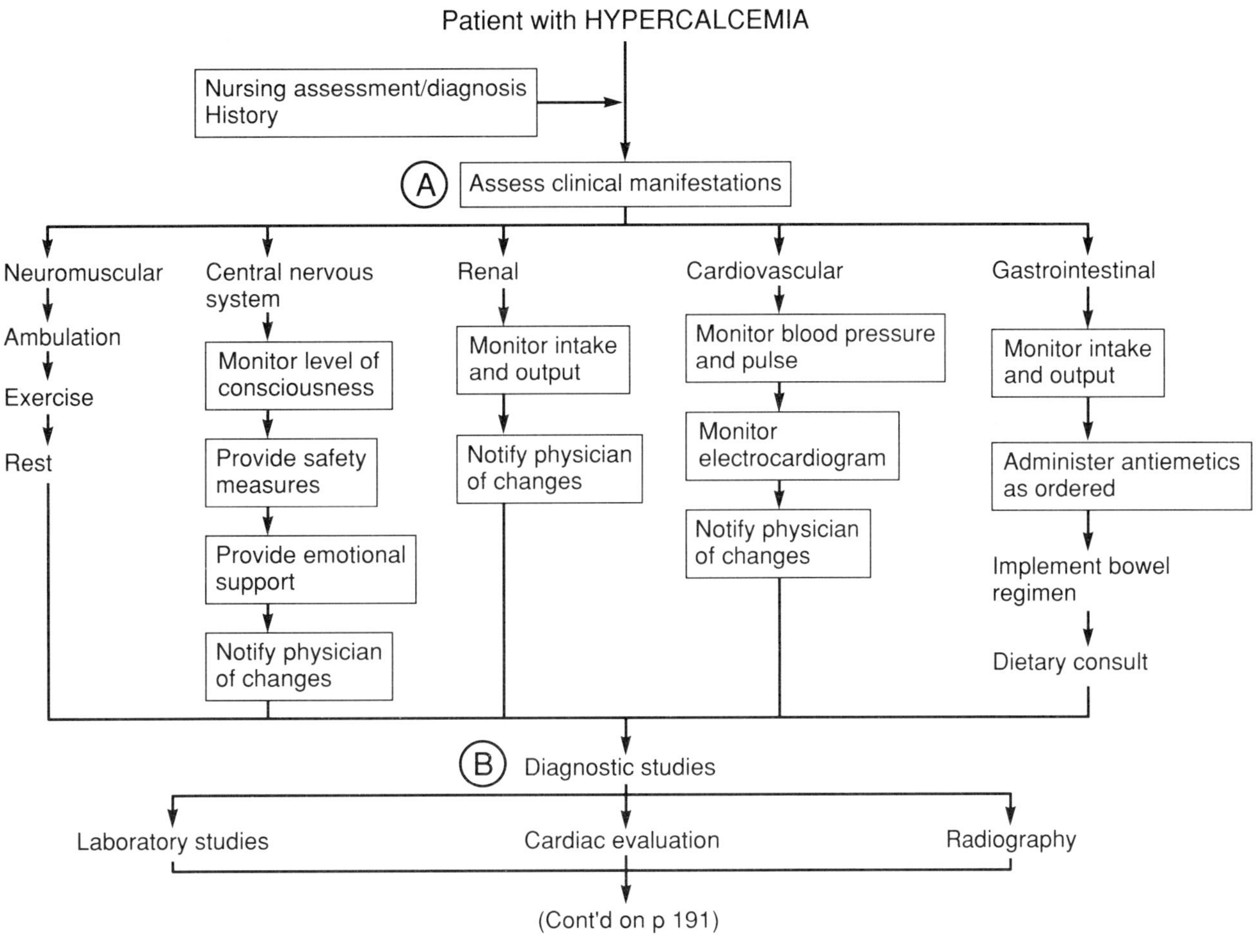
Patient with HYPERCALCEMIA
Nursing assessment/diagnosis
History
A
Assess clinical manifestations
Neuromuscular
Ambulation
Exercise
Rest
Central nervous system
Monitor level of consciousness
Provide safety measures
Provide emotional support
Notify physician of changes
Renal
Monitor intake and output
Notify physician of changes
Cardiovascular
Monitor blood pressure and pulse
Monitor electrocardiogram
Notify physician of changes
Gastrointestinal
Monitor intake and output
Administer antiemetics as ordered
Implement bowel regimen
Dietary consult
B
Diagnostic studies
Laboratory studies
Cardiac evaluation
Radiography
(Cont'd on p 191)

C. Hypercalcemia is categorized according to the serum level, with calcium levels less than 12 mg/dl being mild, 12 to 15 mg/dl being moderate, and above 15 mg/dl being severe hypercalcemia. Treatment depends on the calcium level, severity of the symptoms, and the underlying disease process. If hypercalcemia is mild and symptoms are not present, an aggressive approach is not indicated.

D. In addition to treatment of the cause, moderate hypercalcemia should be treated with a fluid intake of 3 to 5 L per day and a sodium chloride intake of 300 to 400 mEq per day, unless contraindicated by cardiac status. After fluid therapy has been given, loop diuretics such as furosemide may be given to enhance renal excretion of sodium and calcium. If fluid and sodium chloride therapy fail, oral phosphates can be given.

E. *Severe hypercalcemia (hypercalcemic crisis) is considered life-threatening,* and interventions must be implemented immediately. To detect fluid overload and the precipitation of pulmonary edema, the central venous pressure is monitored. For severe or moderate hypercalcemia that does not respond to hydration and diuresis, pharmacologic agents such as mithramycin, glucocorticoids, calcitonin, and phosphates may be given. After calcium has been reduced to a safe level, therapy should be instituted to treat the underlying cause and to prevent recurrence. When the patient is clinically stabilized, further interventions include monitoring for early signs and symptoms of a rising calcium level, promoting ambulation, and implementing isometric exercises if ambulation is not feasible.

F. Patient education should include instructions about the diagnosis, its etiology, the treatment regimen, symptoms to observe for, and appropriate self-care measures. The provision of emotional support to the patient and family is essential.

References

Bilezikian JP. Hypercalcemia. In: Stein JH, ed. Internal medicine. 2nd ed. Boston: Little, Brown, 1987.

Poe CM, Radford AI. The challenge of hypercalcemia in cancer. Oncol Nurs Forum 1985; 12(6):29–32.

Potts JT Jr. Diseases of the parathyroid gland and other hyper- and hypocalcemic disorders. In: Braunwald E, ed. Harrison's principles of internal medicine. 11th ed. St. Louis: McGraw-Hill, 1987.

Singer FR, Fernandez M. Therapy of hypercalcemia of malignancy. Am J Med 1987; 82(Suppl 2A):34–40.

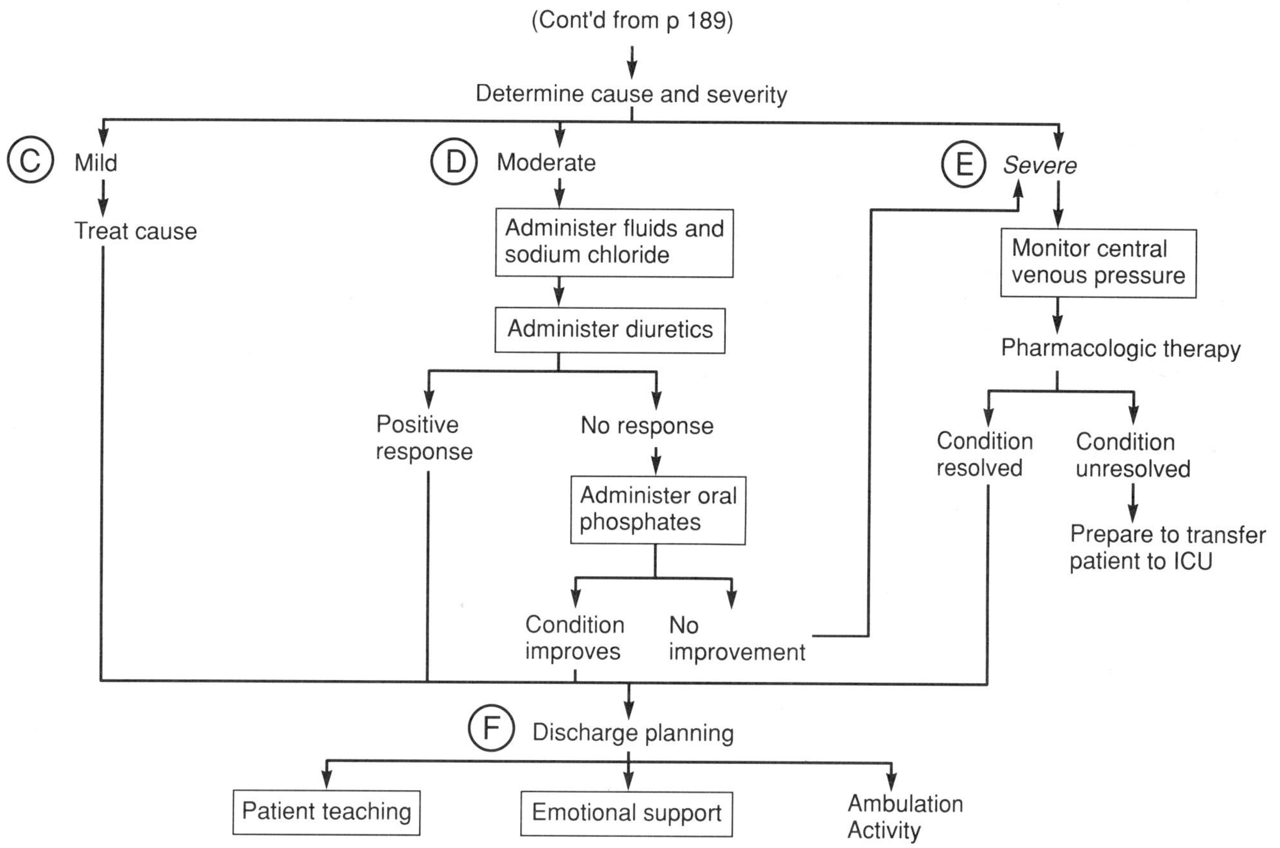
(Cont'd from p 189)
Determine cause and severity
C Mild
Treat cause
D Moderate
Administer fluids and sodium chloride
Administer diuretics
Positive response
No response
Administer oral phosphates
Condition improves
No improvement
E *Severe*
Monitor central venous pressure
Pharmacologic therapy
Condition resolved
Condition unresolved
Prepare to transfer patient to ICU
F Discharge planning
Patient teaching
Emotional support
Ambulation Activity

HYPOCALCEMIA

William B. Marshall

Hypocalcemia is defined as a serum calcium level of less than 8.5 mg/dl, or less than 4.3 mEq/L. Most institutions use the mg/dl standard at a range of 8.5 to 10.5.

A. Dietary calcium is absorbed from the small intestine, and can therefore be decreased as a result of either inadequate intake or decreased absorption. Because of their roles in calcium regulation and metabolism, deficits in parathyroid hormone and vitamin D may predispose to hypocalcemia. Other conditions that may precipitate hypocalcemia include hyperphosphatemia, diminished thyrocalcitonin secretion, hypomagnesemia, malignant bone metastasis or osteomalacia (p 220), acute pancreatitis, renal failure (pp 314, 318), massive transfusions of whole blood or packed red cells, high protein diets, massive subcutaneous infections such as cellulitis, and long-term hyperalimentation therapy.

B. Clinical manifestations of hypocalcemia may be seen in the neuromuscular gastrointestinal, integumentary, and cardiac systems.

C. The increased excitability of the nervous system causes tingling and numbness in the fingers, nose, ears, and/or toes. If calcium is not administered at this time, tetany (painful muscle spasms) and convulsions may occur. Patients who have had thyroid surgery (p 202) should be watched for signs of tetany, as the parathyroid glands could have been removed or damaged by surgery.

D. One of the tests used to determine the presence of calcium deficiency is Chvostek's sign, which is elicited by lightly tapping the finger on the patient's face just anterior to the tragus of the ear. A positive finding, i.e., unilateral twitching of lips or the eyelids, indicates hypocalcemia.

E. Another test for calcium deficit is Trousseau's sign, which is elicited by placing a blood pressure cuff on the arm and inflating it to 20 mm Hg over resting systolic pressure. The cuff remains inflated for 3 minutes to see if carpopedal spasm (hand into palmar flexion) occurs. A positive Trousseau's sign indicates hypocalcemia.

F. Mental status changes may be vague, but can include mood swings, depression, psychoses, confusion, and memory loss.

G. Electrocardiographic (ECG) changes that may be seen with hypocalcemia are extreme bradycardia (p 56); varying degrees of atrioventricular block; lengthened S-T segment; and a lengthened Q-T interval with decreased rate (Fig. 1).

H. Hypocalcemia may enhance the action of the digitalis glycosides, which are used to increase the force of myocardial contraction and to decrease the heart rate. However, hypocalcemia may neutralize the effects of the digitalis and may also exacerbate digitalis-induced bradycardia.

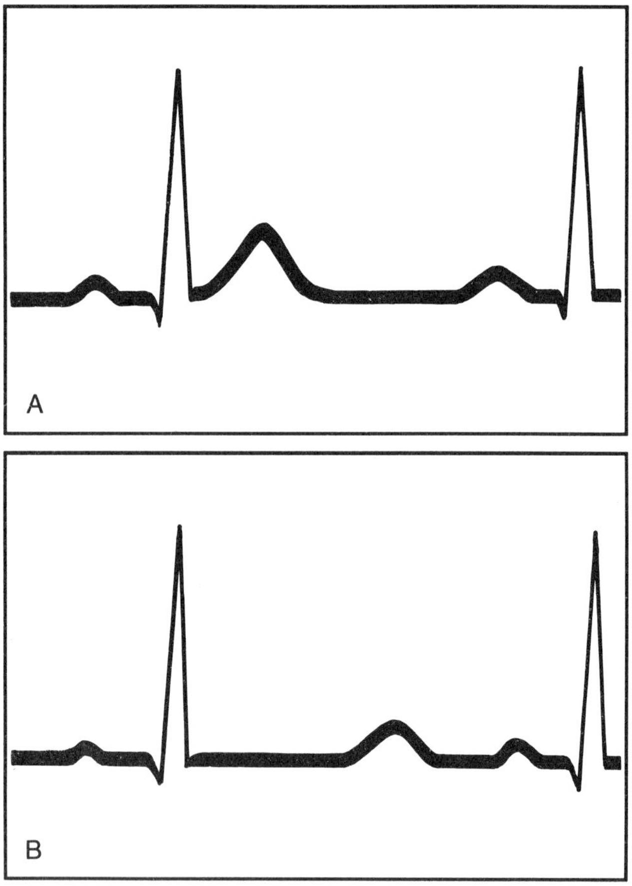

Figure 1 *A.* ECG for patient with normal blood calcium; *B.* ECG changes for patient with hypocalcemia (note long Q-T segment).

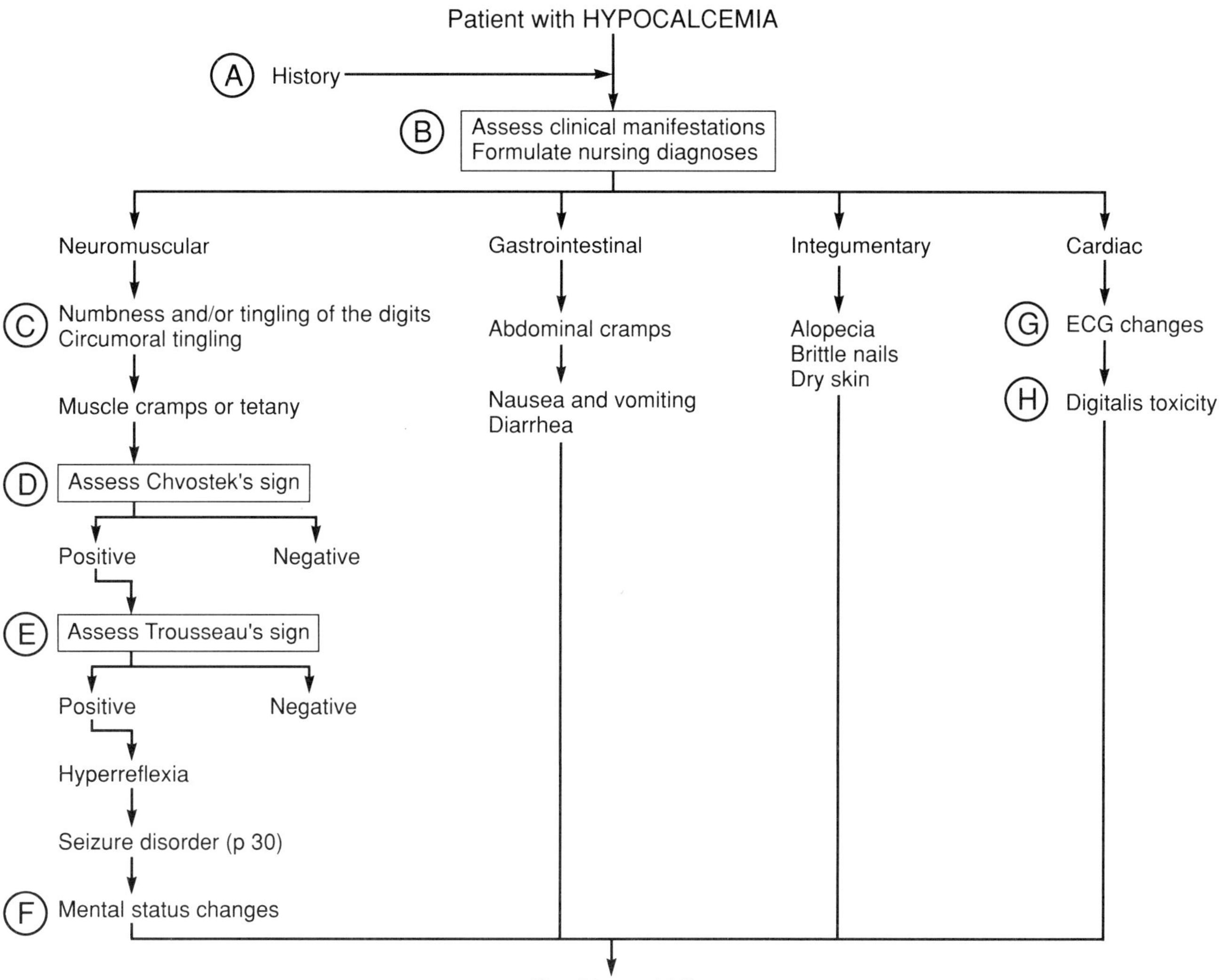

(Cont'd on p 195)

I. Other laboratory findings include decreased serum calcium and elevated serum phosphorus. A Sulkowitch urine test (24-hour sample) shows no precipitation.

J. Chronic or subacute hypocalcemia may be treated simply by increasing dietary intake of calcium. Supplementing the diet with milk and cheeses, and to a lesser extent some meats and vegetables, usually serves to correct the imbalance. However, medicinal supplements may be needed. Calcium carbonate, calcium lactate, and calcium gluconate are commonly utilized. Doses range from 1 to 8 g per day in divided doses. The use of vitamin D supplements may serve to increase the absorption of dietary calcium by the small intestine.

K. Intravenous replacement may be necessary in more acute cases in which symptoms are more pronounced and occur with increased frequency. Commonly used preparations include calcium chloride, calcium gluceptate, and calcium gluconate, depending on the severity of the imbalance. *Calcium preparations given rapidly via the intravenous route may precipitate cardiac arrest.*

L. Phosphorus, magnesium, and potassium must be monitored because of their relationship to calcium. Phosphorus is excreted by the kidneys in an effort to correct hypocalcemia. Hyperphosphatemia may precipitate hypocalcemia. Hypomagnesemia exhibits many of the same neuromuscular symptoms as hypocalcemia and may actually precipitate hypocalcemia. Potassium regulates electrical potential in the skeletal and cardiac muscle cells.

M. The avoidance of foods or pharmacotherapeutics containing phosphates is necessary in order to evaluate and treat hypocalcemia properly.

N. Patients requiring further observation and cardiac monitoring should be admitted to ICU. The lead of choice for monitoring is either MCL1 or MCL6.

References

Byrne CJ, Saxton DF, Pelikan PK, Nugent PM. Laboratory tests. Menlo Park, CA: Addison-Wesley, 1986.

Muir BL. Pathophysiology: an introduction to the mechanisms of disease. New York: John Wiley, 1988.

Price SA, Wilson LM. Pathophysiology: clinical concepts of disease processes. New York: McGraw-Hill, 1986.

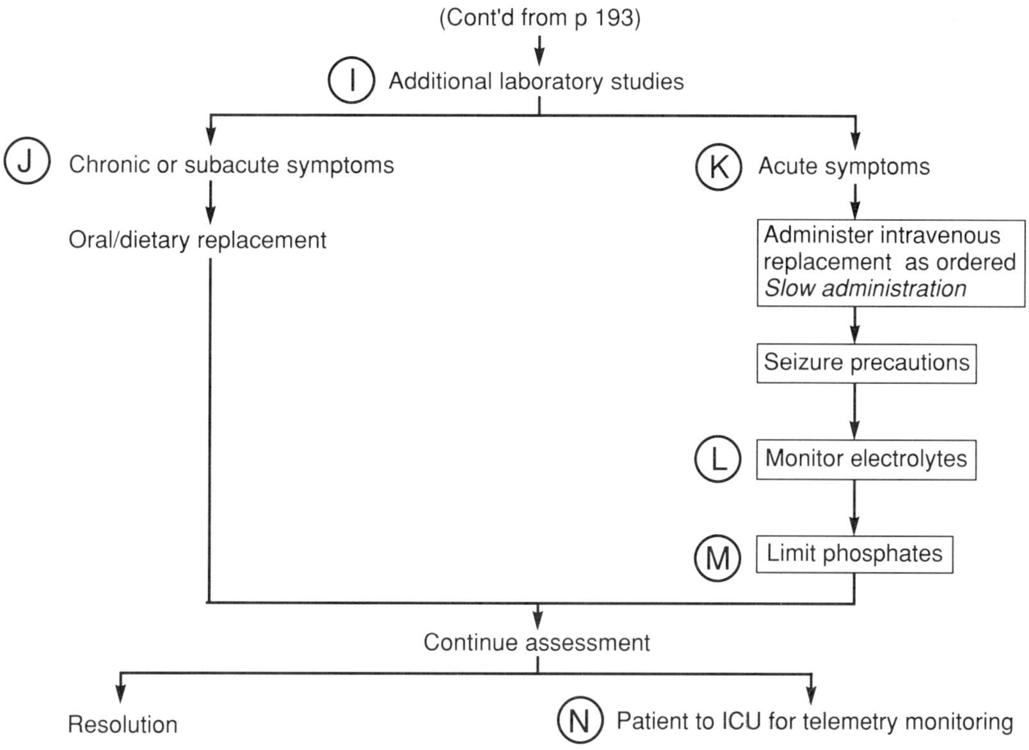
(Cont'd from p 193)
I Additional laboratory studies
J Chronic or subacute symptoms
Oral/dietary replacement
K Acute symptoms
Administer intravenous replacement as ordered
Slow administration
Seizure precautions
L Monitor electrolytes
M Limit phosphates
Continue assessment
Resolution
N Patient to ICU for telemetry monitoring

HYPERKALEMIA

Kathleen H. Toto

Hyperkalemia occurs when serum potassium (K^+) levels are elevated above 5.0 mEq/L. This can be caused by a clinical state, true hyperkalemia, or an error in collection of the sample, pseudohyperkalemia. The most common cause of true hyperkalemia is decreased renal excretion of potassium. Although laboratory values play a vital role in determining electrolyte abnormalities, they cannot substitute for bedside assessment and early detection of conditions that may precipitate dangerous electrolyte imbalances.

A. Nursing assessment of the patient with hyperkalemia includes vital signs, physical assessment, and a complete history including medications the patient is taking and dietary habits. The history and assessment provide valuable information to aid in determining the etiology and severity of hyperkalemia. Inadequate renal excretion is seen in patients with acute and chronic renal failure (pp 314, 318); as a side effect of potassium-sparing diuretics such as spironolactone (Aldactone), triamterene, and amiloride; and in hypoaldosteronism (Addison's disease). Other causes include rapid infusion of intravenous potassium chloride (rate greater than 20 mEq per hour), multiple blood transfusions, and tissue damage as may be seen in patients with burns (p 248), myocardial infarction (p 66), or crush injuries. Dietary intake of potassium is rarely a cause except in the presence of renal failure. Pseudohyperkalemia may occur with hemolysis and thrombocytosis of blood samples.

B. A 12-lead electrocardiogram (ECG) provides useful information in evaluating the cardiotoxic effects of hyperkalemia. The earliest electrocardiographic change seen with hyperkalemia is the development of tall, peaked T waves (Fig. 1). As hyperkalemia becomes more severe, there is prolongation of the P-R interval, flattening of the P wave, heart block, atrial asystole, and prolongation of the QRS complex (Fig. 2).

C. Clinical manifestations of hyperkalemia depend on the degree of serum potassium elevations and the rate of development. These may be seen in several body systems (Table 1).

D. Before the appropriate treatment can be determined, it is necessary to assess the severity of hyperkalemia. This is done by evaluating both the serum potassium level and the ECG. A serum potassium level of less than 6.5 mEq/L with ECG changes limited to tall, peaked T waves is considered mild hyperkalemia. Treatment would be aimed at determining the cause of hyperkalemia and eliminating it if possible.

E. A serum potassium level of 6.5 to 8.0 mEq/L with tall, peaked T waves as the only ECG change is considered moderate hyperkalemia. Treatment includes the administration of a cation exchange resin (Kayexalate) orally or by enema. Serum potassium levels can be reduced by 0.5 to 2.0 mEq/L within an hour. These exchange resins act by binding potassium and eliminating it in the stool. When potassium is bound, sodium is liberated and hypernatremia can result. As a retention enema, the exchange resin should be retained 30 to 60 minutes to be effective. The resin is often dissolved in sorbitol for its cathartic effect.

F. Severe hyperkalemia occurs when serum potassium levels exceed 8.0 mEq/L or if the ECG changes include absent P waves, widened QRS complexes, or ventricular arrhythmias.

G. *Severe hyperkalemia is a medical emergency* and treatment should begin at once. The patient receives continuous ECG monitoring to evaluate the cardiotoxic effects of hyperkalemia. An intravenous (IV) line is established. The initial treatment is directed toward shifting extracellular potassium into the intracellular compartment. This can be accomplished by the administration of hypertonic glucose (ampule of 50 percent dextrose) in conjunction with 5 to 10 units of regular insulin by IV push. An IV infusion of sodium bicarbonate (44 mEq or 1 ampule) also helps to shift potassium into the cell. These measures alleviate the signs and symptoms of hyperkalemia.

H. If the patient exhibits cardiotoxic signs of hyperkalemia, calcium gluconate (10 to 30 ml of a 10-percent solution) should be administered by slow IV infusion. Calcium does not alter serum potassium levels. The primary action of calcium is to counteract the cardiotoxic effects of hyperkalemia. The onset of action of calcium is rapid. Within 1 to 5 minutes the ECG can return to near normal. However, the effect on the ECG is relatively transient. Calcium should be administered cautiously in patients receiving digitalis as it can potentiate digitalis toxicity.

I. It is important to remember that the emergent treatment of severe hyperkalemia does not change total body potassium levels. Over time, potassium leaks back out of the cell and the patient becomes symptomatic again. The next stage of treatment is directed at removing potassium from the body. This can be accomplished through the administration of a cation exchange resin or by dialysis.

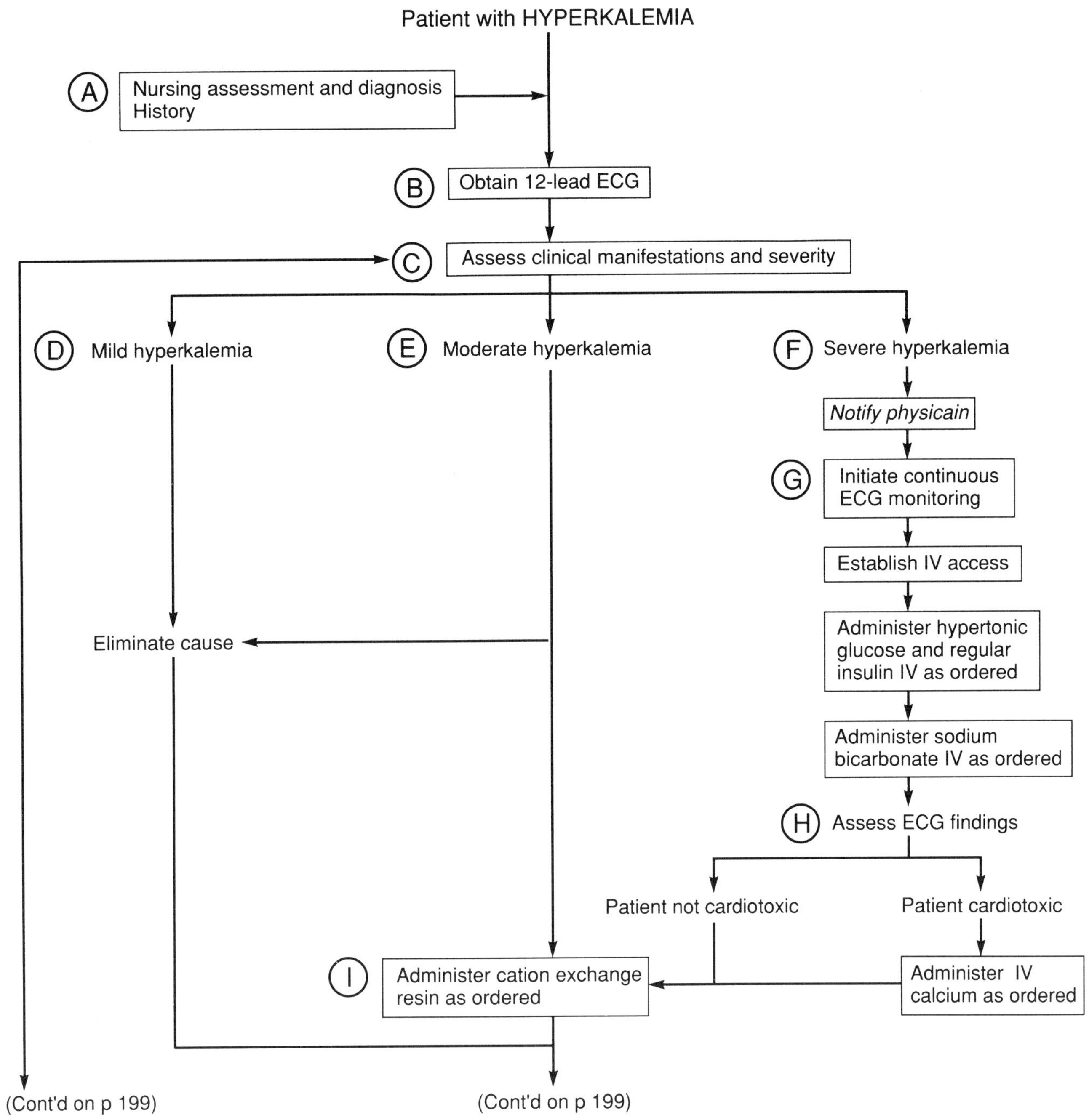

Patient with HYPERKALEMIA
A
Nursing assessment and diagnosis
History
B
Obtain 12-lead ECG
C
Assess clinical manifestations and severity
D
Mild hyperkalemia
E
Moderate hyperkalemia
F
Severe hyperkalemia
Notify physicain
G
Initiate continuous ECG monitoring
Establish IV access
Administer hypertonic glucose and regular insulin IV as ordered
Administer sodium bicarbonate IV as ordered
H
Assess ECG findings
Patient not cardiotoxic
Patient cardiotoxic
Administer IV calcium as ordered
Eliminate cause
I
Administer cation exchange resin as ordered
(Cont'd on p 199)
(Cont'd on p 199)

J. Serum electrolytes should be reassessed after treatment to evaluate the effectiveness of therapy. If the serum potassium levels are within normal limits, the patient should be assessed for recurrence of hyperkalemia. If the patient remains hyperkalemic after treatment, the post-treatment severity of the imbalance should be determined and treatment reinstituted accordingly.

K. Renal function is an important consideration in hyperkalemia. If the patient has acute or chronic renal failure and does not respond to treatment, dialysis must be considered. Both hemodialysis (p 328) and peritoneal dialysis (p 324) effectively lower serum potassium.

L. Recurrence is a major concern. Establishing the underlying cause and initiating treatment to manage this disturbance is essential. Patients must be instructed to recognize signs and symptoms, to understand possible relationships between medications (i.e., cardiac drugs and diuretics), and to maintain regular follow-up with the primary physician.

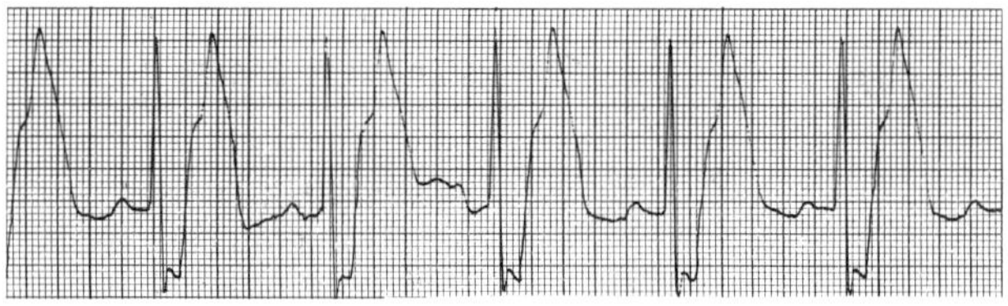

Figure 1 Tall, peaked T waves seen as the earliest ECG change in a patient with hyperkalemia.

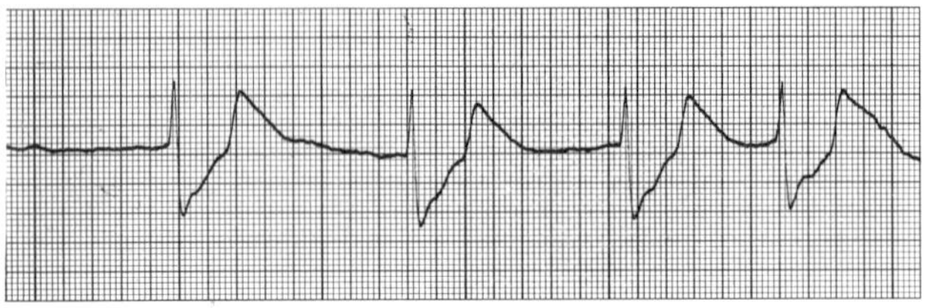

Figure 2 ECG changes seen with more severe hyperkalemia: prolonged P-R internal, flattening P wave, heart block, atrial asystole, and prolonged QRS complex.

TABLE 1 Clinical Manifestations of Hyperkalemia

System	*Manifestation*
Cardiovascular	ECG changes Tall, peaked T waves Shortened Q-T interval Disappearing P waves Lengthening P-R interval Complete heart block Widening QRS complex Asystole
Neuromuscular	Hyperactive deep tendon reflexes Muscle cramps Twitching Paresthesias Ascending paralysis Respiratory arrest
Gastrointestinal	Abdominal cramps Diarrhea Ileus

References

Alpern RJ. Extrarenal potassium regulation: physiology, pathophysiology, and clinical relevance. University of Texas Southwestern Medical School at Dallas: Internal Medicine Grand Rounds, 1987.

Ellis PD. Hyperkalemia. J Emerg Nurs 1979; 5:13–16.

Isselbacher KJ, Adams RD, Braunwald E, Petersdorf RG, Wilson JD. Harrison's principles of internal medicine. 9th ed. New York: McGraw-Hill, 1980.

Maxwell MH, Kleeman CK. Clinical disorders of fluid and electrolyte metabolism. New York: McGraw-Hill, 1980.

Metheny NH. Fluid and electrolyte balance: nursing considerations. Philadelphia: JB Lippincott, 1983.

Toto KH. When the patient has hyperkalemia. RN 1987; 5(4):34–37.

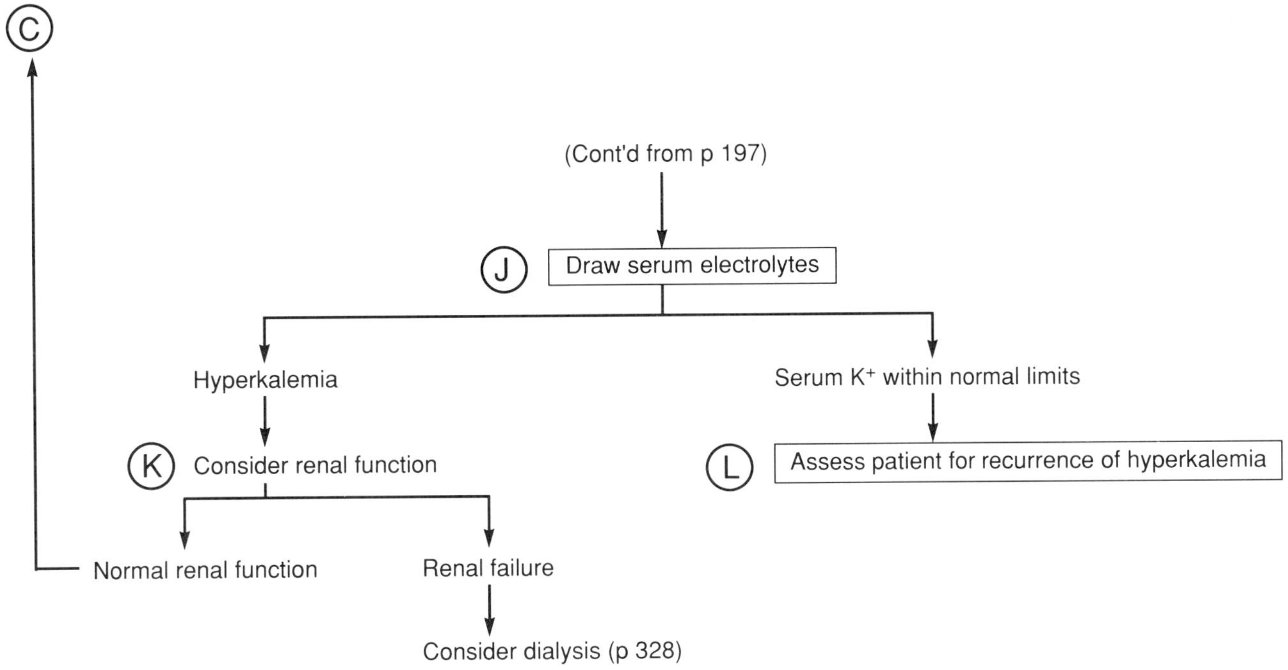
C
(Cont'd from p 197)
J
Draw serum electrolytes
Hyperkalemia
Serum K+ within normal limits
K
Consider renal function
L
Assess patient for recurrence of hyperkalemia
Normal renal function
Renal failure
Consider dialysis (p 328)

HYPOKALEMIA

Kathleen H. Toto

Hypokalemia occurs when serum potassium (K^+) levels fall below 3.5 mEq per liter. Hypokalemia is usually caused by increased renal losses of potassium, but can also occur secondary to gastrointestinal losses, acidosis, excessive diaphoreses, and administration of certain medications.

A. Nursing assessment of the patient with hypokalemia includes vital signs, physical assessment, and a complete history. A complete history provides valuable information to determine the cause of hypokalemia (Table 1). The clinical manifestations of hypokalemia are individualized and depend on the rate at which the hypokalemia develops. Some individuals may be symptomatic with only a mild decrease in serum K^+ levels (Table 2). Conversely, an individual on a starvation diet may have an extremely low serum K^+ and be asymptomatic, since the hypokalemia developed over a prolonged period.

B. Although severe hypokalemia is life-threatening, the treatment of hypokalemia is usually not an emergency, and potassium replacement can often be done with oral agents such as potassium chloride elixir, Slo-K^+, or K^+-Lor. These agents should be taken with meals or with juice, since potassium can be irritating to the stomach. The normal oral dose is 20 to 40 mEq.

C. If the potassium deficit is causing more serious symptoms, intravenous (IV) replacement may be ordered. IV replacement may also be initiated if the patient's gastrointestinal tract is not functional. The physician may order either potassium chloride (KCl) or potassium phosphate (KPhos). IV potassium should not be administered at a rate greater than 20 mEq per hour. Extreme caution should be used and the patient must be placed on a cardiac monitor. Electrocardiographic changes to peaked T waves and prolonged PR and QRS intervals indicate too-rapid infusion. The physician orders the rate of delivery of the potassium as well as the volume of fluid for dilution. Potassium is very irritating to the venous wall, especially when given peripherally. A large vein with at least a 20-gauge needle should be used. A central line should be used when at all possible. In a central line, potassium can be diluted at a concentration of 20 mEq in 50 to 100 ml of fluid. In a peripheral line, 20 mEq should be diluted in 150 to 200 ml of fluid.

D. Assessment of IV sites is important to detect phlebitis secondary to potassium infusion. If the patient complains of burning at the site, the infusion can be further diluted or the rate of administration decreased. If redness develops around the site, the IV infusion should be discontinued and the site treated with warm soaks.

TABLE 1 Causes of Hypokalemia

Increased renal excretion of K^+
Diuretics
Osmotic diuresis
Hormonal imbalances
Primary aldosteronism
Secondary aldosteronism (due to birth control pills, malignant hypertension, etc.)
Cushing's syndrome
Steroid therapy
Diabetic ketoacidosis
Gastrointestinal losses
Excessive nasogastric suction
Vomiting
Diarrhea
Chronic laxative or enema use
Gastrointestinal fistulas
Inadequate intake of K^+
Starvation
Low Na^+ diet
Miscellaneous causes
Alkalosis
Hyperalimentation
Catecholamine infusion

TABLE 2 Clinical Manifestations of Hypokalemia

System	*Signs and Symptoms*
Neuromuscular	Muscle cramps Muscle weakness and fatigue Paralysis
Cardiac	Arrhythmias (premature ventricular contractions, ventricular tachycardia, ventricular fibrillation)
Neural	Lethargy Confusion
Gastrointestinal	Anorexia Abdominal distention Paralytic ileus

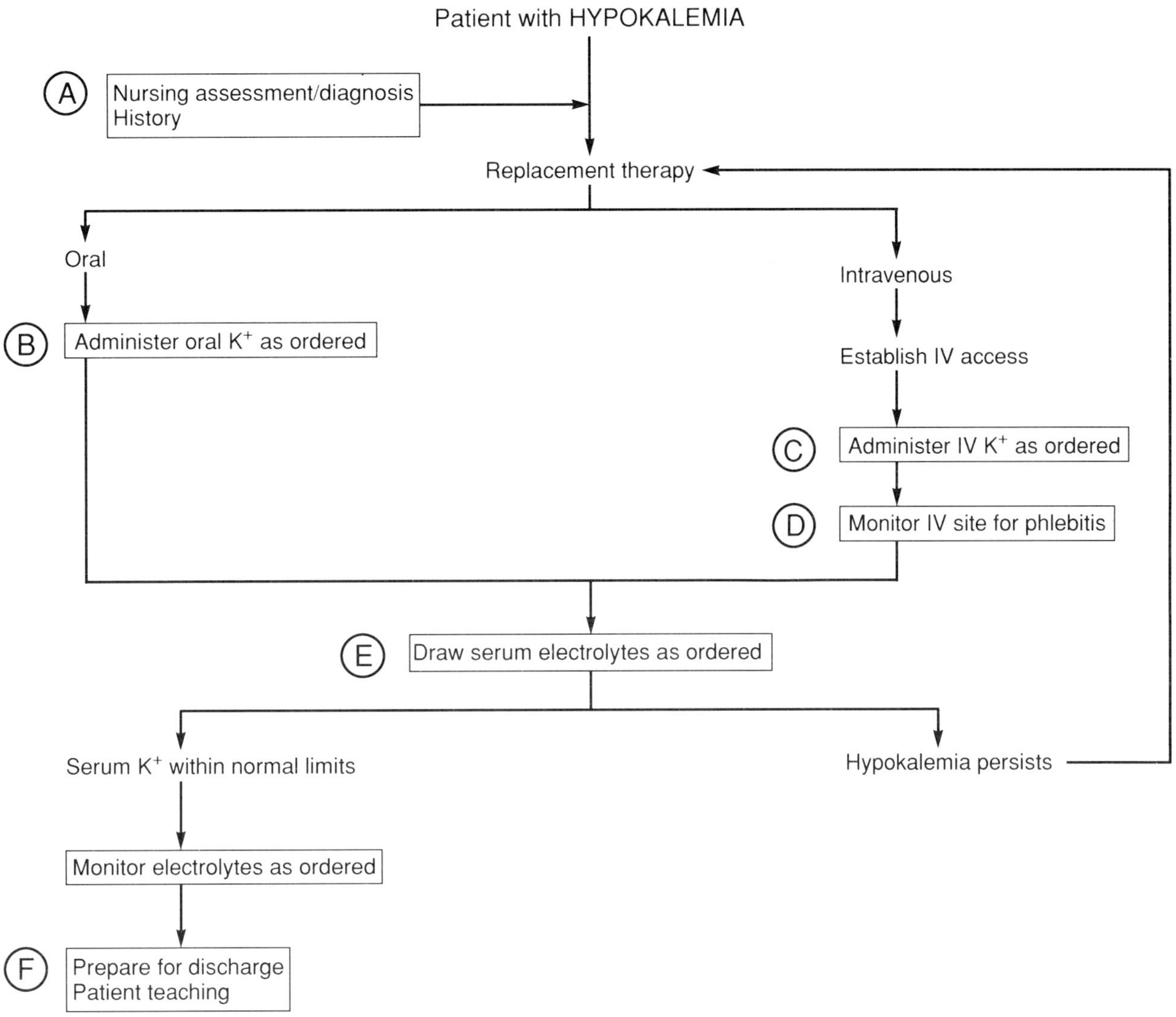

E. After replacement therapy is completed, serum electrolytes may be ordered to assess the patient's potassium level after treatment. The patient should also be assessed for ongoing potassium losses. If the patient remains hypokalemic, additional replacement therapy may be ordered. Treatment is directed at eliminating the cause of the K^+ loss.

F. Patients who are on diuretics should be advised to include in their diet foods high in potassium, such as fruits and vegetables. Muscle weakness, nausea, or vomiting should be reported to the physician.

References

Felver L. Understanding the electrolyte maze. Am J Nurs. 1980 (9):1591.

Maxwell MH and Kleeman, CK. Clinical disorders of fluid and electrolyte metabolism. New York: McGraw Hill, 1980.

Menzel LK. Clinical problems of electrolyte balance. Nurs Clin North Am, 1980; 15(3):5544.

Otakji J. Potassium metabolism disorders. Crit Care Q, 1980; 3(2):55.

Toto KH. When the patient has hypokalemia. RN, 1987; March, 38–42.

THYROIDECTOMY

Diane M. Zintak

Thyroidectomy, removal of the thyroid gland, may be total or partial. Total thyroidectomy is the treatment of choice for cancer of the thyroid. Subtotal thyroidectomy, removal of approximately five-sixths of the gland is performed to correct hyperthyroidism and severe cases of simple goiter. When one-sixth of the funcitoning thyroid is left intact, hormonal replacements may not be necessary; however, individuals undergoing total thyroidectomy must regularly take thyroid replacements for the remainder of life.

A. Patients requiring thyroidectomy most often present with the classic symptoms of hyperthyroidism (p 184). These patients are often tense, anxious, and restless and present a special nursing challenge preoperatively to avoid precipitating thyroid storm (see I). Measures to promote rest, relaxation, and trust are indicated.

B. To minimize the risk of complications, ensure that a euthyroid state exists by administering antithyroid drugs and closely monitoring thyroid function tests. Iodine preparations will reduce the size and excessive vascularity of the thyroid gland, which decreases the risk of hemorrhage. Patients may also be given a high-calorie diet and vitamin supplements to achieve optimal weight and nutritional status before surgery.

C. Besides routine preoperative teaching (p 2), patients must be taught to support the neck postoperatively by placing both hands behind the head during any position change or while coughing. Preventing flexion or hyperextension of the neck decreases strain and tension on the neck muscles and suture line.

D. The primary goals of postoperative nursing care are to decrease strain on the suture line, relieve discomfort from sore throat and tracheal irritation, prevent pooling of respiratory secretions, and prevent or relieve complications. During the first 24 to 48 hours, monitor vital signs closely and report abnormalities to the physician. Elevated pulse and hypotension may indicate hemorrhage and shock (p 70).

E. Dyspnea, tachypnea, stridorous respirations, retraction of neck tissues, increased restlessness, and cyanosis are signs of airway obstruction that may be due to hemorrhage, edema of the glottis, laryngeal nerve damage, or tetany. *Notify the physician immediately* (p 398). Emergency equipment such as suction, a tracheostomy set, and oxygen should be assembled at the bedside before the patient returns from surgery.

F. Check the neck dressing frequently for hemorrhage, not only at the front, but also at the sides and back of the neck, as blood tends to drain posteriorly. Gently support the neck and upper shoulders each time the dressing is checked. Be alert for complaints of a choking sensation, or a feeling that the dressing is tightening, which may indicate bleeding into the tissue. *Loosen the dressing and notify the physician immediately.*

G. Although unnecessary talking is discouraged in order to minimize hoarseness, ask patients to speak every 1 to 2 hours so that the pitch and tone of voice can be evaluated. Because the laryngeal nerves that supply the vocal cords lie just behind the thyroid next to the trachea, slight hoarseness is considered normal. Reassure the patient and family that this hoarseness generally subsides in a few days. However, if the voice changes or if the hoarseness worsens or is accompanied by respiratory difficulty, the physician should be notified.

H. Hypocalcemic tetany (p 192) is a possible complication that may occur if the parathyroid glands, which control serum calcium levels, are accidentally injured or removed during surgery (Fig. 1). Symptoms may develop 1 to 7 days postoperatively. Be alert for signs of muscular twitching or spasms, especially of the hands and feet, and of patient complaints of numbness and tingling of the lips, fingers, and toes. In addition, positive Trousseau's sign or Chvostek's sign is indicative of tetany. *Report the occurrence of any of these symptoms to the physician at once.* Tetany is generally treated by the administration of intravenous calcium gluconate.

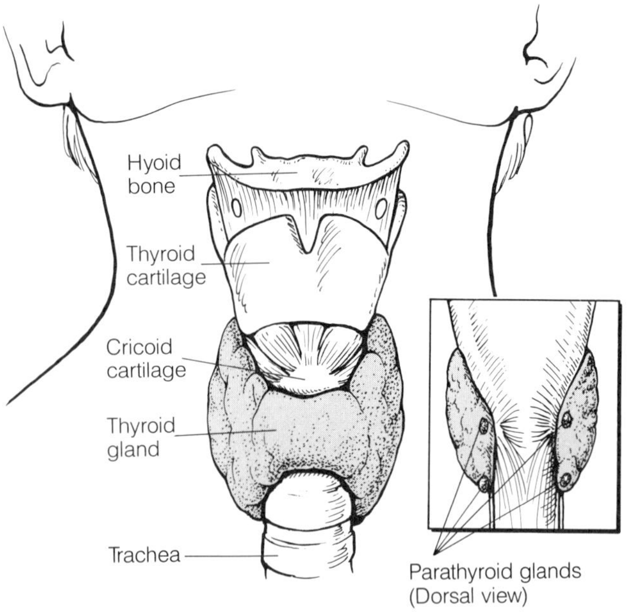

Figure 1 Normal anatomy: thyroid and parathyroid glands.

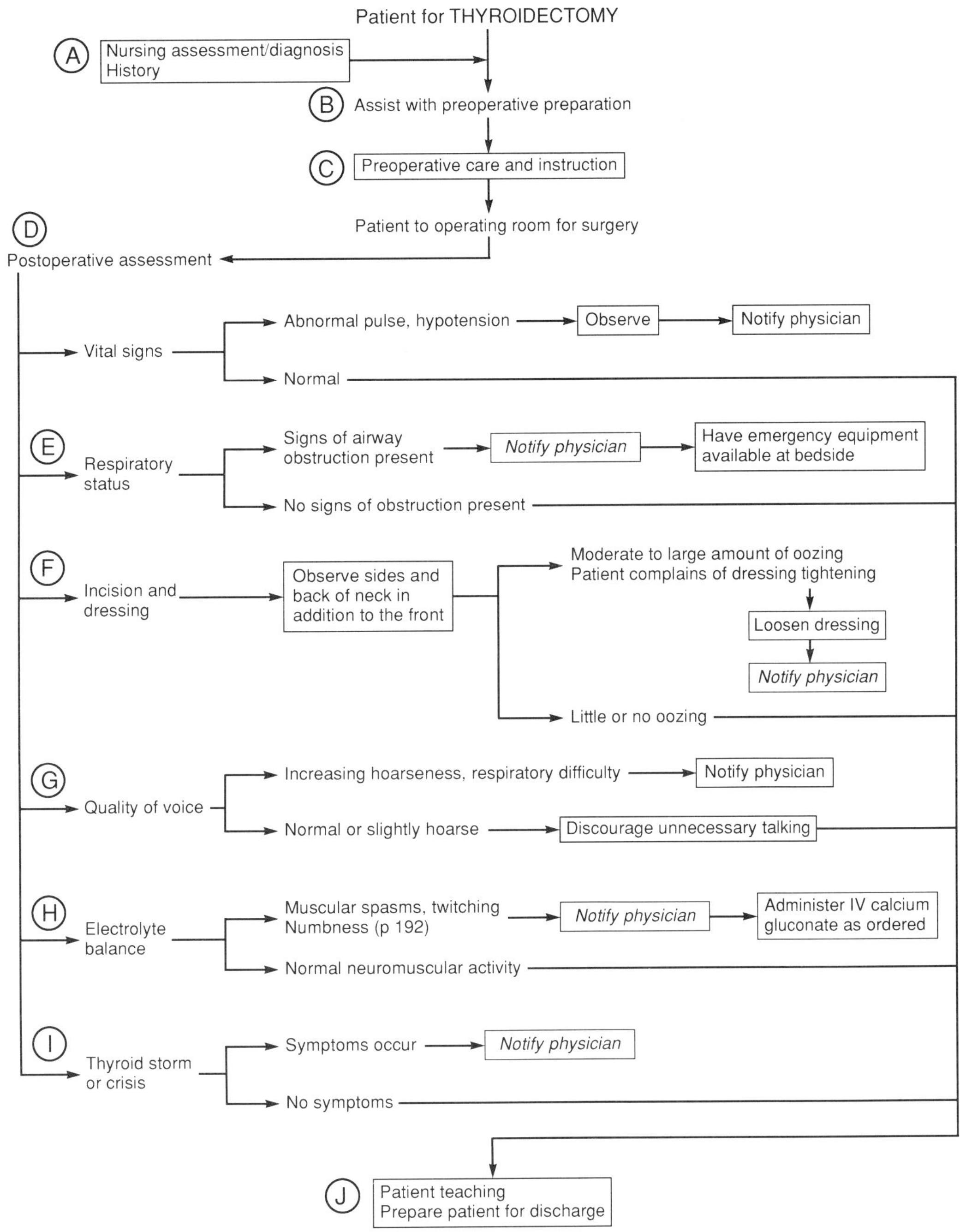

I. Thyroid storm or crisis results from a drastic increase in metabolism due to the sudden release of excessive amounts of thyroid hormones during the surgical procedure. It can be precipitated by emotional stress, infection, or pain. Symptoms include elevated temperature, tachycardia, dehydration, irritability, delirium, shock, and death if not properly treated. Patients may be treated with oxygen and intravenous therapy, sedatives, antithyroid medications, and hypothermia.

J. If there are no complications, patients are discharged with specific instructions related to activity, rest, nutrition, signs and symptoms of hypothyroidism (p 186) and hypocalcemia and when to report these. They must be taught self-administration of thyroid replacement medications, if these are necessary, and care for the surgical incision.

References

Long BC, Phipps WJ. Essentials of medical-surgical nursing. St. Louis: CV Mosby, 1985.

Luckmann J, Sorensen KC. Medical-surgical nursing: a psychophysiologic approach. Philadelphia: WB Saunders, 1987.

Mason MA, Bates GF. Basic medical-surgical nursing. New York: Macmillan, 1984.

Thompson J, McFarland G, Hirsch J, Tucker S, Bowers A. Clinical nursing. St. Louis: CV Mosby, 1986.

MUSCULOSKELETAL SYSTEM

ANKYLOSING SPONDYLITIS

Hazel Harris

A. Ankylosing spondylitis (Marie-Strümpell disease) is a progressive inflammatory disease of the spine and sacroiliac joints that leads to extensive scarring within the joint. The disease begins with synovial inflammation surrounding the joints progressing to ligamental ossification. Progressive ankylosis of the fibrous and bony structures is seen in later stages of the disease process, in which the spinal column becomes ankylosed into a single bony mass. Thus, the disease causes progressive immobility. The hip and shoulder joints may also be involved. Bony changes in the spine are similar to those seen in rheumatoid arthritis. The cause of ankylosing spondylitis is unknown. The disease is much more common in men than women, and usually begins in adolescence or early adulthood.

B. The characteristic symptoms of ankylosing spondylitis are pain and spinal stiffness. The pain may be in the lower back or may radiate into the hips, buttocks, and lumbosacral area. Symptoms vary according to the progression stage of the disease process. Some patients may have pain without stiffness, while others may have stiffness without pain.

C. Diagnosis and treatment are based on radiography and laboratory studies. In early stages the disease process may not be revealed in radiographic examination. Radiographs in later stages of the disease show sacroiliac involvement and some degree of joint erosion and narrowing, with ossification and ankylosis present. The blood sedimentation rate is elevated in most cases, and histocompatibility antigen HLA-B27 is almost always present. The rheumatoid blood factor can differentiate a diagnosis between ankylosing spondylitis and rheumatoid arthritis.

D. If the disease process is diagnosed in the early stage, treatment is directed toward maintaining a straight, erect spine during the entire progression of the disease. This prevents related deformities in later stages of the disease. Additional treatment includes exercise, heat, and anti-inflammatory medication therapy. A spinal osteotomy or other surgical intervention may be required if the disease is diagnosed during a later stage.

E. If the patient has a disability, he or she should be referred to physical and occupational therapy for assistance in adapting to lifestyle changes. The patient should be advised to sleep on a firm mattress and use a small pillow. The nurse should inform the patient about the side effects of medications and the importance of follow-up care.

References

Farrell J. Illustrated guide to orthopedic nursing. 3rd ed. Philadelphia: JB Lippincott, 1986.

Hilt N, Cogburn S. Manual of orthopedics. St. Louis: CV Mosby, 1980.

Ledo KM. Ankylosing spondylitis. Orthopaedic Nursing, 1983; 2(6):39–40.

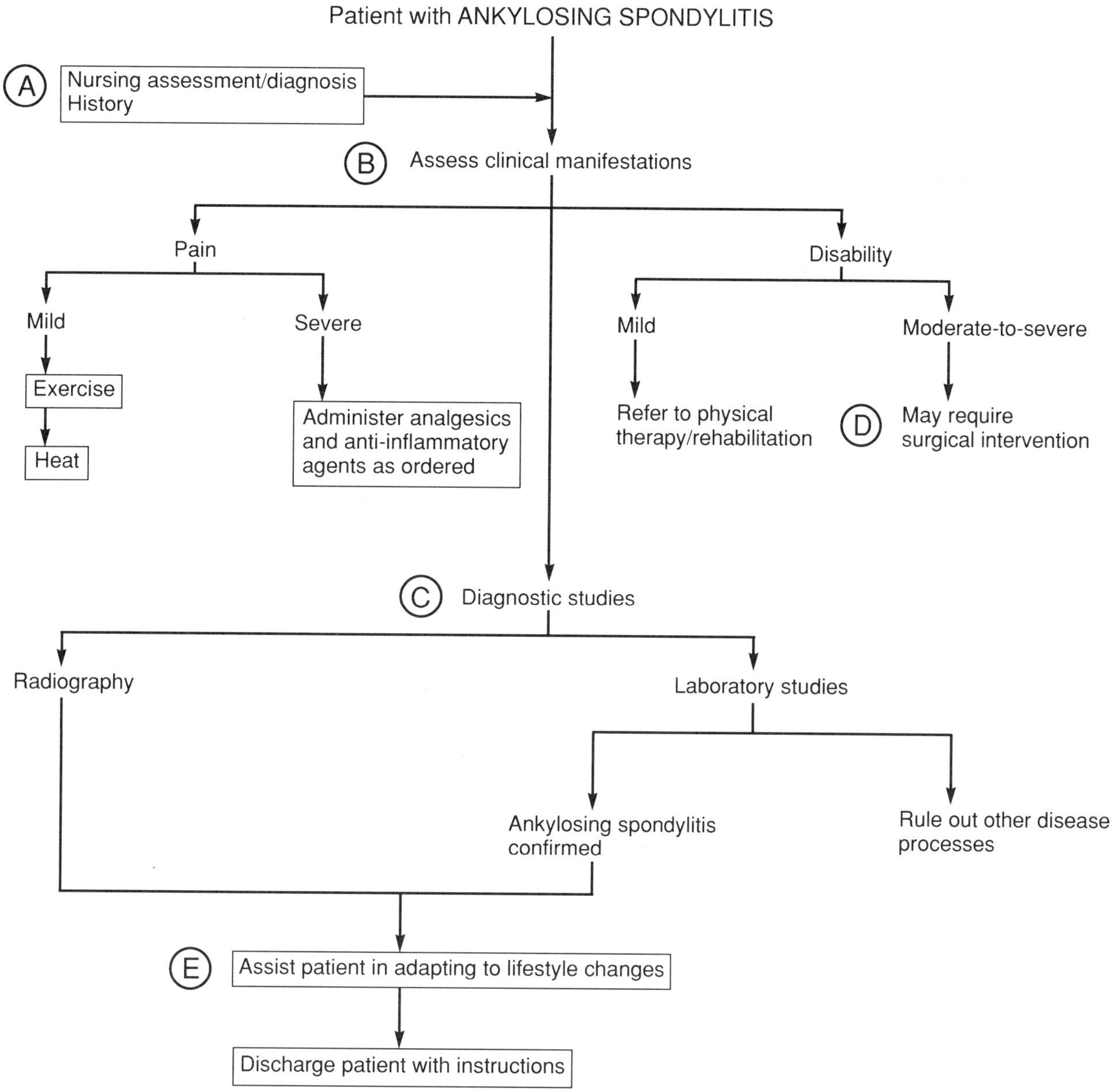
Patient with ANKYLOSING SPONDYLITIS
A
Nursing assessment/diagnosis
History
B
Assess clinical manifestations
Pain
Mild
Exercise
Heat
Severe
Administer analgesics and anti-inflammatory agents as ordered
Disability
Mild
Refer to physical therapy/rehabilitation
Moderate-to-severe
D
May require surgical intervention
C
Diagnostic studies
Radiography
Laboratory studies
Ankylosing spondylitis confirmed
Rule out other disease processes
E
Assist patient in adapting to lifestyle changes
Discharge patient with instructions

BURSITIS

Hazel Harris

Bursitis is an inflammation of a synovial bursa. A bursa is a lubricating sac over a bony surface and beneath the skin, muscle, and tendons, which diminishes friction on movement.

A. Bursitis may result from infection, gout, rheumatoid arthritis, metabolic disease, abnormal tissue growth, trauma and excessive use of a joint. Bursitis develops when there is overstimulation of the synovial membrane, thereby producing excessive fluid and causing distention of the bursa. Bloody synovial fluid is a result of trauma. Gout produces urate crystal in the synovial fluid.

B. Generalized signs and symptoms of bursitis are pain, tenderness, and edema. Movement may be partially or greatly limited. Specific signs and symptoms vary depending on the location of the bursa. Radiographic films may or may not show calcified deposits.

C. Subacromial (subdeltoid) bursitis results when calcium deposits in the bursa located between the shoulder joint and the upper humerus become inflamed. Symptoms include pain radiating to the upper extremity. Subacromial bursitis is seen most commonly in women between the ages of 40 and 50 and those who are less active. A surgical procedure may be indicated if bursitis is unresolved by conservative measures such as heat application, rest, and support. Salicylates (ASA) may be given for pain.

D. Heel bursitis is caused by wearing improperly fitted shoes and continuous irritation of the heel. People who run and walk excessively may be at higher risk. Treatment includes heat, padding, and shoes that fit properly. Steroid injections may be given to relieve the inflammation. Pain may increase temporarily after steroid injections, but within 24 hours the patient should notice pain relief and increased movement.

E. Prepatellar bursitis (housemaid knee) results from excessive use of the knee joint. A mass may be noted on the anterior aspect of the involved knee.

F. Olecranon bursitis is seen in patients with gout, rheumatoid arthritis, and injury or trauma to the elbow. Treatment for prepatellar and olecranon bursitis includes alleviation of pressure over the area. If symptoms continue, aspiration of fluid and/or steroid injections may be indicated. Wrapping the extremity with an elastic bandage helps reduce edema. Antibiotic therapy is implemented and incision and drainage performed if an infection is present. A surgical excision may be indicated for continued recurrence of bursitis.

G. Radiohumeral bursitis is very common among tennis players. Pain spreads from the lateral aspect of the elbow into the forearm. The elbow may need to be immobilized with a sling or cast. Heat application or injections of procaine or steroids may be indicated if immobilization does not relieve the pain. Surgical intervention may be indicated if pain is unresolved by conservative measures.

H. Deep trochanteric bursitis results when the bursa between the gluteus maximus muscle and greater trochanter becomes inflamed. Pain may be present on movement of the hip and radiates down the thigh posteriorly. Tenderness of the hip joint is also present. Treatment includes heat and rest. Antibiotic therapy is implemented if an infection occurs.

I. Superficial trochanteric bursitis results when the bursa between the skin and greater trochanter becomes inflamed. Symptoms include localized tenderness and edema. No pain is present on movement of the hip and leg. Treatment includes heat and rest.

J. Iliopectineal (iliopsoas) bursitis develops when the bursa between the iliopectineal muscle and the anterior surface of the bony prominence becomes inflamed. Pain radiates down the leg anteriorly if the femoral nerve is involved. The patient tends to hold the hip in flexion, abduction, and external rotation for comfort. Treatment includes heat, traction of the lower extremity, and antibiotic therapy if an infection is present.

K. On discharge the patient should be instructed to exercise, but must be cautioned against activities that may cause recurrence of the inflammation.

References

Downing DS, Weinstein A. Ultrasound therapy of subacromial bursitis: a double blind trial. Phys Ther 1986; 66:194–199.

Hilt N, Cogburn S. Manual of orthopedics. St. Louis: CV Mosby, 1980.

Waxman J. Tendonitis and bursitis: diagnostic methods that identify each syndrome. Consultant 1986; 26:97–100, 102, 104.

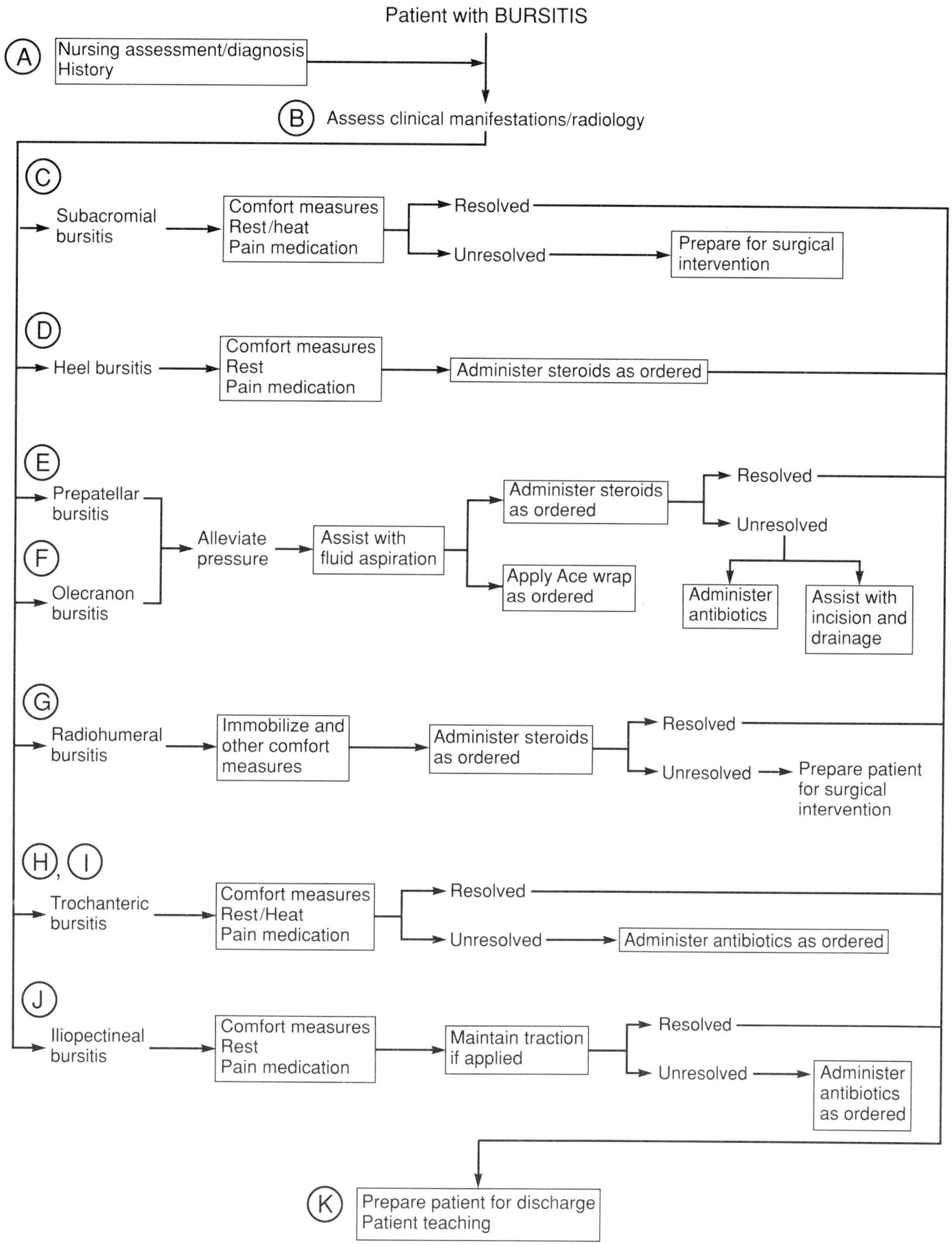

Patient with BURSITIS
A
Nursing assessment/diagnosis
History
B
Assess clinical manifestations/radiology
C
Subacromial bursitis
Comfort measures
Rest/heat
Pain medication
Resolved
Unresolved
Prepare for surgical intervention
D
Heel bursitis
Comfort measures
Rest
Pain medication
Administer steroids as ordered
E
Prepatellar bursitis
F
Olecranon bursitis
Alleviate pressure
Assist with fluid aspiration
Administer steroids as ordered
Apply Ace wrap as ordered
Resolved
Unresolved
Administer antibiotics
Assist with incision and drainage
G
Radiohumeral bursitis
Immobilize and other comfort measures
Administer steroids as ordered
Resolved
Unresolved
Prepare patient for surgical intervention
H, I
Trochanteric bursitis
Comfort measures
Rest/Heat
Pain medication
Resolved
Unresolved
Administer antibiotics as ordered
J
Iliopectineal bursitis
Comfort measures
Rest
Pain medication
Maintain traction if applied
Resolved
Unresolved
Administer antibiotics as ordered
K
Prepare patient for discharge
Patient teaching

PAGET'S DISEASE

Hazel Harris

Paget's disease (osteitis deformans) is a skeletal disease characterized by increased bone resorption (bone loss) alternating with disordered bone construction, which leads to deformity, fractures, and calcium imbalance. Bones most affected by this disease are the skull, pelvis, spine, femur, and tibia. The cause of Paget's disease is unknown. It is more common in men over 45 years of age. The presence of Paget's disease increases the patient's risk of malignant bone tumors.

A. The onset of Paget's disease is insidious. Patients usually complain of pain in the lower back or lower extremities. The pain can vary from a mild ache to severe. The long bones thicken with apparent bowing. Kyphosis, scoliosis, and head enlargement are also clinical manifestations of Paget's disease. Hearing loss may result from the thickening of the skull.

B. Diagnosis and treatment are based on radiography and laboratory studies. Urine calcium, serum phosphorus, and alkaline phosphatase levels are abnormal, but the serum calcium level is normal in Paget's disease. Radiology indicates bowing and thickening of the long bones, thickening of the skull, and an irregular surface between the cortex and medulla.

C. Treatment is symptomatic and supportive and includes aspirin for pain relief, hormones, and vitamins. Suppressive agents such as thyrocalcitonin and mithramycin are also used in the treatment of Paget's disease. If pain is severe, surgery may be performed to relieve stress on the affected joint.

D. Patients with Paget's disease should stay as active as possible, but must be aware of the risk of bone fractures (p 230). These patients also require nutritional counseling regarding a low-calcium diet.

References

Farrell J. Illustrated guide to orthopedic nursing. 3rd ed. Philadelphia: JB Lippincott, 1986.

Hilt N, Cogburn S. Manual of orthopaedics. St. Louis: CV Mosby, 1980.

Ross DC. Paget's disease. Orthopaed Nurs 1984; 3(3):41–44.

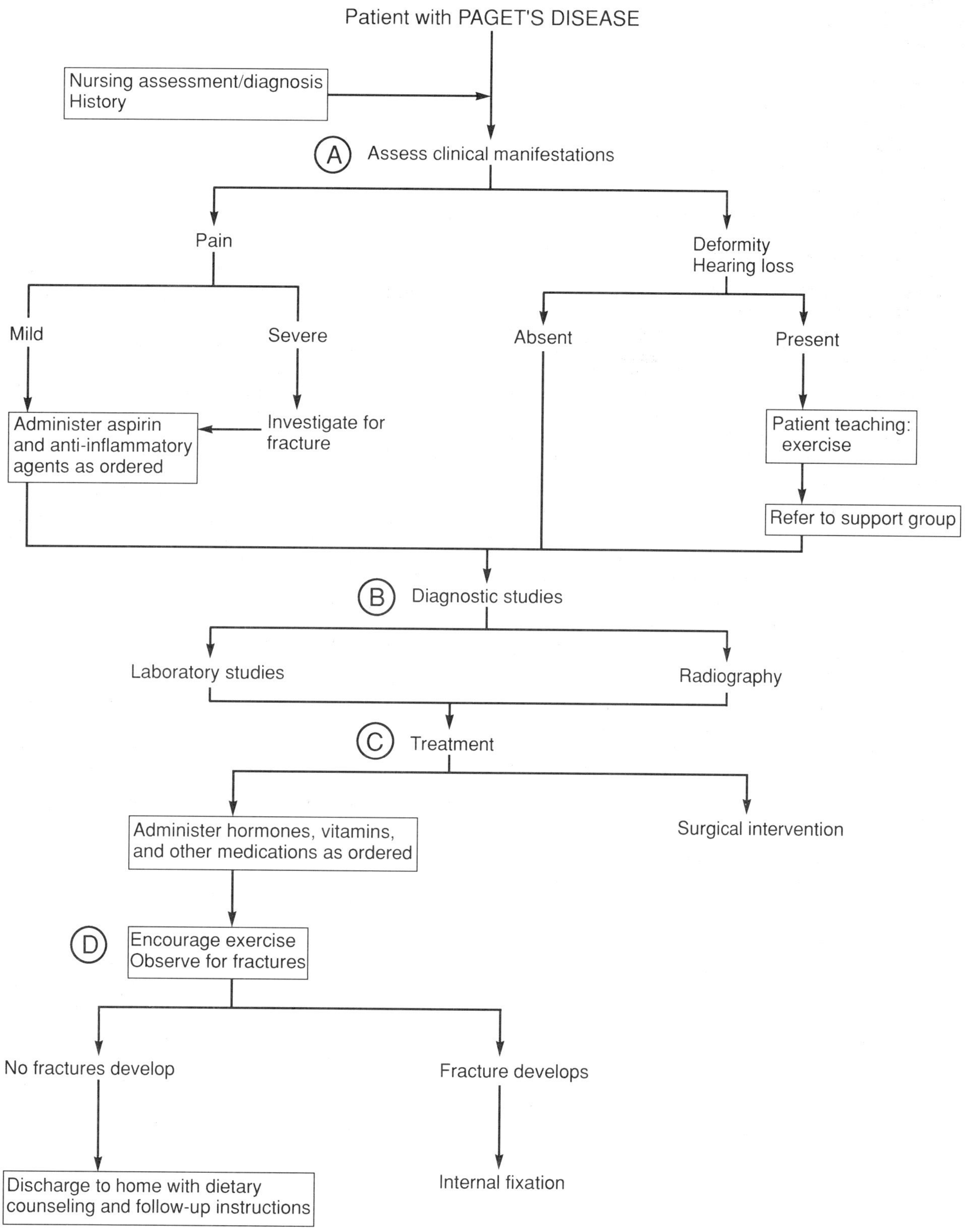

Patient with PAGET'S DISEASE
Nursing assessment/diagnosis
History
A
Assess clinical manifestations
Pain
Deformity
Hearing loss
Mild
Severe
Absent
Present
Administer aspirin and anti-inflammatory agents as ordered
Investigate for fracture
Patient teaching: exercise
Refer to support group
B
Diagnostic studies
Laboratory studies
Radiography
C
Treatment
Administer hormones, vitamins, and other medications as ordered
Surgical intervention
D
Encourage exercise
Observe for fractures
No fractures develop
Fracture develops
Discharge to home with dietary counseling and follow-up instructions
Internal fixation

ARTHRITIS

Joy Gorzeman

Three types of arthritis are osteoarthritis, gouty arthritis, and rheumatoid arthritis.

A. Osteoarthritis, also known as degenerative joint disease (DJD), is commonly seen in 50- to 70-year-old patients. Infections, trauma, and wear and tear on the joints cause inflammation and subsequent deterioration of articular cartilage. The cause of primary osteoarthritis is unknown, although genetics or biochemical abnormalities may be indicated. DJD affects only joints and their surrounding tissue.

B. Unlike DJD, rheumatoid arthritis is a chronic, systemic disease that usually appears in 25- to 50-year-olds and more often in women. The cause of rheumatoid arthritis is unknown, but viral infections, metabolic factors, and the interaction of immunoglobulin G with the rheumatoid factor have been suggested.

C. Gouty arthritis is an inflammation in the joints that results from deposits of uric acid crystals.

D. Laboratory studies in patients with osteoarthritis are essentially normal. In rheumatoid arthritis, the erythrocyte sedimentation rate is elevated, leukocytes are increased, and a positive rheumatoid factor or latex fixation test is present if the disease is severe or long-term. In gouty arthritis, serum uric acid is elevated. Radiology studies in osteoarthritic patients show narrowed joint spaces and often spur formation (new bone). In rheumatoid arthritis, articular erosion is also visible. Synovial fluid aspirated from patients with rheumatoid arthritis shows decreased viscosity and increased turbidity. Fluid of patients with gouty arthritis contains uric acid crystals on microscopic examination.

E. Patients with osteoarthritis complain of pain in the joints, especially the hips, knees, and hands; stiffness; cracking noises with joint movement; and enlargement of the joints. Assessment includes questions about pain—when and where it occurs and what treatments bring relief. Enquire whether the pain has affected the patient's lifestyle. Inspect the joints for limited or slow movement and deformity. Note whether the patient has difficulty standing up after sitting for a time, and observe for limping. Early manifestations of rheumatoid arthritis include fever, fatigue, generalized aching, and weight loss. Morning stiffness is characteristic. As the disease progresses, the aching becomes more localized and the joints become visibly red and swollen, tender, and warm to the touch. Eventually, the fingers taper and there is ulnar deviation of the hand. Joint involvement in rheumatoid arthritis is usually bilateral and symmetric. The course of rheumatoid arthritis varies by individual. Exacerbations and remissions are common. Stress, overexertion, or physical trauma may "trigger" an exacerbation. If untreated, rheumatoid arthritis may relapse, but usually recurs in a more severe form.

F. The goals of intervention are relief of pain and maintenance of joint function. Patients with osteoarthritis and rheumatoid arthritis should be encouraged to balance rest and activities.

G. Inflammation is controlled with salicylates (aspirin). Other medications are added based on the patient's response, including nonsteroidal anti-inflammatory drugs, antimalarials, gold, penicillamine, and cytotoxic or corticosteroid agents. Tylenol or Darvon may give added analgesia, but should not be substituted for aspirin because they do not provide anti-inflammatory properties.

H. An additional supportive measure is application of heat to relieve muscle spasm and stiffness. If heat is not effective, cold application should be tried. Positioning may promote comfort and avoids contracture.

I. Encourage exercise and range of motion to maintain mobility. Excessive exercise should be avoided.

J. Walking aids to assist with weight-bearing should be provided when necessary. Splints may also help to relieve painful joints.

K. Weight should be maintained at a minimum to avoid overstressing the joints.

L. If problems persist, or in cases such as deformity, constant severe pain, or nerve compression, a surgical procedure such as arthroscopy (p 238), realignment, fusion, or joint replacement (p 242) may be indicated.

M. Arthritis patients should be encouraged to be as active as possible. They may need to express feelings about deformity, limitations, and living with a chronic illness that has no cure. Include family in the care planning, which uses a multidisciplinary approach. Patients may benefit from referral to a support group such as The Arthritis Foundation.

N. Compliance with treatment is necessary for the patient to benefit—this is an important part of patient teaching. Other aspects of patient teaching and discharge planning include comfort measures, activity guidelines, methods of joint protection, and balanced nutrition. Ongoing supervision is essential. Patients should monitor their own response to treatment so they can report the effectiveness to their health care providers.

O. The joint swells and becomes extremely tender. The skin over the joint looks red and is hot to the touch. This painful condition occurs more frequently in men

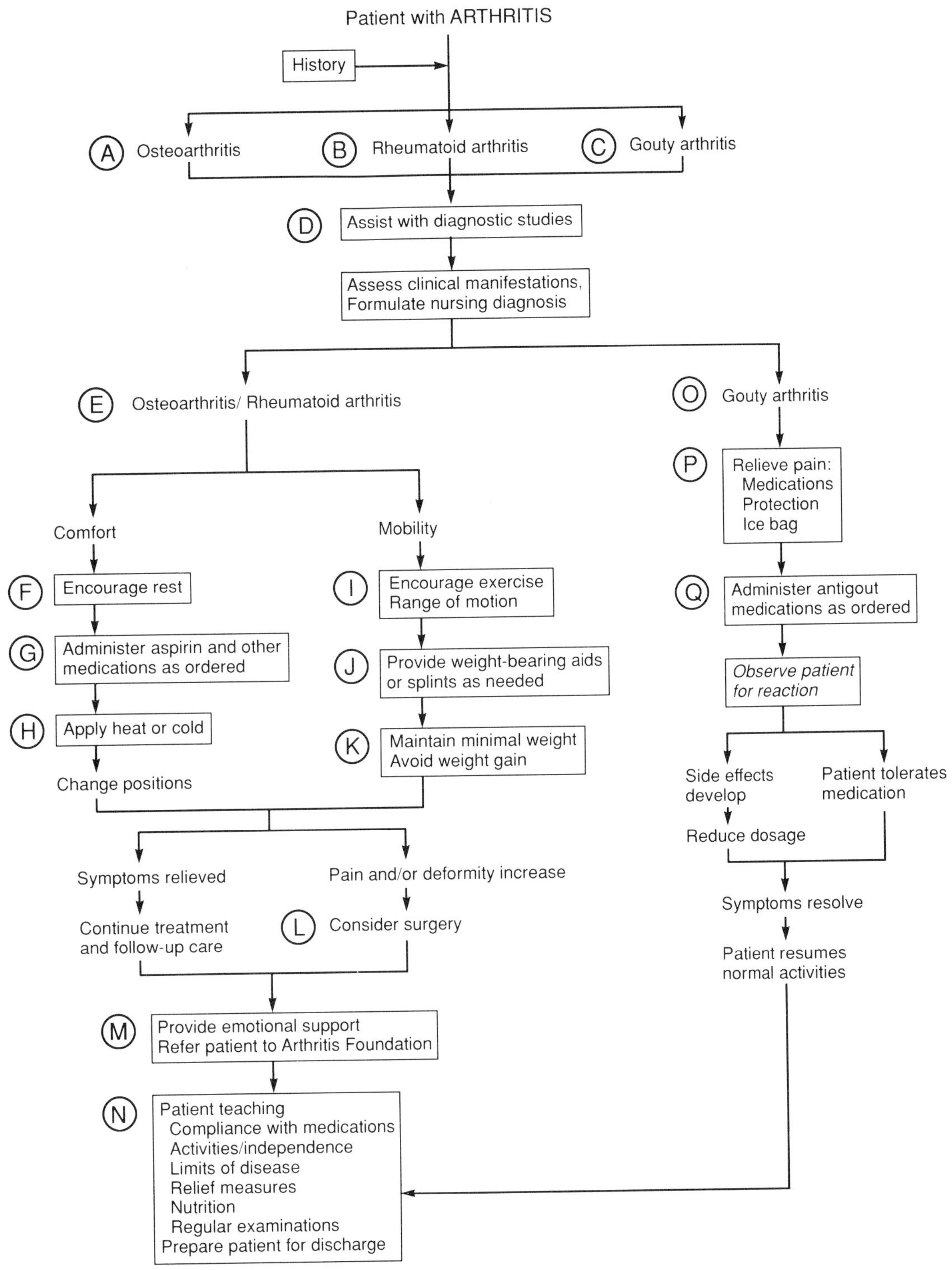

and is commonly seen in the metatarsophalangeal joint of the great toe. Other sites are the ankle and knee.

P. Acute episodes of gouty arthritis usually last 2 to 5 days. The joint should be protected from weight-bearing and pressure during this time. Ice bags may provide some comfort.

Q. Antigout medications such as colchicine are given every hour until a therapeutic blood level is reached. Nausea, vomiting, diarrhea, abdominal pain, and/or muscle weakness should be reported so that the dosage can be reduced. Normal activities should be encouraged when the acute episode subsides.

References

Brunner LS, Suddarth DS. The Lippincott manual of nursing practice. 4th ed. Philadelphia: JB Lippincott, 1986.

Hincker EA, Malasanos L, eds. The Little, Brown manual of medical-surgical nursing. Boston: Little, Brown, 1983.

Luckmann J, Sorensen KC. Medical-surgical nursing: a psychophysiologic approach. 3rd ed. Philadelphia: WB Saunders, 1987.

Phipps WJ, Long BC, Woods NF. Medical-surgical nursing concepts and clinical practice. 3rd ed. St. Louis: CV Mosby, 1987.

Thompson JM, McFarland GK, Hirsch JE, Tucker SM, Bowers AC. Clinical nursing. St. Louis: CV Mosby, 1986.

OSTEOMYELITIS

David L. Lybarger

Acute osteomyelitis is caused by bacteria from superficial infections that are carried in the blood and lodge in the terminal capillary loops of the metaphyseal cortex, causing a purulent necrosing process that emerges into the periosteum. This infection commonly occurs in children, occurs twice as frequently in males as in females, and is most frequently caused by staphylococci.

After the acute phase, the purulent discharge from the necrosing bone spreads through the periosteum and drains through sinus tracts onto the skin's surface. The circulation of the cortex becomes impaired, producing islands of dead bone called sequestra, which may be surrounded by new bone called involucrum and be absorbed or discharged through the sinus; usually surgical removal is required. Continuing necrosis of bone and retention of sequestra cause persistence of the sinus, the orifice of which is surrounded by exuberant granulation tissue (proud flesh).

A. The patient with osteomyelitis usually gives a history of trauma or antecedent infection in the past 3 to 4 weeks, and may present with weakness, malaise, and general signs of sepsis. There is an obvious area of redness, tenderness, edema, and possibly a mass or drainage in the ends of long bones. There is increased pain on movement, and the patient intermittently spikes fevers of 39 to 40°C (101.5 to 104°F).

B. Initial nursing assessment includes evaluation of vital signs, skin and vascular integrity, pain, and impairment of mobility. Self-image and socialization issues should also be evaluated, as well as the degree of support available to the patient from the home environment upon discharge.

C. Testing to confirm the diagnosis of osteomyelitis usually consists of complete blood count (CBC) with differential, erythrocyte sedimentation rate (ESR), blood cultures, and cultures of the drainage or mass. Radiologic studies may not initially reveal destructive processes, but will later (usually in 5 to 10 days) show rarefaction of the involved bone with evidence of formation of sequestrum and involucrum.

D. Closed drainage accomplished by careful dressing changes with or without long-term antibiotic treatment, based on identification of the pathogen, may be satisfactory for new onset or minor recurrences of chronic bone disease. Careful monitoring of the wound site for continued or worsening signs of infection and prompt reporting of the condition of the wound are essential nursing responsibilities, in addition to performing or assisting with dressing changes.

E. Antibiotic therapy in the acute phase should be continued for 2 to 3 weeks following repeated wound cultures while the patient is afebrile. Anti-infective agents are administered according to culture and sensitivity results and patient sensitivity or allergies. They usually include penicillin, erythromycin, ampicillin, and/or cephalothin.

F. Antibiotic therapy may be necessary for 4 to 6 weeks for infections that do not respond promptly and thoroughly to initial treatment and is guided by repeated wound cultures and sensitivity studies.

G. Patients with osteolysis, bone necrosis, and drainage may require surgery. Common surgical correction for osteomyelitis includes removal of sequestrum and bone grafting. Saucerization (bone scraping to remove necrotic tissue) is performed, after which bone regenerates. Bone grafting or metallic fixation may be done. External fixation devices such as the Hoffman apparatus may also be used. Amputation of the limb is seldom necessary now with improved treatment modalities.

H. Supportive care consists of conserving energy and managing pain with analgesia as prescribed (usually aspirin), maintaining bedrest, immobilizing and elevating the affected extremity, using a sling when feasible, and providing activities to divert the patient's attention. Impaired physical mobility may be prevented and/or treated by encouraging range of motion (ROM) exercises and self-care for preservation of function. A wheelchair or crutches may be used to aid in mobility and socialization. Impairment of vascular and skin integrity should be prevented by observing and reporting neurovascular status on a regular basis when changing dressings or splints. Encouraging patient and family interactions and thorough preoperative psycho-

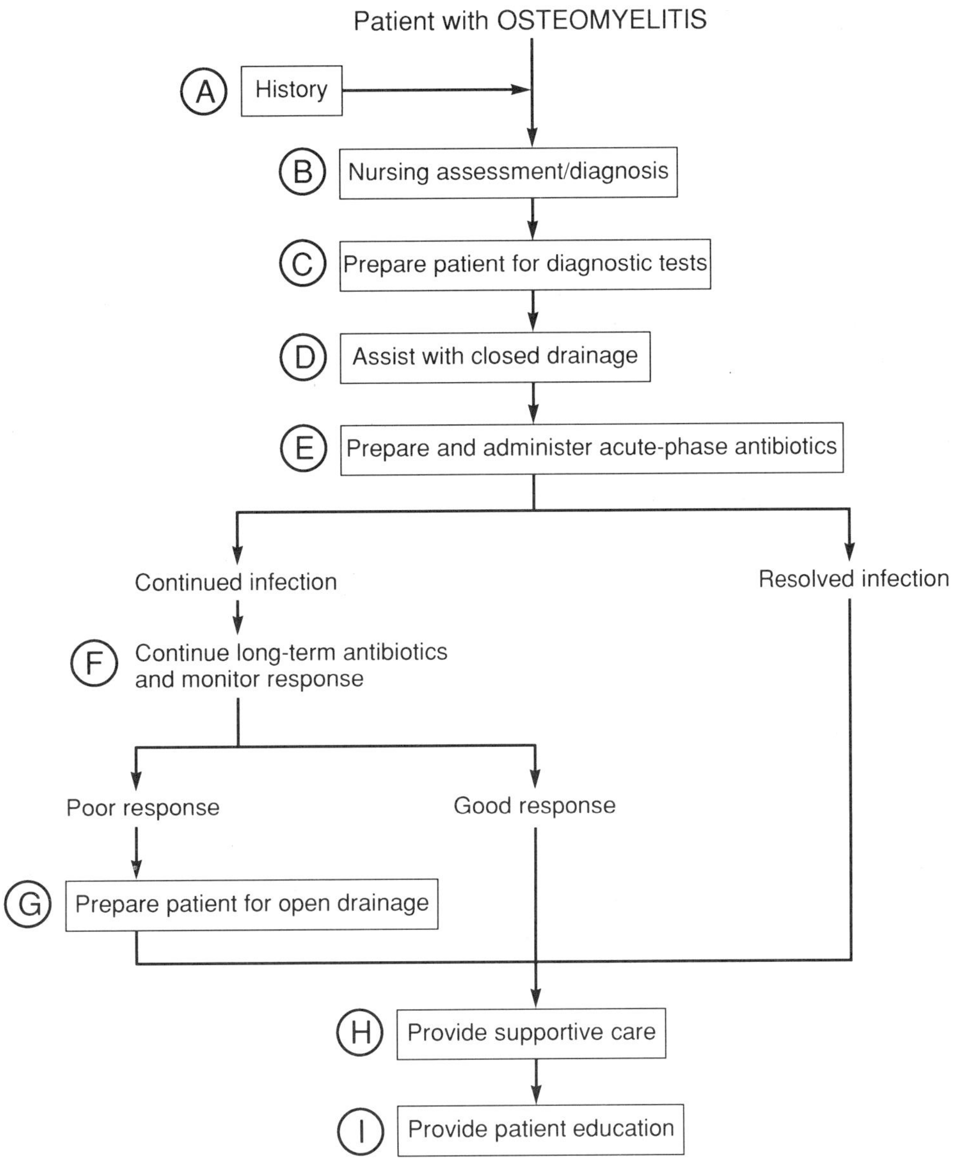

logical preparation should be done to assist the patient in working through any self-concept disturbances related to body image.

I. Patient education should include the disease process, rationale, purpose, and expected outcomes for long-term therapy, signs and symptoms of local or systemic infections that need prompt medical attention, need for continued ROM exercises for strength and mobility maintenance, and referral to local agencies if needed by the patient or family after discharge because of social or environmental factors.

References

Brunner LS, Suddarth DS. The Lippincott manual of nursing practice. 4th ed. Philadelphia: JB Lippincott, 1986.

DeGowin EL, DeGowin RL. Bedside diagnostic examination. 5th ed. New York: Macmillan, 1984:653–654.

Krupp MA, Chatton MJ, Tierney LM, eds. Current diagnosis and treatment. Los Altos, CA: Lange, 1986:525–526.

Mourad LA. Musculoskeletal system. In: Thompson JM, MacFarland GK, Hirsch JE, Tucker SM, Bowers AC, eds. Clinical nursing. St. Louis: Mosby, 1986:458–461.

MUSCULAR DYSTROPHY

Joy Gorzeman

A. Muscular dystrophy is a progressive, hereditary degenerative disease characterized by changes in skeletal muscle fibers as opposed to nerves. The muscles atrophy and the patient experiences symmetric muscle weakness. Sensation remains intact, however. The disease mainly affects the girdle, proximal limbs, and eyes. The cause of muscular dystrophy is unknown. There is some speculation that disturbances in the enzymes related to muscle metabolism may play a role in the etiology of the disease.

B. Diagnosis is mostly based on clinical manifestations and genetic history. Muscle biopsy and/or electromyography may be helpful. Progression of muscular dystrophy varies: some types affect youth, others affect the older population; some types progress rapidly, others show remission. Duchenne muscular dystrophy (DMD) is the most common type. It is a rapidly progressive X-linked recessive disorder in which women are carriers and sons manifest the disorder. Muscle weakness develops starting in the lower extremities and moving upward. Death is usually due to acute respiratory infection. The prognosis is poor, with death occurring before 20 years of age. Patients with these extensive disabilities require much assistance.

C. There is no specific treatment for the progressive muscular dystrophies. The patient should be encouraged to remain active and live as full and normal a life as possible. A regular exercise program is important to prevent contractures and deformities. The use of braces may assist with ambulation.

D. Dietary counseling is helpful to assist the patient in avoiding obesity. The patient should be encouraged to maintain good health and avoid respiratory infections.

E. The patient should seek genetic counseling if he or she plans to have children. Several members of the same family may be affected.

F. Emotional support for the patient and family is a large component of nursing care. They may also benefit from referral to community support groups.

References

Berkow R, ed. The Merck manual of diagnosis and therapy. 15th ed. Rahway, NJ: Merck, Sharp & Dohme Research Laboratories, 1987.

Bullock, B. Normal and altered functions of the muscular system. In: Bullock B, Rosendahl P. Pathophysiology: adaptations and alterations in function. Boston: Scott, Foresman, 1988:631.

Luckmann J, Sorensen KC. Medical-surgical nursing: a psychophysiologic approach. 3rd ed. Philadelphia: WB Saunders, 1987.

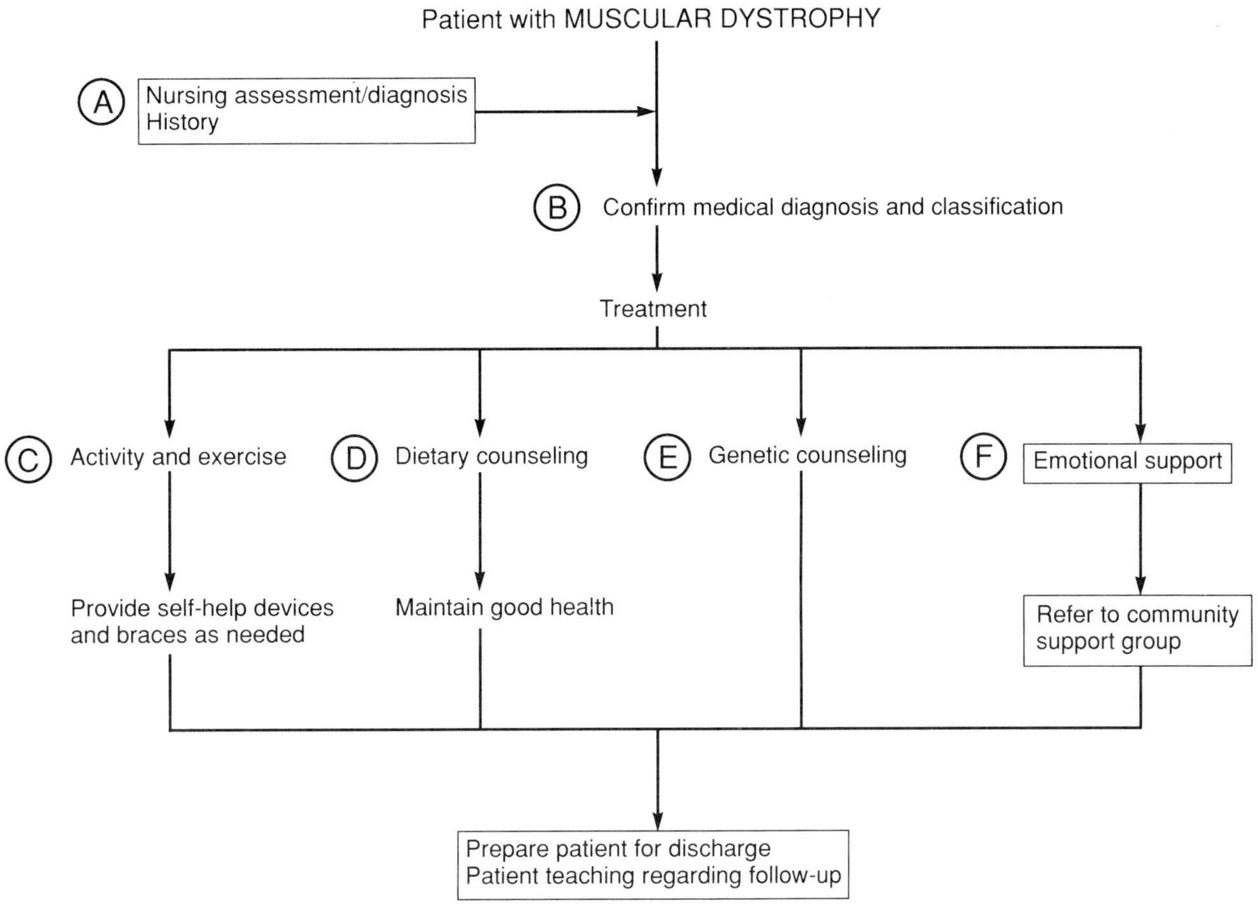
Patient with MUSCULAR DYSTROPHY
A
Nursing assessment/diagnosis
History
B
Confirm medical diagnosis and classification
Treatment
C
Activity and exercise
D
Dietary counseling
E
Genetic counseling
F
Emotional support
Provide self-help devices and braces as needed
Maintain good health
Refer to community support group
Prepare patient for discharge
Patient teaching regarding follow-up

OSTEOPOROSIS

Joy Gorzeman

Osteoporosis is a condition in which there is a reduction in overall bone mass. The bones become porous and fragile, resulting in fractures, vertebral collapse, and skeletal deformity.

A. Osteoporosis is linked to the reduction of the estrogen level after menopause and is commonly seen in white women more than 60 years of age. Other causes include immobilization (p 234); low calcium intake; lack of vitamin D; inadequate protein, vitamins, and minerals; and hyperthyroidism (p 184). Osteoporosis may develop secondary to multiple myeloma (p 312), subtotal gastrectomy (p 166), hypercortisonism, and hypogonadism. Osteoporosis is the twelfth leading cause of death in this country and is the principal cause of fractures in the aged (p 412).

B. The majority of patients with osteoporosis have no symptoms. Those who do present with a dull ache in the lower thoracic or lumbar spine area. If pain is sharp or severe and aggravated by motion, fracture should be suspected. Kyphosis is another clinical manifestation of osteoporosis. Patients can lose from 1 to 6 inches in stature as a result of vertebral compression.

C. Treatment is supportive and empiric. Pain may be relieved by analgesics, heat, and massage. Hyperextension exercises are also helpful. Fractures require orthopaedic attention and support (p 230).

D. Diagnosis and treatment is based on radiologic and laboratory studies. Serum calcium, serum phosphorus, and alkaline phosphatase are normal in primary osteoporosis. If laboratory studies are abnormal, secondary osteoporosis is indicated. Radiographs show increased radiolucency of bones. Bone scans may be done to rule out tumor.

E. Patients with osteoporosis should stay as active as possible, but should avoid lifting and be safety conscious to avoid falls. Osteoporosis patients need dietary counseling; their nutritional requirements include calcium intake and small supplements of vitamin D each day. Calcium therapy requires medical supervision and should include semiannual analysis of urine and serum calcium values. Patients with severe osteoporosis may be placed on estrogen therapy.

References

Brunner LS, Suddarth DS. The Lippincott manual of nursing practice. 4th ed. Philadelphia: JB Lippincott, 1986.

Mugraf C. Nursing's role: the prevention and treatment of osteoporosis. Texas Nurs 1987; January: 11.

Thompson JM, McFarland GK, Hirsch JE, Tucker SM, Bowers AC. Clinical nursing. St. Louis: CV Mosby, 1986.

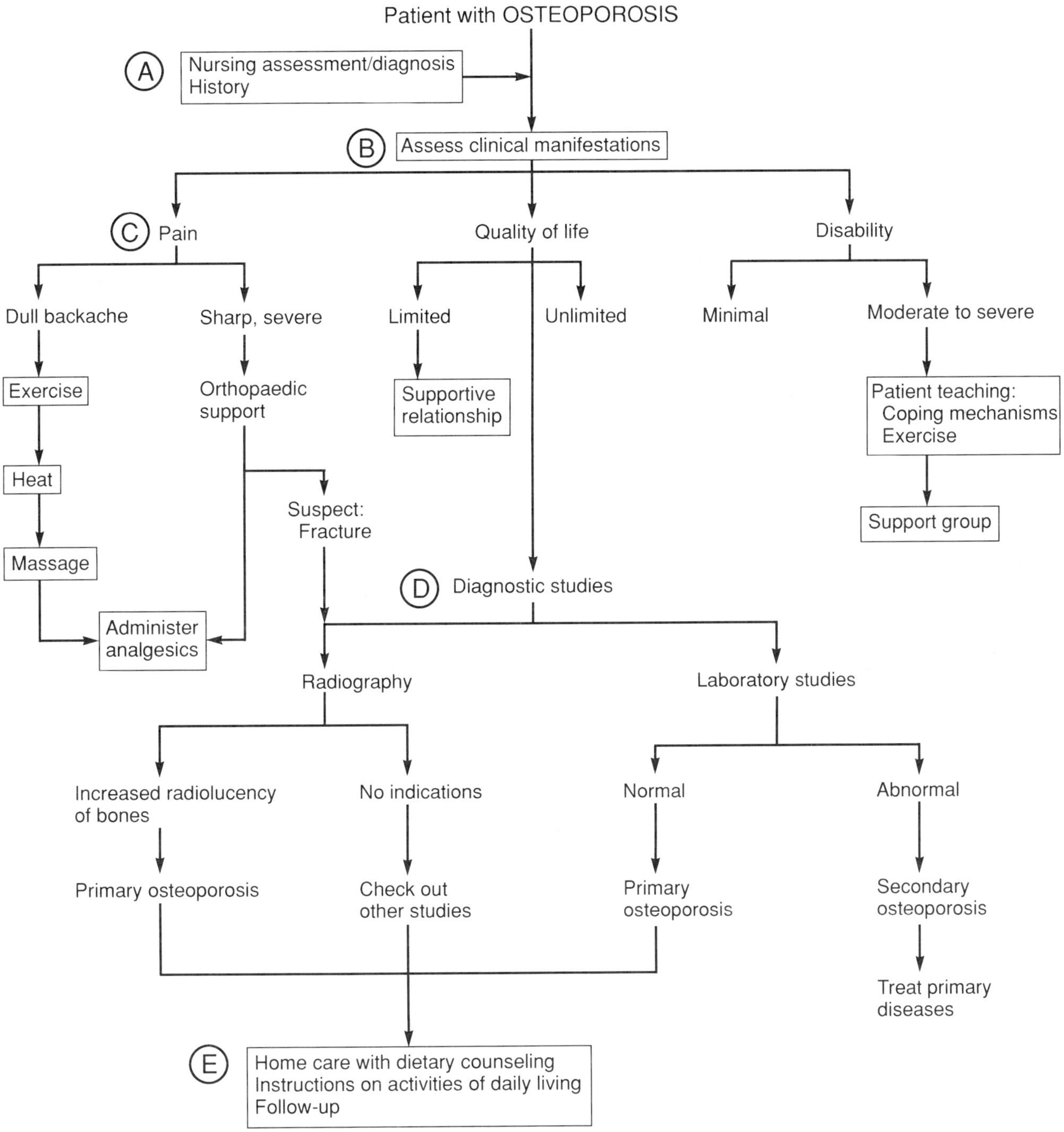
Patient with OSTEOPOROSIS
A
Nursing assessment/diagnosis
History
B
Assess clinical manifestations
C
Pain
Quality of life
Disability
Dull backache
Sharp, severe
Limited
Unlimited
Minimal
Moderate to severe
Exercise
Orthopaedic support
Supportive relationship
Patient teaching:
Coping mechanisms
Exercise
Heat
Suspect:
Fracture
Support group
Massage
D
Diagnostic studies
Administer analgesics
Radiography
Laboratory studies
Increased radiolucency of bones
No indications
Normal
Abnormal
Primary osteoporosis
Check out other studies
Primary osteoporosis
Secondary osteoporosis
Treat primary diseases
E
Home care with dietary counseling
Instructions on activities of daily living
Follow-up

OSTEOMALACIA

Joy Gorzeman

A. Osteomalacia is the adult equivalent of rickets in children. It is a disorder of calcium and phosphorus metabolism caused by a deficiency in vitamin D. The most common causes of vitamin D deficiency are inadequate exposure to sunlight and poor dietary intake.

B. The result of vitamin deficiency is that the bone matrix is not calcified, and the bones become soft, flattened, and deformed. Osteomalacia also occurs in young women who have had frequent pregnancies and lactation and in patients with intestinal malabsorption. Renal disorders and hyperparathyroidism may also cause osteomalacia through interference with absorption of vitamin D. Etiology is important to effective treatment. Osteomalacia must be differentiated from other causes of bone decalcification, such as osteoporosis.

C. Diagnosis is based on the health history and diagnostic tests, such as low serum calcium and increased alkaline phosphatase levels, and radiographs exhibiting general decalcification.

D. Osteomalacia can be cured by oral administration of high levels of vitamin D for 1 month, followed by normal levels of vitamin D and adequate calcium and phosphorus intake. Patients should receive dietary counseling to encourage inclusion of foods such as eggs, milk, and fish.

References

Armstrong ME, ed. McGraw-Hill handbook of clinical nursing. New York: McGraw-Hill, 1979.

Berkow R, ed. The Merck manual of diagnosis and therapy. 15th ed. Rahway, NJ: Merck Sharp & Dohme Laboratories, 1987.

Luckmann J, Sorensen KC. Medical-surgical nursing. 3rd ed. Philadelphia: WB Saunders, 1987.

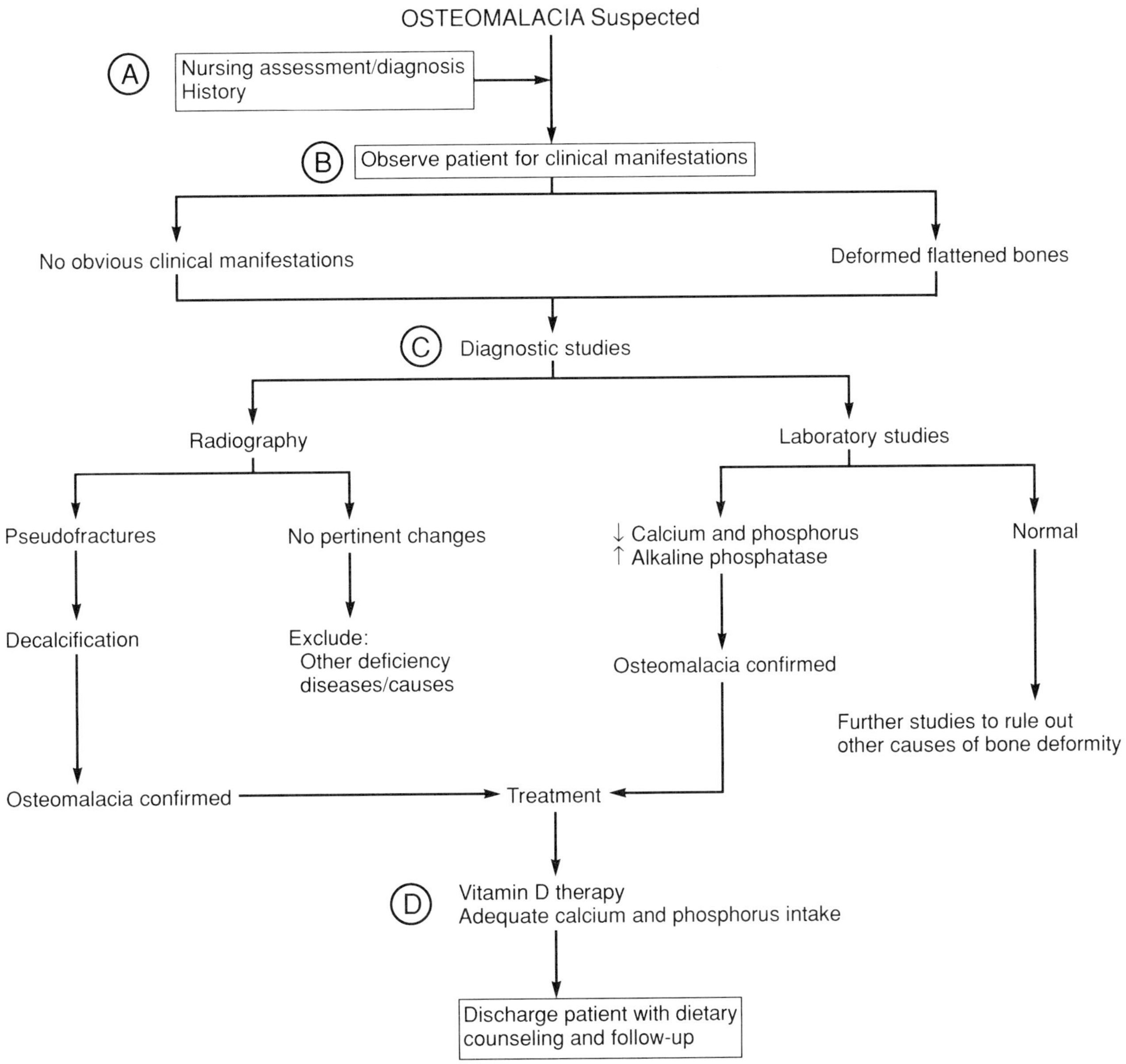
OSTEOMALACIA Suspected
A
Nursing assessment/diagnosis
History
B
Observe patient for clinical manifestations
No obvious clinical manifestations
Deformed flattened bones
C
Diagnostic studies
Radiography
Laboratory studies
Pseudofractures
No pertinent changes
↓ Calcium and phosphorus
↑ Alkaline phosphatase
Normal
Decalcification
Exclude:
Other deficiency diseases/causes
Osteomalacia confirmed
Further studies to rule out other causes of bone deformity
Osteomalacia confirmed
Treatment
D
Vitamin D therapy
Adequate calcium and phosphorus intake
Discharge patient with dietary counseling and follow-up

CARPAL TUNNEL SYNDROME

Barbara Kalo

Carpal tunnel syndrome involves a variety of symptoms caused by compression of the median nerve between the carpal ligament and other structures within the carpal tunnel (Fig. 1). The functions of the wrist, hand, and fingers are affected. This syndrome may occur after a long history of strenuous and repetitive use of the hands, an injury to the wrist, changes in tissue turgor due to aging, or it may occur without any history. One or both hands may be involved. Although splinting may give temporary relief, surgical release of the transverse carpal ligament is indicated and is generally an ambulatory surgical procedure.

A. The initial symptoms are burning, tingling, and numbness in the affected extremity. An aching pain may radiate proximally into the forearm, shoulder, neck, and chest. Patients report that pain is exacerbated by manual activity and can be episodic or constant. Nocturnal symptoms are often reported. A positive Tinel's sign (tingling or shock-like pain on volar wrist percussion) and a positive Phalen's sign (pain on wrist flexion) are other indicators of carpal tunnel syndrome. Muscle weakness or atrophy along the thumb and first and second fingers may be diagnosed with electromyography.

B. Preoperative nursing care includes promoting comfort by elevating the extremity to relieve swelling, and splinting the hand and forearm at night. These conservative measures may have been used by the patient at home before surgery was indicated, along with corticosteroid injections and avoidance of work requiring flexion of the wrist. Preoperative assessment of nerve function and circulation in the affected extremity are necessary for comparison with the postoperative assessment. Patient teaching should include expectations of surgery and the postoperative period. Provide emotional support to alleviate fears about the procedure.

C. Postoperatively, routine procedures such as monitoring of vital signs and assessment are done (p 4).

D. Postoperative nursing care is directed toward preventing infection at the operative site and assessing the neurovascular status of the affected extremity.

E. The affected arm is elevated in a sling, with ice applied to the area for the first 24 to 48 hours to help control swelling. Extension and flexion of the fingers is encouraged to promote circulation.

F. The dressing should be dry and intact. Excess drainage should be reported. If the extremity becomes swollen and the dressing too tight, notify the physician. When the dressing is changed, check the incision for redness, drainage, and other signs of infection.

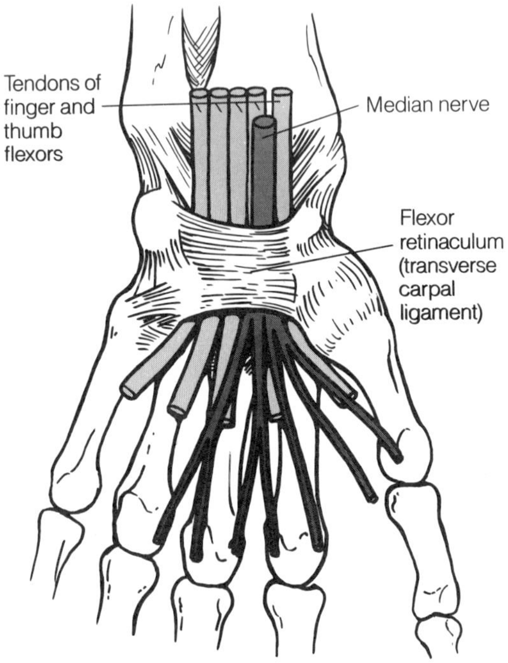

Figure 1 Compression of the median nerve in carpal tunnel syndrome.

G. Medicate the patient for incisional pain as needed. Oral analgesics are usually adequate to alleviate postoperative pain.

H. The patient should be able to tolerate a regular diet, void without difficulty, and tolerate ambulation before discharge.

I. If there are no complications, the patient is discharged with specific instructions regarding dressing changes, wound care, and follow-up care with the physician.

References

Brunner LS, Suddarth DS. Textbook of medical-surgical nursing. 6th ed. Philadelphia: JB Lippincott, 1988.

Krupp MA, Chatton MJ, Werdegar D, eds. Current medical diagnosis and treatment. Los Altos, CA: Lange, 1985.

Thompson JM, McFarland GK, Hirsch JE, Tucker SM, Bowers AC. Clinical nursing. St. Louis: CV Mosby, 1986.

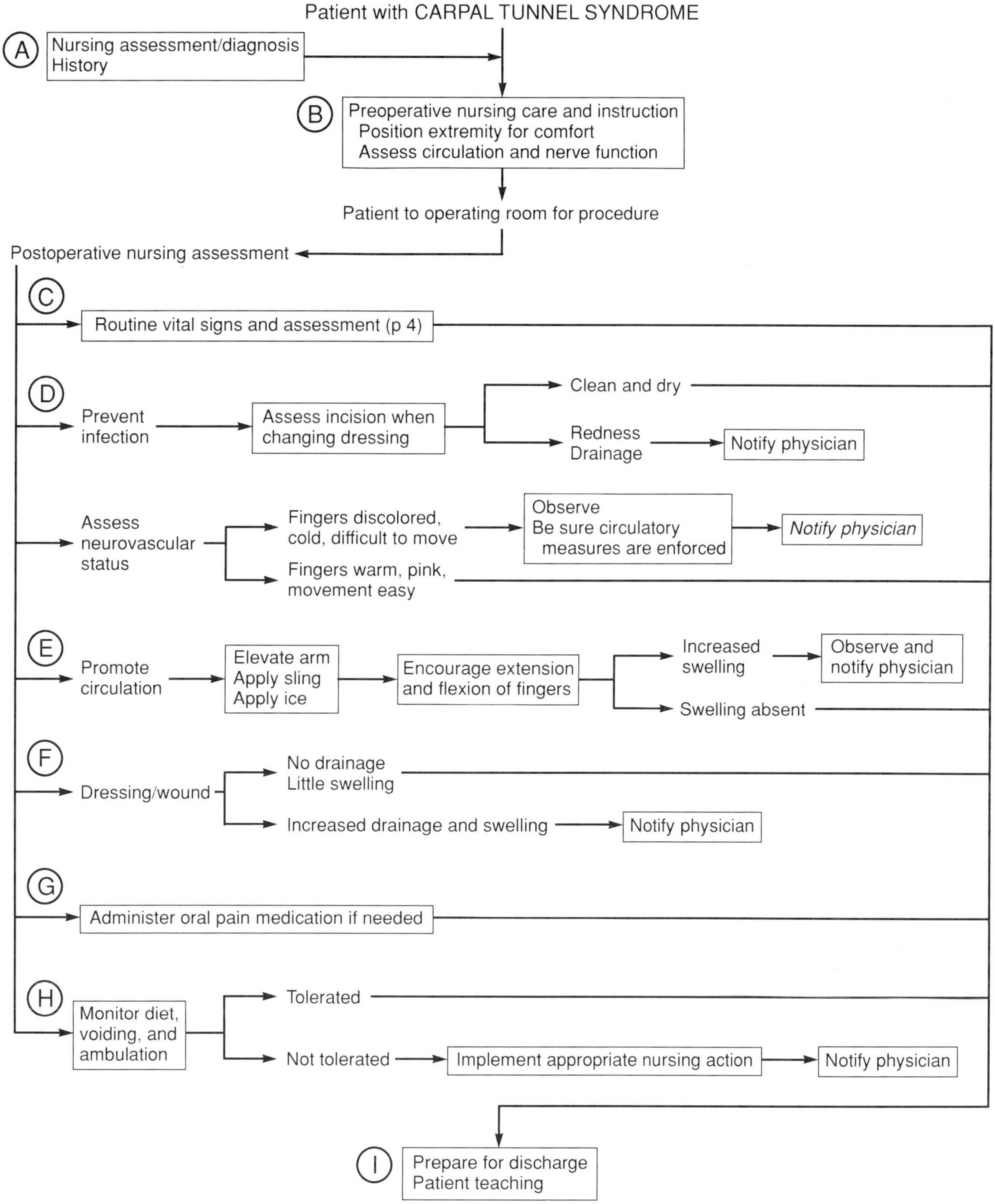
Patient with CARPAL TUNNEL SYNDROME
A
Nursing assessment/diagnosis
History
B
Preoperative nursing care and instruction
Position extremity for comfort
Assess circulation and nerve function
Patient to operating room for procedure
Postoperative nursing assessment
C
Routine vital signs and assessment (p 4)
D
Prevent infection
Assess incision when changing dressing
Clean and dry
Redness
Drainage
Notify physician
Assess neurovascular status
Fingers discolored, cold, difficult to move
Observe
Be sure circulatory measures are enforced
Notify physician
Fingers warm, pink, movement easy
E
Promote circulation
Elevate arm
Apply sling
Apply ice
Encourage extension and flexion of fingers
Increased swelling
Observe and notify physician
Swelling absent
F
Dressing/wound
No drainage
Little swelling
Increased drainage and swelling
Notify physician
G
Administer oral pain medication if needed
H
Monitor diet, voiding, and ambulation
Tolerated
Not tolerated
Implement appropriate nursing action
Notify physician
I
Prepare for discharge
Patient teaching

SCIATIC NERVE INJURY

Jan Metro-Emmert

The sciatic nerve, the longest nerve in the body, is two separate nerves in one sheath: the common peroneal and the tibial. Because of its location and distribution, the sciatic nerve is frequently exposed to internal and external trauma.

A. The possible cause of injury is probed during the history. Most sciatic nerve injuries result from either a herniated intervertebral disk (protruded nucleus pulposus) (p 46) or osteoarthritis of the lumbosacral spine. However, there are many other causes to be considered (Table 1).

B. A complete physical assessment, focusing on the neuromuscular functions, reveals "signs" characteristic of sciatic nerve injury.

C. Motor signs of sciatic nerve injury may include hamstring paralysis (loss of flexion of the leg), paralysis of all muscles of the leg and foot with the resultant "steppage gait" and an inability to stand on heels or toes, and loss of Achilles jerk and plantar flexion. Sensory signs may show loss of sensation to the outer side of the leg and the entire foot.

D. Sciatica (partial nerve injury) is typically severe and burning and is precipitated by the slightest exposure or jarring.

E. Atrophic signs reflect atrophy of the involved muscles, especially those below the knee. However, this sign may be masked by edema.

F. Vasomotor and trophic changes include edema of the leg and foot, dry and discolored skin, plantar hyperkeratosis, ulcerations on the sole of the foot, and toenail changes.

G. A positive Patrick's fabere sign is diagnostic of hip-joint disease. Instruct the patient to place the heel of the painful extremity on the opposite knee. The affected knee remains elevated and when depressed toward the bed causes pain. Thus the acronym f-ab-er-e: pain on *f*lexion, *ab*duction, external *r*otation, and *e*xtension when simultaneously applied.

H. A positive Laseque's sign is diagnostic of sciatic nerve disease. Place stretch on the sciatic nerve by flexing the patient's thigh on the abdomen and extending the leg at the knee. Pain is present with disease. The patient is also unable to fully extend his knee while sitting in a straight chair.

I. Diagnostic studies begin with radiologic examination of the lumbosacral spine. Selective blocking with 1 percent lidocaine is specific to diagnosing this condition. Electromyography measures the velocity of nerve conduction. Other studies are conducted as possible causes are identified.

J. Treatment focuses on the cause. Surgical procedures, medications, and combinations of both are used. Medicines fall into many categories: antibiotics, analgesics, anti-inflammatories, antimicrobials, chemotherapeutic agents, and local anesthetics.

K. Nursing interventions focus on pain relief and maximizing mobility. Analgesia is a priority. There are many agents and routes. Before selection, an extensive pain assessment is done, including site of pain, duration, intensity, current analgesics, side effects of medications, pain tolerance, support, and resources to assist with care of the patient.

L. An interdisciplinary treatment plan is formed based on all data. The choice of analgesic route of administration, type of infusion, and patient and family education are included in the plan. Continuous assessment, management of side effects, and evaluation of the effectiveness of the therapy are vital.

M. When the pain from sciatic nerve injury becomes chronic, surgery (cordotomy, rhizotomy, neurotomy) may be tried. Often the pain returns. All possible means of pain relief should be implemented: analgesia, positioning, comfort measures, relaxation techniques, imaging, biofeedback, and support groups.

N. The nursing goal is to help the patient cope with chronic pain (p 406). It is important to be alert to signs of ineffective coping patterns, especially depression. Maladaptive family dynamics may indicate a need for family counseling.

O. Impaired mobility may be temporary or permanent, depending on the cause and extent of sciatic nerve damage. Measures are taken to maximize the patient's mobility, and support is given to assist in coping with physical limitations.

TABLE 1. Sciatic Nerve Injury

Etiology	*Disease Process*
Herniated intervertebral disk	Trauma, lifting
Lumbosacral osteoarthritis	Aging
Lesions in spinal cord	Trauma, herpes zoster
Vertebral diseases	Tuberculosis, metastasis
Pelvic conditions	Fracture, hip dislocation, pregnancy
Stab or gunshot wounds	Lateral or peritoneal
Polyneuritis	Alcohol, lead or arsenic poisoning, infection, intramuscular injection
Thigh injury	Intramuscular injection
Childbirth injury	Traction on infant's legs
Nerve compression	Tight clothing, crossing legs at knees

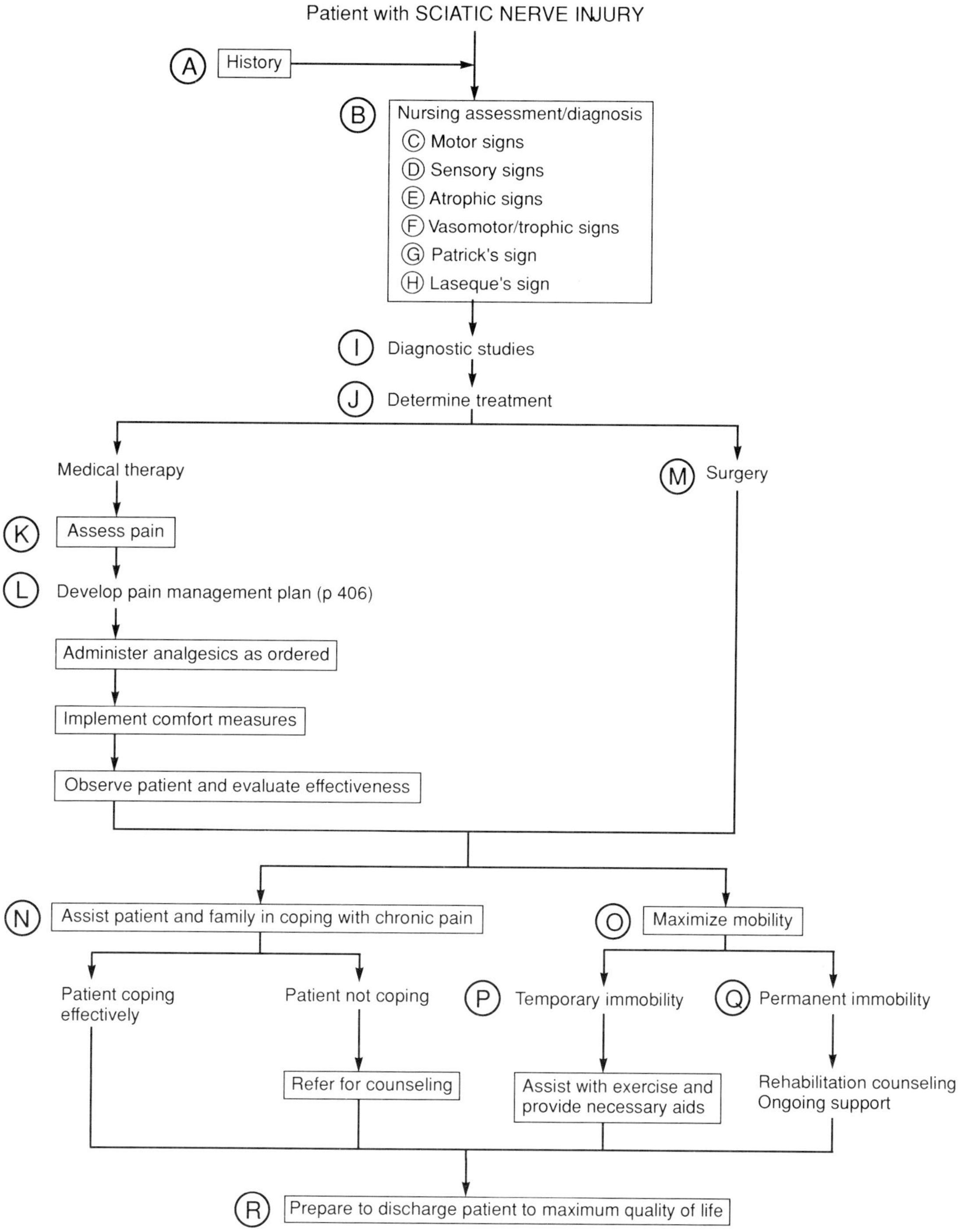

P. Temporary immobility (e.g., patient in traction) necessitates exercising the patient, isometrics, and range of motion and/or active-resistive exercises as indicated (p 234). Aids to mobility such as canes, walkers, and braces can promote increased mobility and decrease pain.

Q. Permanent paralysis or paresis necessitates extensive rehabilitation, including physical therapy, occupational counseling, and support to the patient and family (p 232).

R. Through caring, support, and interventions based on knowledge, the nurse can help the patient and family to achieve the maximum possible quality of life.

References

Chusid JG. Correlative neuroanatomy and functional neurology. 19th ed. Los Altos, CA: Lange, 1985.

Donovan M. Pain control. Nurs Clin North Am 1987; 22:645–648.

Lambert VA, Lambert CE Jr. Psychosocial impacts created by chronic illness. Nurs Clin North Am 1987; 22(3):527–533.

SPRAIN

Nancy A. Young

Accidents produce the most frequent insults to the musculoskeletal system, including soft tissue injuries such as sprains. Sprains and strains commonly occur, usually caused by abnormal stretching forces during vigorous activity or trauma. Whereas a strain involves the stretching of a muscle, a sprain is an incomplete tearing that includes the joint capsule, synovial membrane, and/or ligaments.

A. The nurse interviews the patient to determine the cause of the injury and the degree of severity of the tear. Minor sprains are usually self-limiting, with full function returning in 3 to 6 weeks.

B. More severe sprains warrant radiography to rule out fracture (p 230) or widening of the joint structure and may require surgery. A ligament may pull loose a fragment of bone in an avulsion fracture, or the patient may experience hemarthrosis (bleeding into a joint or cavity) or disruption of the synovial lining.

C. The treatment plan depends on the extent of the injury. Nonsurgical treatment during the acute phase focuses on immobilization of the part with a splint or other appropriate device (p 234), application of ice to reduce edema, and administration of analgesics to control discomfort. Surgical repair is indicated by a complete tear or fracture of the affected part.

D. Upon discharge, the patient should receive information about home care to promote healing of the injured joint as well as advice on techniques for preventing future injury. The joint, protected by casting, taping, or splinting, should be used as tolerated. Movement of joint surfaces maintains cartilage nutrition, and muscle contraction improves circulation and promotes phagocytosis of the hematoma. Warm moist heat applied after the acute phase and elevation of the affected part can reduce swelling. The practice of stretching and warming up prior to vigorous activity can help avert future sprains, as can the use of elastic support bandages or adhesive tape wrapping. Such preconditioning exercises promote slow stretching and protect the joint from quick, traumatic stretches. In addition, a high rate of metabolism improves the oxygenation of muscle fiber during intense work periods.

References

Hilt NE, Cogburn SB. Manual of orthopedics. St Louis: CV Mosby, 1980.

Luckmann J, Sorensen KC. Medical surgical nursing: a psychophysiologic approach. 3rd ed. Philadelphia: WB Saunders, 1987.

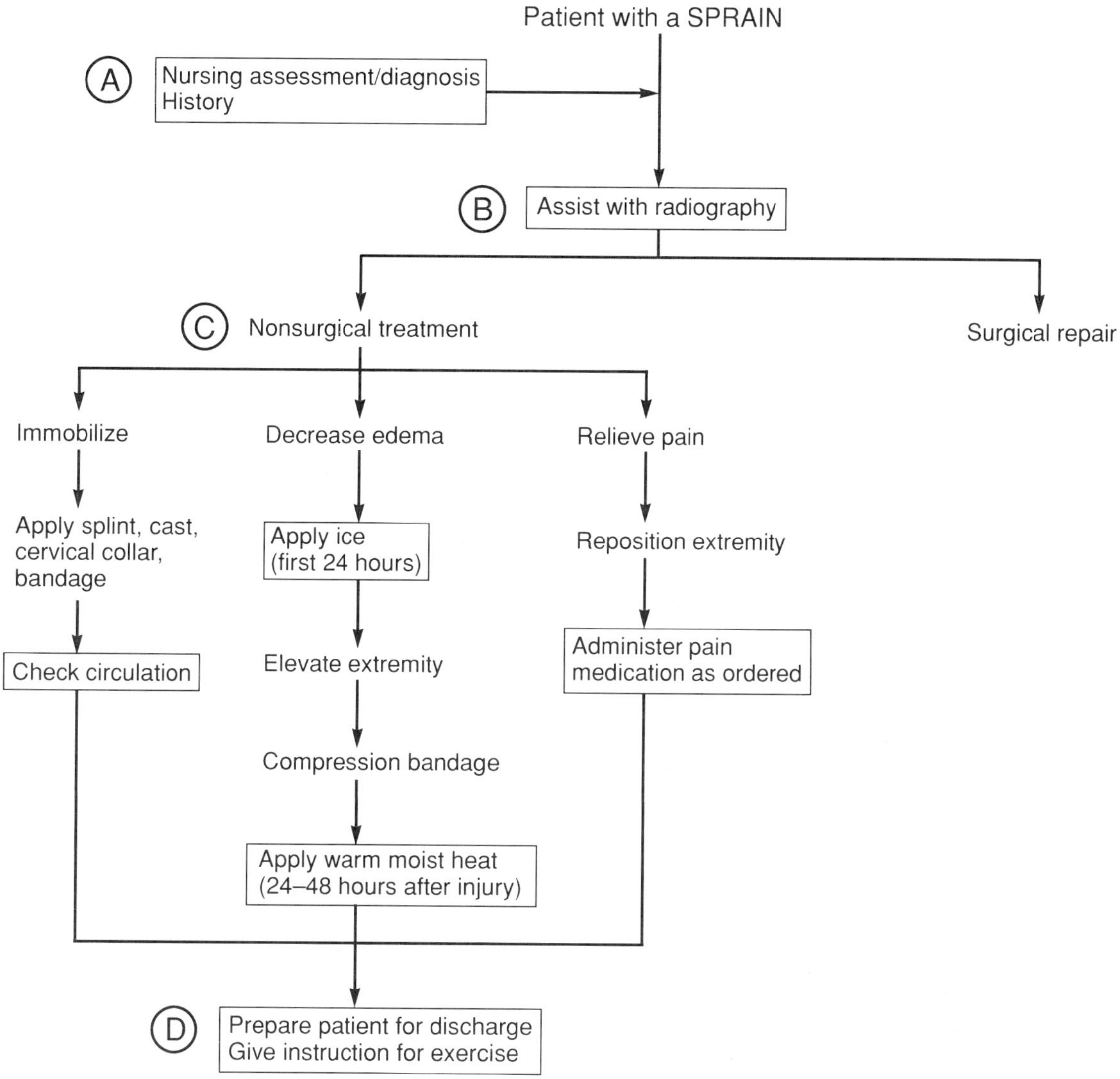
Patient with a SPRAIN
A
Nursing assessment/diagnosis
History
B
Assist with radiography
C
Nonsurgical treatment
Surgical repair
Immobilize
Decrease edema
Relieve pain
Apply splint, cast, cervical collar, bandage
Apply ice (first 24 hours)
Reposition extremity
Check circulation
Elevate extremity
Administer pain medication as ordered
Compression bandage
Apply warm moist heat (24–48 hours after injury)
D
Prepare patient for discharge
Give instruction for exercise

DISLOCATION

Nancy A. Young

A dislocation results during severe injury of the ligamentous structures surrounding a joint. The articular surface of the joint is completely displaced or separated, as opposed to a subluxation in which the joint surface separates partially or incompletely. Dislocations most commonly result from overwhelming force delivered to a joint, disrupting its soft tissues. They may, however, be congenital or occur spontaneously in diseased joints. Moving-vehicle accidents account for most lower extremity dislocations (hip); the upper extremities most often dislocated are the thumb, elbow, and shoulder.

A. A complete history explains the source of the injury, and close observation of the affected part may reveal an asymmetry of the musculoskeletal contour. For example, a hip dislocation presents with a shorter limb on the affected side. The patient complains of other symptoms, such as local pain, tenderness, loss of function of the injured part, and swelling in the affected joint. Radiologic films determine the extent of shifting in the structures; fat cells found in joint aspirations indicate an intra-articular fracture.

B. Dislocations warrant immediate intervention because of the possibility of avascular necrosis (bone-cell death resulting from inadequate blood supply). Open or closed reduction serves to realign the dislocated part of a joint to its appropriate anatomic position. Complete rupture of ligaments requires open reduction. The use of general anesthesia allows muscle relaxation so that the affected bones can be manipulated for closed reduction.

C. Immobilization by taping or use of a sling for 3 to 6 weeks allows torn ligaments and capsular tissue to heal.

D. Although immobilization restricts joint motion, a closely monitored rehabilitation program can prevent the development of contractures. After immobilization, care must be given to assure that active joint stretching remains within certain limits, because the strength of fibrous scar does not equal that of original tissue. The torn capsule and ligament also heal in a shortened position.

E. Discharge teaching focuses on an exercise program that restores the joint to its original range of motion, while avoiding a redislocation. The patient should also understand the signs of impaired circulation in extremities that are taped or wrapped, to allow early identification of problems.

References

Brunner LS, Suddarth DS. The Lippincott manual of nursing practice. 4th ed. Philadelphia: JB Lippincott, 1986.

Luckmann J, Sorensen KC. Medical-surgical nursing: a psychophysiologic approach. 4th ed. Philadelphia: WB Saunders, 1987.

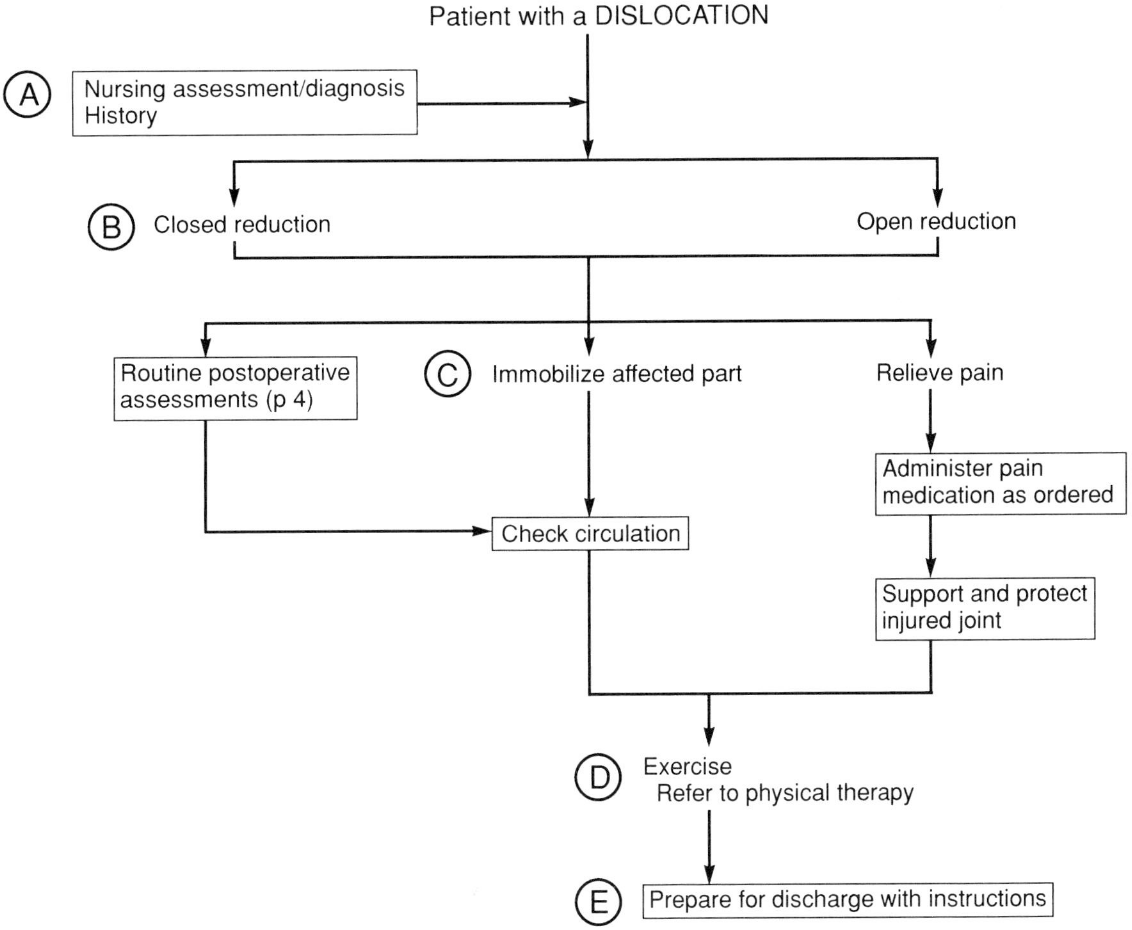
Patient with a DISLOCATION
A
Nursing assessment/diagnosis
History
B
Closed reduction
Open reduction
Routine postoperative assessments (p 4)
C
Immobilize affected part
Relieve pain
Administer pain medication as ordered
Check circulation
Support and protect injured joint
D
Exercise
Refer to physical therapy
E
Prepare for discharge with instructions

FRACTURE

Nancy A. Young

A. Fractures generally result from an accident or traumatic insult to a bone. A person suffering from malnutrition, bone disease, or a previous fracture is also predisposed to fractures. Radiology, bone biopsies, and laboratory studies along with a complete history of recent events, should identify the causative factor(s). Figure 1 shows some of the many types of fractures. Symptoms vary depending on location and severity of the injury and the degree of involvement of surrounding structures.

B. The nurse must monitor vital signs closely to assure adequate tissue perfusion and identify signs of impending shock (p 70). A decrease in blood pressure and a rapid thready pulse indicate a reduction of oxygen to the tissues and may lead to circulatory collapse. A traumatic injury could also impair the function of surrounding nerves, vessels, and organs. Intravenous fluids are given to replace circulating volume. The nurse should also be aware of an increased risk for embolus formation, which can cause circulatory and respiratory collapse (p 116).

C. The patient may experience extreme pain at the time of the injury, which disappears immediately if nerve damage has occurred. Muscle relaxants and analgesics can relieve pain during the recovery period as well as other comfort measures: elevation of the injured part to prevent edema, maintenance of immobility for the injured area, and assessment of casts for jagged edges and traction for sharp pins or wires. The nurse should document the type, location, and intensity of pain before administering medication in order to determine the causative factor(s), and the physician should be notified if pain is severe and prolonged.

D. Most fractures are immobilized during the healing process by applying a cast or traction to the affected part (p 234). The cast assures that bone fragments will realign to prevent or correct deformities and allows earlier weight bearing. A cast cutter should always be available for emergency removal. Traction reduces muscle spasms and pain and prevents possible deformities. Fracture patients require extra physical and emotional support in dealing with their physical limitations.

E. The nurse should assess the affected part for foul odor, drainage, or blood stains, excessively warm areas on the cast, and irritated areas or broken skin. Casts should be inspected for uneven edges, and the skin around traction areas should be cleansed to limit potential contaminants. Changing position and using protective padding promotes tissue perfusion and protects skin integrity over bony prominences. Any signs of infection must be reported to the physician.

F. The patient's decreased mobility due to a fracture contributes to constipation and urinary stasis in the bladder that may result in calculus formation (p 312). The nurse should encourage oral fluid intake and increased amounts of roughage in the diet. Stool softeners, laxatives, or enemas may be necessary. Good perineal hygiene will reduce the chance of meatal contami-

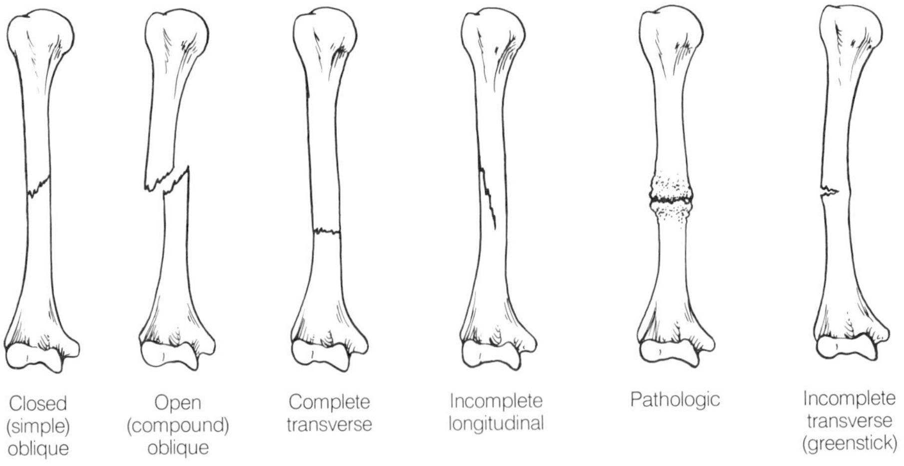

Figure 1 Types of fractures.

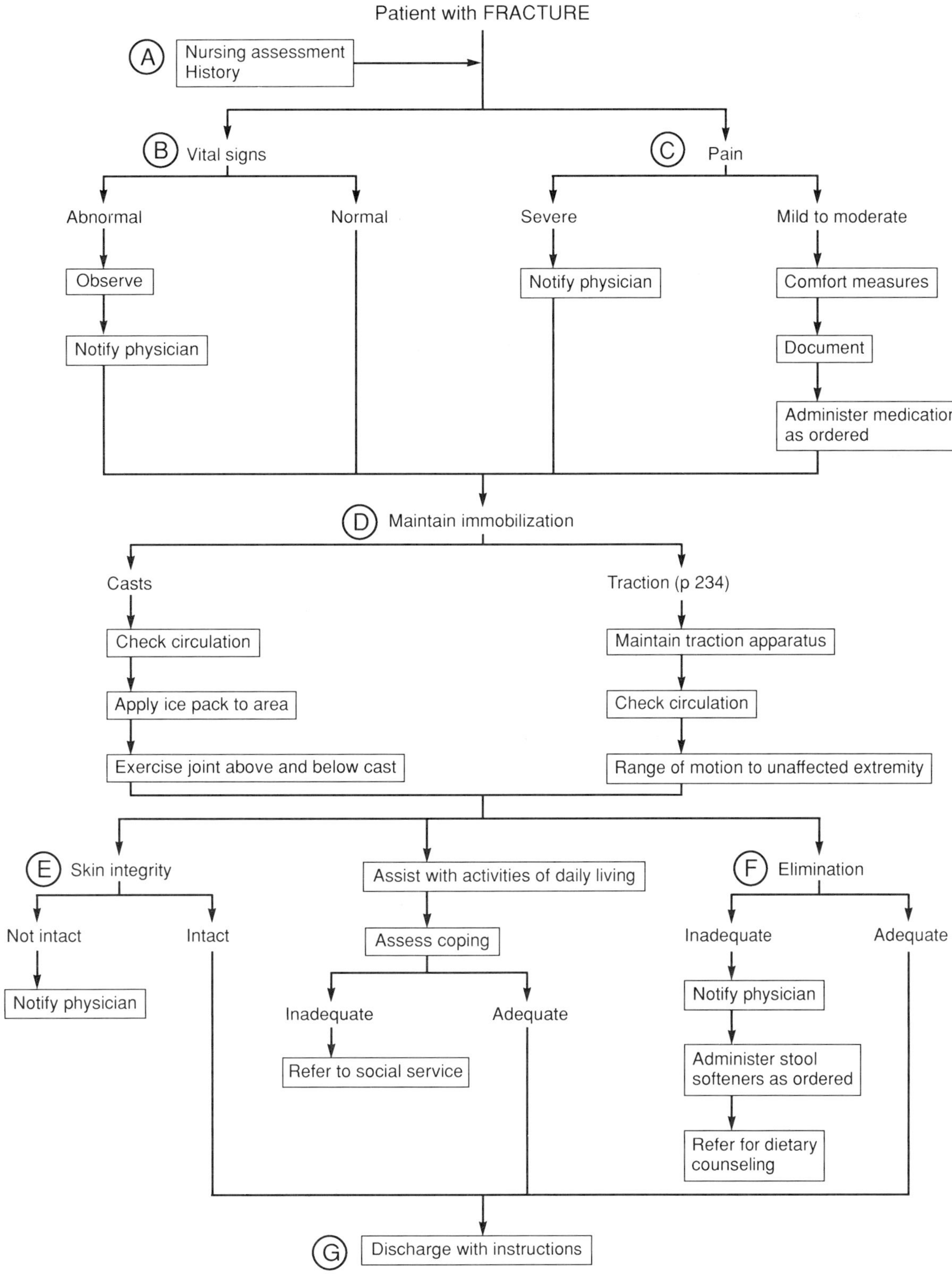

nation. The nurse should report any flank pain or prolonged absence of bowel sounds.

G. Prior to discharge, the patient should be taught the symptoms of infection and compromised circulation. He or she must understand the importance of exercising the joints above and below a fracture and the proper method of ambulation for the particular injury. The patient may need assistance in handling the limitations of activity and changes in body image that occur during healing.

References

Brunner LS, Suddarth DS. The Lippincott manual of nursing practice. 4th ed. Philadephia: JB Lippincott, 1986.

Doenges ME, Jeffries MF, Moorehouse MF. Nursing care plans: nursing diagnoses in planning patient care. Philadelphia: FA Davis, 1984.

Ulrich SP, Canale SW, Wendell SA. Nursing care planning guides. Philadelphia: WB Saunders, 1986.

PARALYSIS

Karen O'Brien

A. Nursing assessment of the paralyzed patient includes history and onset of neuromuscular dysfunction. Explore the patient's understanding of paralysis, and begin discharge planning at admission by assessing the patient's support systems, coping mechanisms, and available resources.

B. Acute immobility involves patients experiencing short-term paralysis such as general or spinal anesthesia. Nursing care is provided during the post-anasthesia period.

C. Patients with intermediate immobility experience paralysis for hours to months and can anticipate future resolution of their symptoms. Examples include head injury, spinal shock, Guillain-Barré syndrome (p 10), and various types of metabolic-induced coma. Nursing care involves supportive measures and prevention of complications.

D. Chronic immobility is found in patients with permanent neurologic deficits resulting from cerebrovascular accident (p 22), spinal cord transection (p 26), severe brain damage due to trauma, spinal tumor (p 40), brain tumor (p 38), and hypoxia. These patients require a prolonged and intensive plan of care.

E. Depending on the extent of paralysis, patients may require support of their vital functions. Monitor all vital signs carefully. Decreased respiratory drive and limited ability to expectorate secretions are common problems. Patients with spinal cord injuries above C4 require ventilatory assistance and frequent suctioning. Paralyzed patients often have an increased incidence of arrhythmias such as atrial fibrillation (p 58). Patients with a recent onset of paralysis should be monitored for life-threatening arrhythmias (p 62) and treated accordingly. Immediately after spinal cord injury, blood pressure is unstable and lowered. Paraplegics and quadriplegics often experience orthostatic hypotension.

F. Pain control is often forgotten when caring for the paralyzed patient. Patients may not be able to verbalize pain because of a tracheostomy tube or dysphagia. Pain is also an indicator of pathology. These patients do not feel pain in the affected areas of their bodies, so they cannot identify potentially dangerous symptoms. For example, a spinal cord injury patient cannot describe increasing abdominal discomfort or pressure or temperature injuries to the skin.

G. Paralyzed patients should be encouraged to participate in activities of daily living. Self-care with assistance promotes feelings of independence and self-worth. Each patient requires an in-depth individualized assessment of the level of assistance needed. A means of communication must be identified immediately—the mode may vary from eye blinks to sophisticated computerized communication systems. If the patient is unable to assist in any part of self-care, allow patient control by permitting choices when possible.

H. Position the patient in proper body alignment to help prevent ankylosis (p 206) and contractures. Place a footboard to prevent foot drop. Wrist-palm splints may be needed to maintain hands in a functional position, and range of motion exercises should be done at least four times a day.

I. Paralyzed patients require a Foley catheter initially. Place a closed drainage system; perform frequent catheter care to prevent infection. Monitor urine output and observe for signs of obstruction. When bladder reflex activity resumes, intermittent catheterization may be helpful in maintaining bladder tone and preventing urinary tract infections. Some patients may be able to learn self-catheterization.

J. Paralyzed patients may suffer from paralytic ileus. Bowel sounds should be auscultated frequently. When flatus and bowel sounds are present, the patient is advanced to an oral diet and a bowel program is begun. The patient's normal bowel habits are assessed and attempts are made to follow this schedule. A suppository or digital stimulation is used to elicit a spontaneous bowel movement. If this fails, impactions are removed manually. Stool softeners, mild laxatives, increased fluid intake, and diet modifications may also be helpful. Finally, enemas may be required if other alternatives fail.

K. Prevent skin breakdown through meticulous skin care. Turn and reposition the patient at least every 2 hours. Keep the skin clean and dry, and observe bony prominences for redness that persists or any breaks in skin integrity. Massage around these areas to promote circulation. Eggcrate mattresses, sheepskins, and flotation beds may also be helpful.

L. Two major pulmonary complications are pneumonia (p 104) and pulmonary emboli (p 116). Paralyzed patients may require frequent suctioning to prevent aspiration and an aggressive pulmonary toilet. An unconscious patient should be placed in a head-down, lateral position so that secretions can drain.

M. Spinal-cord-injured (lesions at or above T6) patients may develop autonomic dysreflexia, *a life-threatening emergency*. Symptoms and treatment are discussed on page 26.

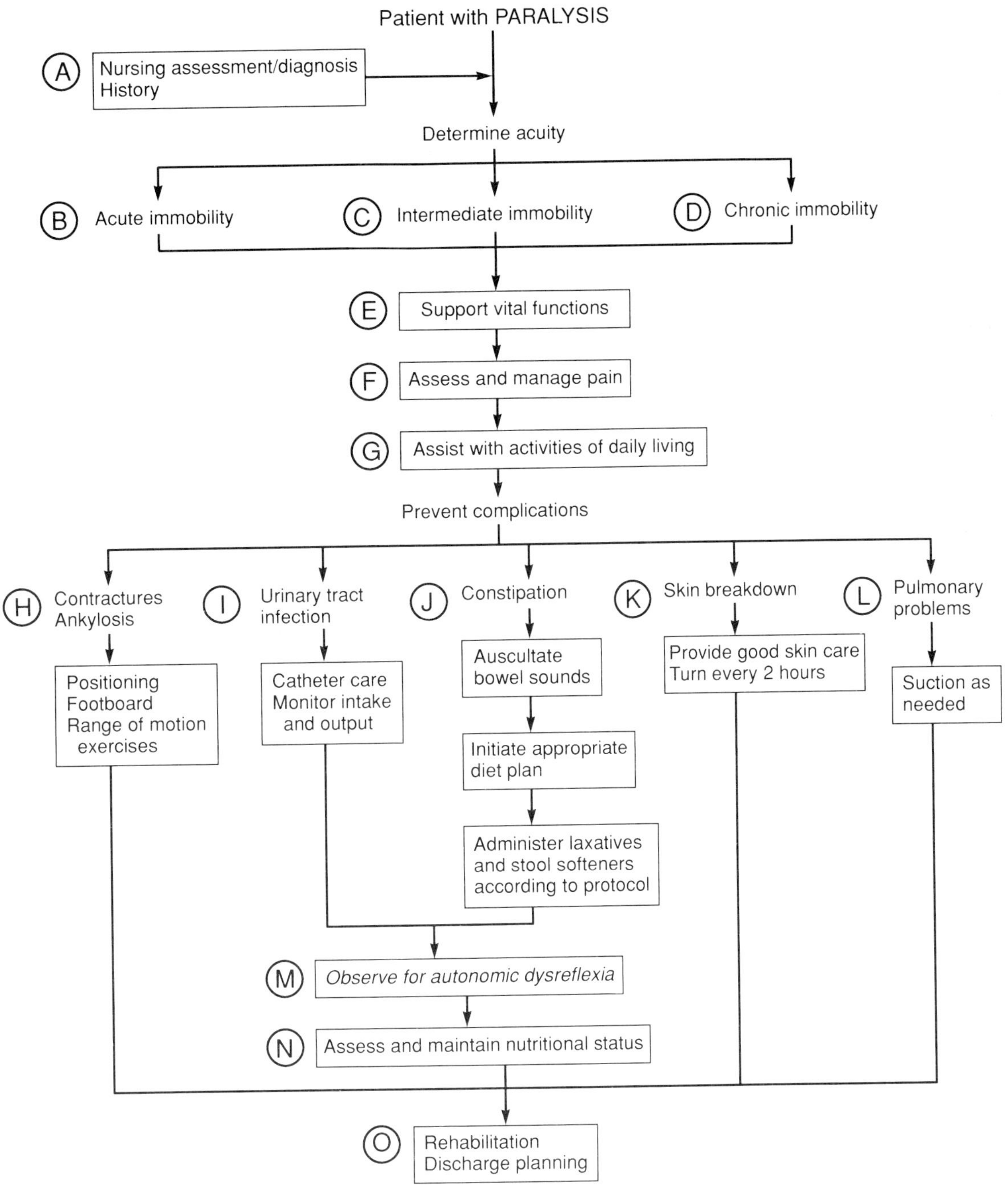

N. The paralyzed patient requires a high-calorie, high-protein diet, sometimes by nasogastric or gastrostomy tube feedings. If the patient can eat, encourage the family to bring favorite foods, because loss of appetite is common.

O. The goal of rehabilitation is to return the patient to the highest possible level of independence. An ongoing multidisciplinary approach is most helpful throughout the hospital stay. The team should include the primary physician, nurse, psychiatrist, physical therapist, occupational therapist, and social worker. Include family and significant others in planning and teaching. The patient may be referred to a rehabilitation center for long-term care.

References

Brunner LS, Suddarth DS. The Lippincott manual of nursing practice. 4th ed. Philadelphia: JB Lippincott, 1986:741.

Hickey J. The clinical practice of neurological and neurosurgical nursing. Philadelphia: JB Lippincott, 1981:131–142, 201–222.

Mitchell PH. Neurologic disorders. In: Kenney M, Packa D, Dunbar S, eds. AACN's clinical reference for critical care nursing. 2nd ed. New York: McGraw-Hill, 1988:971–1028.

Spross JA. Assessment of impaired mobility. In: Baird SB, ed. Decision making in oncology nursing. Toronto: BC Decker, 1988:120.

IMMOBILIZATION

Joy Gorzeman
Leslie C. Hussey

A. Patients with musculoskeletal conditions and injuries may require casts, traction, pins, nails, rods, plates, or grafts to immobilize a joint, realign a fracture, or relieve muscle spasm and pain.

B. Orthopaedic injuries are very painful, so the affected part should be handled gently. Casts, some pins, and traction are applied externally. Casts are the most common method of external fixation and immobilization. Traction is also fairly common and applies force to skin, muscles, and bones and can be applied directly or indirectly. The type of traction depends on the nature of the injury and the patient's age and general condition (Table 1). The amount of weight is determined by the severity of spasm, angulation desired, and general purpose of the traction. Weights may be increased or decreased depending on radiologic studies. Traction should not be used if an open, draining lesion is present. Patients in traction are generally hospitalized because of the specialized equipment and care required (Figs. 1 to 3). Orthopaedic injuries require time to heal, so patients may be in traction (or other method of immobilization) for up to 10 weeks.

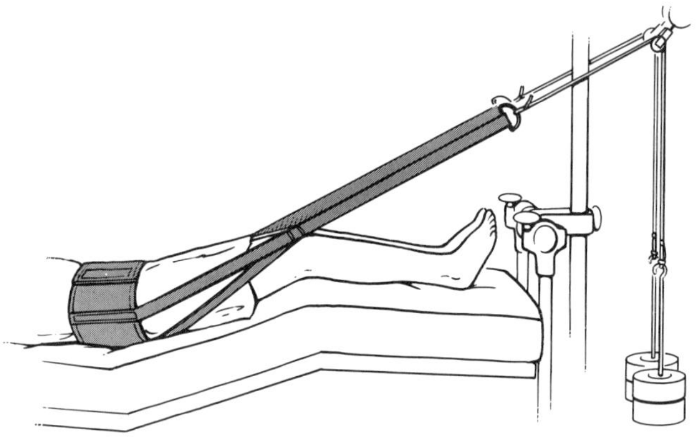

Figure 1 Pelvic belt traction.

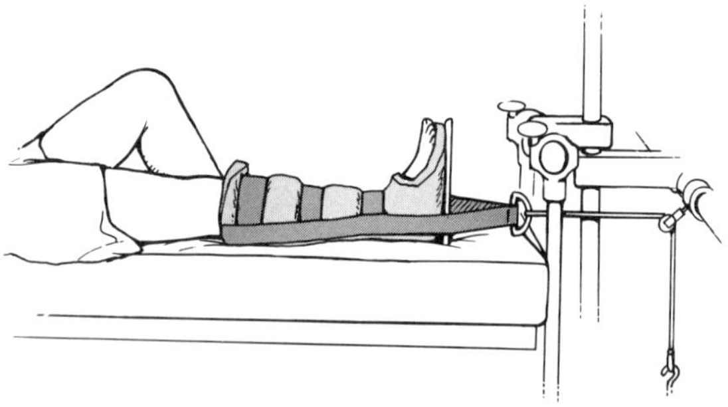

Figure 2 Buck's extension.

TABLE 1 Types and Purpose of Traction*

Type	*Purpose*
Buck's extension and Russel's traction	Preoperative hip fractures Relieves muscle spasms of leg and back
Pelvic belt or girdle	Relieves muscle spasms associated with disc problems
Pelvic sling	Holds fractured pelvic bones
Cervical head halter	Relieves muscle spasms caused by degenerative or arthritic conditions of cervical vertebrae
Dunlop's traction	Realigns fractures of the humerus
Cervical tongs	Realigns fractures of cervical vertebrae Relieves pressure on cervical nerves
Halo-pelvic traction	Preoperative straightening of scoliosis
Steinmann pin	Realigns fractures of the femur

* Adapted from Mourad LA. Musculoskeletal system. In: Thompson J, McFarland G, Hirsch J, Tucker S, Bowers A. Clinical nursing. St. Louis: CV Mosby, 1986:520–522.

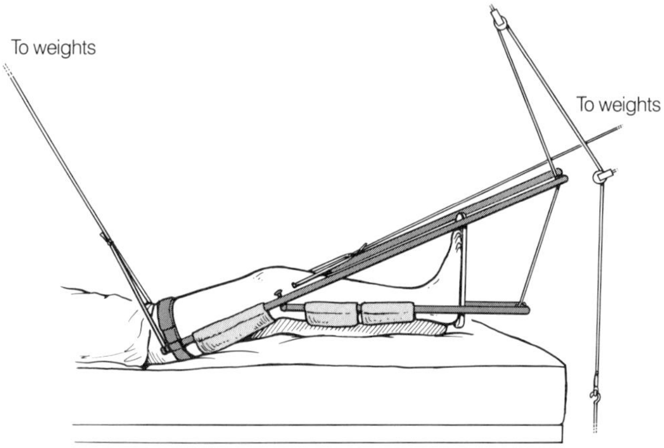

Figure 3 Balanced suspension skeletal traction.

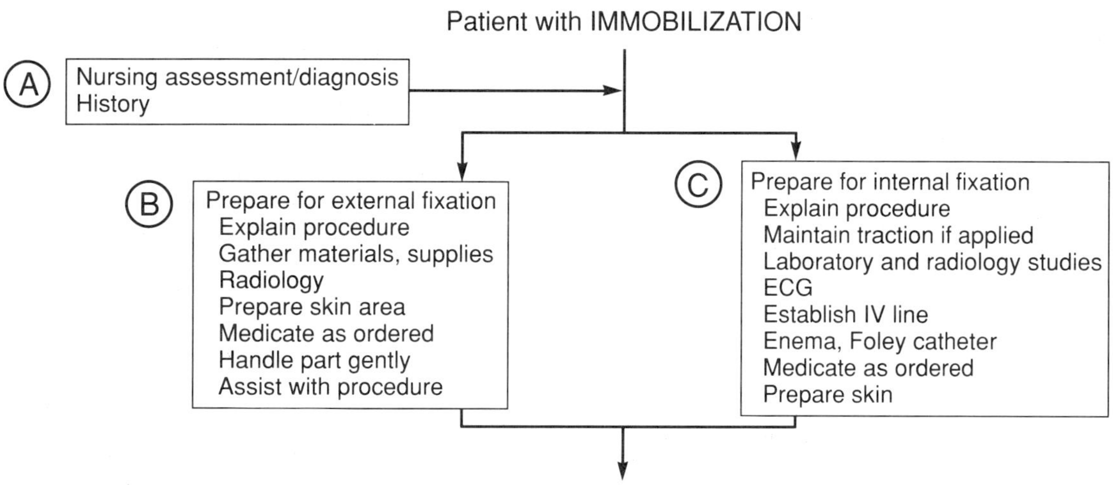

(Cont'd on p 237)

C. Nails, plates and screws, some pins, and bone grafts are internal methods of immobilization that require surgical implantation. Patients undergoing surgery require the usual preoperative treatment, such as laboratory studies, chest films, intravenous (IV) line insertion, and bowel preparation (p 2). If the patient is elderly (e.g., undergoing hip nailing), electrocardiography (ECG) is also done. Patient preparation prior to either external fixation or internal fixation includes a thorough explanation of the procedure. A skin preparation is especially important before insertion of a pin, since these sites are common sources of infection. Preoperative antibiotics are ordered for these patients. Pins are not used for severely comminuted fractures. If the procedure is to be external, all necessary equipment and supplies must be gathered, and the nurse will need to assist with gently holding and positioning the limb.

D. After any immobilization procedure, vital signs should be monitored (p 4). Antipyretics may be given for elevated temperature.

E. The extremity is elevated and ice bags applied. Neurovascular checks should be done every hour the first day, every 2 hours the second day, and every 4 hours thereafter. This includes checking the color and temperature of the skin, observing the site for swelling and drainage, assessing the patient's ability to move adjacent muscles and joints (unless movement is contraindicated), inquiring about numbness or tingling, and assessing pain and peripheral pulses.

F. Analgesics are administered to control pain as ordered the first few days. Pain should subside in about 1 week. Persistent, localized pain should be reported, because associated embolic complications are common.

G. Infection is a common complication of pins, nails, and plates. Antibiotics are administered, and pin sites cleansed with hydrogen peroxide and kept dry. Topical antibiotics may be applied in accordance with institutional protocol.

H. A well-balanced diet that is high in protein and vitamins but low in fat promotes healing. Adequate fluid intake is important to the elimination process and to prevent urinary tract infections.

I. Partial immobilization (casts, most pins, and nails) and almost total immobilization (grafts and traction) affect all body systems and require extensive nursing intervention. Patients should be turned according to guidelines at least every 2 hours to prevent pressure sores. Exercise and range of motion (ROM) to unaffected muscles and joints is extremely important. It is not uncommon for patients in traction to lose weight because of muscle atrophy.

J. Immobilized patients may have difficulties with self-image, especially those who are unable to be productive for a time. Occupational therapy, physical therapy, and social services should be referred. Explain to the patient the purpose of the traction and bedrest, and review the care plan and expected recovery schedule.

K. Discharge instructions should include pin care if applicable, application of a brace if needed, activity and weight-bearing restrictions, problems to report, and follow-up care.

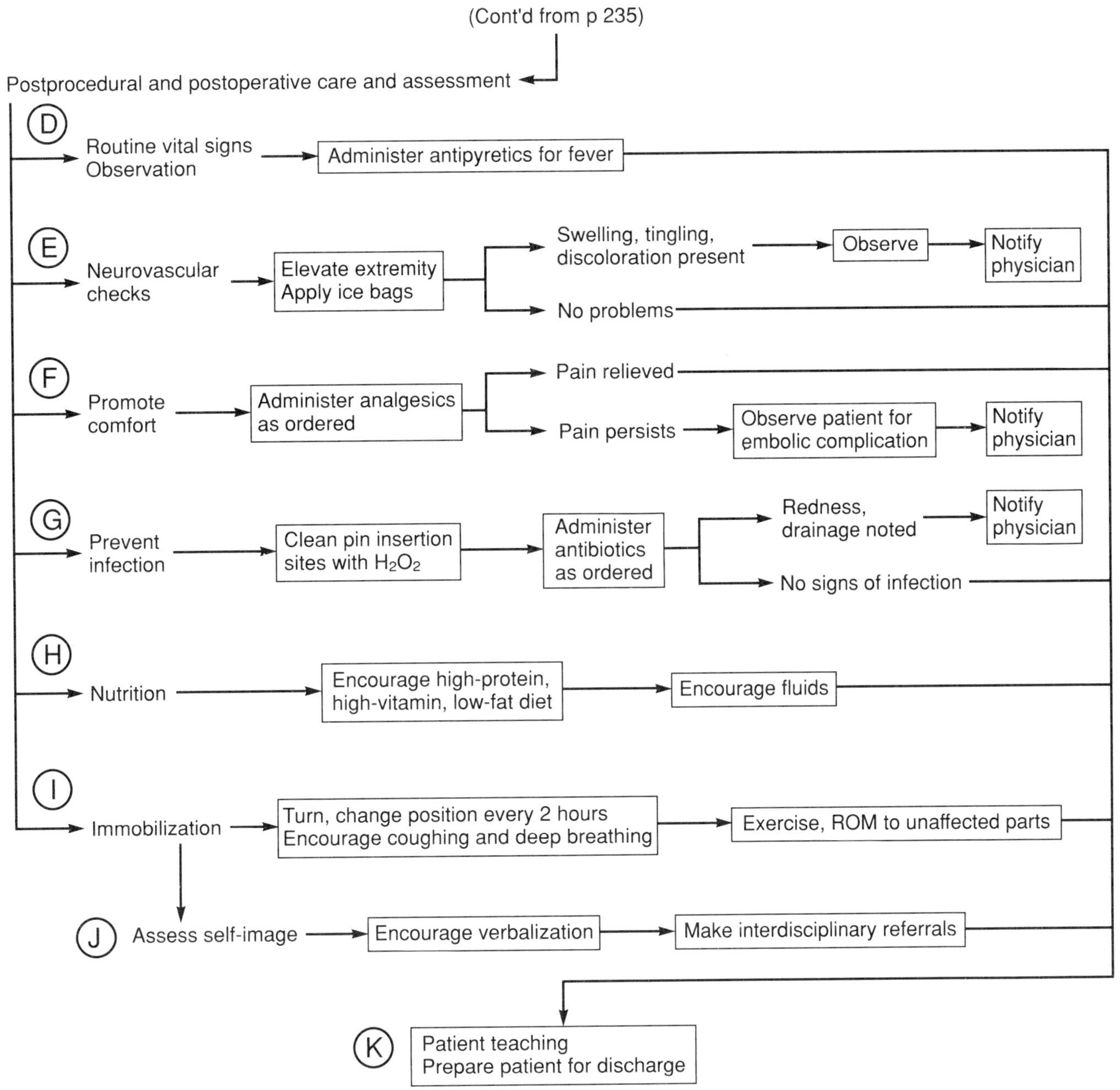

References

Brunner LS, Suddarth DS. The Lippincott manual of nursing practice. 4th ed. Philadelphia: JB Lippincott, 1986.

Luckmann J, Sorensen KC. Medical-surgical nursing: a psychophysiologic approach. 3rd ed. Philadelphia: WB Saunders, 1987.

Morris L, Kraft S, Tessem S, Reinisch S. Nursing the patient in traction. RN 1988; 51(1):26–31.

Rubin M. The physiology of bedrest. Am J Nurs 1988; 88(1): 50–56.

Thompson JM, McFarland GK, Hirsch JE, Tucker SM, Bowers AC. Clinical nursing. St. Louis: CV Mosby, 1986.

ARTHROSCOPY

Hazel Harris

Arthroscopy is a diagnostic examination of the interior surface of a joint permitting visualization with the use of a fiberoptic instrument called an arthroscope. Arthroscopy enables the physician to confirm a diagnosis and surgically correct it at the same time if indicated. The knee is the area most frequently visualized, but arthroscopy may be accomplished in other joints (e.g., shoulder, wrist, elbow, ankle). Arthroscopy is one of the most common diagnostic procedures performed to study the anatomy of the knee. It is a sterile procedure performed in the operating room under local or general anesthesia.

A. Indications for arthroscopy include suspected meniscus injury, ligament tear, chondromalacia, erosion of the surface of the patella and distal femur, and loose bodies in the knee related to arthritis. The patient may experience pain as a result of the injury. The procedure is contraindicated in patients with a bleeding disorder and altered skin integrity (i.e., abscess, abrasion, laceration) making the patient more susceptible to infection.

B. Preoperative teaching includes explanation of the procedure, how it is accomplished, and what to expect after the procedure. Tiny incisions called portals are made around the knee once the patient has been anesthetized. General anesthesia is preferred in case a corrective surgical procedure (i.e., removal or repair of a meniscus, ligament repair, removal of a foreign body or debris from the knee joint) is indicated. Saline solution is injected through one of the portals, causing distention of the knee joint. The arthroscope is inserted, thereby allowing visualization (Fig. 1). Risks of the procedure include infection, damage to a nerve or vessel, hematoma, thrombophlebitis, and possible breakage of the needle in the joint, which would require emergency surgery.

C. Postoperative nursing care includes monitoring of mental status, vital signs, and neurovascular status. The toes should be of equal warmth and color on both feet. Each toe should respond to stimuli.

D. After the procedure, the knee is wrapped with an elastic bandage. Oozing is normal. However, bloody drainage should be reported to the physician.

E. The patient should void without difficulty. If the patient is unable to void in a supine position, he should be assisted to a standing position at the bedside or permitted to ambulate to the bathroom if fully awake and independent on crutches. A one-time catheterization may be necessary.

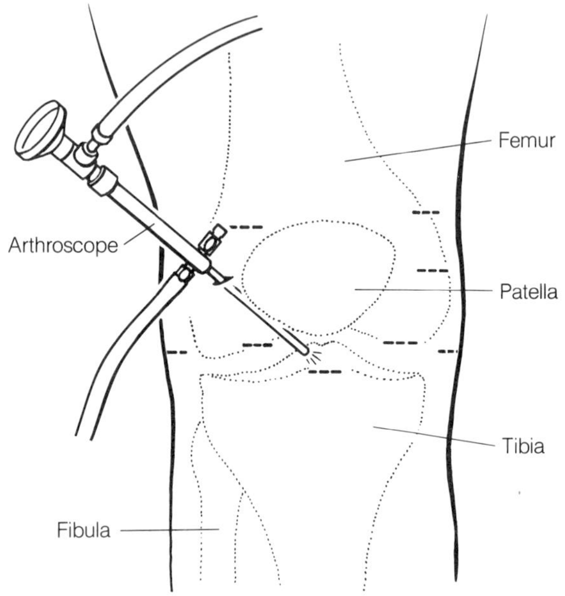

Figure 1 Arthroscope inserted through superolateral portal. Dashed lines indicate portals for additional instruments.

F. Pain is usually controlled by oral analgesia. An ice pack applied to the operative site helps control swelling and discomfort. Elevation also promotes venous return and relieves discomfort.

G. Prior to discharge the patient is instructed in gait training, quadricep settings, and straight leg raising exercises by the nurse and/or physical therapist. The amount of weight bearing for the operated leg depends on the physician's written order. The purpose of the exercises is to increase muscle strength and joint function.

H. If there are no complications, the patient is usually discharged home on the day of surgery with specific instructions in wound care, exercises, and pain medication and an appointment for a follow-up visit. Arthroscopy can also be performed on an outpatient basis. The patient should avoid aspirin, which can cause bleeding into the knee joint.

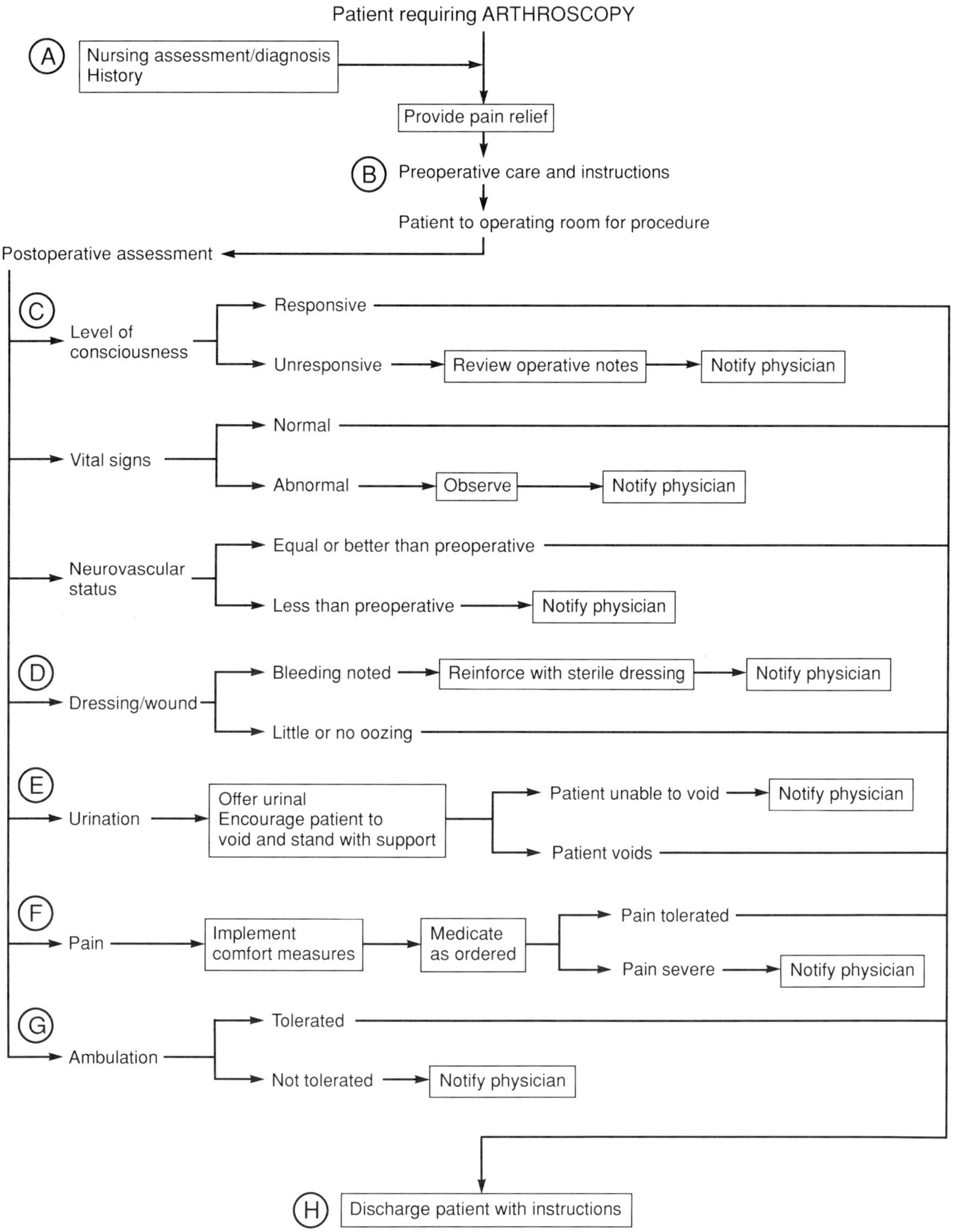

References

Andrews JR, Carson WG Jr, Ortega K. Arthroscopy of the shoulder: technique and anatomy. Am J Sports Med 1984; 12(11):1–7.

Drueke MM. Arthroscopic surgery of the knee. ADRN J 1982; Oct:585–590.

Dutka M. Elbow and wrist arthroscopy: perioperative nursing care. Orthop Nurs 1986; 5(4):29–34.

Farrell J. Illustrated guide to orthopedic nursing. 3rd ed. Philadelphia: JB Lippincott, 1986.

Hilt N, Cogburn S. Manual of orthopedics. St. Louis: CV Mosby, 1980.

MacArthur BJ. Arthroscopy of the shoulder. Orthop Nurs 1986; 5(4):26–28.

MYELOGRAPHY

Barbara Kalo

Myelography is a diagnostic study of the nervous system, which consists of radiography of the spinal cord and vertebral column after the injection of a contrast medium into the subarachnoid space between the fourth and fifth lumbar vertebrae. The fluoroscopic table is tilted and the course of the medium is observed. The contrast medium outlines the subarachnoid space, showing any distortion of the spinal column or spinal dural sac caused by tumors, cysts, herniated intervertebral disks, or other lesions. The contrast medium may be a water-soluble dye, which is absorbed by the body and excreted by the kidneys, or an oil-based medium, which is removed after the procedure by syringe and needle aspiration.

A. A routine nursing admission assessment is done. A history of sensitivity to iodine and iodine-containing substances such as shellfish, topical ointments, or radiographic contrast media is essential. Nursing concerns focus on patient safety and anxiety related to the procedure or implications of test results.

B. An explanation of the procedure is necessary to alleviate fears and to allow the patient to cooperate. Myelography requires that the patient lie in the lateral recumbent position with the knees drawn up as close to the abdomen as possible with the head flexed toward the chest. This position allows the vertebrae to separate for easy insertion of the needle into the subarachnoid space. There is minimal danger of injuring the spinal cord because the injection site is between the fourth and fifth lumbar vertebrae and the cord terminates at the second lumbar vertebrae. The meal prior to myelography is omitted, a preprocedure sedative or anticholinergic is given as ordered, and the patient is instructed to empty the bladder before going to radiology. Inform the patient and family that this diagnostic study may take 1 hour or longer. Prior to the procedure, ensure that the patient or responsible family member signs a consent form.

C. Postprocedure nursing care includes the correct positioning of the patient. If the water-soluble medium (metrizamide) is used, the head of the patient is elevated 15 to 30 degrees to reduce the rate of upward flow of the medium and to minimize the chance of a postmyelography headache. If the oil-based iodine compound (Pantopaque) is used, the patient remains flat in bed for 12 to 24 hours to reduce cerebrospinal fluid leakage and minimize the probability of a headache.

D. Routine procedures such as vital signs, neurologic assessment, and inspection of the injection site are done at least every 30 minutes for the first 4 hours, then every 4 hours for 24 hours.

E. Medicate the patient for postmyelography headache as needed. Usually oral analgesics are adequate to alleviate the pain, along with maintaining the correct position after the procedure and drinking plenty of liquids.

F. Diet is resumed after the procedure with emphasis on drinking large amounts of fluid for rehydration and replacement of cerebrospinal fluid.

G. Assess the bladder for distention. Offer the bedpan or urinal as necessary and encourage oral fluids to help facilitate the process of voiding within 8 hours.

H. Ambulation may be started immediately after the procedure if the water-soluble medium is used. Bedrest is maintained for 12 to 24 hours if the oil-based medium is used, and may be continued for a longer period if the patient experiences a headache when getting up for the first time.

I. The myelogram helps determine the medical management for the patient. Preparing the patient physically and emotionally for further hospitalization, for impending surgery, or for discharge requires specific instructions and teaching.

References

Brunner LS, Suddarth DS. The Lippincott manual of nursing practice. 3rd ed. Philadelphia: JB Lippincott, 1982.

Brunner LS, Suddarth DS, eds. Textbook of medical-surgical nursing. 6th ed. Philadelphia: JB Lippincott, 1988.

Hauseman KA. Myeloscopy. In: Cahill M, ed. Diagnostics. 2nd ed. Springhouse, PA: Springhouse Corporation, 1986: 780–782.

Lewis SM, Collier IC. Medical-surgical nursing: assessment and management for clinical problems. New York: McGraw-Hill, 1983.

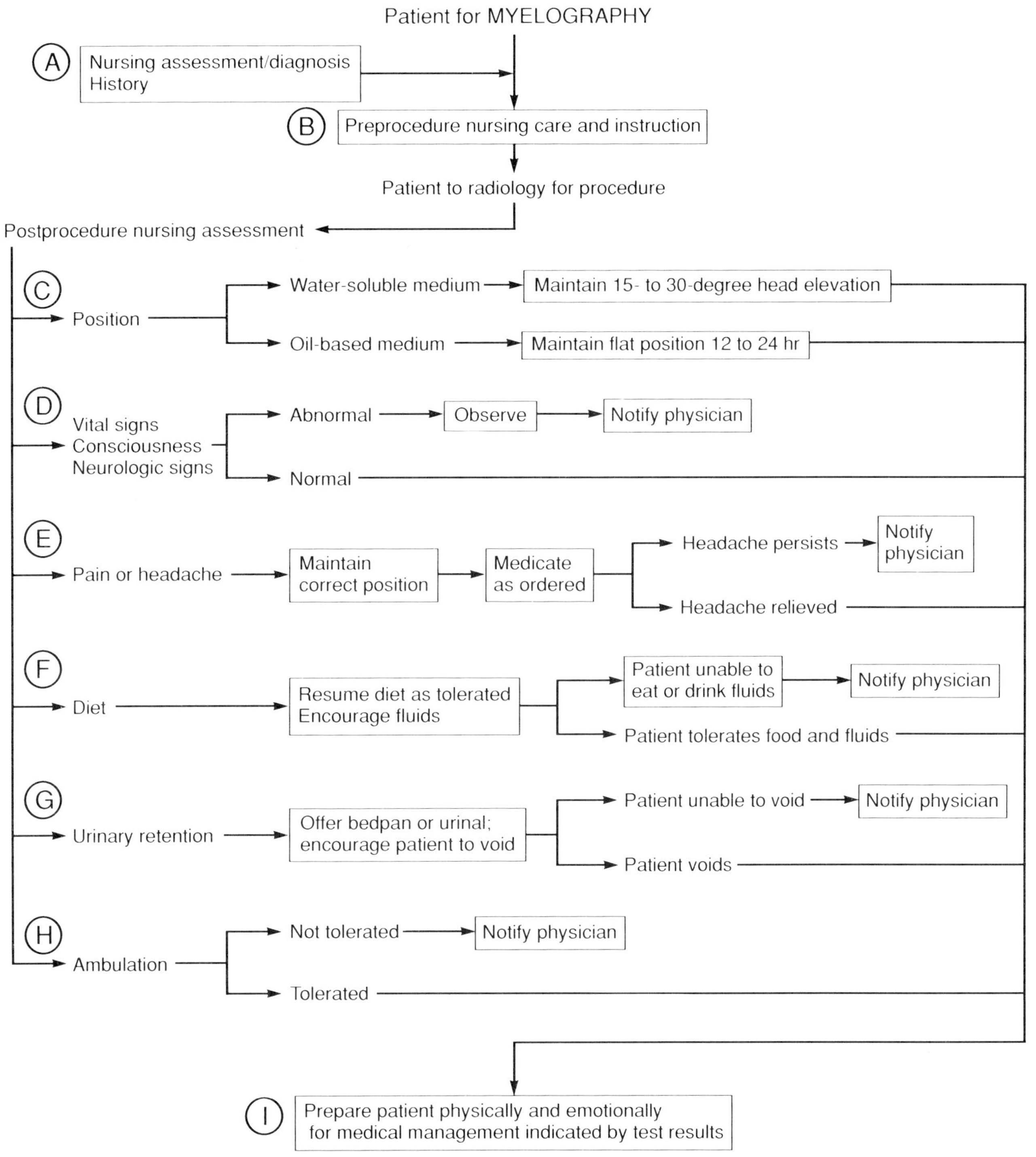
Patient for MYELOGRAPHY
A
Nursing assessment/diagnosis
History
B
Preprocedure nursing care and instruction
Patient to radiology for procedure
Postprocedure nursing assessment
C
Position
Water-soluble medium
Maintain 15- to 30-degree head elevation
Oil-based medium
Maintain flat position 12 to 24 hr
D
Vital signs
Consciousness
Neurologic signs
Abnormal
Observe
Notify physician
Normal
E
Pain or headache
Maintain correct position
Medicate as ordered
Headache persists
Notify physician
Headache relieved
F
Diet
Resume diet as tolerated
Encourage fluids
Patient unable to eat or drink fluids
Notify physician
Patient tolerates food and fluids
G
Urinary retention
Offer bedpan or urinal; encourage patient to void
Patient unable to void
Notify physician
Patient voids
H
Ambulation
Not tolerated
Notify physician
Tolerated
I
Prepare patient physically and emotionally for medical management indicated by test results

TOTAL HIP REPLACEMENT (ARTHROPLASTY)

Joy Gorzeman

Total hip replacement is a surgical procedure in which the femoral head and the acetabulum are both replaced with prostheses (Fig. 1). Although hip replacement is the most common, other joints such as the knee, elbow, shoulder, finger, and ankle can also be replaced.

A. Total hip replacement is usually done in cases of severe arthritis (p 212) in which inflammation or degeneration has caused severe pain and/or limited movement. Other reasons include femoral neck fracture, failure of previous reconstructive surgery, and pathologic fractures caused by metastatic cancer.

B. Total hip replacement surgery is usually elective. Patients are admitted a day before surgery to allow for complete assessment. Patients with renal conditions or bleeding or clotting disorders may be rejected. Surgery is postponed if the patient shows any indication of infection. Skin preparation is important to reduce chances of infection. Radiographs are taken to assist in establishing a proper fit of the prosthesis. Preoperative teaching includes an explanation of the procedure and postoperative activity limitations, such as the use of an overhead trapeze and walking aids. Patients should practice with these devices under the nurse's guidance to assure their comfort and ability in the postoperative period. Patients should also practice coughing and deep breathing in addition to isometric exercises. Prophylactic antibiotics are given intravenously to establish a therapeutic blood level.

C. Total hip replacement requires special operative equipment and conditions. In the past a special cement that was used to hold the prosthesis in place caused inflammatory reactions or hypotension in some patients. Severe or long-term infections resulted in a loosening of the joint and subsequent dislocation. Now, a bone ingrowth prosthesis may be used. This requires more healing time, but decreases the inflammatory response. In patients' whose bone structure is not conducive to this type of implant, somethyl methacrylate (cement) is still used.

D. Postoperative nursing assessment focuses on preventing the two most common complications of total hip replacement: thromboembolic conditions and infection. Vital signs and level of consciousness are checked routinely (p 4). Patients are NPO the first 24 hours and then diet is advanced from clear liquid to regular as tolerated. Fluids and fiber are encouraged to reduce constipation. Frequent neurovascular checks (pulses, color, sensation, and movement) distal to the operative site are essential.

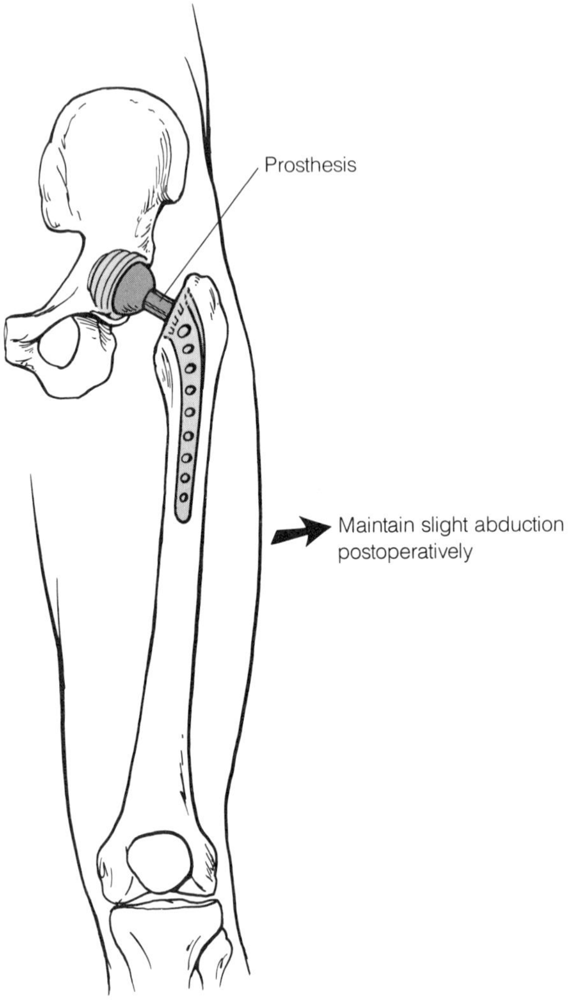

Figure 1 Total hip replacement.

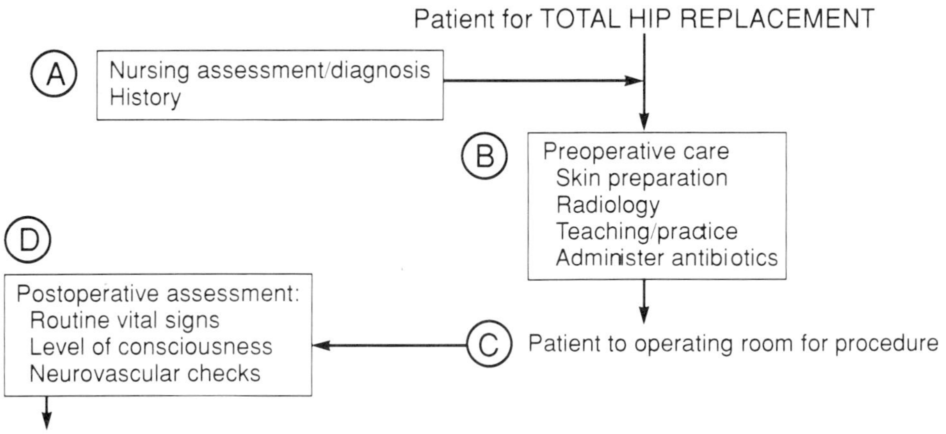

(Cont'd on page 245)

E. Proper positioning is also an important aspect of nursing care because dislocation of the joint can occur. Hip flexion and leg adduction are to be avoided. A pillow placed between the knees may help prevent adduction. An overhead trapeze must be attached to the bed to allow the patient to lift onto the bedpan and change position without putting weight on the affected hip. A fracture bedpan is used to decrease the amount of stress placed on the joint. Patients may be turned onto the unoperated side. The bed should be kept flat most of the time.

F. Dressings should be checked and reinforced as necessary during the first 24 to 48 hours. Subsequent dressing changes are done as needed, using strict aseptic technique. Suction drainage must be monitored and recorded. Excessive or bright red bleeding should be reported. Intake and output must be documented. Any redness, swelling, tenderness, or drainage from the incision must be noted and reported. Elevated temperatures must be monitored. Antibiotics are an important part of postoperative care.

G. Patients should be encouraged to cough and deep breathe. Intermittent positive pressure breathing (IPPB) treatments may be ordered. The cement used to set the prostheses is excreted through the lungs and may cause pink-tinged sputum, which should be observed and recorded. Antiembolism hose are applied, and patients are encouraged to isometrically exercise quadriceps and gluteus daily.

H. Activity or ambulation varies according to physician. Ambulation may begin the first postoperative day. The nurse must assist the patient and give instructions about weight-bearing restrictions. Physical therapy referral may be needed. Long periods of sitting must be avoided, because that position adds stress to the joint.

I. Pain medication is needed the first few days. Proper positioning and maintenance of bladder and bowel function also promote comfort. Complaints of increased discomfort and inability to move the joint should be investigated; this may indicate joint dislocation. A shortened extremity is another verification of dislocation.

J. Discharge teaching includes reinforcement of avoiding positions of extreme internal rotation, adduction, and flexion. Patients are reminded to avoid sitting for long periods and crossing their legs. A raised toilet seat should be used. Straining the joint by heavy lifting, jogging, or jumping should be avoided. Walkers or aids should be used because full weight-bearing is not advised for at least 4 weeks. Support stockings should be worn until full activity is resumed. Isometric exercises should be done daily. Patients should be aware of the need to take antibiotics prophylactically any time there is a risk of infection, such as tooth extraction, surgery, or urinary or renal infection, for the rest of their lives.

References

Brunner LS, Suddarth DS. The Lippincott manual of nursing practice. 4th ed. Philadelphia: JB Lippincott, 1986.

Luckmann J, Sorensen KC. Medical-surgical nursing: a psychophysiologic approach. 3rd ed. Philadelphia: WB Saunders, 1987.

Phipps WJ, Long BC, Woods NF. Medical-surgical nursing concepts and clinical practice. 3rd ed. St. Louis: CV Mosby, 1987.

Putman J. Total hip replacement: helping your patient avoid complications. Nurs Life 1986; 6(2):31–32.

Thompson JM, McFarland GK, Hirsch JE, Tucker SM, Bowers AC. Clinical nursing. St. Louis: CV Mosby, 1986.

(Cont'd from p 243)

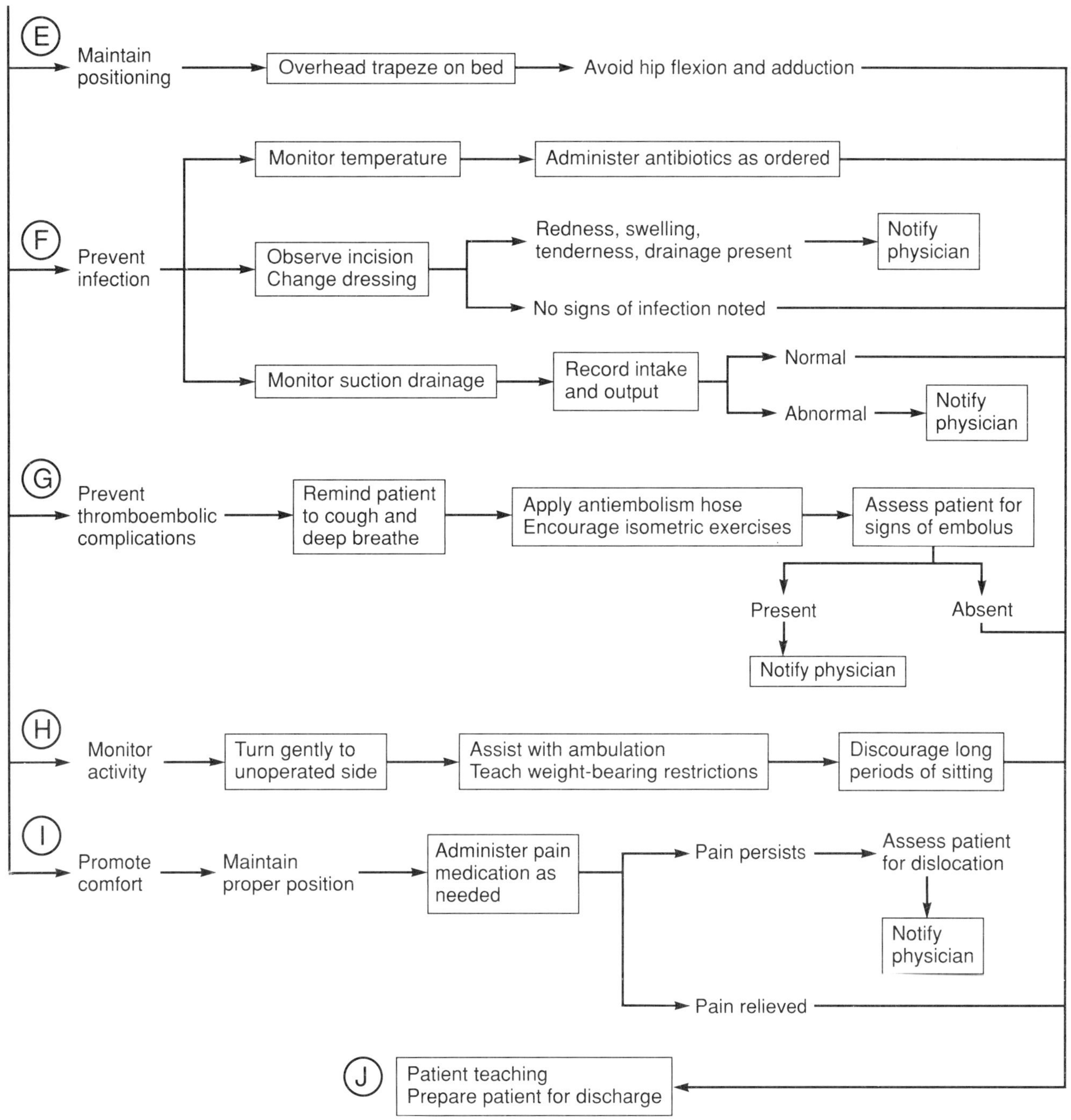

INTEGUMENTARY SYSTEM

BURNS

Karen O'Brien

A. The history of the burn should include time and circumstances of injury, such as causative agent, and other injuries. Past medical history, allergies, and current medication are important. Prehospital and emergency department care should also be noted, including assessment and treatment given before admission to the inpatient setting.

B. The nursing assessment includes percentage and distribution of burns, vital signs, height, and weight. A brief head-to-toe assessment should be performed on admission, which serves as a baseline for future monitoring and may identify abnormalities.

C. Airway assessment and monitoring is of primary importance. Respiratory status may be normal initially, with airway obstruction developing up to 48 hours postburn. Special attention is required for patients with burns around the mouth or neck, singed nasal hairs, oral or nasopharyngeal mucosal injury, voice changes, or if coughing up soot. Prophylactic intubation is the treatment of choice for suspected airway compromise. Nasotracheal intubation with the largest size endotracheal tube possible is preferred. Circumferential chest burns may constrict chest movement and prevent effective respiratory effort. Escharotomy may be required.

D. Major burns require extensive volume replacement because of fluid shifts. Therefore, intravenous (IV) access should be evaluated to ensure the patency of two large-bore IV catheters or a subclavian (central) line. Fluid resuscitation begins as soon as possible after a burn injury and continues on admission to the inpatient area. Initially, lactated Ringer's solution is infused at a volume of 4 cc/kg per percentage of body surface area burned. One-half of the total amount is given in 8 hours, one-quarter in the second 8 hours, and the final quarter during the third 8 hours. Times are calculated from the estimated time of injury. Following the Ringer's lactate infusion, plasma is given at a rate of 0.5 ml/kg per percentage of body surface area burned for 4 to 6 hours, and finally D_5W is infused according to the laboratory test results and vital signs. It is essential that intake and output be monitored strictly.

E. Monitor the need for analgesia frequently. The drug of choice is morphine given IV piggyback. Intramuscular medications are not recommended because of the unpredictable rate of absorption. Always offer pain medication before initiating treatment such as dressing changes.

F. Monitor peripheral pulses carefully on any patient with burned extremities. A Doppler device will probably be required owing to edema. Check radial and pedal pulses hourly. Ask the patient to report sensations of numbness, tingling, or deep pain. If tissue pressure causes neurovascular compromise, permanent damage may occur. Report any change in the patient's neurovascular checks immediately. Elevate burned extremities to decrease tissue trauma.

G. Removal of the eschar (dead tissue), which is necessary to prevent infection and prepare the skin for grafting, may be accomplished in several ways, including surgical excision, immersion of the patient in a Hubbard tank using scissors and forceps to remove dead tissue (p 252), or wet coarse mesh gauze soaks which will adhere to the dead tissue and be removed through frequent dressing changes.

H. Dressing application varies according to the depth and location of the burn. Change dressings frequently, usually in hydrotherapy. Strict aseptic technique must be followed.

I. Skin grafts are applied to full-thickness burn areas (p 254). The face, neck, hands, and areas of motion are usually grafted first to decrease scarring and contracture formation.

J. Infection is a serious complication in the burned patient. When the skin is destroyed, so is one of the body's protective mechanisms. Topical antimicrobials such as 1 percent silver sulfadiazine or Sulfamylon are applied to the burned areas. Monitor the patient's vital signs closely for signs of infection. Special attention must be given to mouth care, Foley catheter care, and general body hygiene. Wound cultures are obtained when indicated, and appropriate subeschar antibiotic therapy initiated.

K. Always consider immobility (p 234) when planning nursing care. Pneumonia (p 104) may be prevented by thorough respiratory care. Make sure the patient's respiratory status (breath sounds, rate, depth, and rhythm) is monitored closely. All burn patients should be instructed to turn, cough, and deep breathe. Pressure sores are prevented by meticulous skin care, careful and frequent position changes, and special beds if needed.

L. Contractures and deformities can be prevented. Body alignment, splints, and supports may be necessary. Physical and occupational therapists should be involved to encourage resumption of activities of daily living as early as possible. Range of motion exercises should be done frequently.

M. Patients who have been burned require prolonged and extensive follow-up. They need encouragement and support to resume independent living. Family, living situation, and change in self-image should be addressed prior to discharge. Appropriate referrals to support groups, home health care, and rehabilitation services must be arranged.

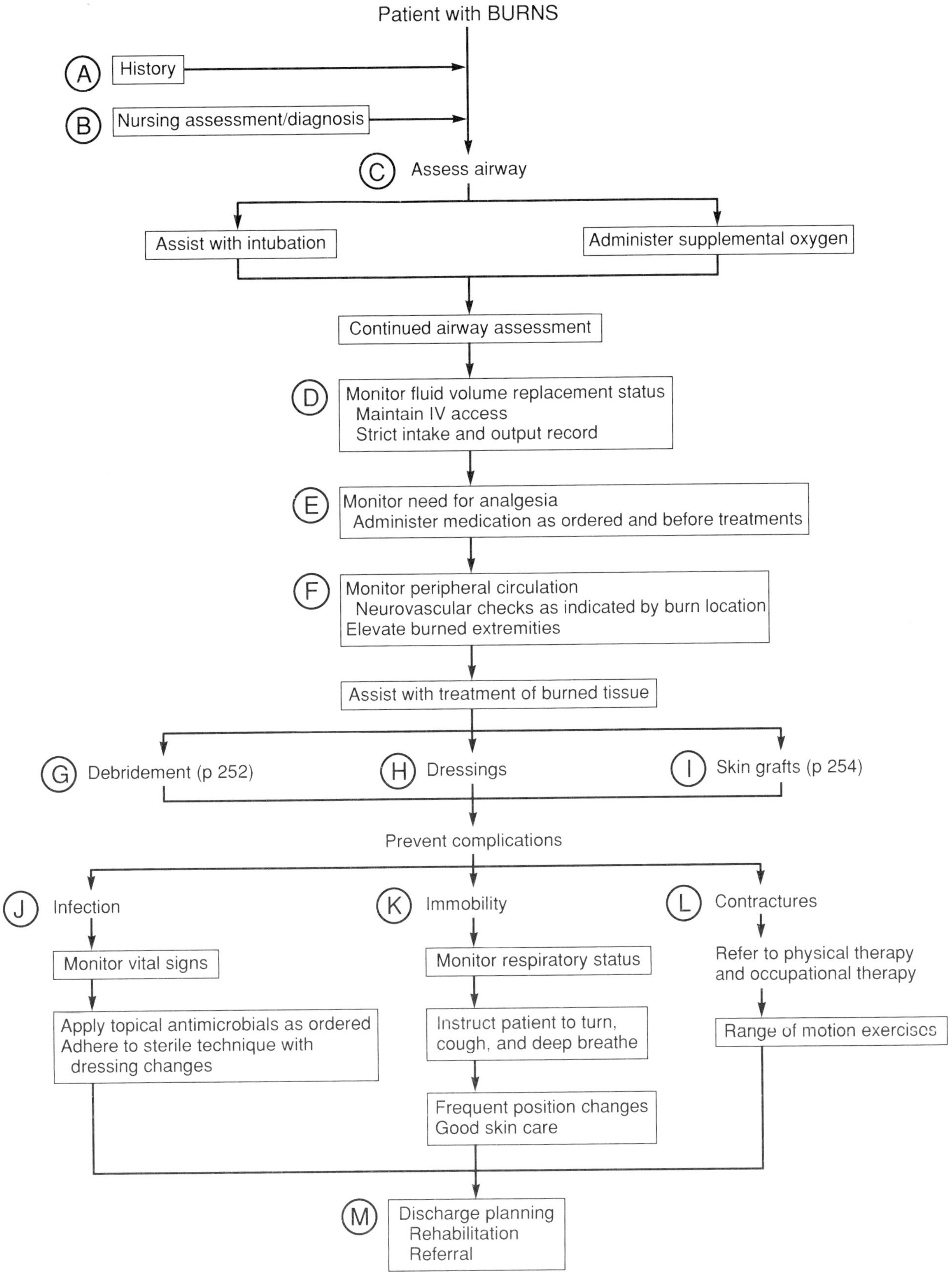

References

Brunner LS, Suddarth DS. Lippincott manual of nursing practice. 4th ed. Philadelphia: JB Lippincott, 1986.

Kinney M, Packa D, Dunbar S. AACN's clinical reference for critical care nursing. 2nd ed. Philadelphia: WB Saunders, 1988.

Mikhail JN. Acute burn care: An update. JEN 1988; 14(1): 9–18.

Morra LB. Burns. In: Mancini ME, ed. Decision making in emergency nursing. Toronto: BC Decker, 1987:66–67.

CARCINOMA OF THE SKIN

Nancy A. Young

Cancer of the skin falls into three major categories: basal cell carcinoma, squamous cell carcinoma, and malignant melanoma (Fig. 1). Basal cell carcinoma, the most common form, arises from the basal cell layer and appears as a small, waxy, translucent nodule with a central depression. This neoplasm grows at a slow rate and rarely metastasizes, which accounts for a 95 percent cure rate with treatment. As with basal cell carcinoma, squamous cell carcinoma occurs most frequently on skin damaged previously by sun exposure or irradiation. It is a cutaneous malignancy, commonly occurring on the face or backs of the hands, invading the dermis and surrounding skin. The probability of metastasis depends on the location and aggressiveness of the original tumor. Malignant melanoma, the most common fatal skin disorder, originates in the melanocytes anywhere on skin, eye, or mucous membrane. Excessive sun exposure remains the largest contributing factor, and the increased mortality rate results from this neoplasm's potential for invasion and metastasis through regional lymphatics and the bloodstream.

A. Malignant lesions are most commonly seen on areas of sun-exposed skin, such as the head and neck. Color of the lesion is important: variegation is suspicious, blue is ominous. The edge of the lesion is usually irregular. Any change in appearance, color, shape, size, or characteristic such as itching, tenderness, or bleeding is an important part of the history and assessment.

B. An early and aggressive initial treatment of basal cell carcinoma can reduce the likelihood of recurrence. Usual approaches include surgical excision, electrodesiccation and curettage, and cryotherapy—the treatment of choice depending on the size, location, and duration of the lesion. Because of its metastatic potential, squamous cell carcinoma should be removed completely by excision or electrodesiccation and curettage. Extensive lesions may require radiation therapy as well. The extent of surgical intervention for malignant melanoma depends on the level of tissue invasion. While wide local excision usually suffices for a primary lesion, a resection of regional lymph nodes should be done with deeply invasive lesions to determine the disease's stage of progression. Chemotherapy (p 408) is indicated if there is metastatic involvement of lymph nodes or other organs.

C. Postoperative care is similar to that for patients following a skin graft (p 254).

D. Patients diagnosed with carcinoma of the skin often express fear and anxiety in varying degrees, depending on the particular type. The nurse should provide appropriate information regarding the treatment and prognosis, and offer the opportunity to ask questions and discuss concerns.

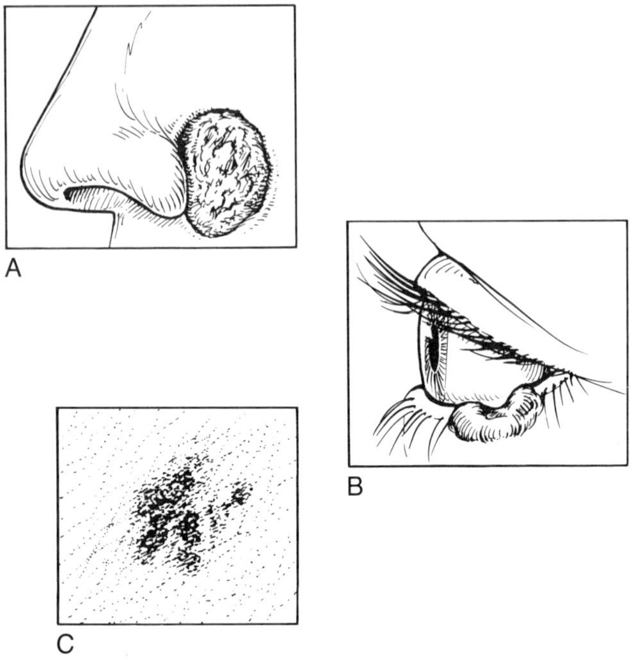

Figure 1 Carcinoma of the skin. *A*. Squamous cell carcinoma characterized by an indurated raised border and ulcerated center. *B*. Basal cell carcinoma characterized by a pearly nodular depressed center. *C*. Malignant melanoma characterized by an irregular border and black or brown color.

E. If the patient does not utilize effective coping mechanisms, referral is made to counseling or community groups that provide contact with other cancer patients at various levels of treatment and recovery. The self-image of these patients may be compromised, depending on the extent of disfigurement from surgical intervention, which could require additional support measures.

F. Discharge teaching for those patients requiring further treatment includes instructions for future therapy as well as the need to undergo reassessment at regular intervals by a health professional. In addition, these patients should understand personal prevention techniques for future episodes: (1) self-examination to monitor pigmented lesions and solicit medical assistance for any changes; (2) limit sun exposure (sun damage is cumulative); and (3) use of sunscreen preparations to protect against damaging ultraviolet rays.

References

Luckmann J, Sorensen KC. Medical-surgical nursing: a psychophysiologic approach. 3rd ed. Philadelphia: WB Saunders, 1987.

Ulrich SP, Canale SW, Wendell SA. Nursing care planning guides. Philadephia: WB Saunders, 1986.

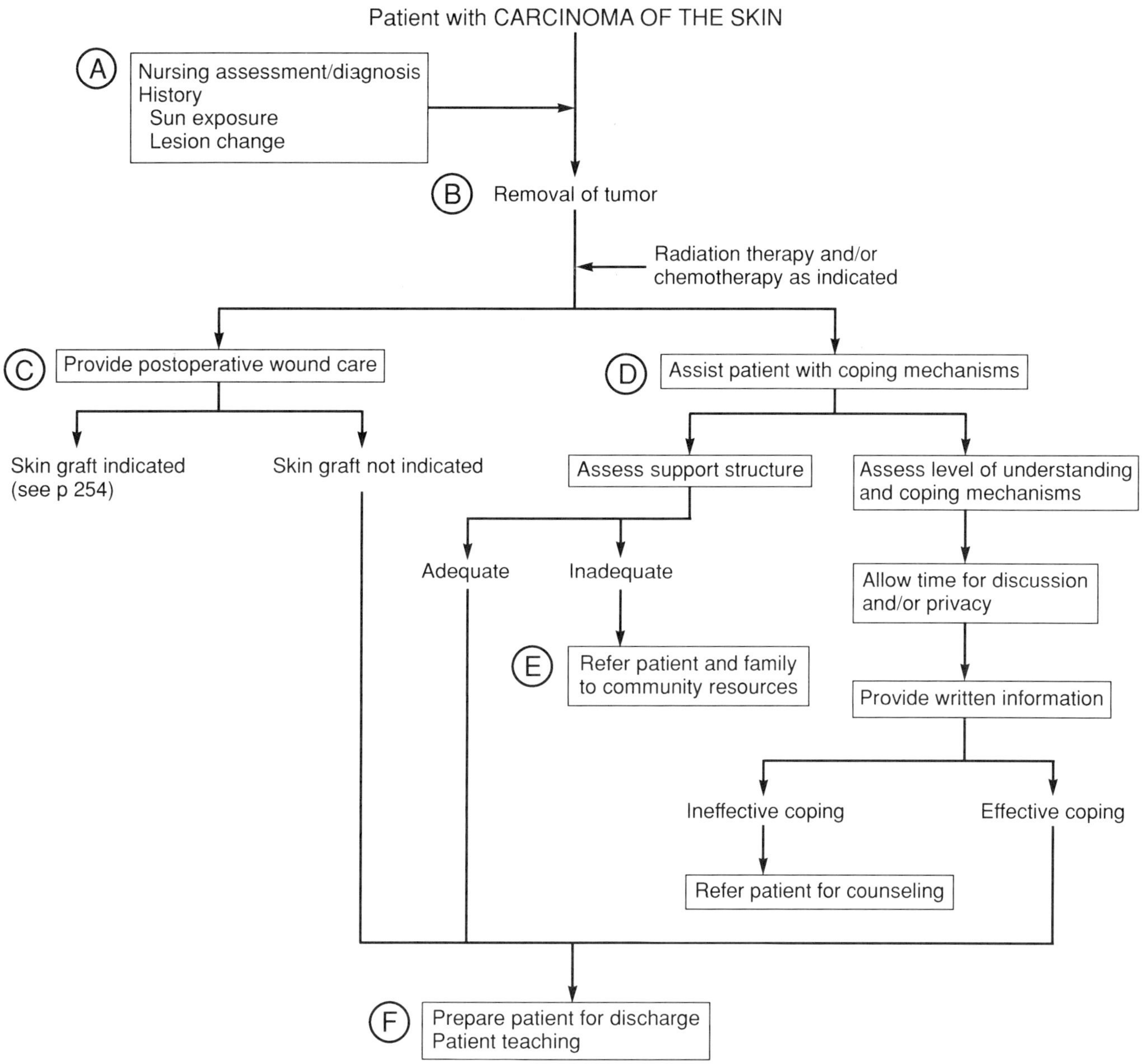
Patient with CARCINOMA OF THE SKIN
A
Nursing assessment/diagnosis
History
Sun exposure
Lesion change
B
Removal of tumor
Radiation therapy and/or chemotherapy as indicated
C
Provide postoperative wound care
D
Assist patient with coping mechanisms
Skin graft indicated (see p 254)
Skin graft not indicated
Assess support structure
Assess level of understanding and coping mechanisms
Adequate
Inadequate
Allow time for discussion and/or privacy
E
Refer patient and family to community resources
Provide written information
Ineffective coping
Effective coping
Refer patient for counseling
F
Prepare patient for discharge
Patient teaching

DEBRIDEMENT

Kendra Ellis

Debridement is a process used to remove eschar, necrotic tissue, and foreign material from a wound. The wound can be traumatic (e.g., burn), or a surgical wound left open because of contamination. An ulcerative wound (e.g., pressure sores) may also be debrided. Debridement removes nonviable tissue, which allows the healing process to begin so that the remaining viable tissue begins granulation and epithelialization. Debridement also removes organisms, decreasing the risk of wound infections.

A. Assess the patient's condition for stability. Pulmonary and hemodynamic status may be affected by the wound or other complications. A decrease in blood pressure and sensorium and pale, cool skin indicate that the patient is in shock (p 70). Stabilization should occur prior to beginning wound care. Determine bleeding times before debridement because of risk of increased blood loss.

B. Assess the wound for depth, contamination, and viability of tissue. Wound depth can involve the epidermal or the dermal layers. It may also involve muscle, bone, and joints. Contamination can be caused by loose debris, foreign material, nonviable tissue, or bacterial organisms. To determine if the tissue is viable, assess the wound for color, extent of damage, and presence of eschar. A purplish-to-black appearance indicates dead tissue. Various degrees of discoloration may indicate nonviable tissue and need further assessment. Debridement is necessary if the tissue is crushed or macerated. Eschar, black leathery skin seen with third-degree burns, is always nonviable and needs to be removed.

C. Surgical debridement is performed on full-thickness injury by removing nonviable tissue with a scalpel, scissors, or electrocautery to expose healthy tissue. Debridement does not go deep enough to remove the elements that assist with regeneration of the epithelium. Surgical debridement has been found to shorten hospital stay and decrease both infection and scar formation. Candidates are evaluated by age, depth and location of injury, cardiopulmonary status, and clotting factors. Surgical debridement can be performed only when the patient is stable.

D. Mechanical debridement involves daily removal of debris until the wound gives the appearance of forming granulated tissue. It may be a combination of hydrotherapy and manual scrubbing of the wound. Hydrotherapy softens the eschar, facilitating removal. Scrubbing with loosely woven gauze increases removal of debris. Dead tissue can be removed with forceps and scissors as needed. This slower process can be performed on unstable patients, but there is an increased risk of wound contamination. It is also very painful.

E. The wet-to-dry dressing is usually used on a surgical wound that was left open because of infection. This process of debridement is sometimes combined with mechanical debridement. A loosely woven gauze, saturated in a solution specified by the physician or agency protocol, is opened to its largest size, loosely packed in the wound, and covered with a dry dressing. The dressing is allowed to dry for 6 to 8 hours. The coarse mesh allows debris to adhere to the gauze, and the wet dressing softens the necrotic tissue. Removal of the dressing rids the wound of the loose necrotic tissue. However, it may also debride healthy tissue.

F. An ulcerative wound is usually a small, deep wound that is contaminated with bacterial organisms. Enzymatic debridement with tissue-specific enzyme (e.g., Travase or Elase) can be used to assist removal of necrotic tissue. The enzymes digest purulent exudates and loosen necrotic tissue. They do not have antimicrobial effects, so may be used in combination with topical agents. Their use should be discontinued when the color of the ulcerative bed changes to pink. Continued use will damage granulated tissue.

G. An occlusive dressing may be applied and kept intact for up to 5 days. Usually a transparent, semipermeable polyurethane film cover is applied to allow observation of the site and exchange of water vapor and oxygen. It also prevents entry of bacteria. This method facilitates liquefaction of the wound, allowing the body's defense mechanisms to remove the necrotic tissue. Studies have shown that a moist environment may increase the rate of epithelialization.

H. As necrotic tissue is removed, the wound appears larger. The presence of granulated tissue indicates that the process of wound healing is beginning. The nurse needs to be able to recognize healthy tissue, because debridement should be discontinued when it appears. Healthy granulated tissue is pink to vivid red. Once granulated tissue is present, capillary buds begin to form a capillary bed over the wound to protect against loss of fluid and entry of bacteria. These capillary buds appear as red, raised bumps.

References

Fowler E. Equipment and products used in management and treatment of pressure ulcers. Nurs Clin North Am 1987; 22:449–461.

Holloway N. Nursing the critically ill adult. Reading, MA: Addison-Wesley, 1984:368.

Pories W. Management of the traumatic wound: debridement. Emerg Med 1986; 18(6):147–148, 153–154, 164–166.

Sieggren M. Healing of physical wounds. Nurs Clin North Am 1987; 22:439–447.

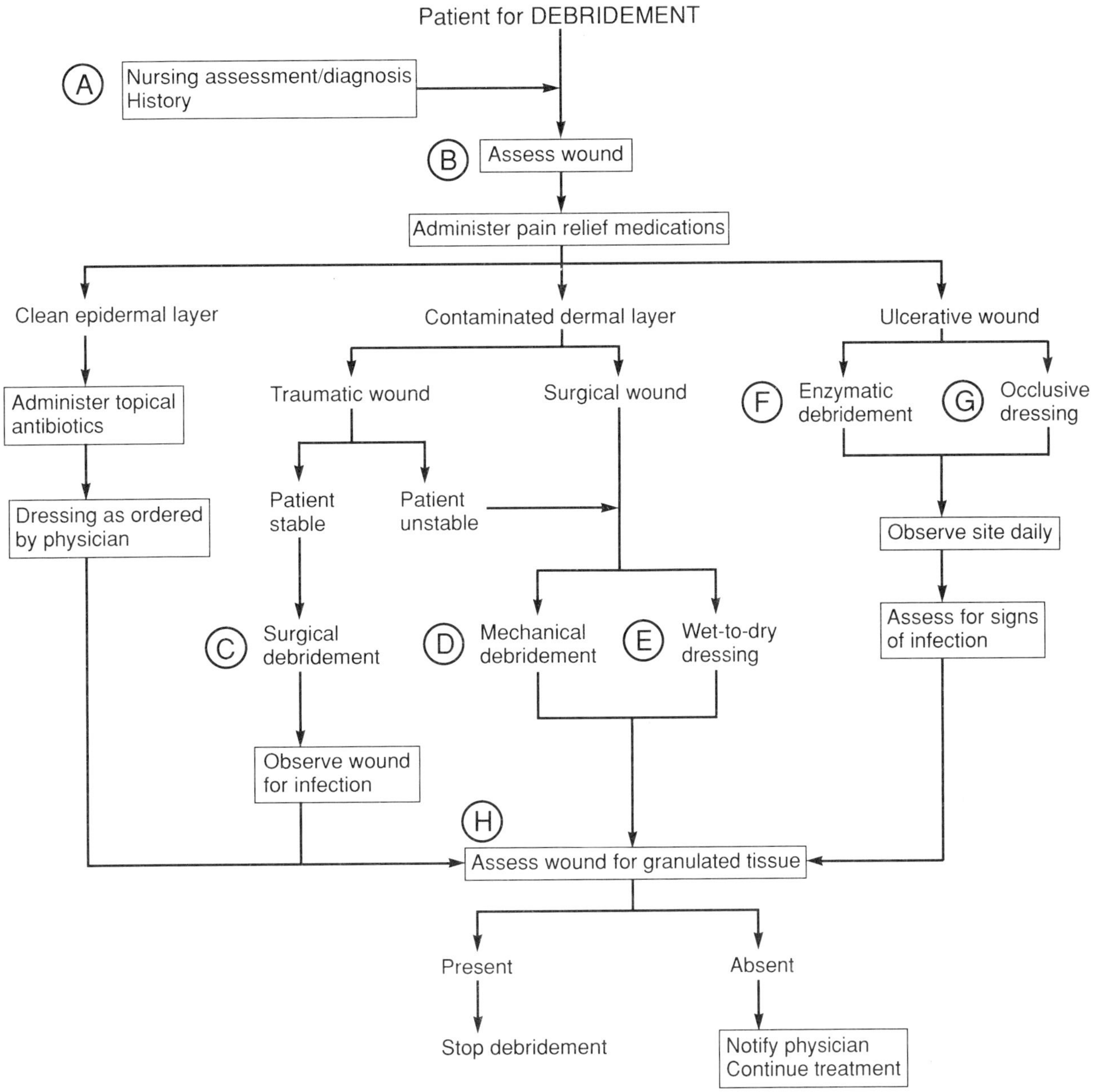

Patient for DEBRIDEMENT
A
Nursing assessment/diagnosis
History
B
Assess wound
Administer pain relief medications
Clean epidermal layer
Contaminated dermal layer
Ulcerative wound
Administer topical antibiotics
Traumatic wound
Surgical wound
F
Enzymatic debridement
G
Occlusive dressing
Dressing as ordered by physician
Patient stable
Patient unstable
Observe site daily
C
Surgical debridement
D
Mechanical debridement
E
Wet-to-dry dressing
Assess for signs of infection
Observe wound for infection
H
Assess wound for granulated tissue
Present
Absent
Stop debridement
Notify physician
Continue treatment

SKIN GRAFT

Susan Cauley

A skin graft is the surgical removal of skin tissue from its blood supply and transfer of a free section of tissue to the recipient site. Full-thickness skin graft contains a full thickness of skin down to the subcutaneous tissue. This type of graft is used frequently for reconstruction of facial defects, since it does not develop unsightly pigmentation and does not contract. Split-thickness skin graft is a graft of approximately one-half the thickness of skin. The skin is removed by a knife or dermatome. Deeper layers of dermis are left intact. This type is used mainly for coverage and closure of skin defects. This type is also referred to sometimes as postage-stamp graft because the graft is cut to pieces the size of postage stamps and placed on the recipient bed, which is surrounded by areas of granulated tissue.

A. It is important to assess the patient's physical and emotional level. Preoperative assessment includes a full systems assessment, including, but not limited to, circulation checks, motor-sensory function, and vital signs.

B. Preoperative nursing care includes promoting comfort, patient teaching, emotional support, and physical preparation. Patient teaching is important and should address appearance of the wound dressings and positioning of the affected area. Physical preparation includes preparing donor and recipient sites, along with routine laboratory and x-ray studies (p 2). Emotionally, the patient needs to be allowed to discuss fears about disfigurement, scarring, or altered body image.

C. Postoperative nursing care is directed at preventing complications and providing opportunity for the graft and donor sites to heal. Routine postoperative vital signs and assessment are done (p 4).

D. Assessment of the vascular supply to the grafted site is critical. Color, warmth, turgor, and capillary refill are assessed. Changes such as sluggish capillary refill, coolness to touch, and no audible pulse with Doppler must be reported to the surgeon immediately.

E. Observe the dressings for bleeding. The dressing usually remains intact until removed by the surgeon. The donor site is covered with a fine mesh gauze. Donor sites are allowed to dry out under a heat lamp for 24 to 48 hours, and the gauze is left intact. The edges of the fine mesh gauze are trimmed away as they separate from the donor site. The wound must be visualized as soon as possible. Blistering, edema, or hematoma at the recipient site should be reported. If infection occurs, antibiotics are administered and wet dressings applied.

F. Encourage the patient to verbalize concerns and fears. Provide the patient with honest answers and obtainable goals to help deal with the surgery and altered body image.

G. It may be necessary to elevate the grafted site, and the part should be immobilized to promote healing. Care should be taken to ensure that the patient is positioned comfortably. Encourage coughing and deep breathing. Pain medication is administered as required, and other pain management techniques may be employed (p 406).

H. If there are no complications, the patient is discharged with specific instructions about applying lubricating lotion to graft sites and donor sites after they are healed and avoiding overexposure to sun.

References

Brunner LS, Suddarth DS. The Lippincott manual of nursing practice. 4th ed. Philadelphia: JB Lippincott, 1986.

Lewis SM, Collier IC. Medical-surgical nursing: assessment and management of clinical problems. 2nd ed. New York: McGraw-Hill, 1987.

Luckmann J, Sorensen KC. Medical-surgical nursing: a psychophysiologic approach. 3rd ed. Philadelphia: WB Saunders, 1987.

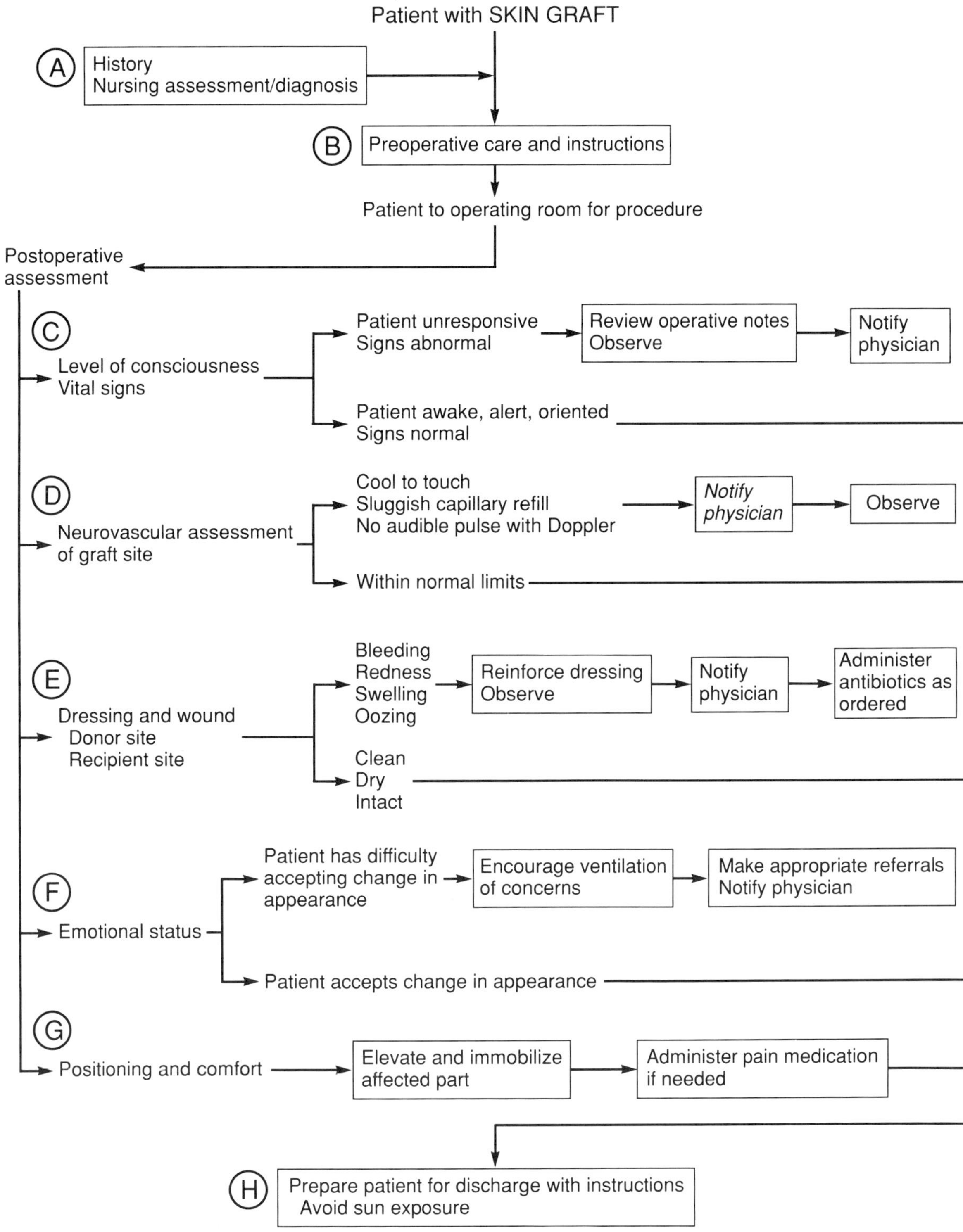
Patient with SKIN GRAFT
A
History
Nursing assessment/diagnosis
B
Preoperative care and instructions
Patient to operating room for procedure
Postoperative assessment
C
Level of consciousness
Vital signs
Patient unresponsive
Signs abnormal
Review operative notes
Observe
Notify physician
Patient awake, alert, oriented
Signs normal
D
Neurovascular assessment of graft site
Cool to touch
Sluggish capillary refill
No audible pulse with Doppler
Notify physician
Observe
Within normal limits
E
Dressing and wound
Donor site
Recipient site
Bleeding
Redness
Swelling
Oozing
Reinforce dressing
Observe
Notify physician
Administer antibiotics as ordered
Clean
Dry
Intact
F
Emotional status
Patient has difficulty accepting change in appearance
Encourage ventilation of concerns
Make appropriate referrals
Notify physician
Patient accepts change in appearance
G
Positioning and comfort
Elevate and immobilize affected part
Administer pain medication if needed
H
Prepare patient for discharge with instructions
Avoid sun exposure

PLASTIC RECONSTRUCTIVE SURGERY

Leslie Rach

Plastic reconstructive surgery is carried out to correct defects, repair tissues and/or structures destroyed by trauma or disease, replace tissue removed by other surgeries, and restore function. Grafting (p 254) is most often used. Implants of bone, wax, metal, ivory, Teflon, and silicone have been used to provide shape.

A. Preoperative assessments establish a database for intraoperative and postoperative comparison and identify potential problems. Preoperative assessment includes a full systems assessment encompassing circulation, motor-sensory function, and vital signs. Promotion of comfort, physical preparation, and emotional support are also important preoperative measures. A potential problem may be the patient's difficulty in dealing with the disfigurement the disease or injury has caused and fears of further damage from surgery. Reassurance and truthful answers help to allay those fears.

B. Preoperative care begins as soon as surgery is planned. The most important aspect is decreasing the patient's anxiety level. Explaining hospital routines, procedures, and treatments is most helpful. Provide time to discuss expectations and goals, and for preoperative teaching (i.e., turning, coughing, and deep breathing, NPO status, postoperative high protein diet, [p 2]). Encourage the support and participation of family and friends.

C. The postoperative goal is to return the individual to an optimal level of functioning as quickly as possible. This includes a full assessment focusing on level of consciousness, airway patency, vital signs, neurovascular assessment, assessment of dressing and wound (if allowed), checking patency and function of drainage devices, level of comfort, urinary retention, and emotional status.

D. Neurovascular status is assessed frequently. Looking at an extremity distal to the surgical site gives a good indication of vascularization and motor sensory changes. Capillary refill time should be 3 seconds or less, and movement and sensation should be comparable to the preoperative assessment within 1 to 2 days. Mark palpable pulses for ease in locating them. If unable to visualize a distal extremity, make windows in the surgical dressing and check vascularization with Doppler's ultrasonography.

E. All areas of the dressings must be visualized. The dressing may appear clean and dry on the top and sides, but next to the surgical site there may be excess drainage. If a small amount of drainage is evident, it can be outlined with ink to assess the rate and amount of further drainage.

F. The wound must be visualized as soon as allowed. Redness, extreme swelling, drainage, foul odor, and unapproximated edges are signs of improper healing or infection. Explain to the patient before the dressing is removed how the wound will look and caution that moderate swelling is to be expected. Also explain that the wound will look better day by day. This will ameliorate depression.

G. Emotional status centers on three areas of concern: the effects of surgery, altered body image, and the future. Encouraging verbalization of these concerns and fears helps the patient to understand and deal with them. Often, preoperative anxieties become postoperative anxieties. Honest answers and attainable goals are most needed. The nurse may consult with the psychiatric liasion nurse to develop a plan of care to assist the patient in dealing with these concerns. Later, referral to a support group may be appropriate.

H. Postoperative rehabilitation continues throughout discharge and into home life. Dressing changes, physical or occupational therapy, and emotional healing will continue to take place. Accepting this new body image is tantamount to healing and cooperating with the prescribed regimen.

I. Teaching is reinforced at the time of discharge. Written instructions are provided and follow-up care is agreed upon. Reinforce the need to return to regular activities slowly. In some cases, limitations are imposed to protect a surgical area. This is a frightening time for patients who must leave a place where trusted people accept their looks. Family involvement during hospitalization is crucial to alleviate those fears.

References

Brunner LS, Suddarth DS. Textbook of medical-surgical nursing. 5th ed. Philadelphia: JB Lippincott, 1984.

Lewis SM, Collier IC. Medical-surgical nursing: assessment and management of clinical problems. 2nd ed. New York: McGraw-Hill, 1987.

Phipps WJ, Long BC. Medical-surgical nursing: concepts and clinical practice. St. Louis: CV Mosby, 1987.

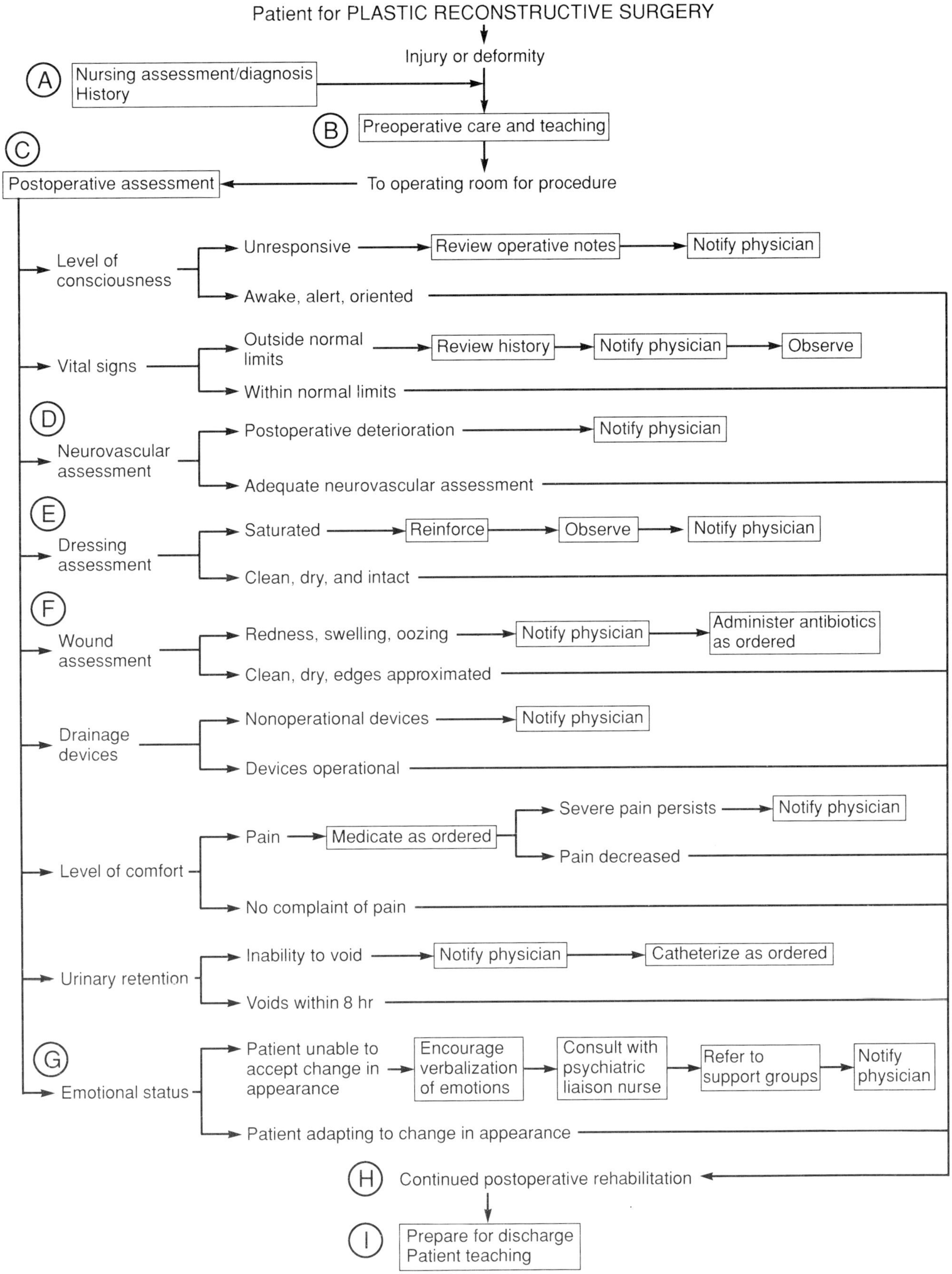
Patient for PLASTIC RECONSTRUCTIVE SURGERY
Injury or deformity
A
Nursing assessment/diagnosis
History
B
Preoperative care and teaching
C
Postoperative assessment
To operating room for procedure
Level of consciousness
Unresponsive
Review operative notes
Notify physician
Awake, alert, oriented
Vital signs
Outside normal limits
Review history
Notify physician
Observe
Within normal limits
D
Neurovascular assessment
Postoperative deterioration
Notify physician
Adequate neurovascular assessment
E
Dressing assessment
Saturated
Reinforce
Observe
Notify physician
Clean, dry, and intact
F
Wound assessment
Redness, swelling, oozing
Notify physician
Administer antibiotics as ordered
Clean, dry, edges approximated
Drainage devices
Nonoperational devices
Notify physician
Devices operational
Level of comfort
Pain
Medicate as ordered
Severe pain persists
Notify physician
Pain decreased
No complaint of pain
Urinary retention
Inability to void
Notify physician
Catheterize as ordered
Voids within 8 hr
G
Emotional status
Patient unable to accept change in appearance
Encourage verbalization of emotions
Consult with psychiatric liaison nurse
Refer to support groups
Notify physician
Patient adapting to change in appearance
H
Continued postoperative rehabilitation
I
Prepare for discharge
Patient teaching

REPRODUCTIVE AND GENITOURINARY SYSTEMS

FEMALE
- Pelvic Inflammatory Disease
- Toxic Shock Syndrome
- Uterine Bleeding
- Fertility Control
- Cancer of the Cervix
- Cancer of the Ovary
- Cancer of the Uterus

REPRODUCTIVE AND GENITOURINARY SURGERIES (FEMALE)
- Mastectomy
- Breast Reconstruction
- Augmentation Mammoplasty
- Reduction Mammoplasty
- Dilatation and Curettage
- Hysterectomy
- Laparoscopy
- Tubal Ligation
- Abortion

MALE
- Prostatic Cancer
- Testicular Cancer
- Bladder Cancer

REPRODUCTIVE AND GENITOURINARY SURGERIES (MALE)
- Transurethral Resection
- Prostatectomy
- Penile Implant

PELVIC INFLAMMATORY DISEASE

Nancy A. Young

Pelvic inflammatory disease (PID) is a chronic or acute infectious condition of the pelvic cavity that may involve the uterus, fallopian tubes, ovaries, pelvic peritoneum, or pelvic vascular system. The causative organisms can gain entrance through sexual contact or nonsexually as a complication from an IUD, abortion, pelvic surgery, or childbirth. The risk of PID increases for individuals with multiple sexual partners and those having previous episodes of PID with resultant damage. Laparoscopy can confirm the diagnosis by visual inspection and collection of inflammatory material. Development of the disease may depend on the immune status of the patient as well as the virulence of the organism.

A. Of the 1 million women treated annually for PID, 25 percent require hospitalization and present with symptoms that may include lower abdominal pain and tenderness, purulent or foul-smelling vaginal discharge, nausea and vomiting, elevated temperature, and general malaise and lethargy. When contemplating hospital admission for the patient, consider the following: severity of disease, suspicion of pelvic abscess, uncertainty of the diagnosis, and failure of outpatient treatment. The nurse needs to rule out disorders with similar symptoms, such as ectopic pregnancy and appendicitis.

B. A high priority in the care of the patient with PID is control of the infectious process to minimize the possibility of septic shock due to circulating bacterial endotoxins. The intravenous infusion of fluids to assist in flushing toxins from the body and the administration of antibiotics promotes healing. The patient should remain in the semi-Fowler's position to facilitate drainage and adhere to a regimen of bedrest to conserve energy. The nurse should monitor vital signs closely and report any indications of deteriorating status. All care providers must follow medical asepsis, strict handwashing, and isolation techniques for handling and disposal of patient linen and equipment. The importance of such procedures should also be explained to the patient.

C. Patients with PID experience varying degrees of pain. Mild and moderate discomfort may respond to comfort measures such as back rubs, heat applied to the abdomen, sitz baths, frequent perineal care, and maintenance of a nonstimulating environment. More intense pain requires administration of analgesics, as ordered by the physician.

D. Indications for surgery include ectopic pregnancy; pelvic, tubal, and ovarian abscesses that may rupture or have ruptured; failure to respond to conservative management; or frequent exacerbations of PID necessitating removal of the site(s) of infection. These patients require hospitalization until they have recovered from the surgical procedure.

E. Attention should be given to the patient's self-concept and emotions that result from contracting PID. Depending on the source of infection, the patient may feel guilty and fear the disease's potential long-term consequences. After assessing the patient's anxiety level, the nurse can provide opportunities to ventilate and offer counseling and support.

F. Patient education prior to discharge should include several topics. The risk factors must be emphasized, such as the use of IUDs, multiple sexual partners, and residual damage from previous episodes of the disease. PID recurs in 25 percent of patients presenting with the first episode. The chance of ectopic pregnancies increases, because PID may partially obstruct the fallopian tube, thus allowing passage of sperm but not ova. Complete obstruction of the tubes by adhesions or strictures results in sterility.

G. The discharged patient should be advised to complete any course of antibiotics, avoid coitus and douching for 1 week after antibiotic therapy, and adhere to a schedule that promotes rest and healthy nutrition. She should also be alerted to the signs and symptoms of recurring episodes.

References

Lewis SM, Collier JC. Medical-surgical nursing: assessment and management of clinical problems. New York: McGraw-Hill, 1983.

Strauss RW, Glimp TH. Sexually transmitted diseases. Top Emerg Med 1985; 7:73–76.

Thompson J, McFarland GK, Hirsch JE, Tucker SM, Bavers AC. Clinical nursing. St. Louis: CV Mosby, 1986.

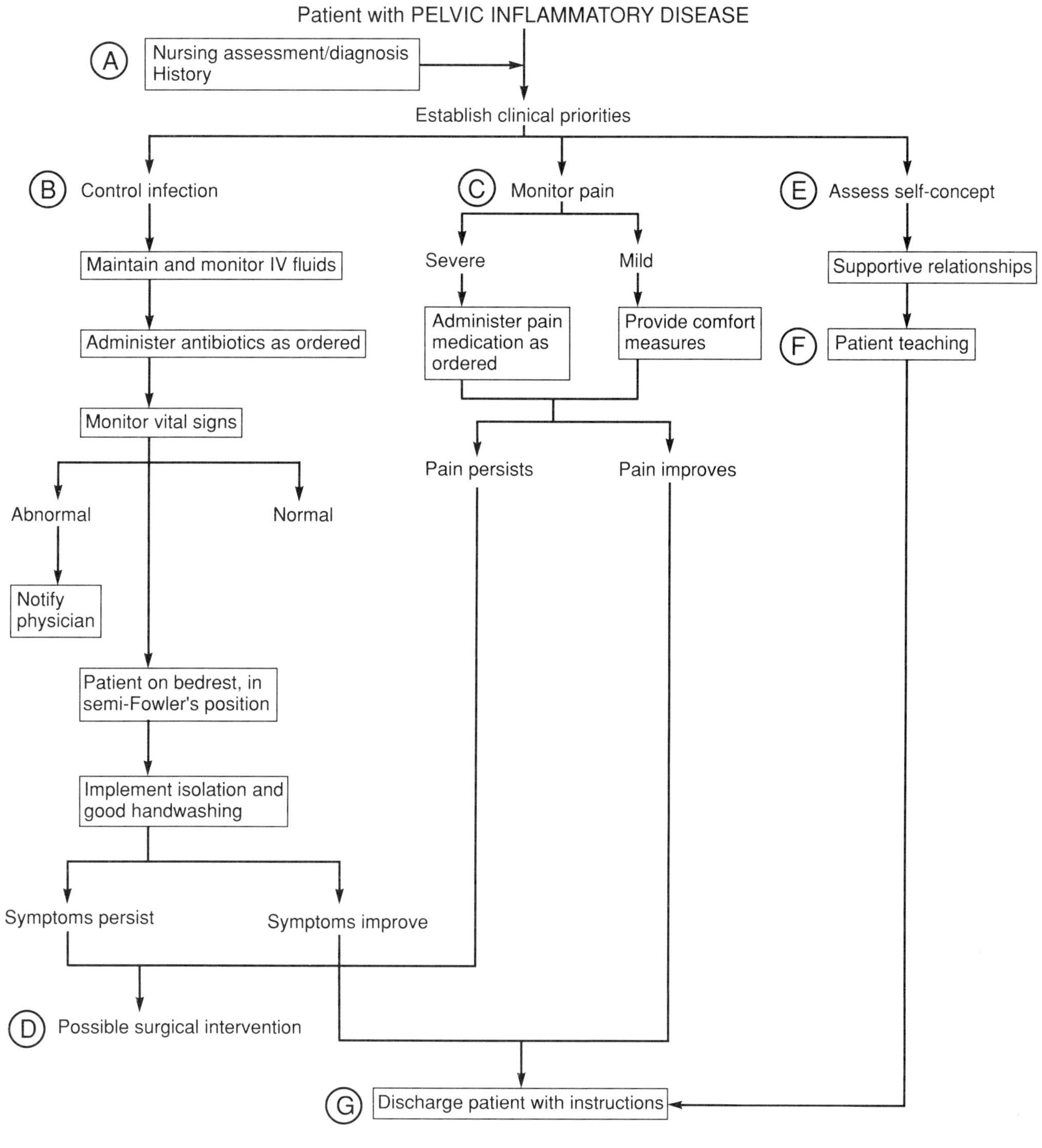

Patient with PELVIC INFLAMMATORY DISEASE
A
Nursing assessment/diagnosis
History
Establish clinical priorities
B
Control infection
Maintain and monitor IV fluids
Administer antibiotics as ordered
Monitor vital signs
Abnormal
Normal
Notify physician
Patient on bedrest, in semi-Fowler's position
Implement isolation and good handwashing
Symptoms persist
Symptoms improve
D
Possible surgical intervention
C
Monitor pain
Severe
Mild
Administer pain medication as ordered
Provide comfort measures
Pain persists
Pain improves
E
Assess self-concept
Supportive relationships
F
Patient teaching
G
Discharge patient with instructions

TOXIC SHOCK SYNDROME

Nancy A. Young

Toxic shock syndrome (TSS) received considerable public attention in 1980 with studies linking the use of certain extra-absorbent tampons with an increased risk of TSS. While TSS can occur in nonmenstruating women, children, and males, the incidence increases in menstruating women using tampons. The exact cause is unknown; however, the presence of *Staphylococcus aureus* has been identified in most cases. Tampon use during menstruation can block the flow of blood, leading to a favorable environment for growth of the bacteria. Other groups at risk include those with infections involving staphylococcus bacteria as a result of skin breakdown, wounds, childbirth, inflammation of the breast, or respiratory infections.

A. The symptoms of a patient with suspected TSS may be confused with those of any viral systemic illness. A thorough history for women should include documentation of the last menstrual period, frequency and type of tampons used, in addition to personal hygiene. The presence of recent or current staphylococcal infections in other patients can help to make a more definite diagnosis.

B. When absorbed into the blood stream, the staphylococcus bacteria release toxins that typically produce symptoms involving three or more of the following systems: gastrointestinal, muscular, renal, central nervous system, hematologic, hepatic, and integumentary. Since a definite diagnosis may be difficult, these symptoms and physiologic changes require close monitoring and prompt attention to reduce the chance of profound shock (p 70).

C. Evaluate vital signs frequently to assess the patient's status. The temperature may exceed 102°F (38.5°C) and changes in pulse and respiratory rate may indicate a worsening condition. Alteration in blood pressure could be a sign of early circulatory overload or inadequate perfusion and should be reported immediately to the physician. Oxygen can be administered as needed to maintain adequate oxygenation to tissues.

D. Cultures of all potential infection sites (vaginal vault, blood, throat, urine, cerebrospinal fluid, and any wound lesions) may identify *Staphylococcus aureus* as the causative agent. Some physicians administer a broad-spectrum intravenous antibiotic; however, this treatment meets with varying success. Careful adherence to universal isolation precautions minimizes the transfer of bacteria to other work areas and limits the challenge to the patient's immune system.

E. The patient's chief complaint may be headaches and/or muscle and joint discomfort. The nurse can attempt comfort measures such as positioning, reducing external stimuli, or massage, but medication may be required.

F. Nausea, vomiting, and diarrhea should be assessed with an accurate intake and output record to evaluate potential fluid and electrolyte imbalances. An intravenous infusion will assist in maintaining adequate levels; however, a nasogastric tube and medication may also be indicated for relief of gastrointestinal discomfort. Any changes in the severity of symptoms or laboratory values must be reported immediately to the physician.

G. Many patients with TSS exhibit a macular erythematous (sunburn-like) rash, especially on their palms, fingers, and toes. The appearance of such a rash should be reported to the physician. The rash usually peels a few days after appearing and lasts 1 to 2 weeks.

H. The nurse must be alert for the symptoms of shock and notify the physician immediately. Hypotension and oliguria are two indicators of a worsening condition, making frequent checking of vital signs and an accurate hourly intake and output by Foley catheter critically important.

I. The patient with TSS can return home once the symptoms have been satisfactorily resolved. Menstruating women should modify or discontinue the use of tampons. Discharge teaching includes use of sanitary pads instead of tampons, especially at night; use of less absorbent tampons; and more frequent changing of tampons throughout the day.

References

Shepard BD, Shepard CA. The complete guide to women's health. Florida: Mariner, 1982.

US Department of Health and Human Services. Recommendations for prevention of HIV transmission in health-care settings. MMWR August 21, 1987; 36(25).

Whettam J. Update on toxic shock: how to spot it and treat it. RN 1984; 47:55–60.

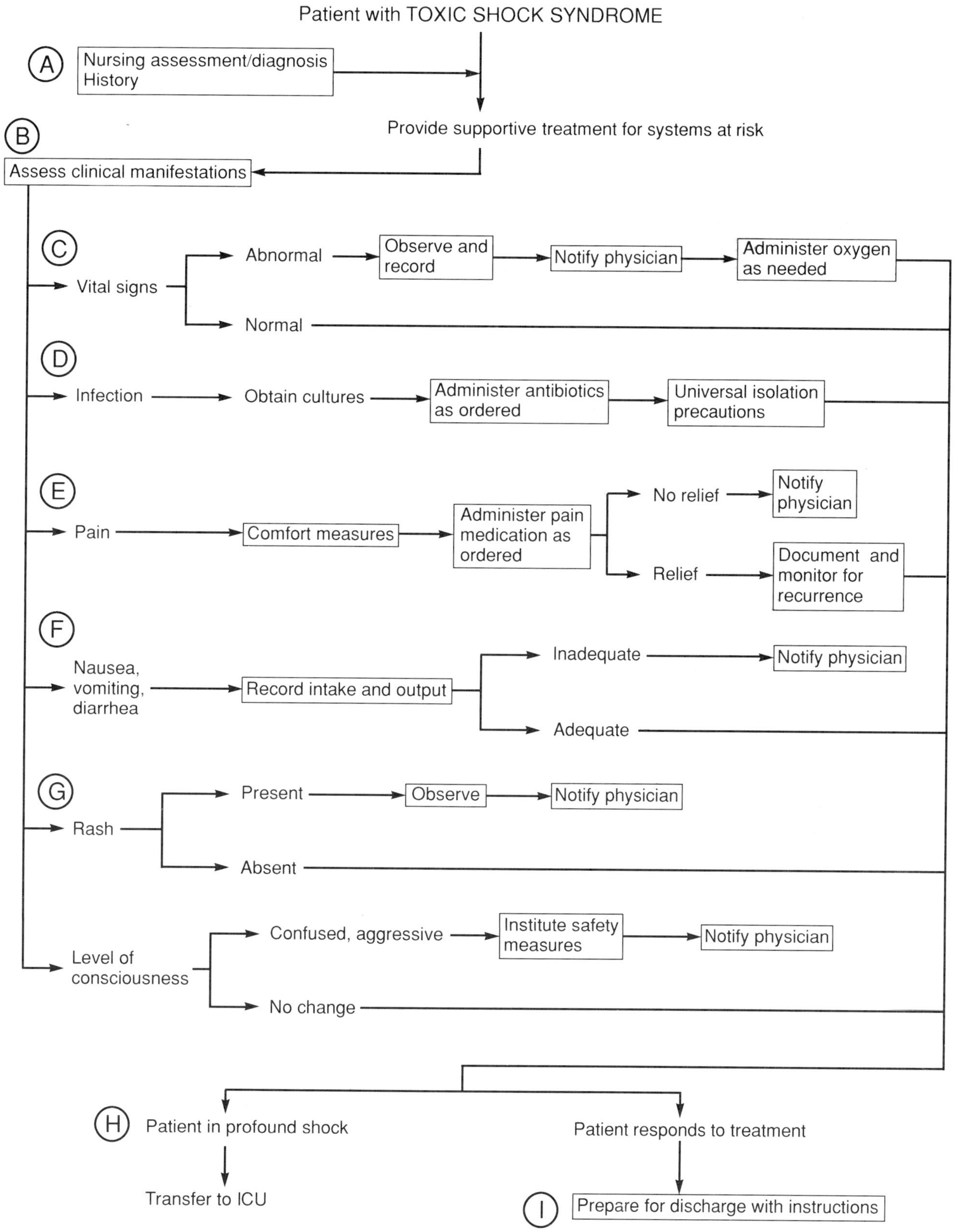
Patient with TOXIC SHOCK SYNDROME
A
Nursing assessment/diagnosis
History
Provide supportive treatment for systems at risk
B
Assess clinical manifestations
C
Vital signs
Abnormal
Observe and record
Notify physician
Administer oxygen as needed
Normal
D
Infection
Obtain cultures
Administer antibiotics as ordered
Universal isolation precautions
E
Pain
Comfort measures
Administer pain medication as ordered
No relief
Notify physician
Relief
Document and monitor for recurrence
F
Nausea, vomiting, diarrhea
Record intake and output
Inadequate
Notify physician
Adequate
G
Rash
Present
Observe
Notify physician
Absent
Level of consciousness
Confused, aggressive
Institute safety measures
Notify physician
No change
H
Patient in profound shock
Transfer to ICU
Patient responds to treatment
I
Prepare for discharge with instructions

UTERINE BLEEDING

Nancy A. Young

Uterine bleeding may be functional (menstruation) or dysfunctional. Factors leading to abnormal genital bleeding generally fit into four major categories: (1) pregnancy-related disorders; (2) ovulatory dysfunction; (3) blood disorders; and (4) genital abnormalities. Treatment varies considerably depending on identification of the cause and whether the problem is acute or chronic, ovulatory or anovulatory.

A. The nurse should collect a thorough menstrual and physical history and description of current symptoms to facilitate formation of a logical diagnostic approach. Vaginal bleeding before age 9 to 10 is usually considered abnormal and postmenopausal bleeding often indicates a malignancy. Anovulatoy uterine bleeding due to hormonal imbalance usually occurs in adolescents or women in their fifth decade. This chapter deals only with disorders *not* related to pregnancy or suspected abuse. All abnormal bleeding indicates an underlying problem.

B. Although most patients complaining of vaginal bleeding do not require immediate hospitalization, hemodynamic instability warrants admission. Once stability has been established, the causative factor(s) determine the treatment approach.

C. A complete gynecologic exam is done. Since multiple procedures, such as vaginal exam and laparoscopy, may be used to diagnose and treat uterine bleeding, provide emotional support to allay patient concerns. Explain the purpose and procedure of each exam thoroughly. Obtain consents as required.

D. Dysfunctional uterine bleeding results from exogenous factors (during administration of hormones) or endogenous factors (response of the endometrium to an abnormal level of circulating hormones). The amount of bleeding varies considerably among patients, thus the treatment ranges from gynecologic referral for a diagnostic work-up to immediate treatment for hypovolemia and surgical intervention.

E. Likewise, the discharge instructions vary, depending on the treatment method for the different causative factors. In cases of suspected violence or abuse, the patient should be referred to the appropriate person or agency for support and follow-up.

References

Ames SW, Kneisl CR. Essentials of adult health nursing. Menlo Park, CA: Addison-Wesley, 1988.

Campbell BF, Tagatz GE. Abnormal uterine bleeding: how to manage acute and chronic episodes. Consultant 1986; 26(8): 153–158, 163.

Gibbons HE. Management of patients with vaginal bleeding. Topics Emerg Med 1985; 7(2):67–72.

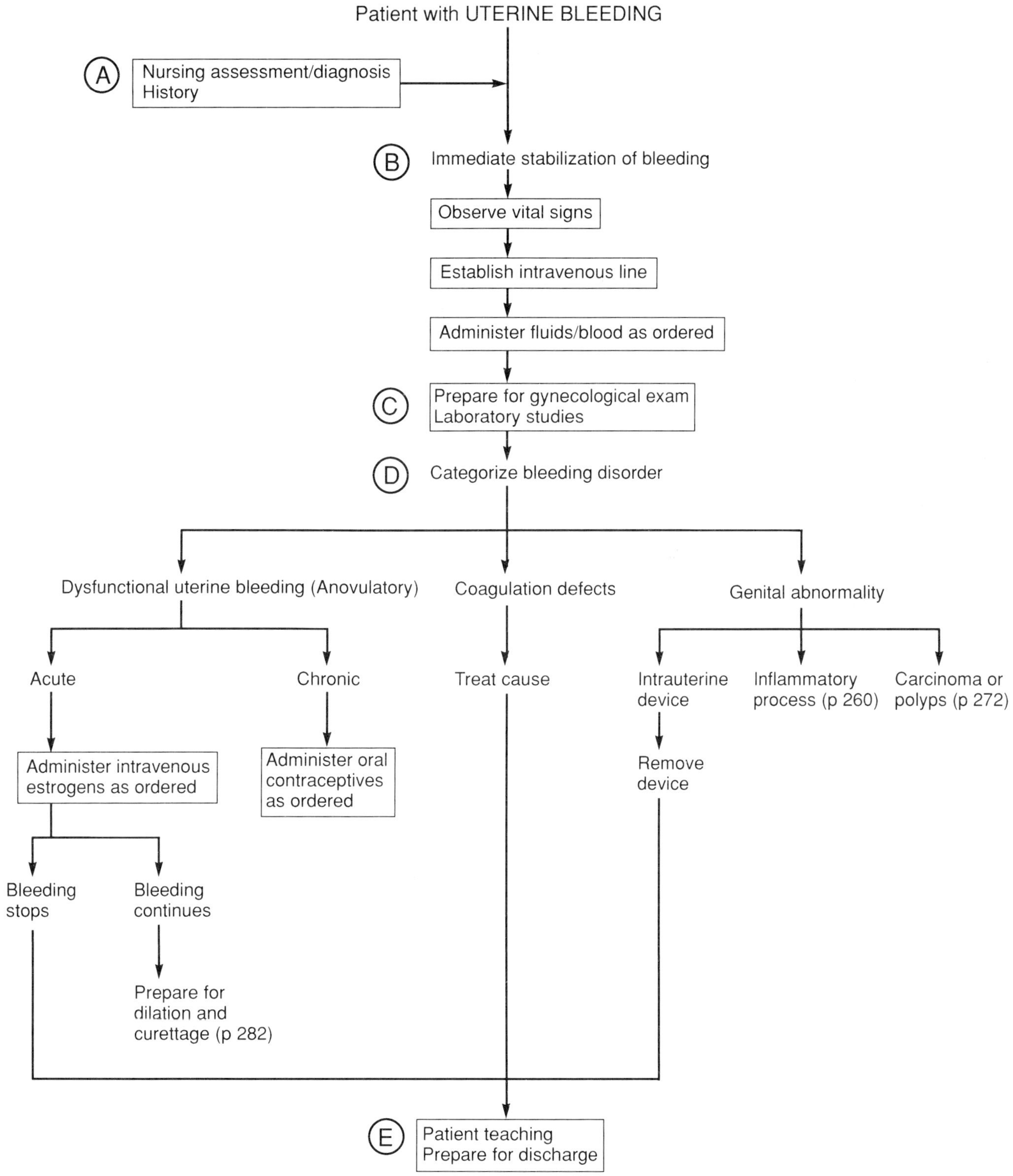
Patient with UTERINE BLEEDING
A
Nursing assessment/diagnosis
History
B
Immediate stabilization of bleeding
Observe vital signs
Establish intravenous line
Administer fluids/blood as ordered
C
Prepare for gynecological exam
Laboratory studies
D
Categorize bleeding disorder
Dysfunctional uterine bleeding (Anovulatory)
Coagulation defects
Genital abnormality
Acute
Chronic
Treat cause
Intrauterine device
Inflammatory process (p 260)
Carcinoma or polyps (p 272)
Administer intravenous estrogens as ordered
Administer oral contraceptives as ordered
Remove device
Bleeding stops
Bleeding continues
Prepare for dilation and curettage (p 282)
E
Patient teaching
Prepare for discharge

FERTILITY CONTROL

Paula K. Ovens
Pamela Y. Donnelly

About 80 percent of sexually active women will become pregnant within 1 year when no contraception is used. Sexually active couples should use effective contraception if they do not wish to have a child. Ideally, contraceptives should be safe, easily available, economical, acceptable, and simple to use. It is important for nurses to know the advantages and disadvantages of the various methods of birth control in order to answer questions and assist patients in making decisions about this issue. A complete gynecologic history and physical examination with follow-up is essential to family planning.

A. One or both members of a couple can use contraception as a temporary measure or sterilization as a permanent measure to prevent pregnancy. Couples should be absolutely sure that future pregnancies are not desired when permanent sterilization is chosen. Although reanastomosis may be possible, it is extremely expensive and not always successful.

B. A condom worn by the male during coitus is a highly reliable method of contraception. The sheath should be placed over the erect penis. The end of the condom should not be applied tightly; the tip should overlap about ½ inch to collect the ejaculate. It must be removed carefully to avoid spilling the contents. Condoms provide considerable but not absolute protection against sexually transmitted diseases. They are inexpensive and readily available. However, the condom may be ineffective if it tears or ruptures during placement or coitus.

C. Contraceptive creams, jellies, suppositories, and foams are spermicidal agents that are applied to the upper vaginal canal. They are not as reliable as other methods, but are easy to use and obtain. The spermicide should be inserted into the vaginal canal no more than 1 hour before sexual intercourse, and each application is effective for one coitus only. These agents may also be used with a condom to increase reliability.

D. The rhythm method is based on abstention from intercourse during ovulation, which occurs approximately 14 days before the onset of menses regardless of the length of time between menstrual cycles. For the woman with irregular menses, the rhythm method is unreliable. Although mothers who are nursing their infants may not ovulate during the first 10 weeks after delivery, breastfeeding is not a reliable method of birth control.

E. Withdrawal has a high failure rate because of the small but active content of the preejaculate secretions. It is not a recommended method of birth control.

F. The diaphragm is a flexible cup-shaped device that is inserted into the vagina and placed over the cervix, keeping the sperm from entering the uterus. Spermicidal cream or jelly should be placed on the diaphragm before insertion. The diaphragm must be fitted by a qualified practitioner. The fitting should be checked at least every 2 years and after each pregnancy. The diaphragm is inserted just before intercourse and should remain over the cervix for 6 to 8 hours after coitus. This device appeals to women who are unable to take oral contraceptives or dislike internal devices.

G. The intrauterine device (IUD) is a plastic or metal coil that is inserted into the uterus during menstruation. A plastic string attached to the IUD enables the woman to check placement periodically. Uterine cramping and slight bleeding is likely to develop soon after insertion and may occur intermittently for several months. Menstrual flow is commonly increased. The IUD may remain in place for 3 to 4 years. IUDs are associated with problems such as ovarium alum, endometriosis, and uterine rupture. Women choosing this method must be advised of all possible side effects and observations to report.

H. The oral contraceptives (OC) most often prescribed consist of a combination of estrogen and progestational agents taken daily for 3 weeks and omitted for 1 week, during which time withdrawal uterine bleeding occurs. Common side effects include nausea, vomiting, fluid retention, headache (p 28), breakthrough bleeding, depression, acne, reduced libido, short or scanty menses, or prolonged, heavy menses. Individualization and proper balance of these two hormones are essential to reduce side effects. Contraindications to OC usage include strong family history of stroke, severe migraines, seizure disorders, cerebral arterial insufficiency, cardiac decompensation, severe diabetes mellitus, severe renal disease, endometrial or breast carcinoma, thromboembolic disease, or sickle cell disease. The benefits of OCs must be weighed against the risks. All women receiving OCs should have an initial gynecologic examination and be reexamined 3 months later. The client is taught to monitor her blood pressure because hypertension (p 80) is an unacceptable side effect. Cigarette smoking increases the risk of cardiovascular side effects and is discouraged.

I. Vasectomy is the permanent method of sterilization for men. The procedure is usually performed in 20 to 30 minutes on an outpatient basis under local anesthesia. A small incision is made in the scrotum, through which the vas deferens are isolated and cut or blocked to

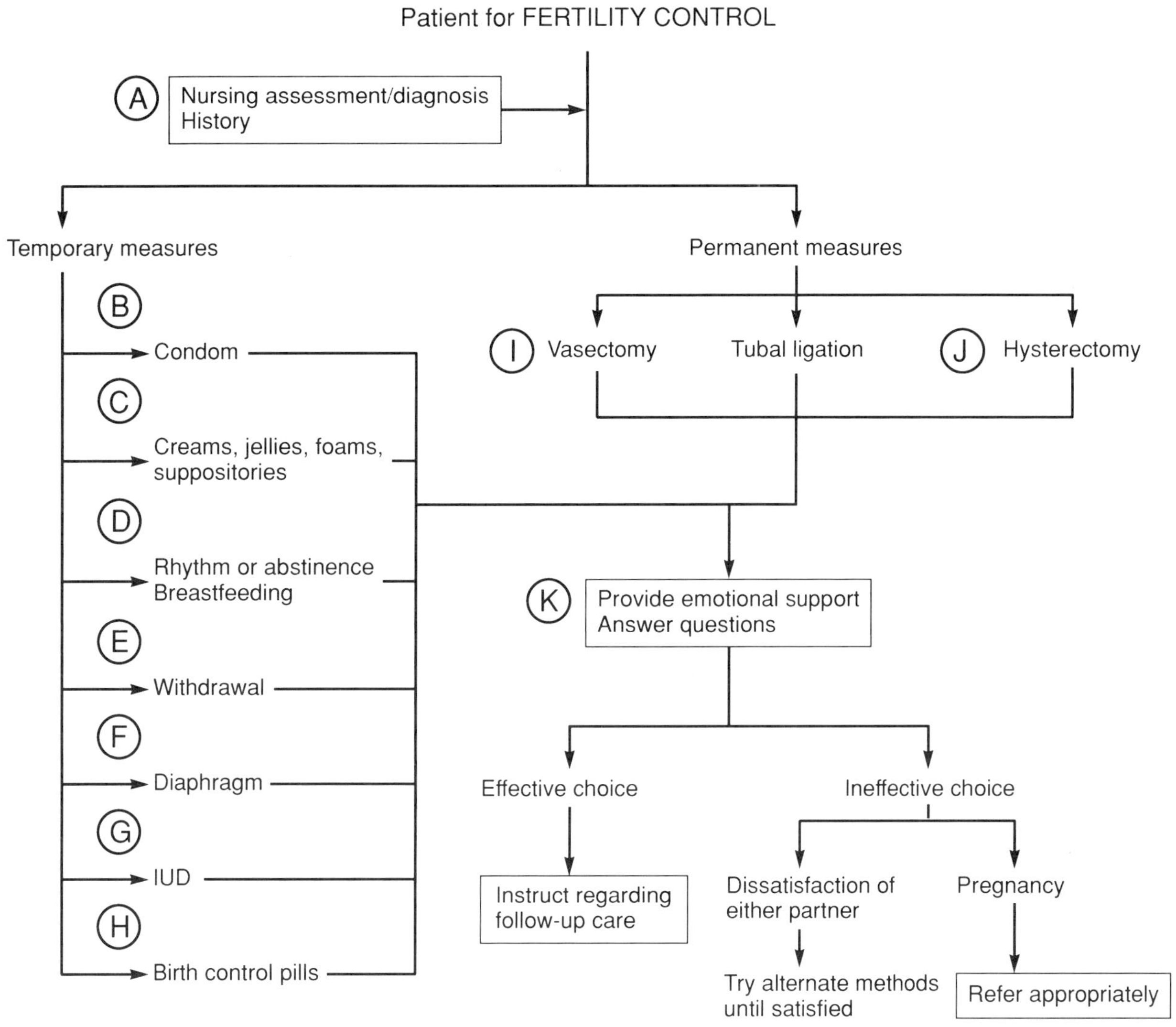

prevent passage of sperm. About 15 to 20 ejaculations are usually required after the procedure before sterility is assured. This is the main disadvantage of a vasectomy. The male is not considered sterile until two sperm-free ejaculates have been produced.

J. Permanent sterility for women is established through bilateral tubal ligation (p 290). A hysterectomy (p 284) also results in sterility, but is done as a treatment for disease, not as a method of fertility control.

K. When counseling a patient about birth control, it is important to give unbiased advice and support the patient's decision without judgment, as this is a private and personal decision.

References

Benson RC. Handbook of obstetrics and gynecology. 8th ed. Los Altos, CA: Lange, 1983:738–753.

Berkow R, ed. The Merck manual. Vol II. 14th ed. Rahway, NJ: Merck, Sharp & Dohme Research Laboratories, 1982:64–69.

Jenson MD, Benson RD, Bobak IN. Maternity care: a nurse and the family. St. Louis: CV Mosby, 1981:66–79.

Pritchard JA, MacDonald PC, Grant NF. Williams obstetrics. 17th ed. Norwalk, CT: Appleton-Century-Crofts, 1985: 811–835.

CANCER OF THE CERVIX

Mary Lindell Marquis

A. Cancer of the cervix is the third most common malignancy in women in the United States. The primary risk factors are early sexual activity, early childbearing, and multiple sex partners. The detection, diagnosis, and eradication of cervical cancer precursors will prevent the development of invasive cervical carcinoma.

B. The cancer precursors, i.e., lesion, dysplasia, or cervical intraepithelial neoplasia (CIN), arise on the cervix. Early detection of dysplasia or CIN by the Pap smear (Papanicolaou screening) allows layers of the squamous epithelium of the cervix to be evaluated. The site where the columnar epithelium and the squamous epithelium meet on the cervix, called the transition zone or squamocolumnar junction, is the origin of most cervical cancer. Early stages of dysplasia and CIN may regress or progress to cancer in situ, and then to invasive carcinoma. The progression from a precancerous lesion to invasive cervical cancer may take 10 to 15 years.

C. Cervical carcinoma is asymptomatic until late in the disease when a bloody watery discharge, occasional spotting after intercourse, or between-menses spotting occurs. Early detection of precursor lesions by the Pap smear are classified in Table 1. When dysplasia is detected on the Pap smear, a colposcopy for diagnosis is indicated. A colposcope, an instrument used to magnify, is utilized to examine and identify abnormal areas on the cervix, and biopsy samples are taken.

D. The goal of treatment is to eradicate abnormal epithelium. The particular treatment indicated is based on the client's desire for future pregnancy, the severity of the dysplasia, and the area of involvement of cervical tissue. Treatments include cryosurgery, laser surgery (p 378), cone biopsy, or hysterectomy (p 284).

E. Cryosurgery destroys the abnormal cells by freezing. The procedure is performed on an outpatient basis. Following this procedure the client experiences a watery vaginal discharge for several weeks, and cervical stenosis can result. This method is not used for large areas or for CIN III.

F. Laser surgery, an outpatient treatment, uses a beam of light to vaporize the tissue. Laser surgery can precisely treat the tissue and results in a moderate amount of vaginal discharge. However, there is a risk of bleeding and pelvic infections with laser surgery.

TABLE 1 Pap Smear Classification

Class I	Normal smear
Class II	Atypical cells
Class III	
CIN I	Mild dysplasia
CIN II	Moderate dysplasia
Class IV	
CIN III	Severe dysplasia to cancer in situ
Class V	Abnormal cells in smear consistent with invasive carcinoma

G. Cone biopsy is performed when the biopsy taken during the colposcopy indicates microinvasion of the epithelium on the cervix and is also performed to rule out invasive cancer. Complications of this outpatient procedure are bleeding, cervical stenosis, infertility, and an incompetent cervix.

H. A hysterectomy is used to treat CIN if no further childbearing is desired.

I. Follow-up after the cyrosurgery, laser, and cone biopsy is essential. Follow-up includes a 1-month postoperative check, repeat Pap smear in 4 months and Pap smears every 4 to 6 months for 1 to 2 years until three to four consecutive negative Pap results are achieved. A follow-up colposcopy may also be recommended. Then Pap smears are repeated every 6 months thereafter. Patients must be made aware of the importance of adhering to these appointments.

References

Beal M. Understanding cervical cytology. Nurse Pract, 1987; 12(3):8, 10, 15+.

Cashavelly B. Cervical dysplasia: an overview of current concepts in epidemiology, diagnosis and treatments. Cancer Nurs, 1987; 10(4):199–206.

Droegemueller W, Herbst A, Mishell D, Stencheuer M. Comprehensive gynecology. St. Louis: CV Mosby, 1987.

Lovejoy N. Precancerous lesions of the cervix: personal risk factors. Cancer Nurs, 1987; 1:10.

Phipps W, Long B, Woods C, Fugate N. Medical-surgical nursing. St. Louis: CV Mosby, 1987.

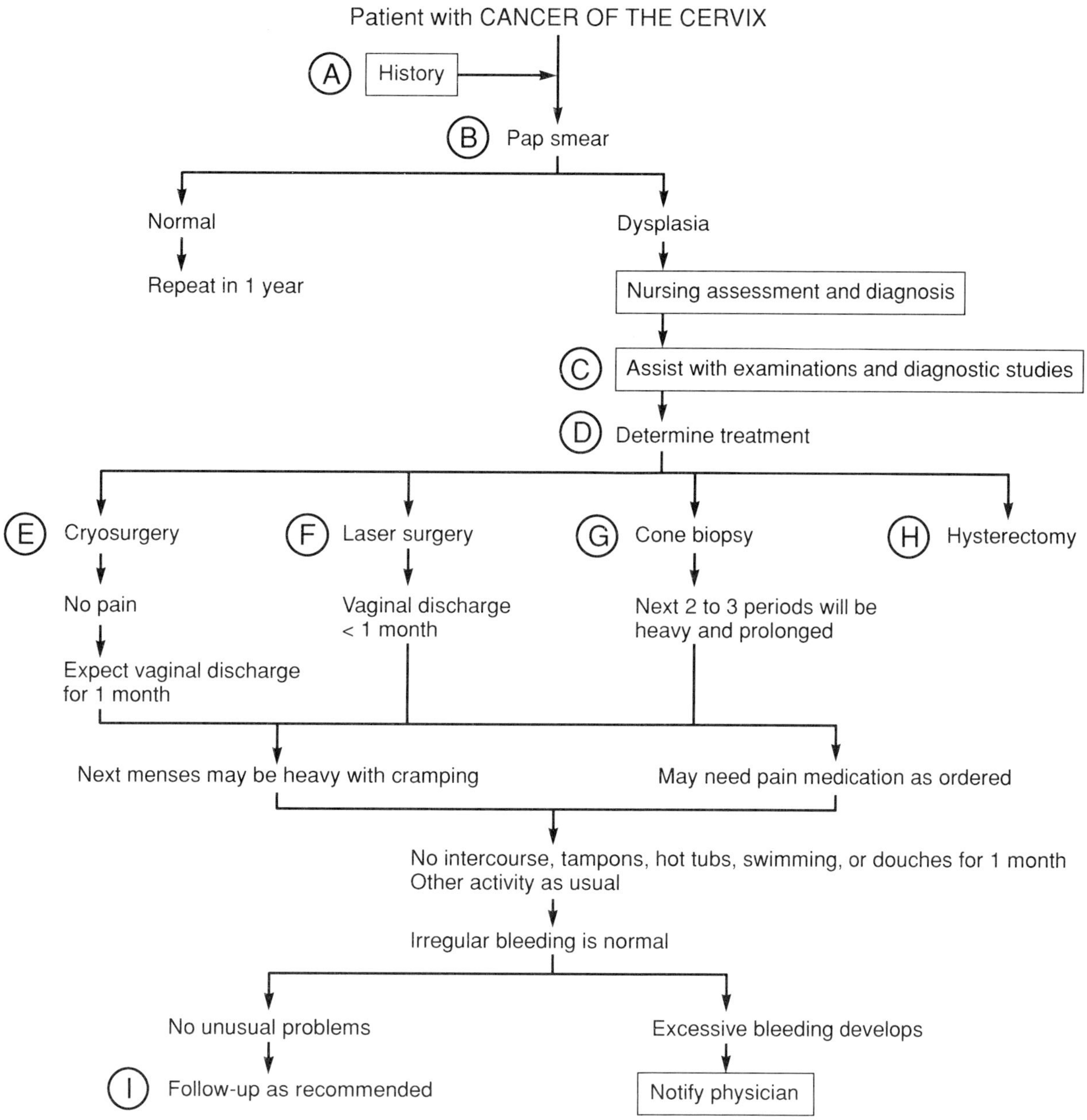
Patient with CANCER OF THE CERVIX
A
History
B
Pap smear
Normal
Repeat in 1 year
Dysplasia
Nursing assessment and diagnosis
C
Assist with examinations and diagnostic studies
D
Determine treatment
E
Cryosurgery
No pain
Expect vaginal discharge for 1 month
F
Laser surgery
Vaginal discharge < 1 month
G
Cone biopsy
Next 2 to 3 periods will be heavy and prolonged
H
Hysterectomy
Next menses may be heavy with cramping
May need pain medication as ordered
No intercourse, tampons, hot tubs, swimming, or douches for 1 month
Other activity as usual
Irregular bleeding is normal
No unusual problems
I
Follow-up as recommended
Excessive bleeding develops
Notify physician

CANCER OF THE OVARY

Mary Lindell Marquis

Ovarian cancer is the second most common malignancy and the most frequent cause of death from genital tract neoplasms. The high death rate is related to late detection of the disease. Ovarian cancer does not cause symptoms until the malignancy is widespread. Three-fourths of all cases are not diagnosed until the cancer has spread beyond the ovary.

A. The cause of cancer of the ovary is thought to be related to frequent ovulation, late menopause, late pregnancy, nulliparity, and living in industrialized countries, the United States and Western Europe. There has also been a familial association. Epithelial adenocarcinoma accounts for 90 percent of all ovarian malignancies. It grows through the capsule of the ovary and spreads into the peritoneal cavity.

B. During a pelvic examination, a physician or nurse practitioner may detect an enlarged ovary. This is followed up with pelvic ultrasonography. The size of the mass and age of the client are considerations in the diagnosis to rule out ovarian cancer. Ovarian cysts are a common occurrence in women under 40 years of age, so it may be decided to observe the enlargement for 2 months and reevaluate. Unless detected on examination, ovarian cancer usually is without symptoms until late in the disease. Late symptoms include enlargement of the abdomen and abdominal bloating and discomfort. Associated symptoms are a change in bowel function, indigestion, and urinary frequency.

C. History, physical examination, and diagnostic studies are performed to determine the structures involved. If late symptoms are present, pelvic ultrasonography, intravenous pyelography, and barium enema are ordered.

D. Surgery is the initial treatment for ovarian cancer. An exploratory laparotomy is performed. The extent of the surgery depends on the amount of spread. One ovary may be removed, but in most cases a total abdominal hysterectomy (p 284) and a bilateral salpingo-oophorectomy is performed. The pelvic lymph nodes and omentum are also removed. Emotional support of the patient and family is extremely important during all phases of diagnosis and treatment.

E. Follow-up treatment with chemotherapy (p 408) or radiation therapy may be given to destroy any remaining cancer cells.

F. A "second look" laparotomy may be performed to surgically reassess clients who have had surgery and chemotherapy.

G. Tumors are found in 50 percent of "second look" laparotomies. For these clients, second-line chemotherapy is initiated.

References

Droegemueller W, Herbst A, Mishell D, Stencheuer M. Comprehensive gynecology. St. Louis: CV Mosby, 1987.

Lamb MA, Bargman C, Brozovich K. Ovarian cancer: patient information booklet. Oncol Nurs Forum 1985; 12(5):83–88.

Phipps W, Long B, Woods C, Fugate N. Medical-surgical nursing. St. Louis: CV Mosby, 1987.

Rubin D. Gynecologic cancer: uterine and ovarian malignancies. RN 1987; 50:52–57.

Rubin S. Ovarian cancer. AORN J 1988; 47(6).

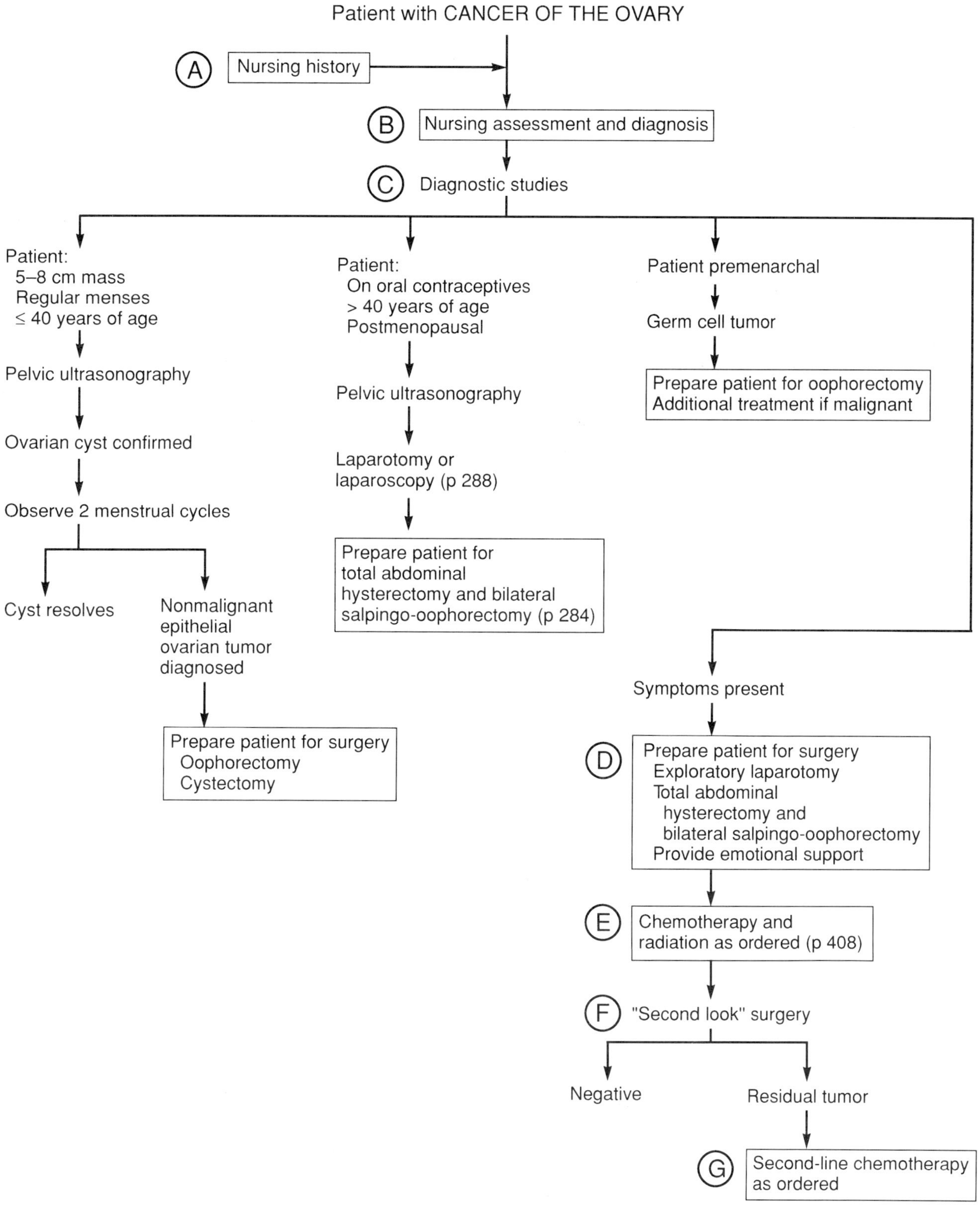
Patient with CANCER OF THE OVARY
A
Nursing history
B
Nursing assessment and diagnosis
C
Diagnostic studies
Patient:
5–8 cm mass
Regular menses
≤ 40 years of age
Pelvic ultrasonography
Ovarian cyst confirmed
Observe 2 menstrual cycles
Cyst resolves
Nonmalignant epithelial ovarian tumor diagnosed
Prepare patient for surgery
Oophorectomy
Cystectomy
Patient:
On oral contraceptives
> 40 years of age
Postmenopausal
Pelvic ultrasonography
Laparotomy or laparoscopy (p 288)
Prepare patient for total abdominal hysterectomy and bilateral salpingo-oophorectomy (p 284)
Patient premenarchal
Germ cell tumor
Prepare patient for oophorectomy
Additional treatment if malignant
Symptoms present
D
Prepare patient for surgery
Exploratory laparotomy
Total abdominal hysterectomy and bilateral salpingo-oophorectomy
Provide emotional support
E
Chemotherapy and radiation as ordered (p 408)
F
"Second look" surgery
Negative
Residual tumor
G
Second-line chemotherapy as ordered

CANCER OF THE UTERUS

Mary Lindell Marquis

Endometrial cancer is the most common malignancy of the female genital tract in the United States. Adenocarcinoma of the endometrium accounts for 95 percent of uterine cancer and is commonly diagnosed between the ages of 50 and 65 years.

A. Endometrial cancer most frequently is the result of hyperplasia of the endometrium. Hyperplasia of the endometrium may be cystic, adenomatous, or atypical. The last two types are considered to be premalignant lesions. The exact cause of hyperplasia is unknown. Estrogen replacement therapy unopposed by progestin has been shown to be a risk factor for hyperplasia. Unopposed estrogen replacement therapy is the administration of estrogen (without the use of progestogens) to control menopausal symptoms, e.g., hot flashes, arterial changes, and osteoporotic changes. Progestogens are known to protect against endometrial hyperstimulation. It is currently recommended that women who have their uterus be treated for menopausal symptoms with an estrogen-progestin combination. Other risk factors for endometrial cancer are obesity, late menopause, nulliparity, hypertension, and diabetes mellitus.

B. There is no reliable screening method for endometrial cancer. Most women are diagnosed after seeking medical help for abnormal bleeding. The diagnosis is made most commonly by either endometrial biopsy or dilatation and curettage (D&C) (p 282). An endometrial biopsy is performed by introducing a small curet into the uterus and taking several specimens of endometrial tissue. A D&C removes endometrial tissue from the entire uterus. Dilators are introduced into the cervical canal, and then curets are used to remove the tissue.

C. An endometrial biopsy is performed in an outpatient setting. Following an endometrial biopsy the patient experiences cramping and vaginal bleeding that should decrease and cease in several days. Sanitary pads should be worn, not tampons. Fever, chills, increased bleeding, or foul odor of vaginal discharge must be reported to the physician. Intercourse is prohibited for 2 days after the procedure. Analgesic medications may be given.

D. The D&C may be an outpatient or short-stay procedure. After the D&C, the patient should expect cramping and vaginal bleeding. The patient is rechecked by the physician in 3 to 4 weeks. Until that time, intercourse, hot tubs, and tampons are prohibited. Activity is restricted, and fever, chills, increased bleeding, or foul odor of vaginal discharge must be reported to the physician. Analgesics are prescribed.

E. The results of the D&C or endometrial biopsy determine the treatment. The patient with hyperplasia without atypia requires long-term follow-up and endometrial biopsy every year.

F. The patient with mild atypia is treated with progestin or an estrogen-progestin combination to prevent menses and thereby prevent build-up and hyperplasia of the endometrium. These women are followed with endometrial biopsies every 6 to 12 months.

G. Women with moderate-to-severe atypia who wish to maintain childbearing ability are treated with progestin therapy, which will cause amenorrhea. Follow-up with an endometrial biopsy is required every 6 months.

H. For those women with moderate-to-severe atypia who do not wish to retain childbearing ability and for older patients, a hysterectomy (p 284) is the recommended treatment.

I. Staging classifications of the International Federation of Gynecology and Obstetrics for endometrial carcinoma are shown in Table 1. Radiation therapy is prescribed postoperatively, at times preoperatively, and as the only therapy for patients unable to undergo surgery. Nurses should review and follow agency protocols and procedures for managing patients with radium implants. Internal radiation using Heyman's capsules to pack the uterus may be prescribed, with a hysterectomy to follow.

References

Droegemueller W, Herbst A, Mishell D, Stencheuer M. Comprehensive gynecology. St. Louis: CV Mosby, 1987.

Phipps W, Long B, Woods C, Fugate N. Medical-surgical nursing. St. Louis: CV Mosby, 1987.

Rubin D. Gynecologic cancer: uterine and ovarian malignancies. RN 1987; 50:52–57.

Whitehead M, Frasier D. Controversies concerning the safety of estrogen replacement therapy. Am J Obstet Gynecol 1987; 156(5):1315.

TABLE 1 Endometrial Cancer Staging Classifications

Stage	*Characteristics*
Stage I	Cancer confined to body of uterus
I A	Uterine cavity ≤ 8 cm
	Substages G1 through G3 subdivide malignancies from highly differentiated adenocarcinoma to undifferentiated tumors
I B	Uterine cavity > 8 cm
	G1 through G3
Stage II	Cancer involves the body of the uterus and the cervix
Stage III	Cancer confined to pelvis
Stage IV	Cancer involves pelvis and mucosa of the bladder and the rectum
IV A	Tumor has spread to nearby organs
IV B	Distant metastasis

* G = Grade

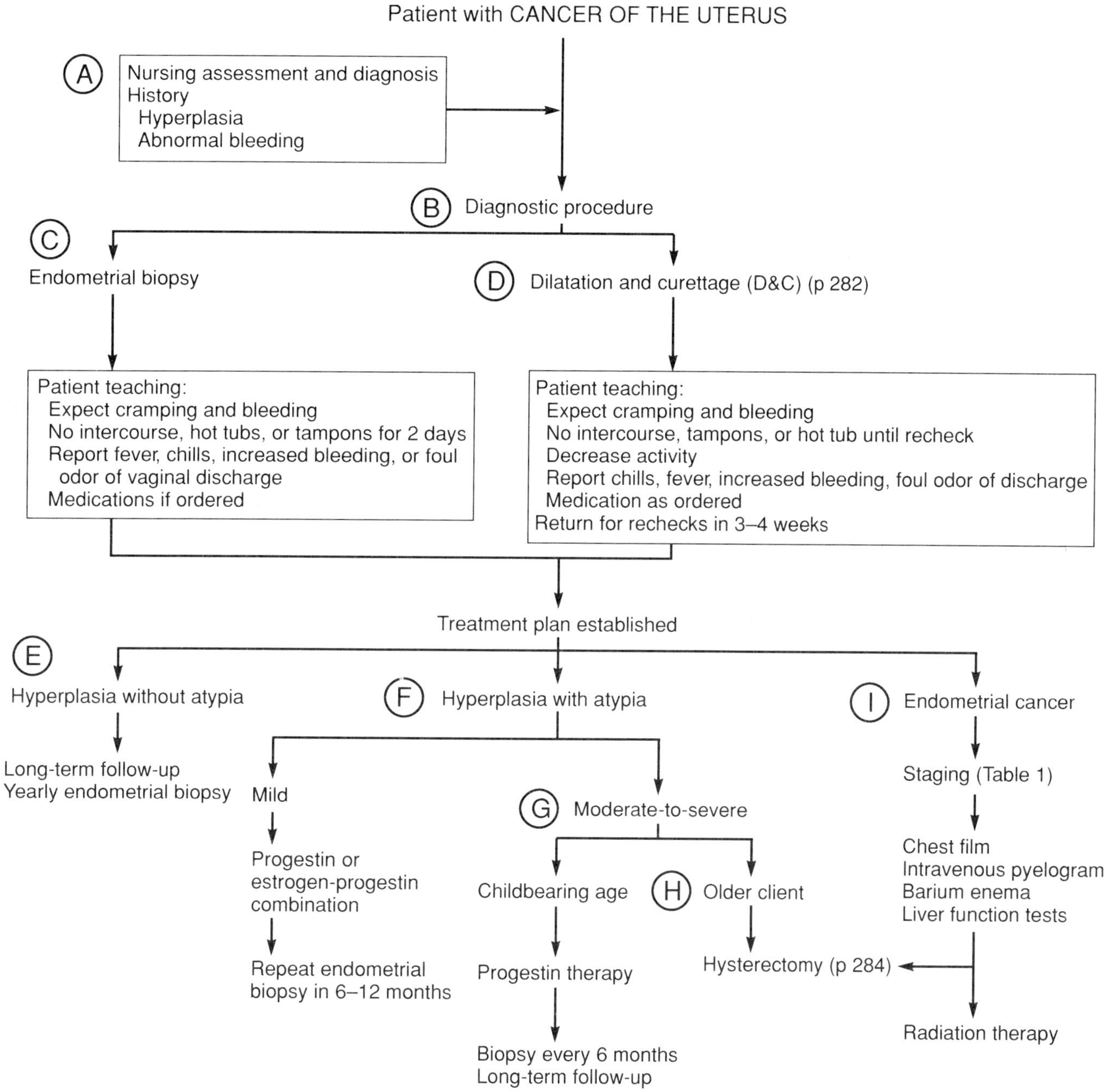
Patient with CANCER OF THE UTERUS
A
Nursing assessment and diagnosis
History
Hyperplasia
Abnormal bleeding
B
Diagnostic procedure
C
Endometrial biopsy
D
Dilatation and curettage (D&C) (p 282)
Patient teaching:
Expect cramping and bleeding
No intercourse, hot tubs, or tampons for 2 days
Report fever, chills, increased bleeding, or foul odor of vaginal discharge
Medications if ordered
Patient teaching:
Expect cramping and bleeding
No intercourse, tampons, or hot tub until recheck
Decrease activity
Report chills, fever, increased bleeding, foul odor of discharge
Medication as ordered
Return for rechecks in 3–4 weeks
Treatment plan established
E
Hyperplasia without atypia
Long-term follow-up
Yearly endometrial biopsy
F
Hyperplasia with atypia
Mild
Progestin or estrogen-progestin combination
Repeat endometrial biopsy in 6–12 months
G
Moderate-to-severe
Childbearing age
Progestin therapy
Biopsy every 6 months
Long-term follow-up
H
Older client
Hysterectomy (p 284)
I
Endometrial cancer
Staging (Table 1)
Chest film
Intravenous pyelogram
Barium enema
Liver function tests
Radiation therapy

MASTECTOMY

Nancy A. Young

Breast cancer is the most common malignancy of American women and the leading cause of death in women ages 39 to 44. Etiologic factors may include heredity, hormonal influences, diet, obesity, cigarette smoking, chemicals, viruses, or glucose intolerance. In spite of advances in cancer research, 23 percent of every 100,000 women die each year from breast cancer. The surgical approach varies, depending on the patient's choice and the extent of tissue invasion.

A. Extensive preoperative teaching helps the patient and her family or friends anticipate and accept her postoperative needs and limitations. Most women express fear of the procedure, since the extent of the disease and the prognosis for the future remain unknown. They may exhibit anxiety about the loss of a body part that changes their self-image and perception of sexuality and attractiveness. The patient should understand fully her particular surgical procedure, the methods for preventing postoperative complications, and common physical sensations and limitations to expect. The nurse further instructs the patient about exercises that reestablish strength and circulation after surgery.

B. Postoperative care focuses on three general areas, the first being prevention of infection. Mastectomy patients may exhibit ineffective breathing due to fear of pain, anesthesia and/or medications, or restrictive dressings. The patient can splint the area to turn, cough, and deep breathe, and assume a semi-Fowler's position with elevation of the affected part in order to facilitate drainage and relieve arm tension. The nurse should check patients with hemovacs or suction for patency of the tubing as well as the amount and type of drainage. Secondly, the patient experiences physical immobility because of removal of muscles, damage to surrounding nerves, and impairment of the lymph system. Finally, the loss of a body part so closely identified with femininity can generate emotions that require additional support.

C. Considering the mastectomy patient's reduced mobility, the nurse must assess circulation by observing hand color and finger movement, as well as testing for tactile sensation. Lymphedema is a common finding that can be minimized by elevating the arm and practicing range-of-motion exercises. Massaging the arm using a lanolin hand cream several times each day can also promote circulation.

D. The nurse can assist a mastectomy patient in dealing with the surgical outcome by providing an opportunity to express her feelings and encourage questions about the incision, scar, and future expectations. The nurse can also watch for signs of depression and offer referral for additional counseling. Most communities have Reach to Recovery volunteers who visit patients and share information about prostheses and home management.

E. Discharge teaching includes several areas. The patient should demonstrate an understanding of hand, arm, and shoulder exercises and the technique of performing self–breast examination. She should be aware of the signs and symptoms of infection and lymphedema and ways to prevent those complications. Information about prostheses, when applicable, can help her decide on a long-term plan and reaffirm the importance of seeking follow-up care.

References

Doenges ME, Jeffries MF, Moorhouse MF. Nursing care plans: nursing diagnoses in planning patient care. Philadelphia: FA Davis, 1984.

Lewis SM, Collier JC. Medical-surgical nursing: assessment and management of clinical problems. New York: McGraw-Hill, 1983.

Ulrich SP, Canale SW, Wendell SA. Nursing care planning guides. Philadelphia: WB Saunders, 1986.

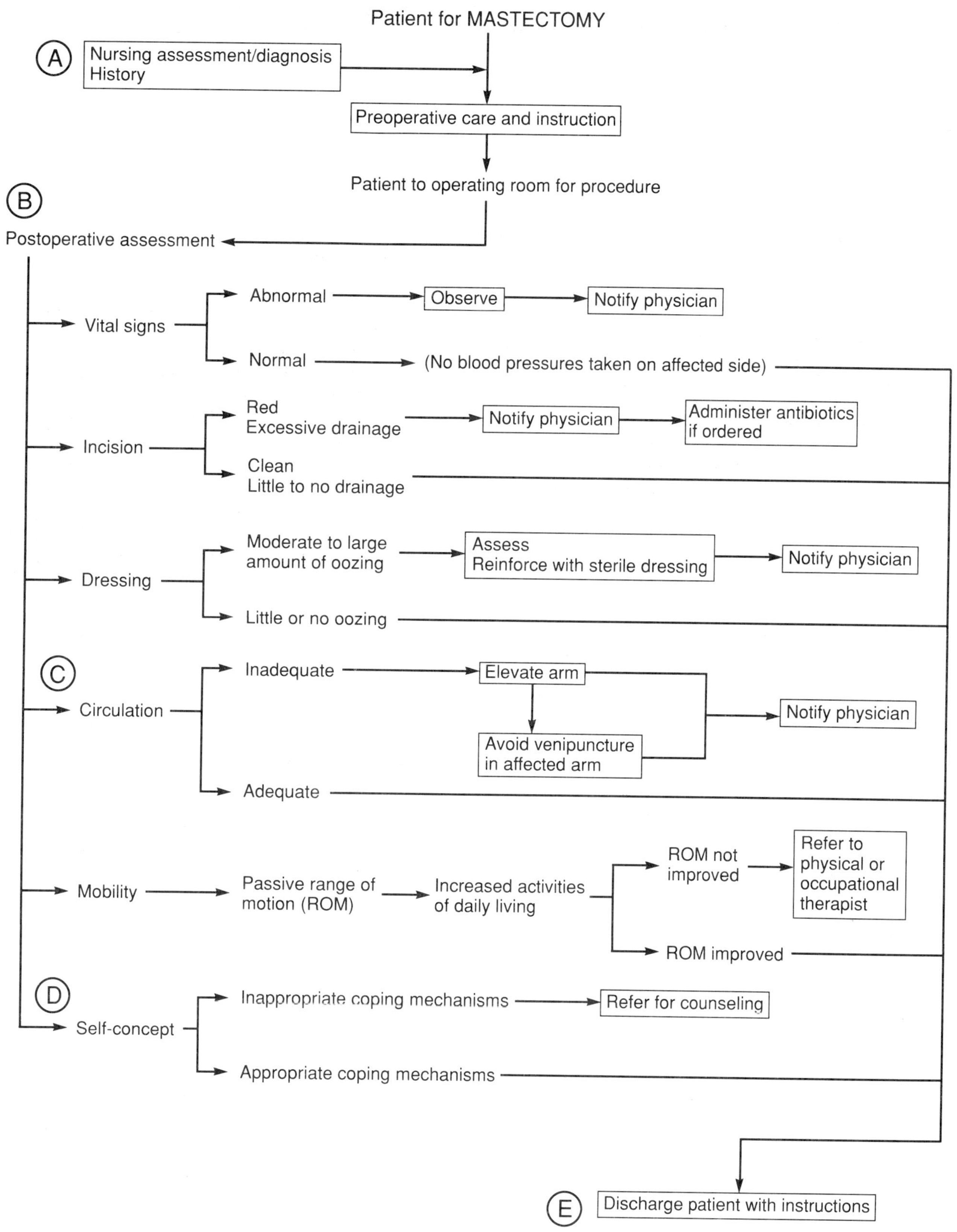
Patient for MASTECTOMY
A
Nursing assessment/diagnosis
History
Preoperative care and instruction
Patient to operating room for procedure
B
Postoperative assessment
Vital signs
Abnormal
Observe
Notify physician
Normal
(No blood pressures taken on affected side)
Incision
Red
Excessive drainage
Notify physician
Administer antibiotics if ordered
Clean
Little to no drainage
Dressing
Moderate to large amount of oozing
Assess
Reinforce with sterile dressing
Notify physician
Little or no oozing
C
Circulation
Inadequate
Elevate arm
Avoid venipuncture in affected arm
Notify physician
Adequate
Mobility
Passive range of motion (ROM)
Increased activities of daily living
ROM not improved
Refer to physical or occupational therapist
ROM improved
D
Self-concept
Inappropriate coping mechanisms
Refer for counseling
Appropriate coping mechanisms
E
Discharge patient with instructions

BREAST RECONSTRUCTION

Chris Kirsch

Breast reconstruction, which is performed on women who have had a mastectomy (p 274), allows a more natural look without an external prosthesis. While there is no medical need to replace breast tissue, the prospect of disfigurement and decreased self-image is often more frightening than the cancer itself. Breast reconstruction can be performed immediately after a mastectomy if the age of the patient and pathologic and clinical evaluations are acceptable. Delayed reconstruction may be necessary if adjunctive chemotherapy and radiation therapy are planned or if the patient's acceptance of the mastectomy is difficult. Methods of breast reconstruction include breast prosthesis (immediate), breast prothesis (delayed), insertion of an expandable silicone sac (delayed), and transverse abdominal island flap (TAIF). For patients having radical mastectomy, TAIF is usually the method of choice. Tissue is transferred from an area of the body where there is excess (abdomen) to an area where needed (chest). Reconstruction is not recommended for women who have other diseases that may impair the healing process, who are undergoing radiation therapy or chest skin grafts, or who have large tumors or extensive nodular involvement. The goals of reconstruction are to establish a close symmetry with the existing breast, to create a breast that is soft and natural, and to construct a pleasing nipple and areola.

A. A thorough nursing assessment is made. The patient's history of cancer and its involvement are important. Cardiac or pulmonary problems will have been verified by electrocardiography (ECG) and arterial blood gases (ABGs). Allergies, medication use, and habits such as smoking are also noted. Use of aspirin must be discouraged for at least 2 weeks before surgery. Smoking is also discouraged for 4 weeks before surgery to reduce the risk of flap tissue loss. Most important for the patient's well-being is psychological support.

B. Ensure that expectations are reasonable. Discuss the possibility of scars around the breast and abdomen, depending on the procedure.

C. Preoperatively, a 24-hour restricted liquid diet aids bowel decompression, which relaxes the abdominal wall, essential if TAIF is the selected method.

D. Postoperatively, routine monitoring is done (p 4). If radical surgery (involving lymph node dissection) has been performed before reconstruction, measure blood pressure in the unaffected arm or leg. Any elevation of temperature should be monitored as possible infection. Most patients, however, will have been on prophylactic antibiotic therapy preoperatively, and broad-spectrum antibiotics are continued for 24 to 48 hours postoperatively.

E. Drains are placed in the breast and abdomen. Drainage should be measured every 30 minutes during the first 24 hours postoperatively. The amount should not exceed 50 ml per hour. Light dressings of 4 × 4s are placed around drains, leaving the operative site exposed for observation. A position of comfort, head elevated 30 degrees and knees flexed, reduces tension on the abdominal incision.

F. The wound flap should be white to pale pink. The breast will be cold to touch for the first hour, becoming gradually warmer. Should the breast become mottled or remain cold to touch, notify the physician. Surgery may be required to return circulation to the flap. Oxygen is given by face mask or cannula to further aid oxygenation of the flap. Hematoma, the most common complication, generally forms within 48 hours; should this occur, notify the physician. If a prosthesis has been used, the patient may be returned to surgery for removal of the prosthesis, evacuation of the hematoma, irrigation and coagulation of the operative site, and reinsertion of a prosthesis with application of elastoplast. If no prosthesis has been used and TAIF has been done, coagulation of bleeders is generally all that is necessary. Edema, tissue discoloration, and foul odor indicate flap failure in TAIF. *Notify the surgeon immediately*. The patient may shower after drains are removed. Careful cleaning of the umbilicus and incision sites with hydrogen peroxide is necessary.

G. Response to pain varies and must be assessed accordingly. The patient's discomfort with a prosthetic insertion may be handled with a mild nonaspirin pain medication. For the patient with TAIF, narcotics may be offered for the first 24 to 48 hours, followed by nonnarcotic analgesics. Antiemetics, as needed to prevent nausea, reduce strain on the abdominal sutures. Light, small, and frequent meals to decrease distention and flatus are encouraged.

H. Ambulation is encouraged within the first 24 hours postoperatively. TAIF patients incur a tightness and pulling in the abdominal wall and should walk leaning forward with flexed knees for the first 5 to 7 days. Prosthetic patients generally experience no difficulty ambulating.

I. Discharge instructions depend on the type of surgery. If an implant prosthesis has been used, the patient will have started massage of the area several times per day

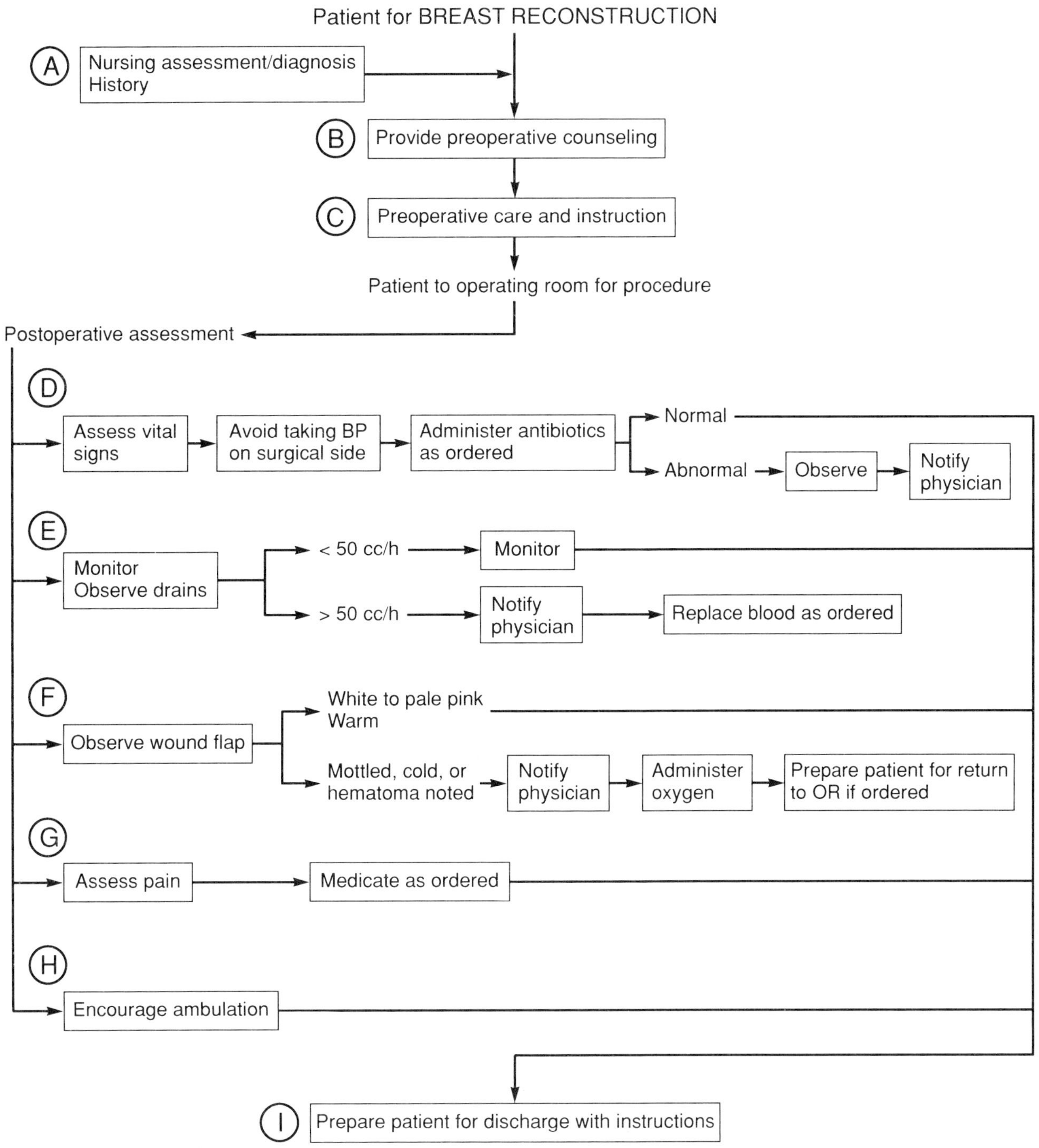

to soften the prosthesis and limit the possibility of capsular contraction. In the patient with TAIF, to ensure adequate circulation, the reconstructed breast should not be massaged and no bra worn for approximately 3 weeks. Strenuous exercise should be avoided. Instruct the patient not to raise the affected arm above shoulder level for 1 month and not to lift objects that weigh more than 5 pounds for at least 6 weeks. Even with preoperative counseling, some patients experience a reactive depression because of disappointment with the results, adjustment to lifestyle, or grief over cancer diagnosis. Continued psychological counseling is advised; referrals to support groups are of assistance.

References

Berger K, Bostwick J. A woman's decision, breast care, treatment and reconstruction. St. Louis: CV Mosby, 1984.

Dinner M. Postmastectomy reconstruction. Surg Clin North Am 1984; 64:1193–1207.

Hutchinson H. TAIF: new option for breast reconstruction. Nursing 1986; 16:52–53.

Kneisl CR, Ames SW. Adult health nursing: a biopsychosocial approach. Menlo Park, CA: Addison-Wesley, 1986.

Solomon J. The good news about breast reconstruction. RN 1986; 49(11):47–54.

AUGMENTATION MAMMOPLASTY

Chris Kirsch

Mammoplasty is surgical change of the size and/or shape of the breast. Augmentation mammoplasty is a surgical procedure in which the size of the breasts is increased by insertion of a prosthesis. Most prostheses consist of a thin, seamless Silastic enveloped filled with dextrin, silicone fluid, or saline. Silicone is the most popular prosthesis because it feels normal to palpation and looks and behaves more naturally. Size varies from 70 to 600 ml of fluid, depending on the needs and desire of the client.

A. Most women seeking augmentation mammoplasty do so within the realm of psychological need. Women with aplasia, hypoplasia, asymmetry, or secondary atrophy may suffer a deep sense of inadequacy that may seriously interfere with courtship and marriage, cause unhappiness with their sex life, and lead to low self-esteem. Assessment should include the patient's perception of the functional and emotional significance of this body part.

B. Preoperative instruction is given regarding routine postoperative care such as coughing, deep breathing, turning, and early ambulation. Skin is usually scrubbed with povidone-iodine solution the evening before surgery. The laboratory work-up is minimal.

C. Routine postoperative procedures such as vital signs and systems assessment are done (p 4). Any elevation in temperature may be an indication of infection. The physician is notified and antibiotic therapy initiated.

D. Mammoplasty patients can ambulate as soon as they recover from anesthesia; however, arm and shoulder movements are restricted. Activities involving elevation of the arms over the head (such as brushing hair) or pectoral muscles (lifting) must be restricted.

E. Pressure dressings are maintained for 5 to 7 days with a bulky circumferential figure-eight bandage, leaving the nipples exposed so they can be checked for swelling or hematoma. The dressing is checked further for bleeding and to ensure that it is intact. Dressings are tighter across the upper lateral quadrants because bleeding vessels are more likely to originate there.

F. Pain is associated with various reconstructive procedures and may range from mild to severe. Assess the individual patient's response to pain and provide pharmacologic and/or nonpharmacologic therapy. Aspirin is not advised because of its anticoagulant effect. Psychological support and teaching methods to reduce anxiety and stress are of great value.

G. Patients are instructed to begin breast exercises about 6 weeks postoperatively. The exercise helps to maintain an open and wide retromammary pocket and ensure soft breasts. Instruct the patient to place the right hand under the breasts, push up firmly, hold for a count of ten and release five consecutive times to soften and stretch the capsule's fibers. Capsule formation is a frequent complication that causes excessive firmness of the breast and is treated with steroid injection or a capsulotomy.

H. This procedure is frequently done on a day-surgery basis. If there are no complications, the patient is discharged with instructions to note color and size of her breasts and report any change that may occur. A tight-fitting supportive brassiere without underwire should be worn continuously. Instructions include (1) no lifting for at least 2 to 3 weeks while the wounds heal; (2) no participation in activities such as golf, tennis, and swimming for about 6 weeks; and (3) sleeping on the back, not on the sides or stomach for 6 weeks. Patients should be encouraged to schedule follow-up appointments to ensure proper healing.

References

Beale S. Augmentation mammoplasty: the surgical-psychological effects of the operation and prediction of the results. Ann Plast Surg 1984; 8:279–297.

Finn KL. Augmentation mammoplasty: the cosmetic surgery with a lift. Nursing 1979; 42(2):60–63.

Georgiada NC. Reconstructive breast surgery. St. Louis: CV Mosby, 1976:254–317.

Koch SJ. Augmentation mammoplasty. Am J Nurs 1980; 80(8):1480–1484.

Luckmann J, Sorensen KC. Medical-surgical nursing: a psychophysiologic approach. 3rd ed. Philadelphia: WB Saunders, 1987.

Walsh KC. Breast augmentation: your patients adjustment to new body image. Today's OR Nurse 1986; 8(9):20–26.

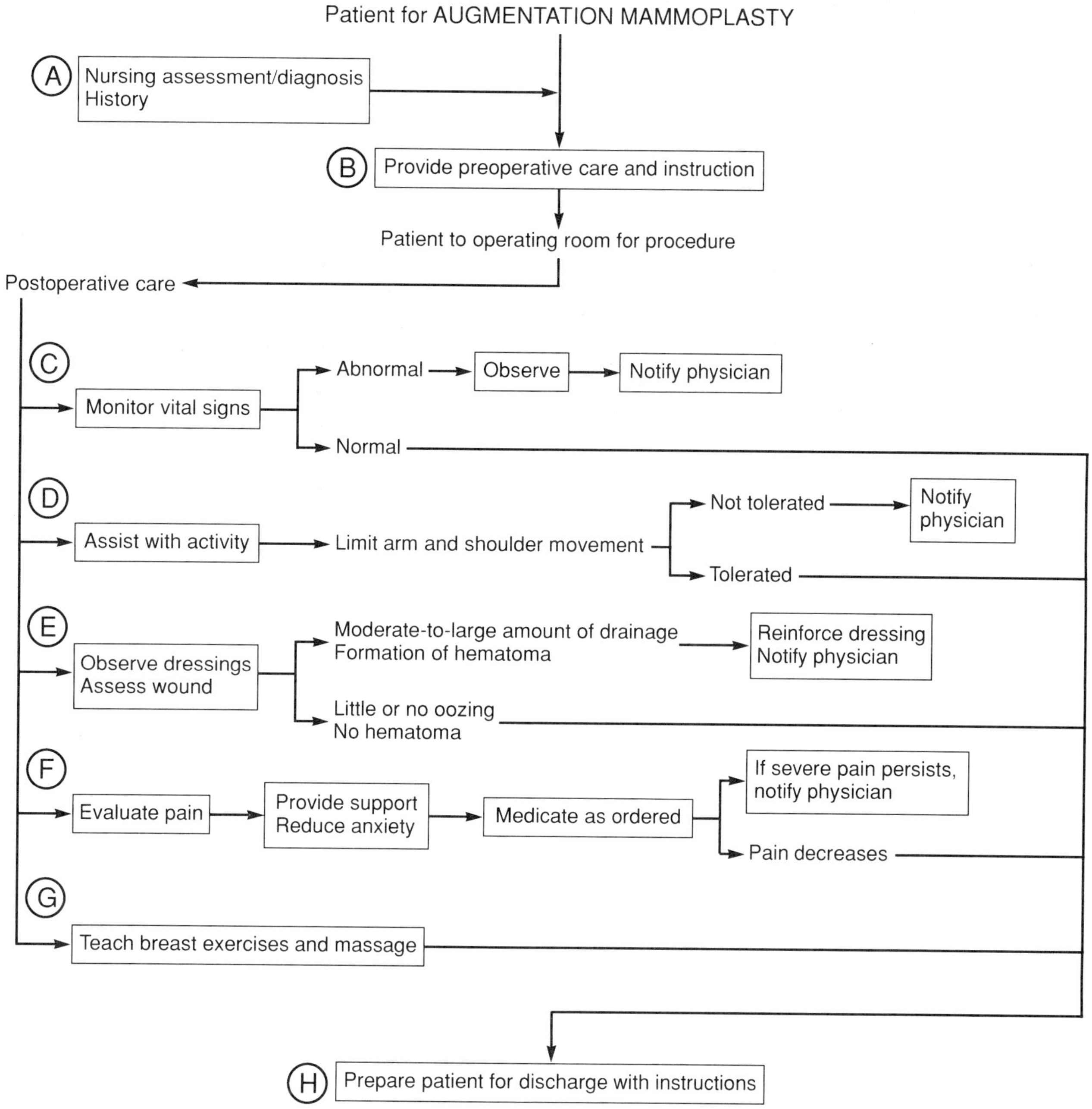
Patient for AUGMENTATION MAMMOPLASTY
A
Nursing assessment/diagnosis
History
B
Provide preoperative care and instruction
Patient to operating room for procedure
Postoperative care
C
Monitor vital signs
Abnormal
Observe
Notify physician
Normal
D
Assist with activity
Limit arm and shoulder movement
Not tolerated
Notify physician
Tolerated
E
Observe dressings
Assess wound
Moderate-to-large amount of drainage
Formation of hematoma
Reinforce dressing
Notify physician
Little or no oozing
No hematoma
F
Evaluate pain
Provide support
Reduce anxiety
Medicate as ordered
If severe pain persists, notify physician
Pain decreases
G
Teach breast exercises and massage
H
Prepare patient for discharge with instructions

REDUCTION MAMMOPLASTY

Chris Kirsch

A. Reduction mammoplasty may be performed in women with extremely large breasts. Large breasts may cause back pain and shoulder discomfort. Pendulous breasts limit physical activity and make fitting of clothing difficult. While the cause of gigantomastia is unknown, hormonal imbalances and familial tendencies have been implicated. In this operation the surgeon makes an incision beneath the breast and a similar curved incision in the skin of the anterior breast. The nipple is transplanted to a new location after redundant tissue is excised. The remaining skin edges are approximated with sutures and the nipple sutured to its new location. Drains are placed in the incision and remain for 1 to 2 days.

B. As in breast augmentation, women seeking breast reduction do so within the realm of psychological need. The nurses' role should be one of emotional support and protection of privacy at all times. A clear understanding that biological function is lost and breast feeding is no longer possible must be made known to patients prior to surgery.

C. Patients receive routine preoperative preparation (p 2) similar to that of the patient undergoing breast augmentation.

D. Initial postoperative care follows that for breast augmentation (p 4).

E. A light compression dressing is in place and must be examined frequently to assure that it is intact, and for bleeding, swelling, discoloration, or extensive hematoma. Drains must be closely observed for patency. Drainage, color, and consistency are also recorded. Drains are generally removed in 24 to 48 hours.

F. The patient must be offered psychological support with respect to her nipple, which may be black and covered by a dry scab. This is to be expected, and after approximately 10 to 14 days, the nipple regains a viable blood supply in its new location.

G. Pain medication is needed initially. Excessive pain may indicate hematoma and should be reported to the physician immediately.

H. Prior to discharge, patients are instructed to wear a brassiere during the night for the first 2 postoperative weeks. Follow-up visits to monitor healing are essential. Breast surgery patients must continue monthly breast self-examination postoperatively. Any unusual findings should be reported promptly to the physician.

References

Brunner LS, Suddarth DS. Textbook of medical-surgical nursing. 6th ed. Philadelphia: JB Lippincott, 1988:1141.

DiNoble C. Reconstructing a self-image: reduction mammoplasty. Today's OR Nurse, 1985; 7(11):18–21.

Georgiadi NG. Reconstructive breast surgery. St. Louis: CV Mosby, 1976.

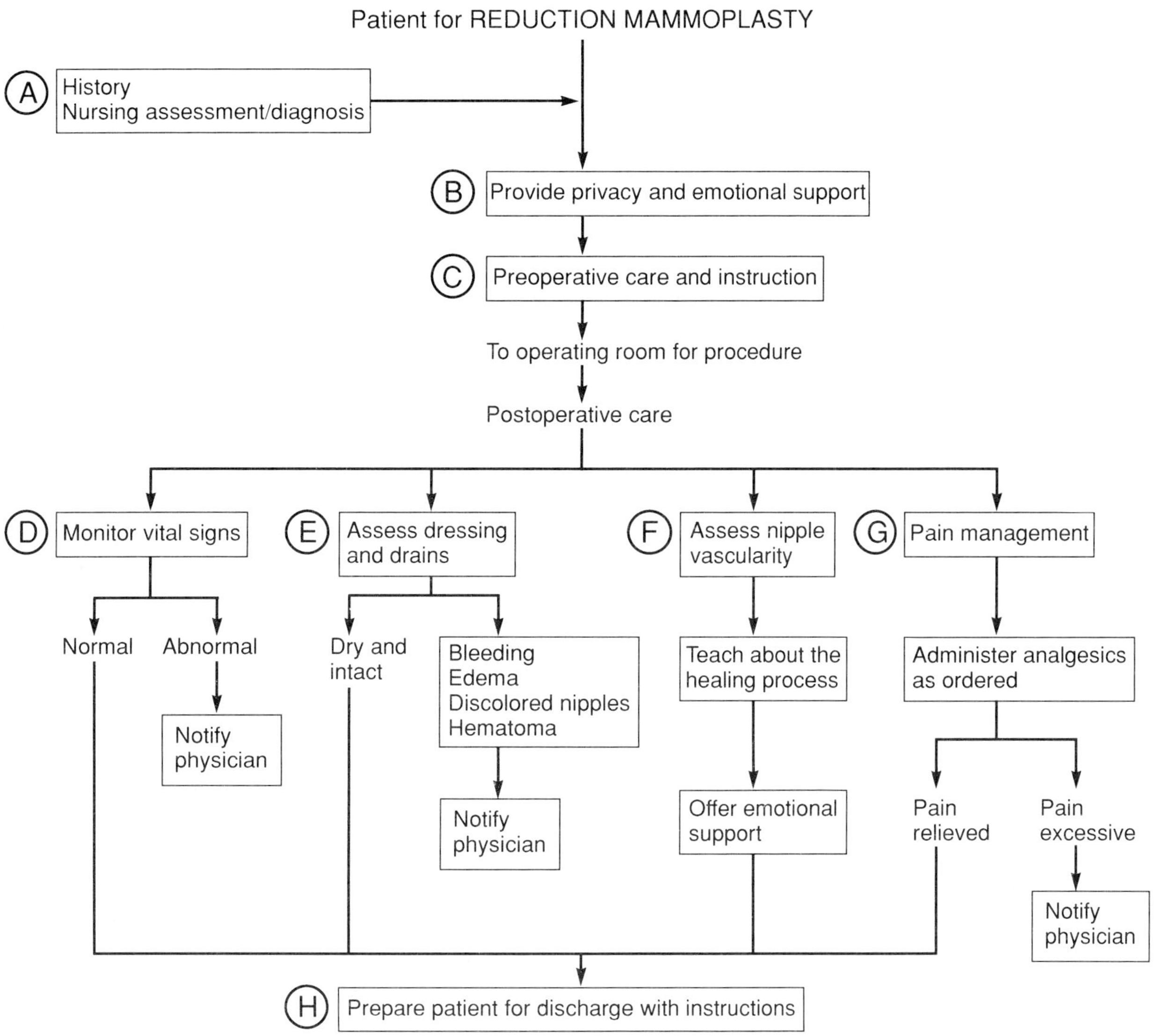
Patient for REDUCTION MAMMOPLASTY
A
History
Nursing assessment/diagnosis
B
Provide privacy and emotional support
C
Preoperative care and instruction
To operating room for procedure
Postoperative care
D
Monitor vital signs
Normal
Abnormal
Notify physician
E
Assess dressing and drains
Dry and intact
Bleeding
Edema
Discolored nipples
Hematoma
Notify physician
F
Assess nipple vascularity
Teach about the healing process
Offer emotional support
G
Pain management
Administer analgesics as ordered
Pain relieved
Pain excessive
Notify physician
H
Prepare patient for discharge with instructions

DILATATION AND CURETTAGE

Nancy A. Young

Dilatation and curettage (D&C), the most frequently performed gynecologic procedure, involves a widening of the cervical canal and scraping of the uterine lining. Indications for a D&C as a therapeutic measure include induced abortion, incomplete spontaneous abortion, removal of hydatidiform mole, retention of placental pieces, and/or correction of excessive or prolonged bleeding from other causes. A D&C can also serve as a diagnostic tool in identifying lesions of the endocervix (p 268) or endometrium.

A. The reasons for performing a D&C vary; therefore, a thorough history should be taken to include a complete menstrual history: menarche and, if applicable, menopause; frequency and duration of menstrual periods; date of last menstrual period; amount of flow; symptoms; and any other bleeding abnormalities. Patient assessment varies because the procedure may be performed on an emergency basis (for hemorrhage or acute pain) or as elective surgery.

B. Preoperative nursing care depends also on the status of the patient. Whenever possible, the nurse should explain the steps involved in the procedure and expectations after surgery. The D&C patient generally requires emotional support, and comfort measures are important for those experiencing pain.

C. The patient may experience some vaginal bleeding; therefore, the number and degree of saturation of vaginal pads should be checked frequently in the first 24 hours. Nursing care includes close monitoring of fluid intake and urine output, because vaginal and cervical packing can exert pressure on the urethra. Excessive bleeding, increased fatigue, changes in blood pressure, and blood counts that could indicate anemia (p 340) and hypovolemia should be reported to the physician. An intravenous line and/or administration of blood products may be indicated to replace fluid volume, and oxytocin may be given to improve uterine contractility.

D. Postoperatively, the patient may experience some cramping and discomfort that should resolve with mild analgesics. Extreme or persistent pain could indicate perforation of the uterus or other trauma and should be reported before administering medications that may mask the symptoms.

E. Postoperative emotions of the D&C patient vary depending on the reason for surgery. Women having therapeutic abortions (p 292) may experience a wide range of feelings from relief to guilt and sadness. The patient with a spontaneous abortion or removal of hydatidiform mole may express shock and disbelief at first and then grief and anger or guilt and blame if the pregnancy was not planned. Women with possible carcinoma usually display fear and anxiety about the possible outcome. For each patient, the nurse can encourage verbalization of feelings and offer a listening and supportive environment and/or the opportunity for privacy to grieve. The patient needs information on short-term physical care and the long-term indications of her diagnosis. In some cases, the nurse can refer patients for additional health care services (infertility, genetic counseling) or to support groups.

F. Most patients are discharged the first day postoperatively. Discharge teaching includes signs and symptoms of infection and potential hemorrhage. The patient should avoid tampons, douches, tub baths, and sexual intercourse for 2 to 3 weeks. She can expect a vaginal discharge and should avoid strenuous activity for at least 1 week. Women with a hydatidiform mole should be followed for at least a year and avoid pregnancy during that period. Rh-negative mothers receive RhoGAM after termination of pregnancy.

References

Lewis SM, Collier JC. Medical-surgical nursing: assessment and management of clinical problems. New York: McGraw-Hill, 1983.

Spillacy WN. Clinical obstetrics and gynecology. Philadelphia: Harper & Row, 1983.

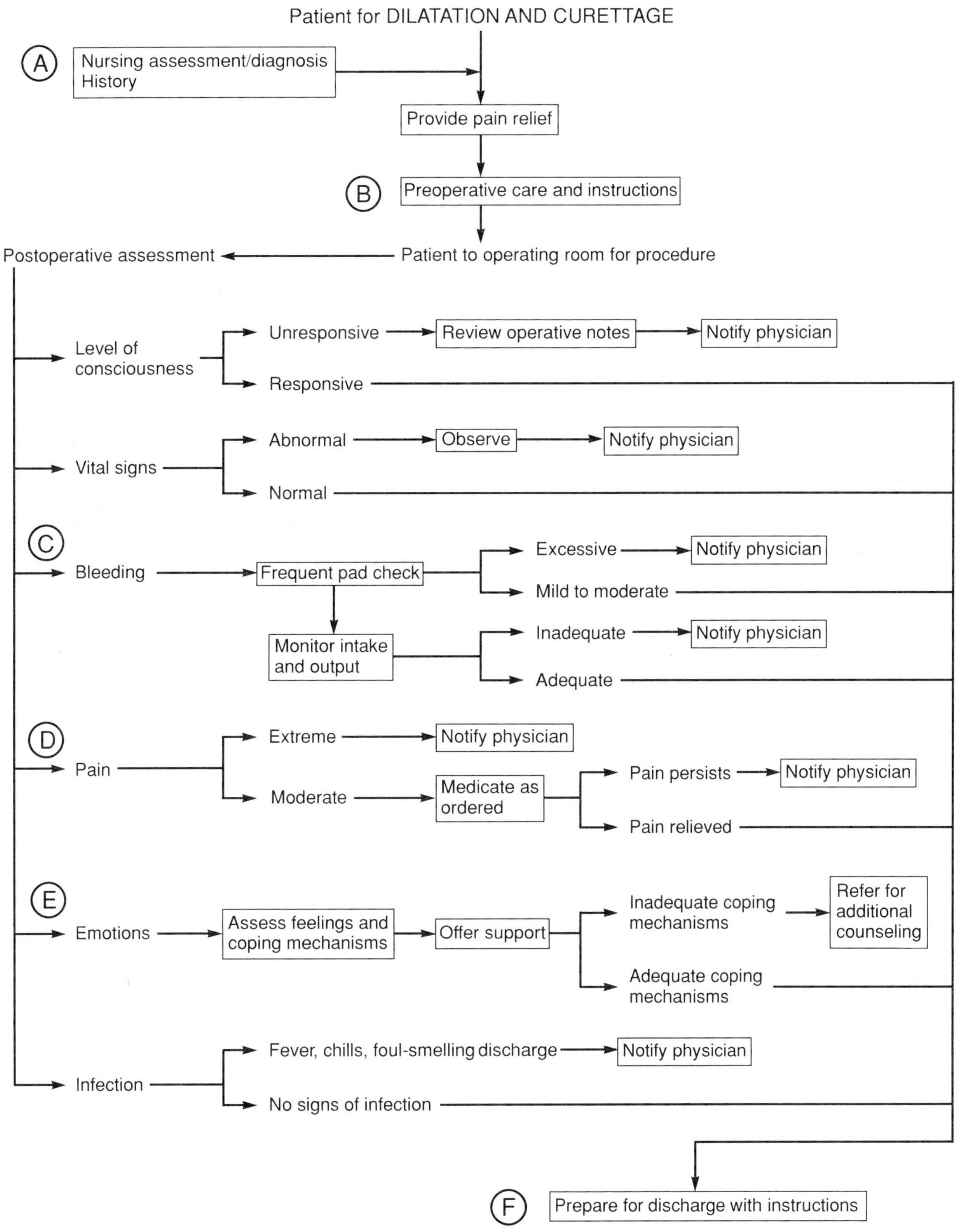
Patient for DILATATION AND CURETTAGE
A
Nursing assessment/diagnosis
History
Provide pain relief
B
Preoperative care and instructions
Patient to operating room for procedure
Postoperative assessment
Level of consciousness
Unresponsive
Review operative notes
Notify physician
Responsive
Vital signs
Abnormal
Observe
Notify physician
Normal
C
Bleeding
Frequent pad check
Excessive
Notify physician
Mild to moderate
Monitor intake and output
Inadequate
Notify physician
Adequate
D
Pain
Extreme
Notify physician
Moderate
Medicate as ordered
Pain persists
Notify physician
Pain relieved
E
Emotions
Assess feelings and coping mechanisms
Offer support
Inadequate coping mechanisms
Refer for additional counseling
Adequate coping mechanisms
Infection
Fever, chills, foul-smelling discharge
Notify physician
No signs of infection
F
Prepare for discharge with instructions

HYSTERECTOMY

Paula K. Ovens
Pamela Y. Donnelly
Joy Gorzeman

Hysterectomy is the surgical removal of the uterus. The procedure may be indicated to aid in the diagnosis and treatment of endometriosis, fibroids, pelvic inflammatory disease (p 260), dysfunctional uterine bleeding (p 264), and cancer (p 272). There is controversy about the number of hysterectomies performed and whether some may be done unnecessarily. Women may wish to seek a second opinion before consenting to surgery.

A. These women usually have a history that includes painful menstruation, irregular menses, and/or infertility. Usually they have consulted their physician and tried other treatments before consenting to surgery. Depending on the cause, some women may look forward to relief of their symptoms, while others will regret the loss of the reproductive organs.

B. Women undergoing hysterectomy may experience hormonal imbalances. They may exhibit depression and heightened emotional sensitivity to people and situations. Preoperative preparation should include listening to the patient's fears and concerns. The patient and/or significant other may have questions about reproductive and sexual functions. Patients need to be told they will no longer have menstrual periods. Additional preparation should include information about anesthesia (spinal or general); an enema; a preoperative pubic area shave; and for vaginal hysterectomies, a douche and prophylactic antibiotics. Other preparation is similar to that for other general surgeries (p 2). In the assessment process these patients may have had many of the following tests and procedures: Papanicolaou smear, endometrial biopsy, coloscopy, curettage, and cone biopsy. Laboratory studies also need to be done. If invasive cancer is suspected, intravenous pyelography (IVP) and barium enema may be ordered.

C. The surgery can be performed vaginally or abdominally. The approach used depends on the disease process and the patient's and physician's preferences. The vaginal approach is often used if repair of cystocele or rectocele is needed. This approach has some advantages over the abdominal, including: (1) shorter procedure with very little anesthesia, (2) a quicker recovery period, and (3) usually less discomfort. Because infection is a greater risk in the vaginal approach, prophylactic antibiotics are given preoperatively. A total hysterectomy (removal of the entire uterus and cervix) is almost always done abdominally and is most common. When the fallopian tubes are removed (salpingectomy) and ovaries are removed (oophorectomy) in addition to the uterus and cervix, the procedure is called hysterectomy with bilateral salpingo-oophorectomy or panhysterectomy. Partial hysterectomy is removal of the uterus only and leaves the cervix in place. This procedure is no longer as common as in the past.

D. Postoperative care is the same as that for most other major surgeries (p 4) and is almost the same for either the vaginal or abdominal approach. The abundant blood supply in the pelvic area predisposes to a high risk of bleeding after hysterectomy, especially during the first 24 hours.

E. The patient who has had the vaginal approach has a perineal pad. A small to moderate amount of pink, yellow, or brown serous drainage is normal. Even a small amount of frank blood may be normal. However, heavy bleeding should be reported to the physician. Bleeding accompanied by a distended abdomen, referred shoulder pain, and shock indicates the need to return to surgery.

F. Abdominal dressings (abdominal approach) should be assessed frequently. Excessive bleeding or drainage should be documented and reported. A drain inserted during surgery may increase drainage. The incision should be assessed during dressing changes. Persistent seepage of serosanguinous drainage increases the risk of wound dehiscence. A heat lamp may help a slow-healing incision. Vaginal drainage must also be carefully monitored.

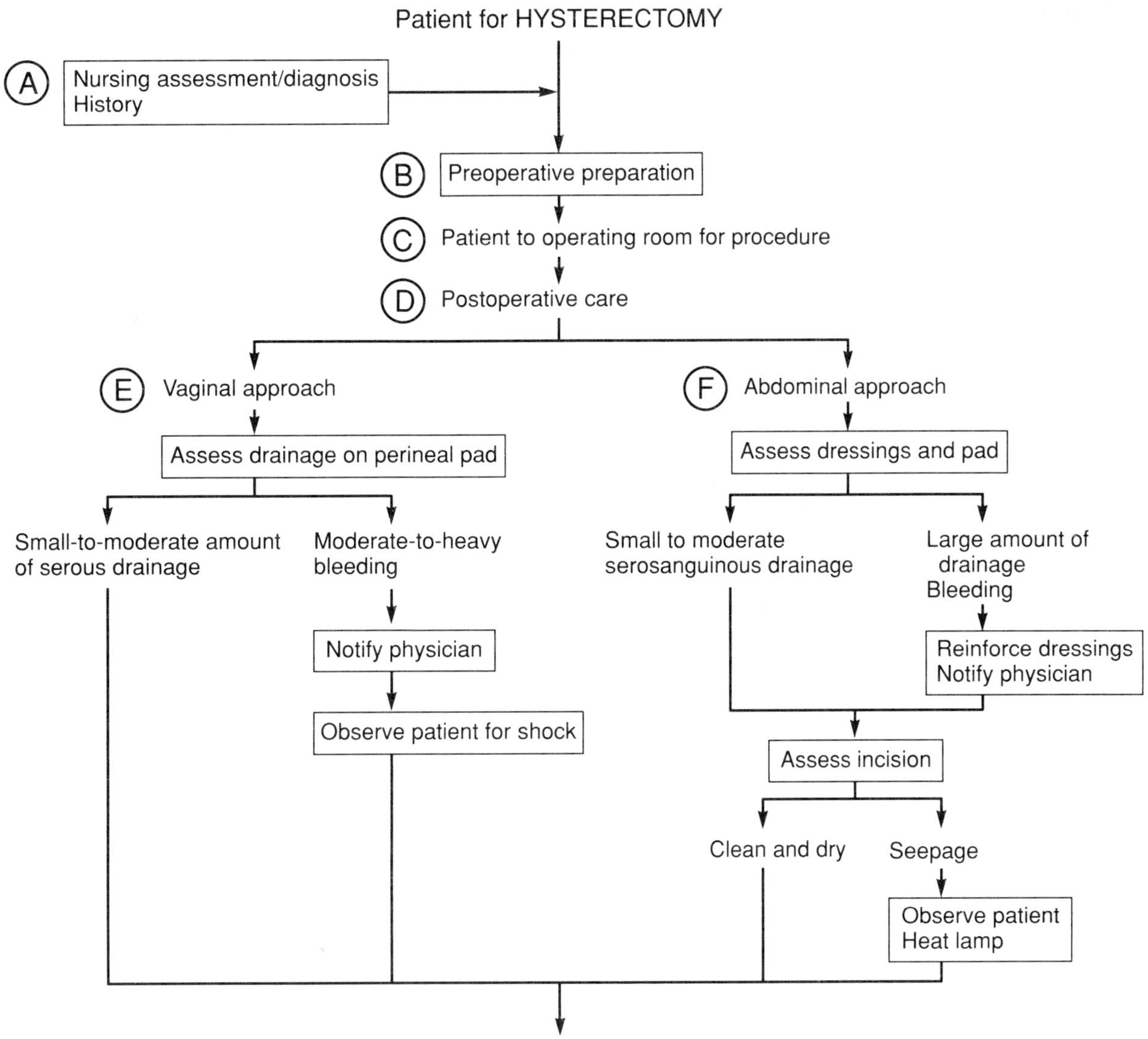

(Cont'd on p 287)

G. Aseptic technique should be maintained with catheter care, and output should be recorded after the catheter is removed. Decreased output together with low or lateral back pain may indicate accidental ligation of a ureter during surgery and warrants close observation. Urinary infections are more common after vaginal hysterectomies.

H. Gastrointestinal function is slower to return in patients with abdominal hysterectomies. Diet may be increased as tolerated, based on return of intestinal peristalsis. Ambulation may relieve gas pains related to gastrointestinal function. All patients should be ambulating within 12 hours following surgery.

I. Other postoperative considerations for patients with either approach include prevention of complications and thrombophlebitis, pain management, ambulation, and discharge teaching. Patients must be encouraged to turn, cough, and deep breathe to prevent respiratory complications. Abdominal splinting with pillows may relieve discomfort related to coughing. Early ambulation helps prevent thrombophlebitis. Antiembolic hose may also benefit patients at higher risk for developing circulatory complications. Pain may be relieved by sitz baths, back rubs, and/or heating pads. Pain medication may be given as needed.

J. Discharge teaching includes instructions to avoid lifting and other strenuous activities (vacuuming) for 6 to 8 weeks. Douching and sexual intercourse are discouraged for at least 4 to 6 weeks. Fever, bleeding, or increased drainage should be reported to the physician. Showers are permitted, but tub baths are discouraged until healing is complete. Follow-up care and clearance for activities are essential. If the patient is placed on hormone replacement therapy, medication instructions should be reinforced. The patient and family should also be reminded that hormonal changes may cause mood swings and crying spells. Emotional support is needed during these adjustments. If cancer or other disease processes are present, chemotherapy or other treatment may be needed.

References

Benson RC. Handbook of obstetrics and gynecology. 8th ed. Los Altos, CA: Lange, 1983:446.

Berkow R, ed. The Merck manual. 14th ed. Rahway, NJ: Merck, Sharp and Dohme Research Laboratories, 1982: II:70.

Jenson JD, Benson RD, Bobak IN. Maternity care: a nurse and the family. St. Louis: CV Mosby, 1981:76, 401.

Luckmann J, Sorenson KC. Medical-surgical nursing: a psychophysiologic approach. 3rd ed. Philadelphia: WB Saunders, 1987:1786–1788.

Pritchard JA, MacDonald PC, Gant NF. Williams obstetrics. 17th ed. Norwalk, CT: Appleton-Century-Crofts, 1985: 879–881.

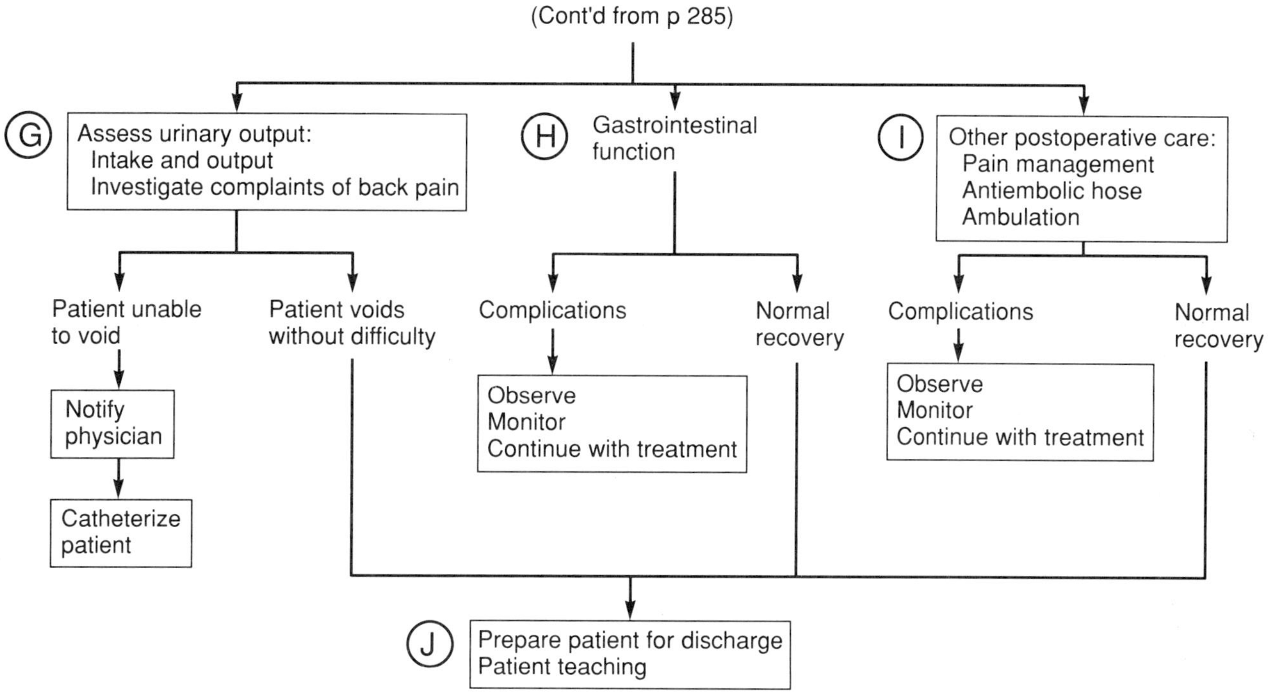
(Cont'd from p 285)
G
Assess urinary output:
Intake and output
Investigate complaints of back pain
Patient unable to void
Notify physician
Catheterize patient
Patient voids without difficulty
H
Gastrointestinal function
Complications
Observe
Monitor
Continue with treatment
Normal recovery
I
Other postoperative care:
Pain management
Antiembolic hose
Ambulation
Complications
Observe
Monitor
Continue with treatment
Normal recovery
J
Prepare patient for discharge
Patient teaching

LAPAROSCOPY

Paula K. Ovens
Pamela Y. Donnelly

Laparoscopy is a surgical procedure used to diagnose, evaluate, and/or treat many gynecologic conditions. The procedure involves inserting a metal cannula into the abdomen via a stab wound beneath the umbilicus, which allows the physician to visualize the pelvic cavity directly. Very small instruments can then be passed through the cannula as needed. Laparoscopy may be used to diagnose the cause of pelvic pain, presence of an unruptured ectopic pregnancy, and to confirm the extent of endometriosis or pelvic inflammatory disease (PID) (p 260). Infertile patients may benefit from laparoscopy. This is also the method for performing a tubal ligation (p 290). Most often this procedure is elective and performed as day surgery.

A. A woman may present with varying clinical symptoms. The nursing history and assessment must include the client's reproductive history (menstrual, gynecologic, and obstetric). Menstrual history includes age at menarche and menopause if applicable, date of last menstrual cycle, usual amount of flow, and presence of dysmenorrhea, menorrhagia, or metrorrhagia. The nurse seeks gynecologic data regarding presence and characteristics of vaginal discharge, vaginal pruritus, and type of birth control used. Preventive health practices such as routine breast and Pap smear examinations should be queried. Obstetric data should reflect the number of pregnancies, births, abortions, miscarriages, or stillbirths. Questions related to the client's sexual attitudes and practices may also be explored if appropriate. The client should be questioned about prior surgeries because adhesions and scarring interfere with passage of the laparoscope.

B. Preadmission nursing instructions should be provided when the procedure is scheduled (usually 2 days or more before surgery). The instructions should include not eating or drinking anything after midnight the night before surgery, removing nail polish, and taking a complete bath with bacteriostatic soap (e.g., PhisoHex) the night before surgery.

C. Preoperative nursing care includes (1) providing time for the patient to discuss psychological or emotional concerns related to surgery; (2) providing positive support for their decision to proceed with the procedure; (3) answering questions about anesthesia; (4) ensuring adequate decompression of the abdomen (emptying of the bowel and bladder); and (5) patient teaching regarding the expectations after surgery (turning, coughing, deep breathing, ambulation, expected normal incisional pain, pain medication, and discharge).

D. Postoperative nursing care is directed at preventing complications secondary to anesthesia. Vital signs and other assessments are done at least every 15 minutes and more frequently if indicated.

E. Observe the Band-Aid or small abdominal dressing. Report moderate to large amounts of oozing to the physician immediately. Little to no bleeding should be observed. Cramping and feeling bloated are common after laparoscopy. Shoulder pain may also be experienced.

F. Administer pain medication as needed. Encourage the patient to cough and deep breath.

G. Check the patient's bladder for distention. If the patient has not voided within an hour postoperatively, notify the physician. The patient must void prior to discharge.

H. The timing of ambulation depends on the type of anesthesia used. Frequently, general anesthesia is preferred for this procedure. Early ambulation (within 4 to 6 hours) is encouraged since same-day discharge is common.

I. If there are no complications, the patient is discharged with specific instructions. The Band-Aid should be left in place for 3 to 4 days, but is replaced if it gets wet when showering. Swimming and tub baths are allowed in 5 to 6 days. After 3 to 4 days, the incision can be treated as any other cut. Full physical activity is allowed as soon as the patient feels up to it.

References

Benson RC, ed. Handbook of obstetrics and gynecology. 8th ed. Los Altos, CA: Lange, 1983.

Billings DM, Stokes LG, eds. Medical-surgical nursing: common health problems of adults and children across the lifespan. 2nd ed. St. Louis: CV Mosby, 1987.

Egdahf RH, ed. Manual of gynecologic surgery. 2nd ed. Masterson and Byron, 1986.

Hulka JF Textbook of laparoscopy. Orlando: Grune & Stratton, 1986.

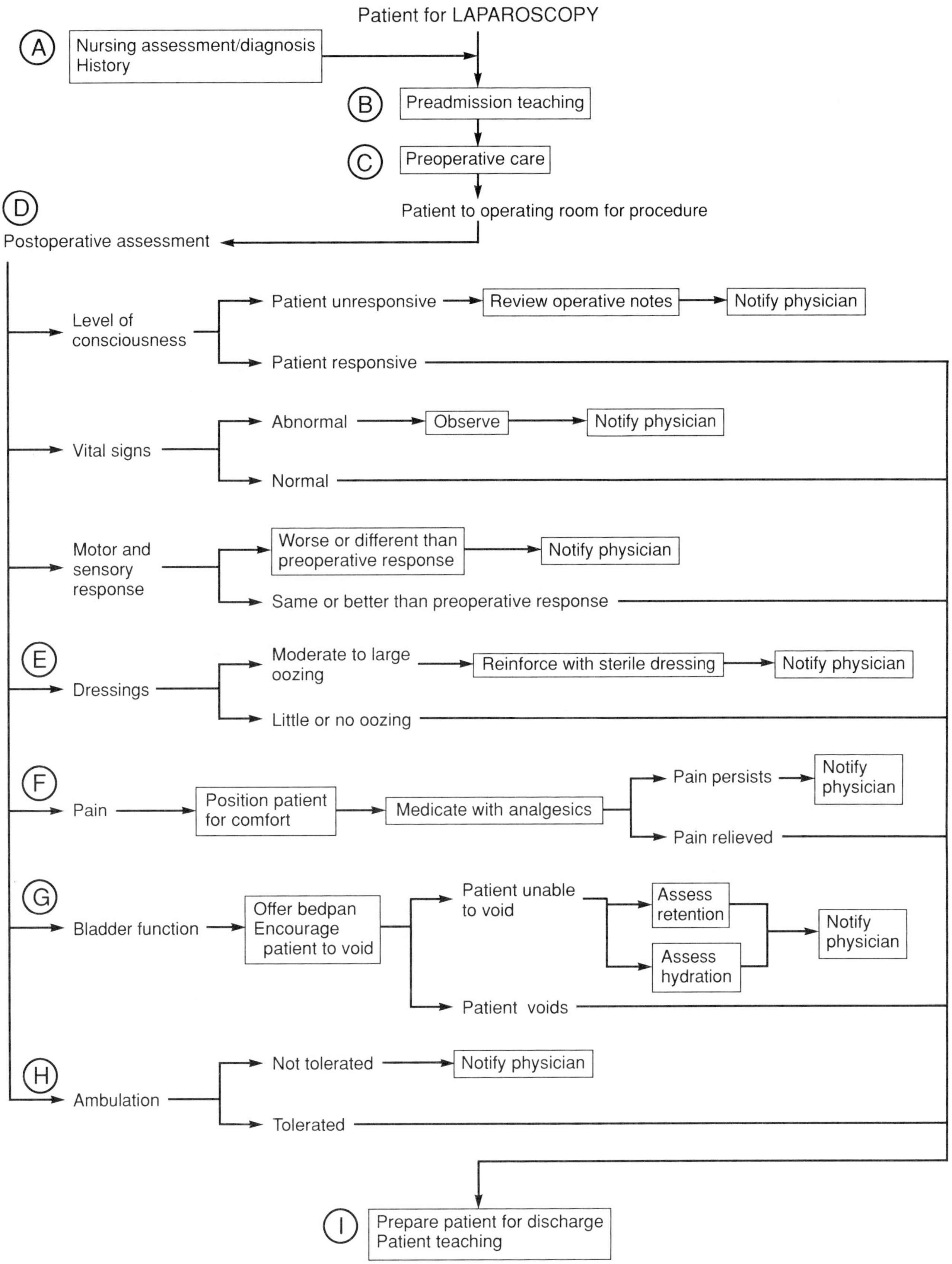
Patient for LAPAROSCOPY
A
Nursing assessment/diagnosis
History
B
Preadmission teaching
C
Preoperative care
Patient to operating room for procedure
D
Postoperative assessment
Level of consciousness
Patient unresponsive
Review operative notes
Notify physician
Patient responsive
Vital signs
Abnormal
Observe
Notify physician
Normal
Motor and sensory response
Worse or different than preoperative response
Notify physician
Same or better than preoperative response
E
Dressings
Moderate to large oozing
Reinforce with sterile dressing
Notify physician
Little or no oozing
F
Pain
Position patient for comfort
Medicate with analgesics
Pain persists
Notify physician
Pain relieved
G
Bladder function
Offer bedpan
Encourage patient to void
Patient unable to void
Assess retention
Assess hydration
Notify physician
Patient voids
H
Ambulation
Not tolerated
Notify physician
Tolerated
I
Prepare patient for discharge
Patient teaching

TUBAL LIGATION

Paula K. Ovens
Pamela Y. Donnelly

Bilateral tubal ligation is a surgical procedure performed on women to prevent conception. The procedure disrupts tubal patency, preventing fertilization of ova. Tubal sterilization is often done on an outpatient basis ("band-aid surgery") or in-hospital during the postpartum period. The fallopian tubes may be approached by abdominal incision, by laparoscopic visualization (p 288), or through the vagina. The technique used is determined by patient and physician preference in addition to history. Tubal sterilization should always be considered irreversible. Restitution of tubal continuity is technically feasible, but the success rate is unknown. If any doubts exist regarding the desire for future childbearing, the procedure should not be performed.

A. The woman requests permanent sterilization because (1) she does not want any more children or (2) she has a disease process that would complicate a pregnancy, possibly leading to a life-threatening condition.

B. Preoperative nursing care includes providing time for the patient and spouse to discuss psychological and emotional implications of permanent sterilization, providing positive support for the decision, answering questions about the surgery, and giving instructions about postoperative care.

C. Postoperative nursing care is directed at preventing complications such as hemorrhage, infection, and pulmonary embolism (p 116). Vital signs and assessments are done at least every 15 minutes and more frequently if indicated.

D. Abdominal dressing(s) (abdominal incision, laparoscopic approach) should be observed for bleeding. Moderate to large amounts of bleeding should be reported to the physician immediately. The perineal area should be examined for any bleeding if a vaginal tubal ligation was performed. Normally, minimal bleeding should be seen.

E. Pain medication should be administered as needed. Encourage the patient to cough and deep breathe. Positioning may also promote comfort.

F. Check the patient's bladder for distention. If the patient has not voided within 4 hours postoperatively, the physician should be notified.

G. The timing of ambulation depends on the type of anesthesia used. All patients should be ambulating within 12 hours after the procedure.

H. If there are no complications, the patient is discharged with specific instructions to include signs and symptoms of wound infection that should be reported immediately. Explain that libido will not be affected. Sexual intercourse can resume usually within 1 week or as tolerated. Condoms and foam should be used until the first menses following surgery, unless midcycle tubal ligation was performed. Full activity is allowed as tolerated.

References

Benson RC. Handbook of obstetrics and gynecology. 8th ed. Los Altos, CA: Lange, 1983:448–453.

Berkow R, ed. The Merck manual. 14th ed. Rahway, NJ: Merck, Sharp, & Dohme, 1982:69.

Jenson MD, Benson RD, Bobak IN. Maternity care: a nurse and the family. St. Louis: CV Mosby, 1981:75–76.

Pritchard JA, MacDonald PC, Gant NF. Williams obstetrics. 17th ed. Norwalk, CT: Appleton-Century-Crofts, 1985:827–831.

Tucker SM. Female reproductive system. In: Thompson JM, MacFarland GK, Hirsch JE, Tucker SM, Bowers AC. Clinical nursing. St. Louis: CV Mosby, 1986:997–1000, 1029.

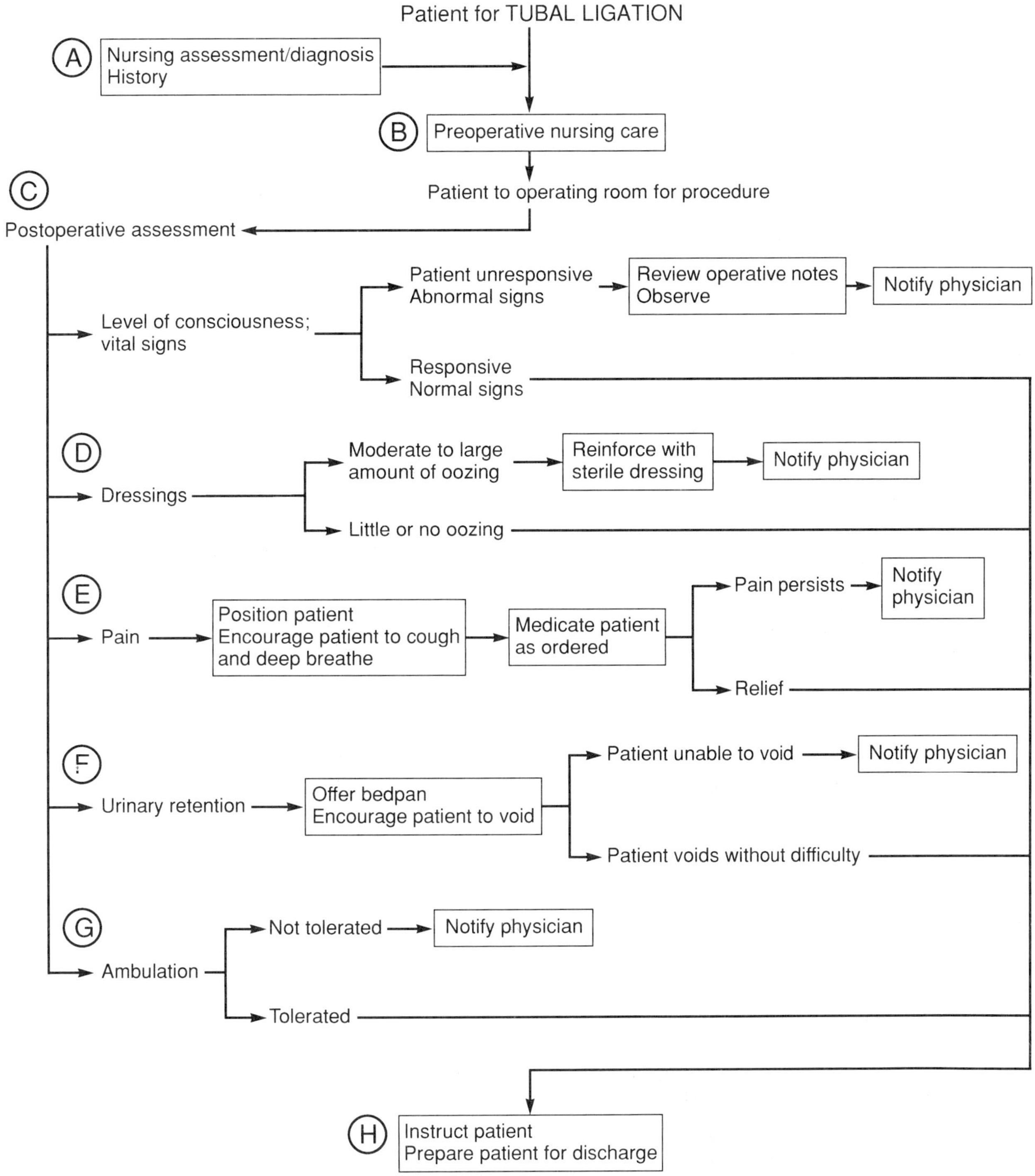
Patient for TUBAL LIGATION
A
Nursing assessment/diagnosis
History
B
Preoperative nursing care
Patient to operating room for procedure
C
Postoperative assessment
Level of consciousness; vital signs
Patient unresponsive
Abnormal signs
Review operative notes
Observe
Notify physician
Responsive
Normal signs
D
Dressings
Moderate to large amount of oozing
Reinforce with sterile dressing
Notify physician
Little or no oozing
E
Pain
Position patient
Encourage patient to cough and deep breathe
Medicate patient as ordered
Pain persists
Notify physician
Relief
F
Urinary retention
Offer bedpan
Encourage patient to void
Patient unable to void
Notify physician
Patient voids without difficulty
G
Ambulation
Not tolerated
Notify physician
Tolerated
H
Instruct patient
Prepare patient for discharge

SPONTANEOUS ABORTION

Nancy A. Young

Abortion is the termination of pregnancy prior to the twentieth week of gestation, before the fetus has attained viability outside the uterus. Some providers also use the criterion of a birth weight of 500 g (1.1 pounds). (Spontaneous interruption of a pregnancy between 20 and 28 weeks is commonly referred to as a miscarriage.) Abortion represents the most common emergency in early pregnancy, with one pregnancy in every five to seven terminating in spontaneous abortion. The factors that predispose to spontaneous abortion include abnormal development of ova or sperm cells, defects in fetus or placenta, low progesterone levels, uterine abnormalities or incompetent cervix, acute infections, environmental or workplace hazards, and maternal systemic diseases.

A. Considering the variety of causes for spontaneous abortion, the nurse should document a thorough history and assess each hospitalized patient carefully before determining a care plan. History should include the data of the last menstrual period, amount of bleeding, abdominal cramping, and passage of tissue. The patient should be questioned regarding familial history of miscarriage, recent injury or fall, and past gynecologic history. Women who habitually miscarry (three or more times) should investigate treatment for the possible causes through referral to appropriate resources. A septic abortion occurs from unskilled instrumentation of, or chemicals introduced into, the uterus to induce abortion. The septicemia and endotoxic shock that result can lead to death (p 70) unless early appropriate medical treatment is instituted.

B. The nursing assessment includes vital signs, a pregnancy test, and initiating a pad count to assess bleeding. In a threatened abortion (less than 24 weeks' gestation), the patient usually complains of mild abdominal cramping and vaginal spotting or bleeding. The cervix remains undilated (Fig. 1A).

C. The treatment for spontaneous abortion varies. Some women who threaten to abort may respond to management with bedrest and tocolytic drugs, but others progress to inevitable expulsion of the fetus.

D. The patient with an incomplete or inevitable abortion has abdominal pain accompanied by frank bleeding, a dilated cervix, and possible expulsion of fetal tissue (Fig. 1B). Patients may experience labor and require emotional and physical support during this time. The potential for infection can be reduced by adhering to aseptic conditions for all examinations, administering antibiotics as ordered, and observing for any signs of infection. Most women express grief with a pregnancy loss and require emotional support. Grief may be accentuated for those with a missed abortion who have carried the dead fetus for a period of time before delivery (Fig. 1C). Prompt passage of the fetus reduces the possibility of developing disseminated intravascular coagulation (p 348) or infection.

E. Incomplete abortions (fetus expelled but placenta and membranes retained) (Fig. 1D) require a dilatation and

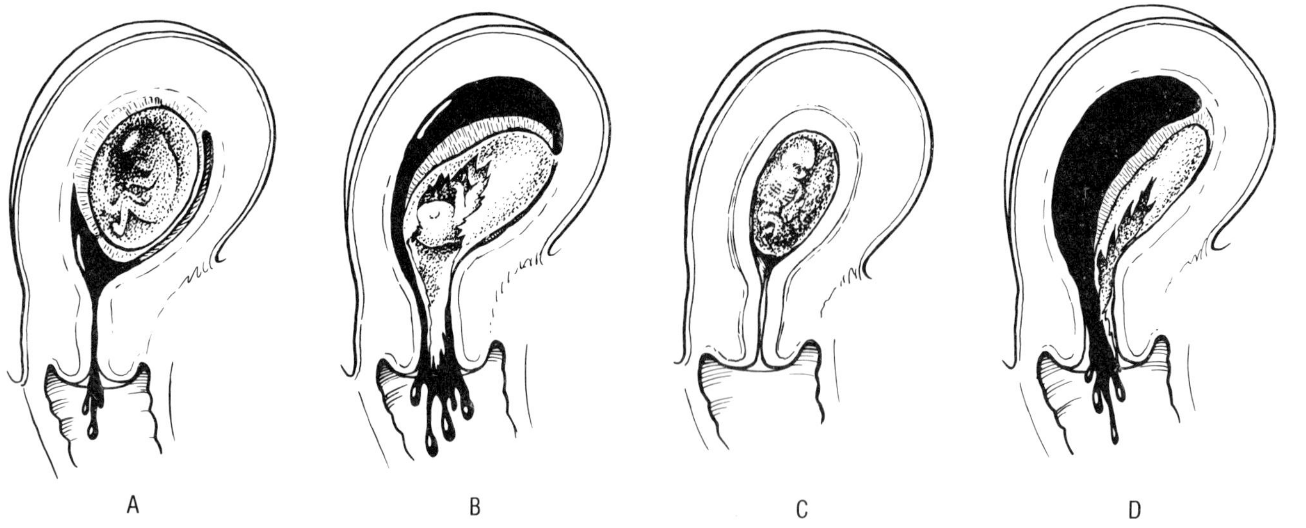

Figure 1 Types of abortion: *A*, threatened; *B*, inevitable; *C*, missed; and *D*, incomplete.

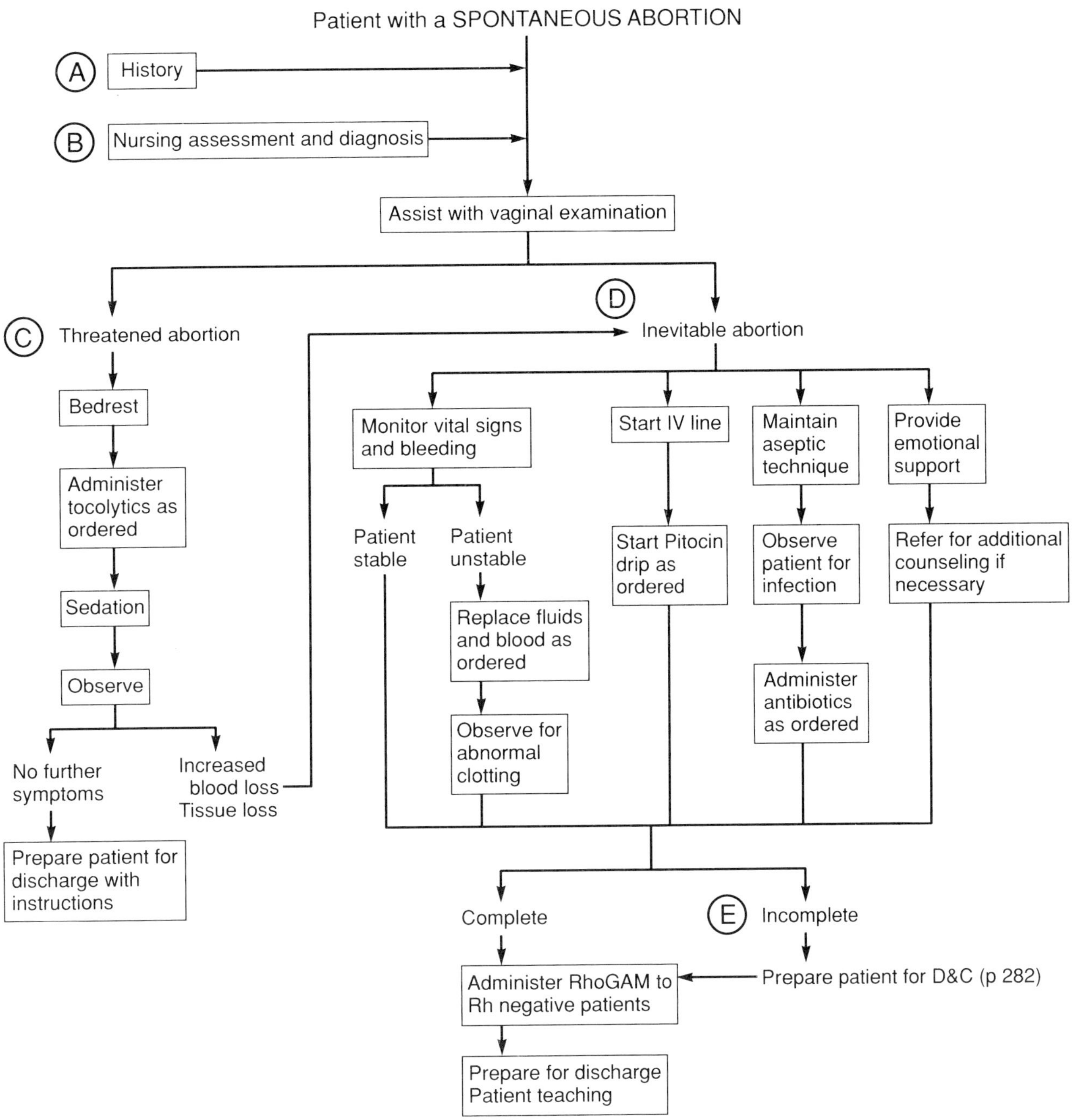

curettage (D&C) (p 282). Oxytocin may be prescribed to contract the fundus before a D&C is performed. Mothers with Rh negative blood receive RhoGAM prior to discharge. The nurse should instruct the patient about signs of potential infection and bleeding abnormalities. Women who require services for treatment of the causes of abortion or additional emotional support should be appropriately referred.

References

Brunner LS, Suddarth DS. The Lippincott manual of nursing practice. 4th ed. Philadelphia: JB Lippincott, 1988.

Hopper B. Abortion. In: Mancini ME, ed. Decision making in emergency nursing. Toronto: BC Decker, 1987:136–137.

Warner CG. Emergency care assessment and intervention. St. Louis: CV Mosby, 1983.

PROSTATIC CANCER

Joy Gorzeman

A. Cancer of the prostate is the second most common cause of death from cancer in men. It is most commonly seen in men over 50 years of age. Several factors may be related to the cause of prostatic cancer, including familial tendency, a history of multiple sex partners, premature cessation of sexual activity, and environmental factors. Studies have shown that the younger the patient, the more aggressive the cancer. Early diagnosis leads to a much higher treatment success rate. Many prostate tumors are found during the rectal examination of a routine physical. This makes annual physical examinations imperative for men over 40 to 50 years of age. Clinical manifestations of prostatic cancer are similar to those of prostatitis: urinary frequency, dysuria, slow stream, and sometimes urinary retention. Some patients complain of low back, hip, and leg pain. This may indicate metastasis to the bones.

B. Once a prostatic nodule has been found, further diagnostic studies are done to identify the extent of the disease. Laboratory studies show an increased serum acid phosphatase level if the cancer has spread outside the prostate. An elevated alkaline phosphatase level goes along with bone metastasis.

C. Radiologic studies include a bone scan and skeletal films to detect metastasis. Other tests such lymphangiography and pelvic lymphadenectomy may be done to determine the spread of the cancer.

D. Actual diagnosis of prostatic cancer is made through biopsy.

E. The method of treatment depends on how far the cancer has advanced. A radical prostatectomy (p 302) is usually successful if the cancer is localized in the prostate area. Other interventions include radiation therapy, hormone therapy, and chemotherapy (p 408).

F. Radiation therapy may be done by external beam or implant. The patient may experience side effects, such as diarrhea, loss of appetite, and impotence.

G. Hormone (endocrine) therapy is utilized when the cancer is inoperable or if there are signs of metastasis after surgery. In addition, an orchiectomy will probably be performed. The purpose of hormone therapy is to suppress and/or eliminate the main source of androgen production, thus slowing progression of the disease. Patients on hormone therapy should be aware of the possible side effects of the medication. Nausea and enlargement of the male breast are common. Fluid retention and cardiovascular problems should be reported to the physician immediately.

H. Chemotherapy (cytotoxic drugs) is not usually effective for prostatic cancers, but may be tried as a palliative treatment for advanced cancers.

I. As with other chronic illnesses, the patient and family will need emotional support as they adjust to a life-threatening disease that will indeed affect their lifestyle. Depending on the type of treatment, the patient will be discharged with instructions for medical follow-up.

References

Brunner LS, Suddarth DS. The Lippincott manual of nursing practice. 4th ed. Philadelphia: JB Lippincott, 1986.

Luckmann J, Sorensen KC. Medical-surgical nursing: a psychophysiologic approach. 3rd ed. Philadelphia: WB Saunders, 1987.

Phipps WJ, Long BC, Woods NF. Medical-surgical nursing: concepts and clinical practice. 3rd ed. St. Louis: CV Mosby, 1987.

Thompson J, McFarland G, Hirsch J, Tucker S, Bowers A. Clinical nursing. St. Louis: CV Mosby, 1986.

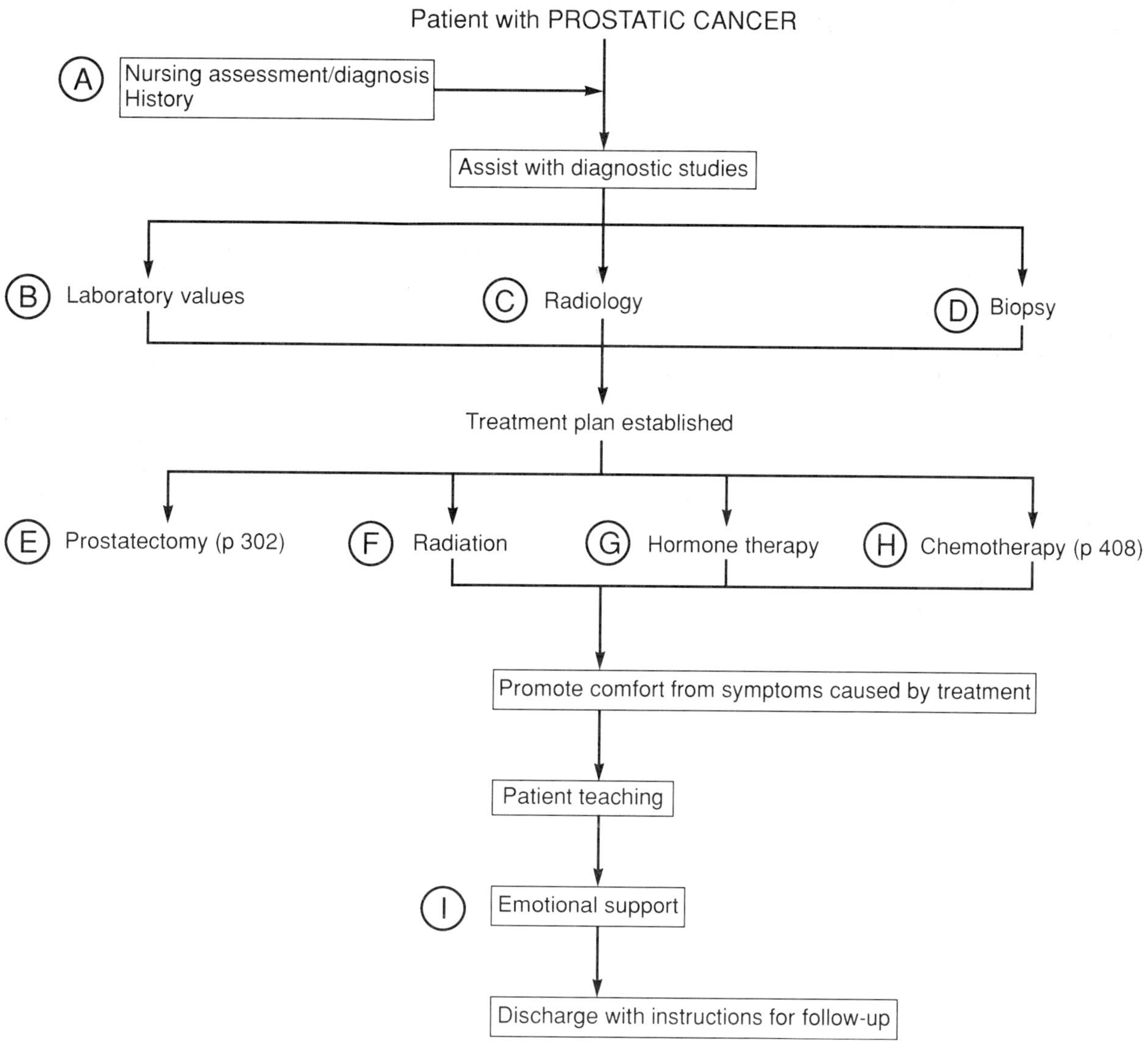
Patient with PROSTATIC CANCER
A
Nursing assessment/diagnosis
History
Assist with diagnostic studies
B
Laboratory values
C
Radiology
D
Biopsy
Treatment plan established
E
Prostatectomy (p 302)
F
Radiation
G
Hormone therapy
H
Chemotherapy (p 408)
Promote comfort from symptoms caused by treatment
Patient teaching
I
Emotional support
Discharge with instructions for follow-up

TESTICULAR CANCER

Nina McIntosh

Testicular cancer represents only 1 percent of all cancers diagnosed in men, yet it is the leading cause of death from cancer in males between 20 and 40 years of age. The cause is unknown; however, the incidence of these tumors is much higher in males who have had cryptorchidism, a developmental defect in which the testes fail to descend into the scrotum. If detected early, the overall cure rate is very good with certain cell types.

A. Testicular tumors may have a slow or rapid onset, depending on the type. The patient may have a lump in his scrotum, enlargement, or a heavy feeling in one testicle. He may also have some swelling of the scrotum from an accumulation of fluid or blood. Only about 20 percent of cases involve any pain. Back pain or gynecomastia is associated with metastasis. *Note: Because of the increased risk, it is extremely important to assess for a history of cryptorchidism.*

B. Laboratory studies are done to rule out other conditions that might cause the symptoms associated with testicular cancer. Patients with malignant testicular tumors often have elevated alpha-fetoprotein and human chorionic gonadotropin blood levels. A chest film is taken to look for signs of mediastinal or pulmonary involvement. Computerized tomographic (CT) scanning is done to look for visual evidence of tumors in the mediastinum, lungs, lymphatic chains, and abdomen.

C. An orchiectomy is done to excise the primary tumor and to establish the diagnosis. Although orchiectomy reduces the patient's sperm count by 50 percent, it does not affect his ability to have normal intercourse or reproduce. However, additional treatments can further decrease fertility. Therefore, the patient should be informed of the option to store his sperm in a sperm bank before surgery.

D. Postoperative physical care is routine (p 4). Check vital signs frequently for the first 24 hours, and observe the wound for signs of infection.

E. Encourage the patient to cough and deep breathe, and take measures to decrease the pain and discomfort. The inguinal incision should be supported (hold a pillow tightly against it) and pain medication given as ordered. Ambulation is encouraged within 24 hours after surgery. Observe the patient closely for urinary retention.

F. Testicular cancer strikes primarily young men, at a time when they are trying to establish and maintain young families. Give the patient the information needed to maintain a realistic sense of sexual capacities. The strain is difficult on a young couple. There are many support groups that can help.

G. Seminomatous tumors account for 40 percent of testicular tumors. If the patient has no evidence of metastasis from earlier diagnostic work-ups, radiation therapy is usually given as a precaution. The patient starts daily radiation in the hospital and continues it as an outpatient.

H. Nursing care focuses on emotional support and controlling side effects. Radiotherapy commonly causes skin irritation, fatigue, mild nausea and vomiting, and decreased red and white blood cells and platelets. The patient should be instructed not to apply any creams, lotions, or powders not approved by the radiologist. He should wear loose-fitting clothing to avoid friction on sensitive skin. Bland foods, small meals, and antiemetics help control nausea and vomiting. Blood counts should be monitored closely. The patient should be told there will be no sperm for up to 18 months following the radiation treatments.

I. Lymphadenectomy is the most common type of surgery for removing tumors that have metastasized to the retroperitoneal lymph nodes. Because of pain and fear of breaking open the abdominal sutures, these patients need extra support and encouragement postoperatively. The patient still has erections, but may develop retrograde ejaculation and a low sperm count.

J. The patient who has a nonseminoma tumor or whose cancer has spread beyond the retroperitoneal lymph nodes will probably receive chemotherapy (p 408). Eighty percent of these patients obtain complete remissions, and 70 to 75 percent are cured. The side effects from chemotherapy are unpleasant and sometimes seem unbearable to these young men. The patient needs a great deal of support and understanding. The patient may become infertile because of a low sperm count and damaged sperm. Chemotherapy also lowers the blood counts, exposing the patient to increased risk of infection and bleeding.

K. Once remission occurs, the patient must be encouraged to return for regular follow up. The anxiety of waiting for possible recurrence during this time may cause depression, hostility, or withdrawal. Support mechanisms are imperative at this point.

References

Burns N. Nursing and cancer. Philadelphia: WB Saunders, 1982.

Casey MP. Testicular cancer: the worst disease at the worst time. RN 1987; 50(2):36–40.

Managing the patient with testicular cancer (case study). Nursing 1986; 16(8):42–45.

Thompson J, McFarland G, Hirsch J, Tucker S, Bowers A. Clinical nursing. St. Louis: CV Mosby, 1986.

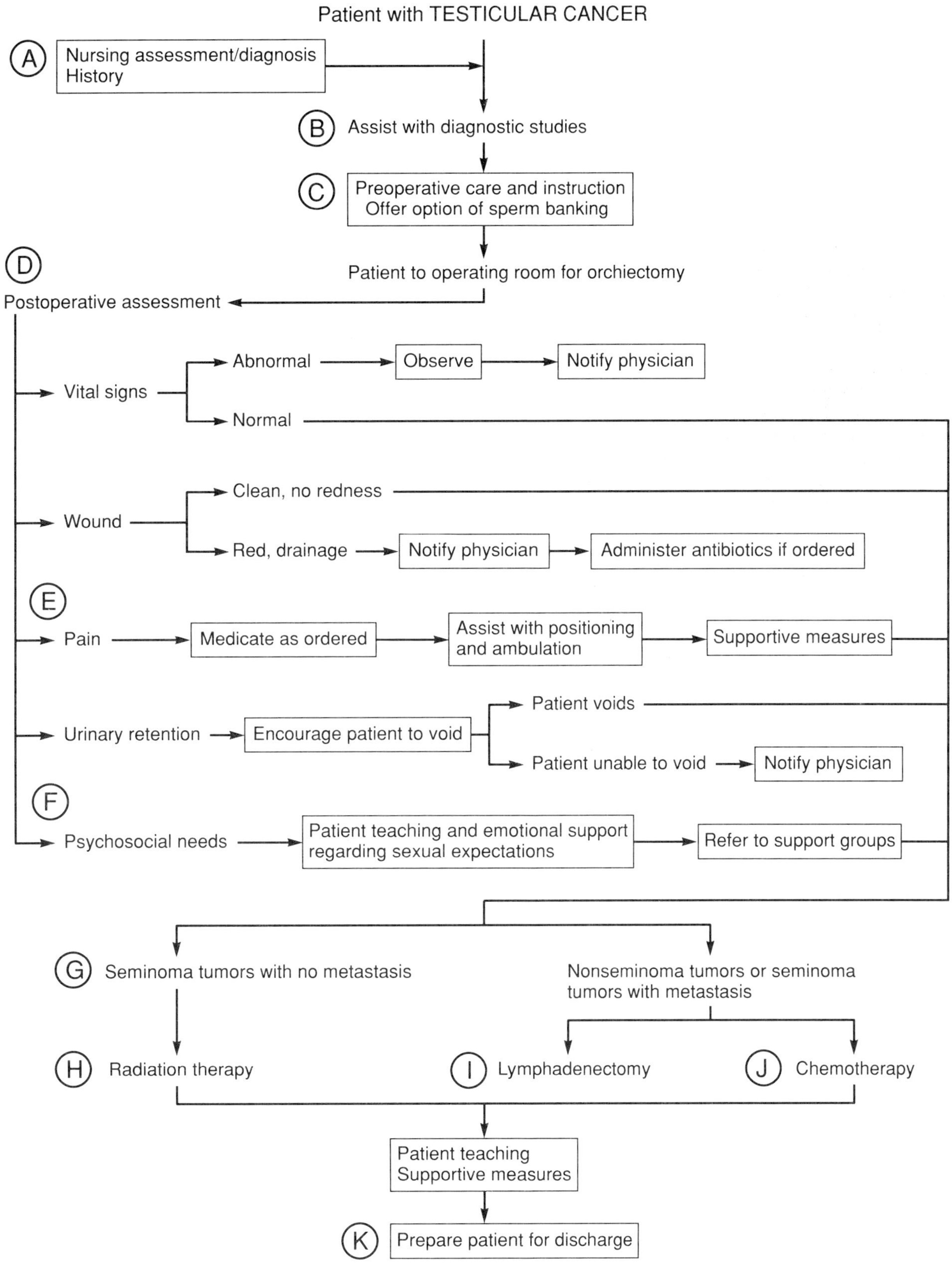
Patient with TESTICULAR CANCER
A
Nursing assessment/diagnosis
History
B
Assist with diagnostic studies
C
Preoperative care and instruction
Offer option of sperm banking
Patient to operating room for orchiectomy
D
Postoperative assessment
Vital signs
Abnormal
Observe
Notify physician
Normal
Wound
Clean, no redness
Red, drainage
Notify physician
Administer antibiotics if ordered
E
Pain
Medicate as ordered
Assist with positioning and ambulation
Supportive measures
Urinary retention
Encourage patient to void
Patient voids
Patient unable to void
Notify physician
F
Psychosocial needs
Patient teaching and emotional support regarding sexual expectations
Refer to support groups
G
Seminoma tumors with no metastasis
Nonseminoma tumors or seminoma tumors with metastasis
H
Radiation therapy
I
Lymphadenectomy
J
Chemotherapy
Patient teaching
Supportive measures
K
Prepare patient for discharge

BLADDER CANCER

Rosemary Keller

A. A history of cigarette smoking and exposure to carcinogens in the work environment such as dyes, rubber, leather, ink, or paint is strongly correlated with a diagnosis of bladder cancer. Chronic bladder infections and chronic schistosomiasis (parasite infection) are also risk factors.

B. Bladder cancer most often occurs in males, 50 to 70 years old. Gross, painless hematuria is the most common symptom. Bleeding is usually intermittent and may be microscopic. Other symptoms include bladder irritability, frequency, urgency, and dysuria. Urine cytology is recommended for workers exposed to carcinogens. Any change in micturition or lower back pain should be explored for metastasis.

C. Laboratory tests should include a complete blood count (CBC) and chemistry profile (SMA 12). Tumor markers such as serum carcinoembryonic antigen (CEA) levels are frequently elevated in metastatic and late-stage disease. Excretory urography is helpful in detecting the tumor or revealing ureteral obstruction. Cystoscopy allows visualization of the tumor, with biopsy or resection. Bimanual palpation is performed under anesthesia to determine the presence or absence of tumor invasion into the muscle or serosa. Chest films, pelvic tomographic scan, skeletal survey, and liver and bone scans should be done to stage invasive lesions.

D. The most important factors in predicting prognosis are the depth of penetration of the tumor into the bladder wall and the presence or absence of metastasis. Tumors may spread to regional lymph nodes, pelvic tissues, bone, liver, and lungs. Treatment of bladder cancer depends on the grade of the tumor, the stage of growth, and the patient's age and physical, mental, and emotional status.

E. Patients diagnosed with superficial, low-grade tumors are treated with transurethral resection (p 300). Because of the possibility of recurrence, the patient should be followed with cytology and cystoscopy periodically for the rest of his life.

F. Topical chemotherapy (Thiotepa, doxorubicin, 5-fluorouracil) given by bladder instillation may be done. Fluid intake is limited for 2 hours during the procedure. After the treatment, fluid intake is increased and the patient is encouraged to void in order to flush the drug from the bladder. Side effects include severe bladder irritability, myelosuppression, and renal failure if there is reflux.

G. High-stage, high-grade tumors require more aggressive treatment. Treatment includes radiation alone with curative intent, radical cystectomy with urinary diversion, or preoperative irradiation followed by surgical excision.

H. Simple cystectomy or radical cystectomy is done for invasive or multifocal bladder cancer. Radical cystectomy in the male involves removal of the bladder, prostate, seminal vesicles, and immediate adjacent perivesical tissues. In the female, it involves removal of the bladder, lower ureters, uterus, tubes, ovaries, anterior vagina, and urethra. One method of urinary diversion is the ileal conduit. Urine is diverted by transplanting the ureters to a section of the terminal ileum with an exit through the abdominal wall. An ileostomy bag is used to collect the urine.

I. Patients often experience anxiety related to the anticipated losses of love, body image, and security. In addition, these patients must adapt to an external appliance, a stoma, alteration in toileting habits, and sexual impotence. The nurse can support the patient by encouraging an expression of fears and concerns and exploring alternative ways to cope with the stresses imposed by multiple losses. Explain the surgical procedure to the patient and family.

J. Postoperative nursing diagnoses and interventions include alteration in bladder elimination related to urinary diversion. Check urine volume hourly. Output less than 30 cc per hour may indicate obstruction with possible backflow or leakage from the anastomosis. Encourage high fluid intake to flush the ileal conduit and prevent mucus from congealing. A catheter may be inserted to check for possible stasis or residual urine from a tight stoma.

K. Impaired skin integrity (potential) is related to outcome of surgery. Inspect the stoma for bleeding, adequate vascular circulation, urine irritation caused by an ill-fitting appliance, and skin sensitivity to appliance adhesive. Evaluate the stoma for complications such as wound infections, dehiscence, urinary leakage, ureteral obstruction, small bowel obstruction, and stomal gangrene.

L. Assisting patients to improve their self-concept and allowing them to ventilate feelings enhances their ability to cope. Encourage the patient and partner to share their feelings about this loss. Assist them to explore alternative ways of expressing sexuality. Provide male patients with information about penile implants (p 304). Refer for sexual counseling if additional assistance is required.

M. Assess the knowledge deficit concerning management of urinary function. Provide instruction for the patient and family on all phases of management of the ostomy and opportunities to practice and demonstrate skills. Patient teaching includes information relating to appliance selection, determining stoma size, changing the appliance, skin care, odor control, connecting a leg bag to the appliance, and cleaning and deodorizing

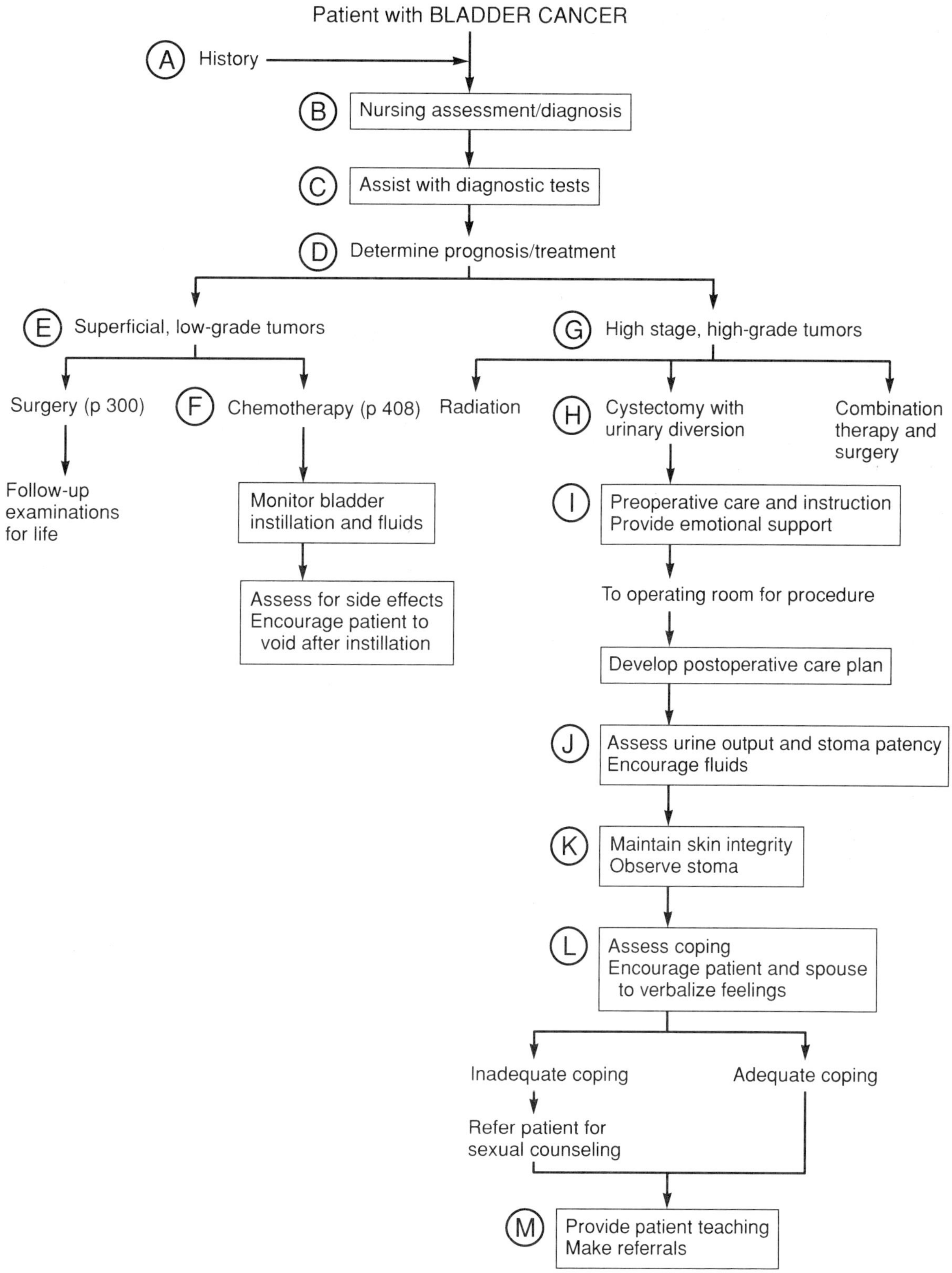

the appliance. Assist patients to resume their usual lifestyle and independence. Initiate a referral to the American Cancer Society Ostomy Visitation Program.

References

Folk-Lighty ME, Dillon LS. Renal and urologic problems. In: Lewis SM, Collier IC. Medical-surgical nursing: assessment and management of clinical problems. New York: McGraw-Hill, 1983:1096–1097.

Groenwald SL. Cancer nursing principles and practice. Boston: Jones & Bartlett, 1987.

Rubin P. Clinical oncology: a multidisciplinary approach. 6th ed. New York: American Cancer Society, 1983:205–209.

Smeltzer SC. Management of patients with renal and urinary disorders. In: Brunner LS, Suddarth DS. Textbook of medical-surgical nursing. 6th ed. Philadelphia: JB Lippincott, 1988:1059–1066.

TRANSURETHRAL RESECTION

Leslie Hussey

Transurethral resection (TUR) is the surgical removal of the prostate. It is the most common procedure used to treat benign prostatic hypertrophy. In TUR a resectoscope is passed through the urethra. Tiny pieces of prostate tissue are cut away. The bladder is continually irrigated with normal saline during the procedure.

A. The patient presents with a history of difficulty urinating and possibly recurring urinary tract infections. If benign prostatic hypertrophy (BPH) is severe, hematuria can develop from overstretching of the bladder. The enlarged prostate causes nocturia, difficulty initiating a stream, and progressive reduction in force and size of the urinary stream. If the prostate becomes very large, it can completely obstruct urination causing back pressure into the urinary system.

B. Preoperative nursing care must include explicit, thorough explanation of all procedures. The patient often has concerns about impotency, sterility, and urinary incontinence. Assure the patient that although infertility does occur, sexual potency will not be affected by the surgery. Describe tubes and drains he will have postoperatively. Reassure him that even though he may experience some pain and/or bladder spasms, he will be given medication to relieve these symptoms.

C. Postoperatively, the bladder is irrigated with a normal saline solution. Irrigation may or may not be continuous. Irrigating the bladder prevents clot formation. Bright red blood in the drainage bag indicates hemorrhage. The physician should be notified immediately and the patient must be observed for shock (p 70).

D. Other complications include possible urinary tract infections and urethral stricture from the rectoscope and/or catheter. It is important to use aseptic technique when handling the urinary drainage system.

E. Antispasmodics such as belladonna and opium suppositories may be ordered to relieve bladder spasms. Administer pain medication as ordered.

F. Because the patient was in the lithotomy position during surgery, he is predisposed to deep vein thrombosis. Elastic bandages or antiembolic stockings may be used to facilitate venous return. The patient is generally ambulated the first day postoperatively.

G. The Foley catheter is removed when the urine is clear. Observe the patient for urinary retention. "Dribbling" may occur at first. The patient should be assured that this is normal and will soon decrease.

H. Discharge instructions should include information about the patient's activities. He should avoid any strenuous exercise or heavy lifting for at least 6 weeks, as these activities could cause bleeding. The patient may resume sexual activity in 6 to 8 weeks. He should maintain an adequate fluid intake, and stool softeners may be taken as prescribed. It is important that the patient report any urinary infection, incontinence, or difficulty in voiding to his physician.

References

Luckmann J, Sorensen KC. Medical-surgical nursing: a psychophysiologic approach. 3rd ed. Philadelphia: WB Saunders, 1987:1851–1854.

Kneisl C, Ames S. Adult health nursing: a biopsychosocial approach. Reading, MA: Addison-Wesley, 1986.

Thompson J, McFarland G, Hirsch J, Tucker S, Bowers A. Clinical nursing. St. Louis: CV Mosby, 1986.

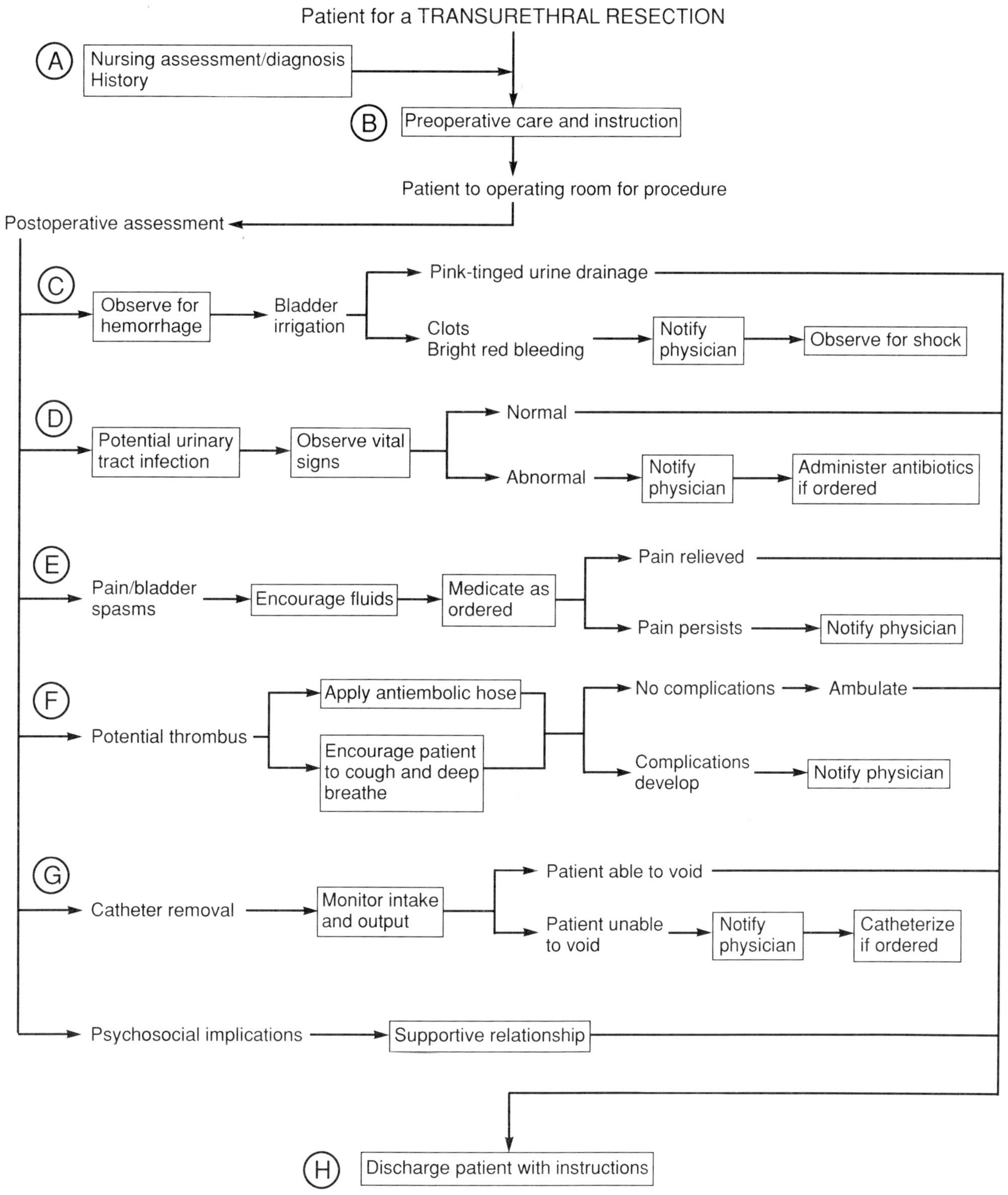
Patient for a TRANSURETHRAL RESECTION
A
Nursing assessment/diagnosis
History
B
Preoperative care and instruction
Patient to operating room for procedure
Postoperative assessment
C
Observe for hemorrhage
Bladder irrigation
Pink-tinged urine drainage
Clots
Bright red bleeding
Notify physician
Observe for shock
D
Potential urinary tract infection
Observe vital signs
Normal
Abnormal
Notify physician
Administer antibiotics if ordered
E
Pain/bladder spasms
Encourage fluids
Medicate as ordered
Pain relieved
Pain persists
Notify physician
F
Potential thrombus
Apply antiembolic hose
Encourage patient to cough and deep breathe
No complications
Ambulate
Complications develop
Notify physician
G
Catheter removal
Monitor intake and output
Patient able to void
Patient unable to void
Notify physician
Catheterize if ordered
Psychosocial implications
Supportive relationship
H
Discharge patient with instructions

PROSTATECTOMY

Joy Gorzeman

A. Prostatectomy is the excision of part or all of the prostate gland. This surgical procedure is approached from one of four routes: (1) transurethral, (2) suprapubic, (3) retropubic, or (4) perineal. A transurethral prostatectomy (p 300) is a closed procedure that is most commonly performed on patients with benign prostatic hypertrophy, when a small amount of tissue needs to be resected. The suprapubic approach is an open procedure that is used when a larger mass of tissue needs to be resected. The retropubic approach is a similar procedure, but the bladder is not opened. A perineal prostatectomy is done when there is confirmed or suspected cancer of the prostate.

B. Preoperative preparation for a prostatectomy should include emotional support, as most patients have questions about impotence and incontinence. Patients undergoing radical perineal prostatectomy usually experience both of these problems. Patients undergoing the other procedures should not experience impotence, although reproductive capability may be affected. Incontinence usually improves over time. A patient undergoing the perineal approach needs a bowel preparation. Monitor fluid intake and output of all these patients to assess renal function and ensure a positive hydration status. Other preoperative care is similar to that preceding any major surgery (p 2).

C. Postoperatively all patients return with a urethral catheter, which may or may not be attached to an irrigation system. The urine may be red the first 24 hours and tinged with pink for a few days. Report bright red bleeding to the physician immediately, because hemorrhage and shock are the most common complications following prostate surgery. Changes in pulse and/or respiration could also indicate hemorrhage or shock (p 70) in the early postoperative period.

D. In addition to observing the color of the urinary drainage, the nurse must be sure the catheter remains patent. Kinked tubing can cause an obstruction, which may result in pain. An obstruction to urine flow may also precipitate an infection. Pulling and tugging on the catheter causes irritation and should be avoided.

E. Fluid intake and output should be documented accurately. This documentation is continued after the catheter is removed to assist in assessing for signs of urinary retention. Dribbling and even incontinence are not unusual at first. Perineal exercises help strengthen the sphincter muscles and reduce the dribbling.

F. Also included in the intake and output record is the amount and color of drainage on the dressings. A cystotomy drain, which may be inserted during surgery, increases the amount of drainage. The dressing needs to be changed frequently to prevent skin breakdown.

G. Observe the incision each time the dressing is changed. Aseptic technique must be used to decrease the risk of infection. Report redness or drainage around the incision to the physician. If an infection develops, antibiotics are ordered. Use of a heat lamp may help to keep the area dry. Vital signs must be monitored on a regular basis. An increase in temperature may indicate an infection.

H. As with any surgical procedure, some pain is to be expected in the incisional area postoperatively. Patients with prostatectomy may also experience bladder spasms. Pain medications and/or antispasmodics should relieve the discomfort. Sitz baths may help promote comfort.

I. Ambulation should be started as early as possible. Sitting for prolonged periods should be avoided, because it increases intra-abdominal pressure, which increases the risk of bleeding.

J. Upon discharge, the patient should be advised to avoid heavy lifting, vigorous exercise, sexual intercourse, straining, and driving for about 6 weeks. Prostatectomy patients should include a lot of fluids in their diet (unless restricted by another health problem) and should be reminded that alcoholic beverages cause urinary burning. Advise the patient of the importance of follow-up visits, and tell him to notify his physician if he notices bleeding or a decrease in the urinary stream. Patients with dribbling or incontinence should be encouraged to continue exercises to strengthen the perineal muscles.

References

Luckmann J, Sorensen KC. Medical-surgical nursing: a psychophysiologic approach. 3rd ed. Philadelphia: WB Saunders, 1987.

Phipps WJ, Long BC, Woods NF. Medical-surgical nursing: concepts and clinical practice. 3rd ed. St. Louis: CV Mosby, 1987.

Thompson J, McFarland G, Hirsch J, Tucker S, Bowers A. Clinical nursing. St. Louis: CV Mosby, 1986.

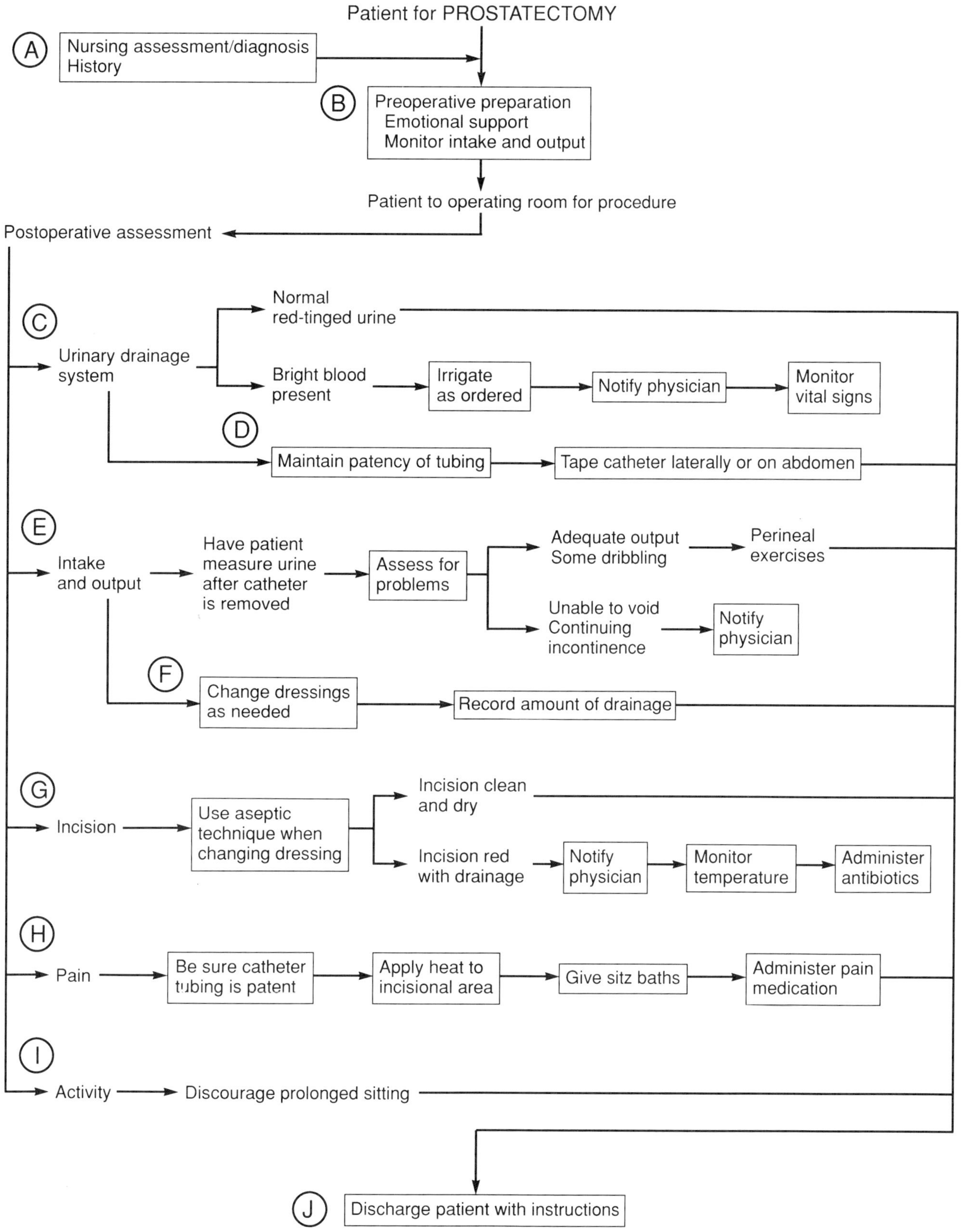
Patient for PROSTATECTOMY
A
Nursing assessment/diagnosis
History
B
Preoperative preparation
Emotional support
Monitor intake and output
Patient to operating room for procedure
Postoperative assessment
C
Urinary drainage system
Normal red-tinged urine
Bright blood present
Irrigate as ordered
Notify physician
Monitor vital signs
D
Maintain patency of tubing
Tape catheter laterally or on abdomen
E
Intake and output
Have patient measure urine after catheter is removed
Assess for problems
Adequate output
Some dribbling
Perineal exercises
Unable to void
Continuing incontinence
Notify physician
F
Change dressings as needed
Record amount of drainage
G
Incision
Use aseptic technique when changing dressing
Incision clean and dry
Incision red with drainage
Notify physician
Monitor temperature
Administer antibiotics
H
Pain
Be sure catheter tubing is patent
Apply heat to incisional area
Give sitz baths
Administer pain medication
I
Activity
Discourage prolonged sitting
J
Discharge patient with instructions

PENILE IMPLANT

Chris Kirsch

Traditionally, impotence has been viewed as having a psychogenic etiology in 90 percent of cases. Today, although impotence in the elderly male may be related to psychological factors as much as to general health, it is evident that disease processes may cause impotence at any age. Consequently, although every effort is made to treat those who are suffering from psychogenic impotence, prosthetic implantation is the treatment of choice for physiologic impairment. There are two basic types of surgically implanted penile prostheses—semirigid and inflatable.

A. Factors that impair erectile capability include long-term use of drugs for the treatment of cardiovascular disease and hypertension; adrenergic drugs; diabetes and other systemic disorders related to arteriosclerotic vascular disease; spinal cord injuries; and prostatic surgeries using the perineal approach.

B. Diagnosis is made from hematologic studies for serum testosterone level and biochemical profile (BCP) 20 test. The testosterone level indicates whether impotence is related to a low hormone level, the BCP evaluates general well-being, and a glucose tolerance test rules out diabetes. Nocturnal penile tumescence monitoring or a Dacomed snap gauge study may help to differentiate psychogenic from organic impotence.

C. Patients should be encouraged to discuss the various types of penile implants prior to admission. Whenever possible, the client's sexual partner should participate in the decision about the type of device to be used. Patient teaching should include expectations after surgery and when sexual activity may resume. Encourage the patient to practice deep breathing, coughing, and ankle exercises to minimize possible complications. Patients should expect intravenous (IV) therapy, urinary catheter, and an ice bag to the scrotum. Explain that the penis and scrotum may be painful, discolored, and edematous for several days postoperatively and that they should request pain medication if needed. Physical preparation includes Betadine showers several days preoperatively, enema, catheterization, and prophylactic antibiotic therapy. Demonstrate the function of the selected device and explain possible complications and trouble-shooting. Provide emotional support related to self-esteem and self-image.

D. Postoperative nursing care is directed at preventing complications such as infection. Place the patient in a true Trendelenburg position for the first 18 hours after surgery to minimize swelling. A Foley catheter to prevent urinary retention remains in place until penile edema subsides.

E. Routine postoperative vital signs and assessment are done (p 4).

F. A small gauze dressing is present over the operative site, and although blood loss is minimal, checks should be made every 2 hours and the dressing changed as necessary. If a wound drain is present in the scrotal sac, 30 ml of clear, nonfoul drainage per day is considered within normal limits. Culture suspicious drainage and notify the physician. Drains are usually removed within 24 to 48 hours. Prophylactic antibiotics are generally continued for 10 to 14 days until healing is assured.

G. Pain is controlled with selected parenteral narcotics for the first 24 hours and then with oral agents. Drugs of choice may be intravenous Dilaudid every 4 to 6 hours and then oral Percodan or Percocet every 4 hours. After 24 hours very little medication is required. An ice pack may be placed to reduce scrotal swelling. Nausea, if present and discomforting to the patient, may be controlled by antiemetics. If no drain is present, sitz baths may be offered for mild discomfort.

H. Ambulation is generally not a problem and should be encouraged within 24 hours postoperatively.

I. The inflatable prosthesis is tested during placement in the operating room, but it is not inflated again until the first visit to the physician's office.

J. Patients are instructed to wear loose-fitting underwear and to avoid strenuous physical activity. Intercourse is discouraged for 4 to 6 weeks after surgery. Encourage patients and partners to call the physician's office with questions about the implant. Scheduled follow-ups are essential to prevent complications and assure functioning of the device.

References

Brunner LS, Suddarth DS. Impotence. In: Brunner LS, Suddarth DS, eds. Textbook of medical-surgical nursing. 6th ed. Philadelphia: JB Lippincott, 1988:1168–1169.

Gregory JG. Impotence: the surgical approach. Surg Clin North Am 1982; 62:981–997.

Healy PF. Surgical approaches to male reproductive system dysfunction. In: Ames SW, Kneisl CR, eds. Adult health nursing: a biopsychosocial approach. Reading, MA: Addison-Wesley, 1986:1968–1971.

Weigel J. Inflatable penile prosthesis: troubleshooting and management of complications. Am Urol Assoc Update Series, 1987; 6(34).

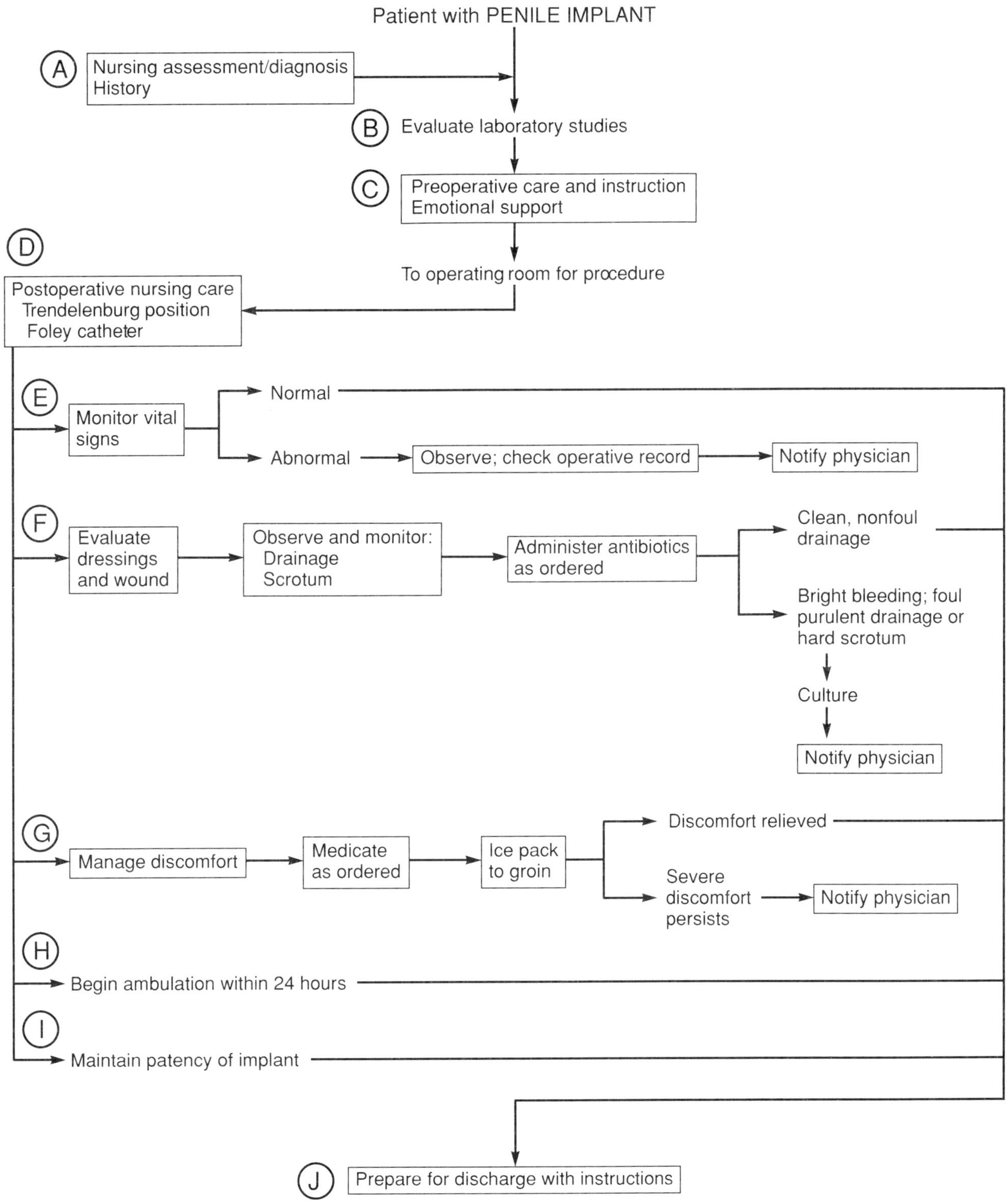

Patient with PENILE IMPLANT
A
Nursing assessment/diagnosis
History
B
Evaluate laboratory studies
C
Preoperative care and instruction
Emotional support
To operating room for procedure
D
Postoperative nursing care
Trendelenburg position
Foley catheter
E
Monitor vital signs
Normal
Abnormal
Observe; check operative record
Notify physician
F
Evaluate dressings and wound
Observe and monitor:
Drainage
Scrotum
Administer antibiotics as ordered
Clean, nonfoul drainage
Bright bleeding; foul purulent drainage or hard scrotum
Culture
Notify physician
G
Manage discomfort
Medicate as ordered
Ice pack to groin
Discomfort relieved
Severe discomfort persists
Notify physician
H
Begin ambulation within 24 hours
I
Maintain patency of implant
J
Prepare for discharge with instructions

RENAL SYSTEM

GLOMERULONEPHRITIS

Joy Gorzeman

Glomerulonephritis (GN) is a disease that causes an inflammatory reaction in the glomeruli of the kidney. It may be acute, latent, or chronic. Causes include immunologic reactions, such as lupus (p 352); hypertension (vascular injury [p 30]); diabetes mellitus (p 176); and disseminated intravascular coagulation (p 348). Antibodies of the patient react with circulating antigens that arise from the toxic products of the infecting organism. Immune complexes are formed and lodge in the glomeruli, causing inflammation and subsequent damage to the glomerular membrane in both kidneys.

A. Acute glomerulonephritis most commonly follows a *Streptococcus* infection (usually respiratory or skin) and is often seen in preschool and grade-school children. Sore throats and upper respiratory infections should be treated promptly. Cultures should be obtained and antibiotics administered when appropriate to help prevent GN. Most children and about half the adults with acute glomerulonephritis recover completely; a small percentage (1 to 2 percent) develop end-stage renal failure. Total recovery may take as long as 2 years. The severity of the illness is not related to the prognosis.

B. Laboratory studies and urinalysis show proteinuria, hematuria, elevated serum creatinine and urea nitrogen, increased urine specific gravity, and elevated antistreptolysin O titer (from reaction to *streptococcus* infection).

C. Clinical manifestations result from damage to the glomeruli, which eventually causes scarring and depression of renal function. Early signs and symptoms include anorexia, weakness, shortness of breath, and mild headache. Dependent edema, hypertension, and decreased urine output may be present.

D. Treatment includes long-term antibiotic therapy (several months); penicillin is the drug of choice. Patients must avoid exposure to infection, since any infection may reactivate nephritis.

E. Patients are put on bedrest until clinical manifestations disappear.

F. Dietary protein should be reduced if blood urea nitrogen and creatinine levels are elevated. Carbohydrates should be increased to provide energy and reduce catabolism of protein. A low sodium diet helps decrease fluid retention.

G. Intake and output should be measured. Fluid control should also control hypertension. If not, antihypertensive medication may be necessary.

H. Patients are assessed for edema, and the daily weight is recorded. If severe fluid overload is present, diuretics are ordered.

I. Vital signs should be taken frequently. Observe the patient for signs of chronic renal failure (p 318).

J. When ambulation is allowed, proteinuria and hematuria must be monitored. If they increase, bedrest is reinstituted. Patients may become depressed at this perceived setback and should be allowed to express their concerns and feelings. Diversional activities are encouraged.

K. If ambulation is tolerated, the patient is discharged. Instructions include the rationale for treatment, dietary and medication instructions, and suggestions for avoiding infections and fatigue. Stress the importance of follow-up care. Hematuria, edema, or headaches should be reported to the physician immediately.

L. Although chronic glomerulonephritis (CGN) may follow the acute disease, usually the patient has no history of glomerulonephritis. The course of CGN is varied, with slow progression of the disease in some patients and rapid progression in others. Symptoms that may cause a patient to seek medical care include weakness, fatigue, blurred vision, headaches (especially in the morning), and/or dyspnea. Other signs include nocturia, edema, and weight loss. In the early stages of CGN, urinalysis shows albumin, casts, and blood, although renal function tests may be normal. As more glomeruli scar and fewer nephrons are functioning, hematuria and proteinuria decrease and the nonprotein nitrogen level in the blood increases.

M. Since the cause of CGN has not been identified, preventive measures cannot be taken. Steroid therapy may be tried, although the results are not known. Treatment is symptomatic and supportive. CGN patients should be monitored for congestive heart failure (p 68) and pulmonary edema (p 114).

N. Patient teaching should include instruction in preventing infections; eating a well-balanced low protein, low-salt, high-carbohydrate diet; medication regimen; importance of follow-up visits; and reporting exacerbations of symptoms to the physician. Pregnant women with CGN should be under close medical supervision because they are at increased risk for spontaneous abortion and toxemia.

References

Brunner LS, Suddarth DS. The Lippincott manual of nursing practice. 4th ed. Philadelphia: JB Lippincott, 1986.

Hincker EA, Malasanos L, eds. Little, Brown manual of medical-surgical nursing. Boston: Little, Brown & Co, 1983.

Phipps W, Long B, Woods N. Medical-surgical nursing: concepts and clinical practice. St. Louis: CV Mosby, 1987.

Thompson JM, McFarland GK, Hirsch JE, Tucker SM, Bowers AC. Clinical nursing. St. Louis: CV Mosby, 1986.

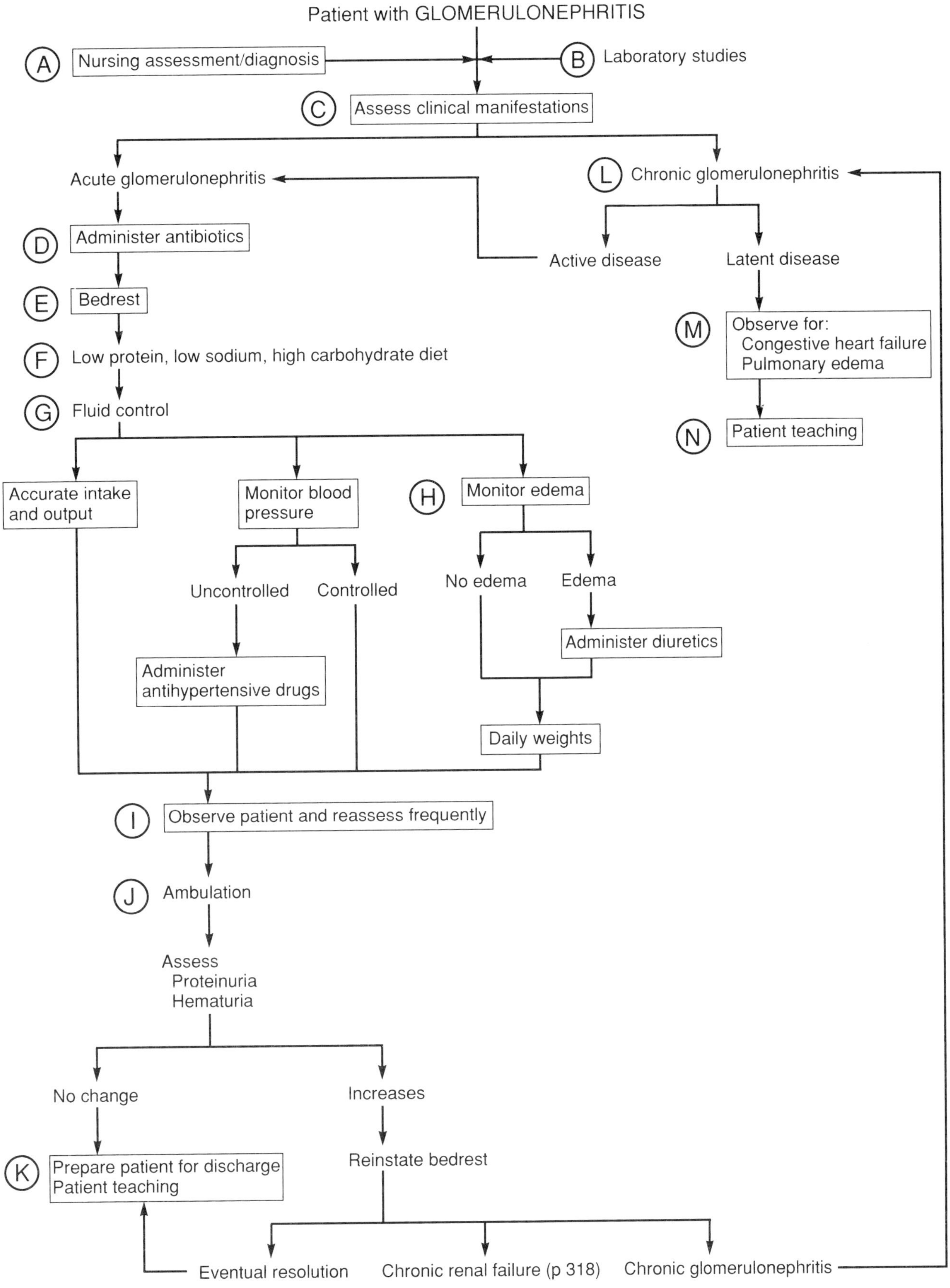
Patient with GLOMERULONEPHRITIS
A
Nursing assessment/diagnosis
B
Laboratory studies
C
Assess clinical manifestations
Acute glomerulonephritis
L
Chronic glomerulonephritis
D
Administer antibiotics
Active disease
Latent disease
E
Bedrest
M
Observe for:
Congestive heart failure
Pulmonary edema
F
Low protein, low sodium, high carbohydrate diet
G
Fluid control
N
Patient teaching
Accurate intake and output
Monitor blood pressure
H
Monitor edema
Uncontrolled
Controlled
No edema
Edema
Administer diuretics
Administer antihypertensive drugs
Daily weights
I
Observe patient and reassess frequently
J
Ambulation
Assess
Proteinuria
Hematuria
No change
Increases
Reinstate bedrest
K
Prepare patient for discharge
Patient teaching
Eventual resolution
Chronic renal failure (p 318)
Chronic glomerulonephritis

PYELONEPHRITIS

Diane M. Zintak

Pyelonephritis is an inflammation of the kidney caused by a bacterial infection. Most infections are acute and generally begin in the lower urinary tract and then ascend into the kidneys, where inflammation, fibrosis, and scarring may occur as a result of the infectious process. This is especially true in chronic pyelonephritis, in which renal tissue becomes permanently damaged because of repeated infection and inflammation. This, then, can lead to renal failure.

A. Acute pyelonephritis may cause mild, easily ignored symptoms or may even be asymptomatic except for bacteriuria. More typically, chills and fever, nausea, flank pain on the affected side, fatigue, anorexia, or headache are experienced. Percussion or deep palpation over the costovertebral angle usually elicits marked tenderness. The patient may also describe burning, frequency, or urgency with urination for several days. The nurse must determine the onset and duration of these symptoms and any previous treatment of the patient. The nurse should also be aware that pyelonephritis is most commonly associated with (1) pregnancy; (2) obstruction, instrumentation, or trauma of the urinary tract; and (3) chronic health problems such as diabetes (p 176), analgesic abuse, polycystic kidney disease, and hypertensive kidney disease.

B. Diagnostic procedures begin with a urinalysis, which generally reveals urine that is cloudy and foul-smelling along with bacteriuria, pyuria, and possible hematuria. Before antibiotic therapy is initiated, it is essential that a urine culture and sensitivity tests be done to determine the causative organism, so that appropriate antibiotics may be selected. *E. coli* is the most common organism identified in pyelonephritis, although other causative organisms include *Proteus, Enterobacter, Pseudomonas, Klebsiella, Staphylococcus,* and *Streptococcus.*

C. Other diagnostic procedures such as intravenous pyelography (IVP), abdominal and kidney-ureter-bladder (KUB) films, and cystoscopy are done to determine whether any renal or urologic abnormality, obstruction, calculus, or other potentiating factors are present. Surgical, pharmacologic, or other interventions may be required to correct any contributing factor.

D. Treatment is directed at eliminating the bacterial infection and providing symptomatic relief. Appropriate antibiotics, as determined by the urine culture and sensitivity tests, are given. Depending on the severity of the infection, the initial intervention may involve parenteral antibiotics for 3 to 5 days until the person is afebrile, with oral antibiotics continuing for 2 to 4 weeks. The patient must be instructed to complete the full course of antibiotics.

E. Increasing fluid intake to 3,000 ml per day in persons capable of excreting this amount of fluid is desirable to flush out the urinary tract, prevent stasis of urine, and inhibit further bacterial growth.

F. Bedrest is encouraged during the acute phase, and analgesics or external applications of heat may be used to promote comfort.

G. The patient is reassessed and the urine recultured 2 weeks after drug therapy has been discontinued and every month thereafter for the next several months. A chronic or recurring infection without symptoms may occur, requiring a prolonged course of antibiotic therapy. For reinfection, alternative antibiotic therapy specific for the new causative organism must be initiated.

H. After discharge, antibiotic therapy is necessary for a specified period after symptoms subside or after urine culture becomes negative. Emphasize the importance of continuing these medications in spite of feeling asymptomatic, maintaining an adequate fluid intake, and voiding frequently. Personal hygiene should also be reviewed to minimize the potential for recurrence of a urinary tract infection. Review the signs and symptoms of recurrent pyelonephritis that warrant immediate attention.

I. Chronic pyelonephritis may develop when all bacteria are not eliminated from the urine during an acute infection or when underlying disease or obstruction is not identified and corrected. In early stages of chronic pyelonephritis, the patient may be asymptomatic or have only mild symptoms such as fatigue, headache, anorexia, and weight loss. The disease may be discovered incidentally when the person is being eval-

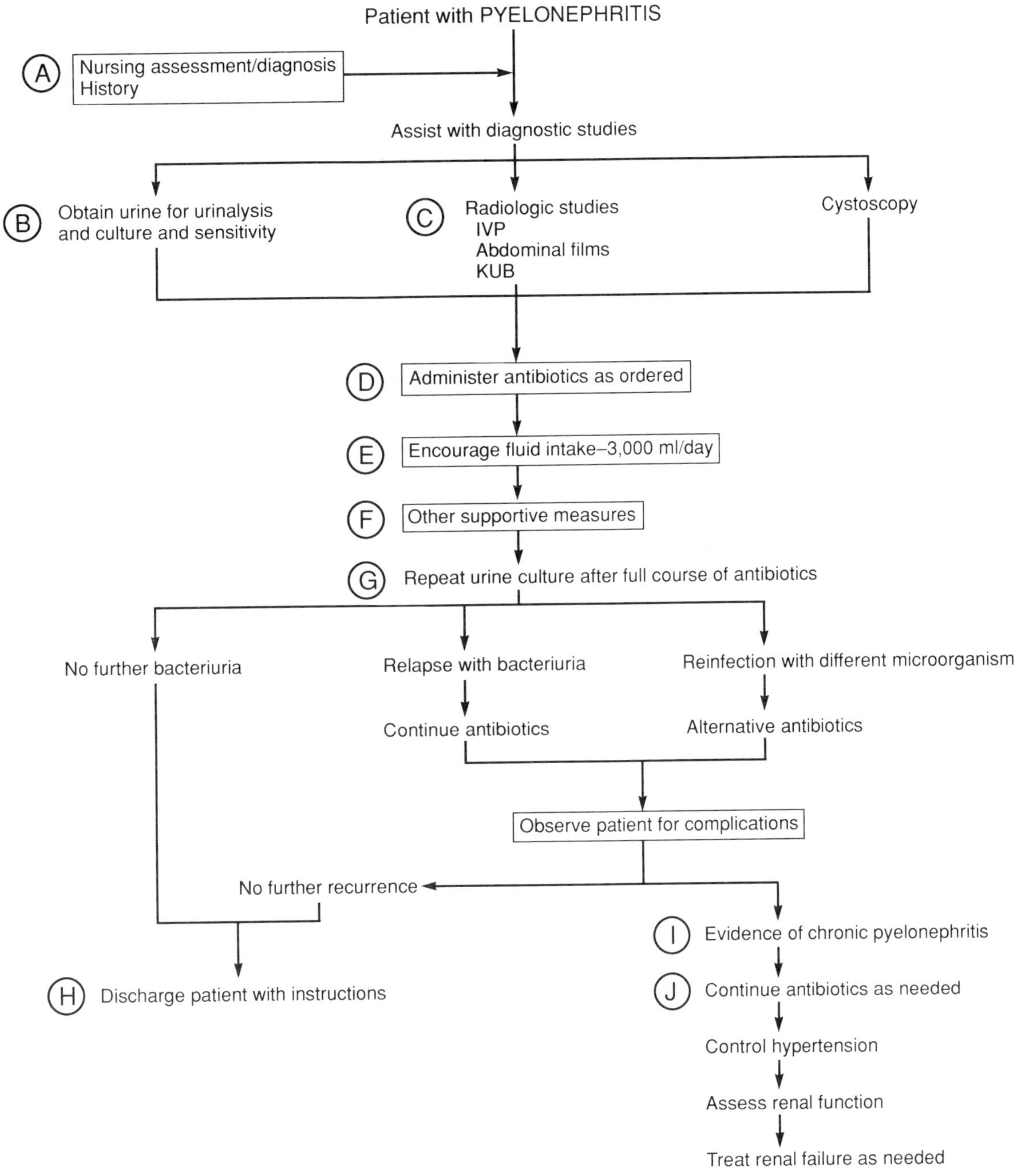

uated for hypertension (p 80), the most frequent manifestation of the disease. Upon further examination, the patient may also be found to have abnormal amounts of protein and white blood cell casts in the urine and elevated serum levels of blood urea nitrogen (BUN) and creatinine. The patient is generally uremic and anemic, and may be acidotic.

J. Specific antibiotic therapy is prescribed for the bacteriuria, and efforts must be made to control hypertension. The degree of renal failure must be evaluated and uremia treated accordingly. A discussion of the care of the patient with chronic renal failure is found on page 318.

References

Long BC, Phipps WJ. Essentials of medical-surgical nursing. St. Louis: CV Mosby, 1985.

Luckmann J, Sorensen KC. Medical-surgical nursing: a psychophysiologic approach. 3rd ed. Philadelphia: WB Saunders, 1987.

Reller LB. The patient with urinary tract infection. In: Schrier RW, ed. Manual of nephrology: diagnosis and therapy. Boston: Little, Brown, 1985:97–111.

Richard CJ. Comprehensive nephrology nursing. Boston: Little, Brown, 1986.

RENAL CALCULI

Joy Gorzeman

A. A patient with kidney stones may be admitted for observation and/or surgery. The history may play an important role in determining the cause of the stones. Precipitating factors in stone formation include infection, dehydration, immobilization (p 234), hypercalcemia (p 188), vitamin A deficiency, excessive intake of tea, and heredity. If the patient has not had a complete blood count, urinalysis culture, and chemistry studies, these will be done on admission. Other diagnostic studies include kidney-ureter-bladder (KUB) films and intravenous pyelograms (IVP).

B. The most common symptom of kidney stones is pain in the renal area. The pain may radiate anteriorly and downward. External heat and ambulation may relieve the pain; however, severe pain may require the administration of narcotic analgesics (p 406). The patient may experience nausea and vomiting caused by renal-intestinal reflexes and anatomic location.

C. A patient with kidney stones is also susceptible to urinary tract infection.

D. The pain and procedures may cause the patient to be anxious. Keeping them informed helps to allay anxiety.

E. All urine must be strained through gauze. If the stone is passed it can be analyzed and appropriate therapy initiated.

F. Once the stone is passed, the pain is relieved and the patient can be discharged. Teaching should include a prescribed diet (based on stone analysis). Excessive vitamin D intake must be avoided and high fluid intake maintained.

G. If the radiograph indicates the stone is too large to pass, or if the stone is producing obstruction, unremitting pain, infection, or progressive renal damage, surgery is indicated.

References

Luckmann J, Sorensen KC. Medical-surgical nursing: a psychophysiologic approach. 3rd ed. Philadelphia: WB Saunders, 1987.

Armstrong ME, Dickason EJ, Howe J, Jones DA, Snider MJ, eds. McGraw-Hill handbook of clinical nursing. New York: McGraw-Hill, 1979.

Thompson J, McFarland G, Hirsch J, Tucker S, Bowers A. Clinical nursing. St. Louis: CV Mosby, 1986.

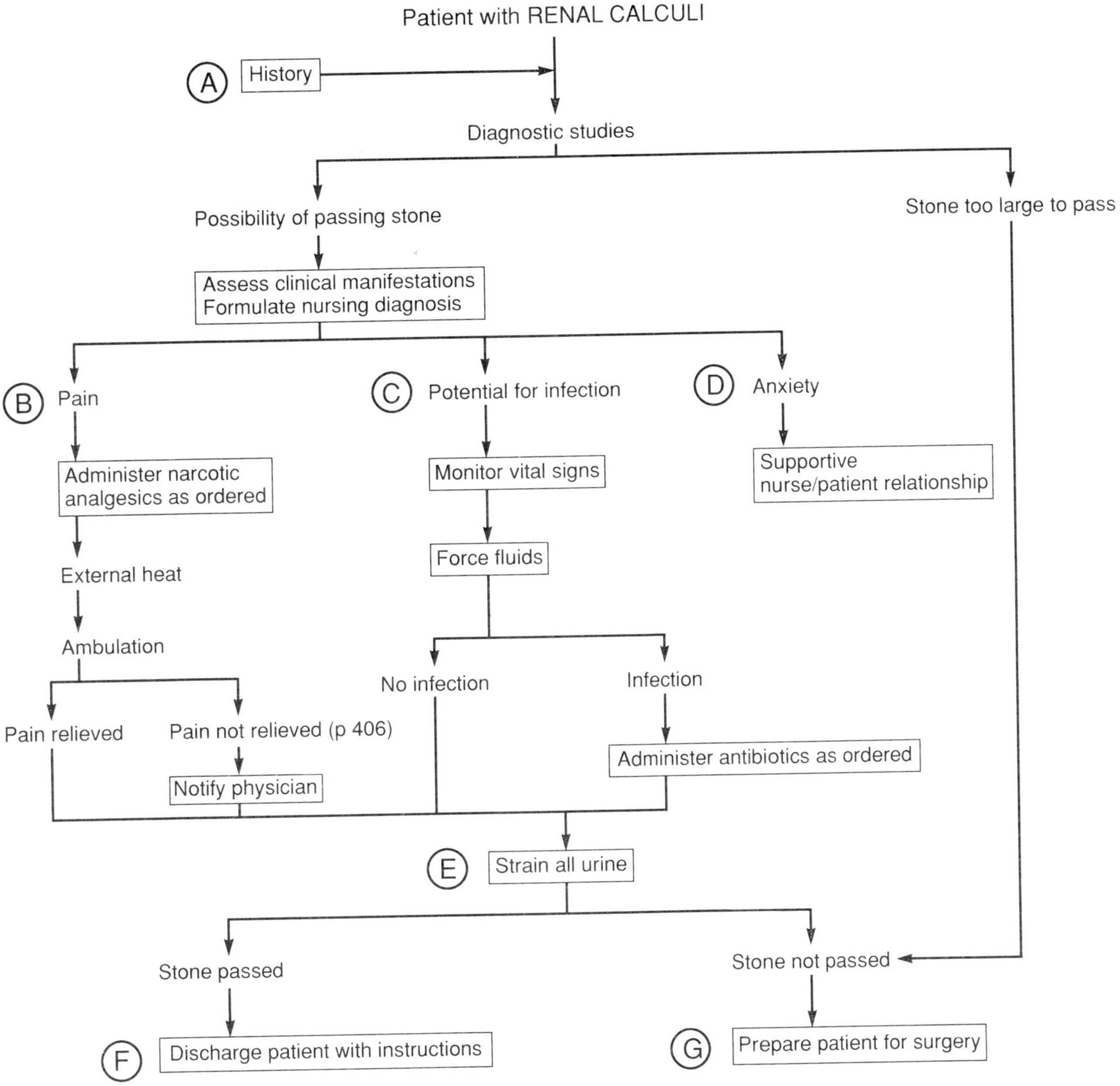

Patient with RENAL CALCULI
A
History
Diagnostic studies
Possibility of passing stone
Stone too large to pass
Assess clinical manifestations
Formulate nursing diagnosis
B
Pain
C
Potential for infection
D
Anxiety
Administer narcotic analgesics as ordered
Monitor vital signs
Supportive nurse/patient relationship
External heat
Force fluids
Ambulation
No infection
Infection
Pain relieved
Pain not relieved (p 406)
Administer antibiotics as ordered
Notify physician
E
Strain all urine
Stone passed
Stone not passed
F
Discharge patient with instructions
G
Prepare patient for surgery

ACUTE RENAL FAILURE

Kathleen H. Toto

Acute renal failure (ARF) can be defined as a rapid deterioration in renal function characterized by a progressive or sudden decline in urine output and elevation of serum creatinine and urea. Acute renal failure may be reversible or irreversible.

A. Obtaining a complete history from a patient with newly diagnosed acute renal failure is important in order to determine precipitating factors and provide direction for treatment. Key information to be obtained includes a family history of hereditary diseases such as glomerulonephritis (p 308), diabetes mellitus (p 176), or polycystic kidney disease and a medication history indicating use of nephrotoxic drugs, over-the-counter drugs such as nonsteroidal anti-inflammatory agents (e.g., Advil, Nuprin), prescription drugs (antibiotics), street drugs (amphetamines), or other nephrotoxic agents such as ethylene glycol (antifreeze). Establish the onset of symptoms such as frequency and urgency of urination, color and quantity of urine, and incontinence. The nursing assessment includes vital signs and a complete physical assessment. Respiration rate may be increased as a result of metabolic acidosis and volume overload. The blood pressure may be elevated or low, depending on the volume status. Fever may be present because of the increased susceptibility to infection that occurs with ARF. Cardiovascular assessment includes blood pressure, pulse tilt, evidence of peripheral edema, pericardial friction rub, and an S_3 heart sound. Rales, wheezing, tachypnea, cyanosis, and apprehension may be discovered during the respiratory assessment. Neurologic assessment includes level of orientation, unusual behavior, and occurrence of seizure activity. The patient should also be assessed for internal or external bleeding sites. A Foley catheter should be inserted to monitor urine output. Urine output of less than 400 cc per 24 hours (oliguria) is a key sign.

B. Laboratory data should include serum and urine electrolyte and creatinine levels, blood urea nitrogen (BUN), a complete blood count with differential, arterial blood gas values (ABGs), serum amylase and lipase levels, urine for specific gravity and protein, and a toxicology screen. Common electrolyte imbalances seen in ARF include hyperkalemia (p 196), hypocalcemia (p 192), hyperphosphatemia, and hypermagnesemia. Metabolic acidosis is often present. Serum creatinine and urea levels are elevated and the bicarbonate is usually low. Diagnostic procedures may include an abdominal film (kidney, ureters, bladder), abdominal ultrasonography, intravenous pyelography (IVP), and possibly a kidney biopsy. Explain these procedures before they are done. Informed consent is required for IVP and kidney biopsy.

C. ARF can be divided into three major categories according to the etiology of the renal dysfunction: prerenal, intrarenal, and postrenal. Prerenal causes of ARF are attributed to events that occur before the blood reaches the kidney for filtration or an inability of the cardiovascular system to perfuse the kidneys adequately. The kidneys are functionally intact. Potential causes of prerenal failure include volume depletion, myocardial infarction, sepsis, hypotension, and anaphylaxis. With stabilization, the kidney can resume normal function.

D. Intrarenal failure occurs when there is actual damage to the kidney itself, specifically the nephrons. The diagnosis of intrarenal failure is one of exclusion, eliminating prerenal and postrenal causes of oliguria and azotemia. The two forms of intrarenal failure include glomerulonephritis and acute tubular necrosis (ATN). ATN accounts for approximately 75 percent of all cases of acute renal failure. ATN is a form of intrarenal failure that can be divided into two categories: ischemic ATN and nephrotoxic ATN. Ischemic ATN occurs when there is a significant decrease in blood flow to the kidney as in traumatic injury, sepsis, or shock (p 70) state. Nephrotoxic ATN occurs secondary to the administration or ingestion of agents that are toxic to the renal tubules, such as aminoglycoside antibiotics (tobramycin, gentamicin), radiographic contrast dye, cephalosporin antibiotics, ethylene glycol, and many others. The clinical course of ATN can be divided into sequential stages (Table 1). Intrarenal failure may be reversible depending on the extent of damage.

E. Postrenal or obstructive failure is caused by disruption of the normal flow of urine from the urinary tract. The obstruction can occur anywhere in the collecting system of the kidneys, the ureters, the bladder, and the urethral meatus. Function will be regained with prompt correction of the obstruction. Causes of postrenal failure include mechanical obstructions such as kidney stones (p 312), blood clots, prostatic hypertrophy (p 302), Foley catheter obstruction, urethral strictures, and functional obstructions that may occur with diabetic neuropathy, pregnancy, or spinal cord disease. Medical treatment of ARF varies depending on the etiology.

F. Assessment of the patient in ARF is an ongoing process. After the initial assessment, the nurse performs a more in-depth assessment focusing on the complications of ARF that can affect almost every body system (Table 2). Many of these complications of ARF are related to uremia.

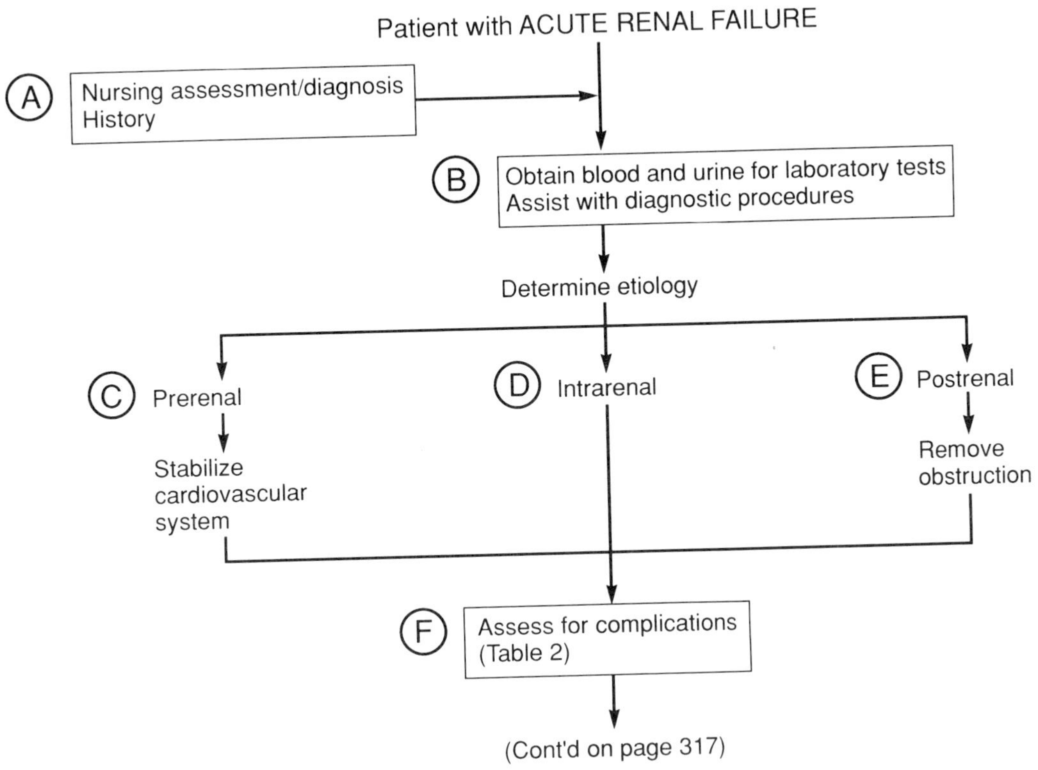
Patient with ACUTE RENAL FAILURE
A
Nursing assessment/diagnosis
History
B
Obtain blood and urine for laboratory tests
Assist with diagnostic procedures
Determine etiology
C
Prerenal
Stabilize cardiovascular system
D
Intrarenal
E
Postrenal
Remove obstruction
F
Assess for complications (Table 2)
(Cont'd on page 317)

TABLE 1 Clinical Stages of Acute Tubular Necrosis

Stage	*Duration*	*Signs and Symptoms*	*Treatment*
Oliguric	Begins a short time after causative event and may last 8–14 days	Urine output <400 cc/24 hr The patient is at risk for volume overload and electrolyte imbalances.	Diuretics to increase urine output The patient may require dialysis (p 328) during this stage.
Diuretic	5–7 days	Urine output increases and BUN begins to fall. Urine output may be as high as several liters per day and is rich in electrolytes.	Volume and electrolyte replacement as indicated according to serum and urine electrolytes
Recovery	1–2 weeks and up to 3–6 months	Urine output and serum electrolyte concentrations gradually return to normal or near normal depending on the extent of residual renal damage Stable BUN and creatinine levels indicate maximum recovery	Monitor electrolytes and creatine/BUN

TABLE 2 Complications of Acute Renal Failure

Body System	*Signs and Symptoms*	*Nursing Action*
Cardiovascular	Hypertension Hypotension S_3 heart sound Pericardial friction rub Arrhythmias	Monitor blood pressure Strict intake and output Vital signs Daily weights Breath and heart sounds ECG, CVP as ordered
Neurologic	Lethargy Confusion Agitation Seizures Unusual behavior	Reorient prn Restraints as ordered Seizure precautions
Metabolic	Acidosis Hyperkalemia Hyperphosphatemia Hypocalcemia Hypermagnesemia Hyponatremia	Monitor electrolytes Consider medication interactions (Amphogel rather than Maalox)
Hematologic	Bleeding tendencies Anemia Thrombocytopenia	Observe for bruising, melena, and bleeding Minimize invasive procedures Avoid unnecessary trauma
Immunologic	Decreased resistance to infection Poor wound healing	Good handwashing Aseptic technique for dressing changes, etc. Observe for signs of infection Private room
Gastrointestinal	Nausea and vomiting Anorexia Abdominal pain	Monitor intake and output Antiemetics as ordered Dietary consult

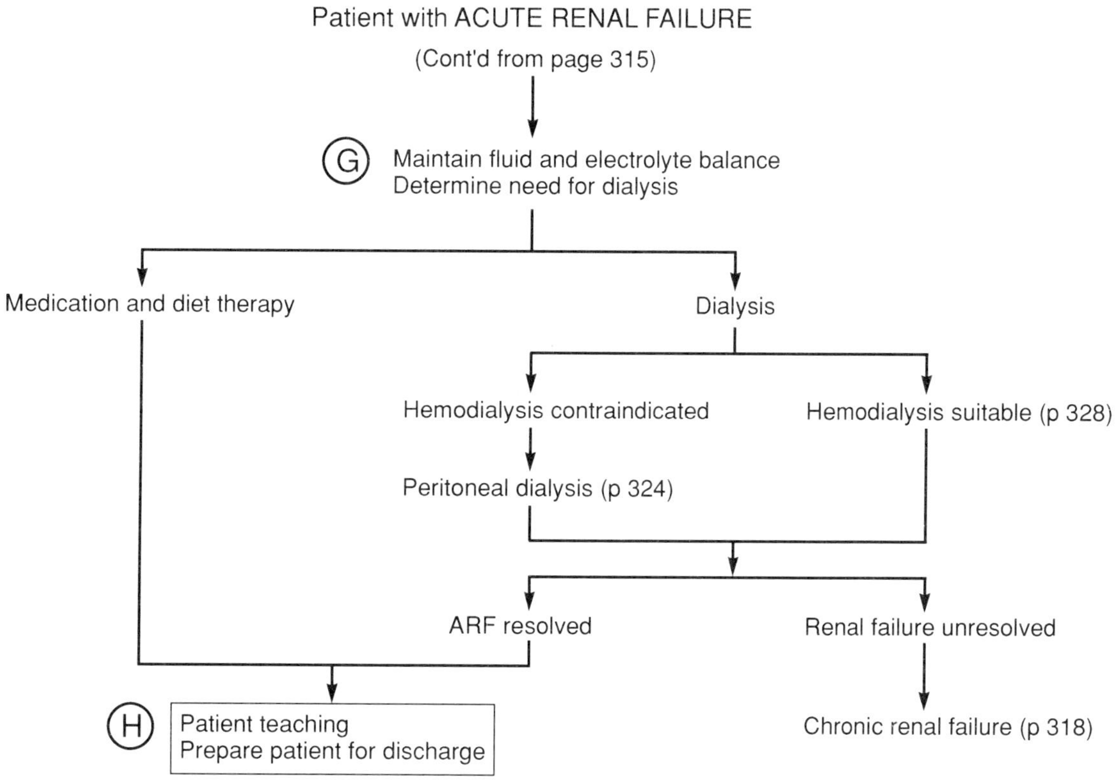

G. The goal of treatment for patients with ARF is to maintain fluid and electrolyte homeostasis until the kidneys are able to regain complete or partial function. Peritoneal dialysis (p 324) or hemodialysis (p 328) may be used to replace function temporarily or to manage the following complications: hyperkalemia (p 196), volume overload, pericarditis (p 76), severe metabolic acidosis, seizures or coma, hyperphosphatemia, and symptomatic uremia.

H. Education of the patient and family is important in any acute disease. Many patients with acute renal failure fear never regaining function of their kidneys and being on dialysis indefinitely. Throughout hospitalization, the patient and family should have tests, procedures, and the rationale for performing them explained. The patient should be reassured that ARF does not necessarily proceed to chronic renal failure (CRF) (p 318). Discharge teaching should include an explanation of the nature of the disease process, dietary restrictions, information about the medication regimen, symptoms that may require medical attention (edema, decreased urine output, nausea and vomiting, anorexia, signs of infection), and the importance of follow-up health care.

References

Bullock B. Renal failure and uremia. In: Bullock B, Rosenthal P, eds. Pathophysiology: adaptations and alterations in function. Boston: Scott, Foresman, 1988:464–467.

Gross M, Gehr M, Flamenbaum W. Acute renal failure. In: Flamenbaum W, Hamburger RJ, eds. Nephrology: An approach to the patient with renal disease. Philadelphia: JB Lippincott, 1982:505–547.

Hekelman FP, Ostendarp CA. Nephrology nursing: perspectives of care. New York: McGraw-Hill, 1979.

Isselbacher KJ, Adams RD, Braunwald E, Petersdorf RG, Wilson JD, eds. Harrison's principles of internal medicine. 9th ed. New York: McGraw-Hill, 1980.

Toto KH. Acute renal failure. In: Mancini ME, ed. Decision making in emergency nursing. Toronto: BC Decker, 1987:148–149.

CHRONIC RENAL FAILURE

Susan Nussle

Chronic renal failure (CRF) results when irreversible damage to both kidneys has occurred and renal function has decreased to less than 10 to 15 percent. When the kidneys cannot regulate the body's internal environment, a multitude of changes occur. These changes are related to the accumulation of toxins, which alter the function of various organ systems, and to fluid and electrolyte abnormalities. Hemodialysis (p 328) or peritoneal dialysis (p 324) is essential to maintain the proper fluid and electrolyte balance of the body and to remove the "uremic" toxins.

A. The nursing history should include determination of compliance with fluid and diet restrictions, prescribed medications, and meeting regularly scheduled dialysis treatments. The general history should include the nature of the renal disease and mode of dialysis. The most common causes of renal disease are glomerulonephritis (p 308); hypertension (p 80); diabetes (p 176); collagen vascular disease, including systemic lupus erythematosus (p 352); intravenous drug abuse; and polycystic kidney. If the patient is receiving hemodialysis, the last date of dialysis and the dry weight (the weight obtained at the end of each dialysis treatment) should be determined. The most common reasons for hospital admissions for CRF patients are access problems; noncompliance with regularly scheduled dialysis treatments, resulting in volume overload and uremic manifestations; and pericarditis.

B. Nursing assessment begins with vital signs and evaluation of the history and then focuses on the effects of uremic toxins on every body system (see Table 1).

TABLE 1 Effects of Uremic Toxins on Body Systems

System	*Manifestation*
Neurologic	Lethargy Fatigue Confusion
Cardiovascular/ pulmonary	Hypertension Congestive heart failure Pulmonary edema Hyperkalemia Pericarditis
Gastrointestinal	Nausea Vomiting Anorexia Gastrointestinal bleeding
Integumentary	Yellow-gray, dry skin Pruritus
Hematologic	Anemia Bleeding tendencies
Other	Renal osteodystrophy Metabolic acidosis Increased risk of infection

C. Noncompliance with scheduled dialysis treatments often results in volume overload and the need for emergent dialysis in the hospital setting. Clinical signs of volume overload include peripheral edema, dyspnea, rales, tachypnea, hypertension, jugular venous distention, and the presence of an S_3 heart sound. Comparison of the present weight with the baseline or "dry" weight is also an excellent method of fluid assessment.

D. Pericarditis (p 76) is another complication that occurs in CRF patients. It is often manifested by chest pain that is usually relieved by leaning forward, low-grade fever, possible hypotension, and a pericardial friction rub (a scratchy "leathery" sound heard best with the stethoscope's diaphragm over the left mid-to-lower sternal border). However, some patients are completely asymptomatic except for a friction rub. Treatment consists of intense dialysis until the condition improves.

E. Pertinent laboratory tests include a complete blood count, electrolyte and creatinine levels, and a blood urea nitrogen (BUN) level. Typical findings in a renal patient include a low hemoglobin and hematocrit; low bicarbonate levels; elevated BUN, creatinine, and uric acid levels; low serum calcium and elevated serum phosphate levels; and hyperkalemia. *Hyperkalemia results in electrocardiogram changes (p 196), progressing to cardiac arrest and death if not corrected by emergent dialysis.* Elevated BUN and creatinine leads to the clinical state of uremia if not corrected by dialysis.

F. A permanent vascular access site (p 328) should be assessed for patency on admission and every shift thereafter. Patency can be determined by either palpating for a thrill (buzzing sensation) or listening with a stethoscope for a bruit (buzzing sound). The site should also be assessed daily for signs of infection, such as redness, swelling, or purulent drainage. No blood pressure measurements, placement of intravenous lines, or needle sticks should be performed on the access arm.

G. A clotted access that is surgically declotted within the first 24 hours can potentially continue to be used for hemodialysis. If declotting is impossible, a temporary device (i.e., a double-lumen subclavian catheter) is used for dialysis until a new permanent access has matured.

H. Signs and symptoms of an infected access include redness, pain, purulent drainage, and swelling along the access site. Fever and positive blood cultures are present if the infection is systemic. Treatment is with antibiotics, although the infection is often difficult to eradicate and the access must be removed. Again, a temporary device is placed and used for dialysis until a new permanent access has matured.

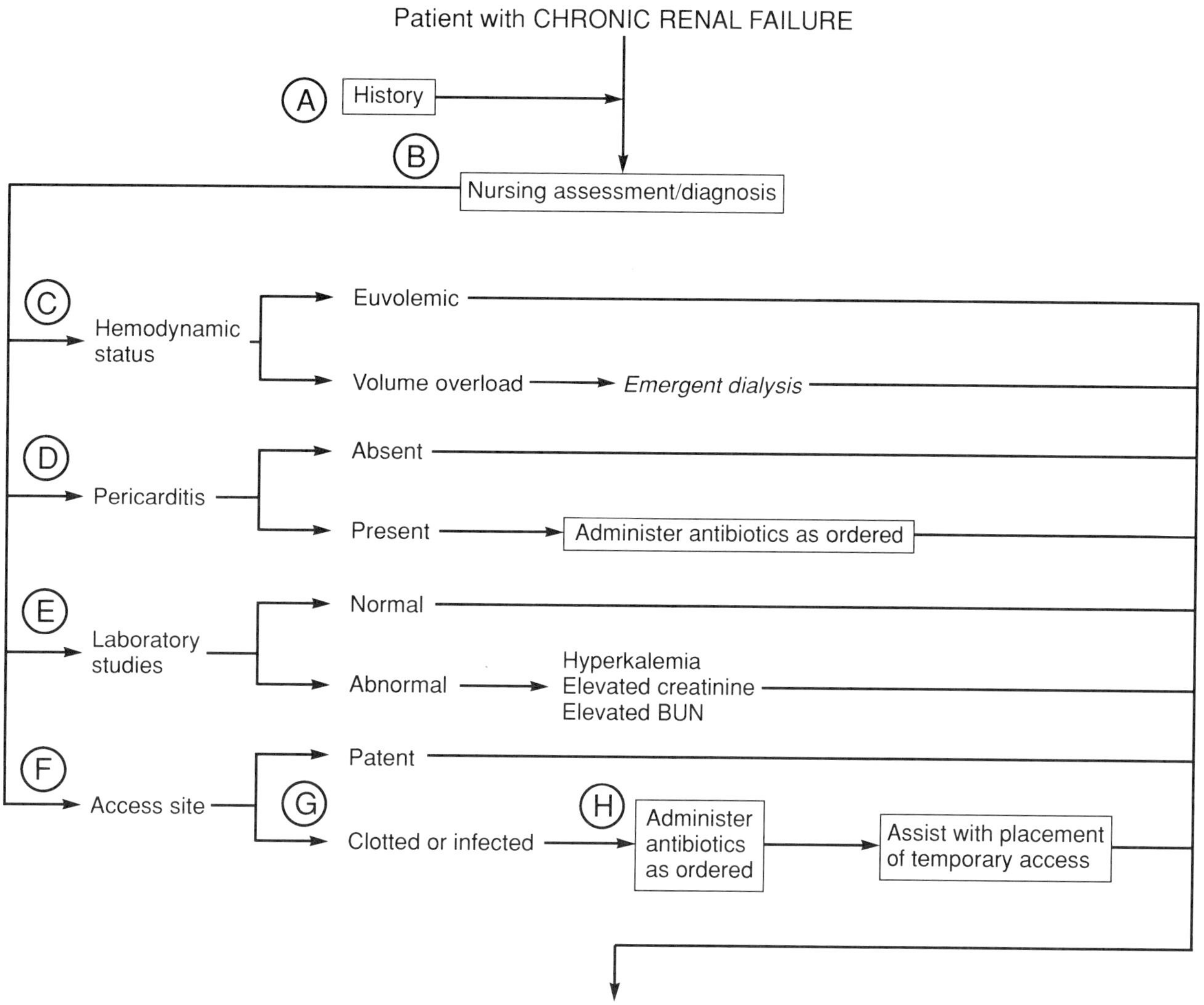

(Cont'd on page 321)

TABLE 2 Guidelines for the Care of a CRF Patient

Maintain fluid balance; promote stable hemodynamic status
Monitor intake and output
Restrict fluid intake
Daily weights
Assess for edema
Auscultate breath sounds
Monitor blood pressure and pulse
Administer antihypertensive medications
Maintain electrolyte balance
Monitor electrolyte levels (especially sodium, potassium, calcium, phosphate, bicarbonate)
Low-sodium and -potassium diet
Administer phosphate-binding medications (i.e., Amphojel, Basaljel)
Administer oral alkalizing agents (i.e., Shohl's solution) to control acidosis
Provide symptomatic relief from the effects of anemia and abnormal clotting activity
Minimize blood loss (avoid collection of unnecessary blood specimens)
Avoid fatigue
Avoid bruising or trauma to skin
Prevent bleeding (use a soft toothbrush, avoid constipation)
Promote maximal level of functioning
Avoid immobilization as it promotes bone demineralization
Administer analgesics for pain related to renal osteodystrophy
Maintain good oral hygiene to counteract decreased appetite related to nausea and vomiting
Use lanolin-base lotion on skin or administer antipruritic medication to alleviate dryness and itching
Provide safe environment for confused patient
Prevent infection by aseptic technique with nursing procedures
Monitor for signs of infection (character of sputum, erythema or drainage from access, temperature elevation)
Maintain good nutritional status through adequate protein, calorie, and vitamin intake

I. Routine care of the CRF patient is complex and requires continuous assessment by the nurse. See Table 2 for nursing care guidelines.

J. Discharge planning for the CRF patient on dialysis includes instruction for medications, access care, diet and fluid restrictions, and reinforcement of basic knowledge about the condition. Support is vital in encouraging patients to meet regularly scheduled dialysis treatments, comply with the fluid and diet limitations, and take the prescribed medications.

References

Hahn K. The many signs of renal failure. Nursing '87 1987; August:34–41.

Lancaster LE. Core curriculum for nephrology nursing. Pitman, NJ: Anthony J. Jannetti, 1987.

Lancaster LE. Renal failure: pathophysiology, assessment and intervention. Part I. Nephrol Nurse 1983; 5(2):38–51.

Lancaster LE. Renal failure: pathophysiology, assessment and intervention. Part II. Nephrol Nurse 1983; 5(3):30–38.

Richard CJ. Comprehensive nephrology nursing. Boston: Little, Brown, 1986.

Patient with CHRONIC RENAL FAILURE

(Cont'd from page 319)

↓

Maintenance hemodialysis (p 328)

↓

(I) Routine nursing care (Table 2)

- ↓ Patient stable
  - ↓ (J) Discharge patient home with instructions
- ↓ Patient unstable
  Complications with access
  - ↓ Continue hospitalization with treatment and observation

RENAL ARTERY STENOSIS

Kendra Ellis

Renal artery stenosis is defined as a partial occlusion of one or both renal arteries and their major branches. The narrowing of the artery is usually caused by atherosclerosis, but may also be caused by fibrous dysplasia or neoplasm. The progression of the lesion can result in arterial dissection, occlusion, or thrombosis. This disease is prevalent in whites, and found in twice as many men as women.

A. The partial occlusion of the renal artery results in a decrease in renal perfusion. The decreased blood flow to the kidneys causes the release of renin, which triggers the response of the angiotensin system, resulting in vasoconstriction. It also stimulates the production of aldosterone. Secondary hypertension is caused by vasoconstriction and sodium and water retention. Hypertension (p 80), the most common and important symptom in renal stenosis, can damage the kidneys. The patient may present with hypertension, decreased urine output, pain in the flank area, and an abdominal bruit. Hyponatremia and a high urine specific gravity may also be present.

B. The diagnosis of renal artery stenosis is made based on the presenting symptoms and renal tests. The presence of collateral circulation and unilateral small kidney is suggestive of stenosis. The diagnostic renal tests include renal flow scan, intravenous pyelography (IVP), and renal arteriography. Although renal arteriography is the most specific diagnostic test, the risks include embolization (p 116) caused by invasive manipulation of the catheter through the diseased arteries.

C. Hypertension may be controlled with medication and diet restrictions. The types of medication include antihypertensives, vasodilators, and diuretics, but renal function must be continually assessed with these medications. A drop in renal perfusion may occur when the patient is normotensive. Fluid and sodium restrictions are used to decrease the circulating blood volume, thus decreasing the blood pressure.

D. If stenosis greatly inhibits circulation or becomes occlusive, surgical intervention is required. Preoperatively, the patient needs to have adequate hydration. Fluid replacement and adequate diuresis help maintain renal function prior to surgery. Accurate fluid intake and output need to be assessed and recorded. A Foley catheter is recommended.

E. Nephrectomy (p 332) is the removal of one kidney. This surgery can be performed when the stenosis involves only one kidney; the contralateral kidney must be normal. A nephrectomy is also considered when medical therapy is ineffective and revascularization is contraindicated (i.e., complete renal artery occlusion or renal atrophy).

F. Renal artery bypass or revascularization involves anastomosis between the renal artery and other major arteries, such as the splenic artery or aorta. This allows the blood flow to bypass the site of stenosis. Either the saphenous vein or prosthetic material may be used for the bypass graft. Indications for revascularization are severe refractory hypertension, low predicted surgical risk, altered renal function, and/or renal ischemia. The increased perfusion to the kidneys decreases renin production and relieves hypertension.

G. Percutaneous transluminal angioplasty (PTA) is the mechanical dilatation of a stenotic arterial lesion. It widens the lumen by disrupting the plaque and stretching the medial layer of the artery. It is the alternative for a patient who would be at high risk for surgery. PTA is performed with a local anesthetic and has a low morbidity risk. Complications include: trauma of the artery, resulting in embolization; hemorrhage, if the vessel wall is ruptured; or excessive bleeding from the femoral artery puncture site. Pressure to the site is necessary for at least 20 minutes.

H. The patient is taken to the ICU for at least 24 hours after surgery. Initially, the blood pressure may remain high. The administration of Nipride (a potent vasodilator) and continual blood pressure monitoring may be needed to prevent damage to the graft. Prophylactic antibiotics may be given, and the patient's white blood cell count and temperature must be monitored continually. Paralytic ileus is usually present postoperatively, owing to manipulation of the bowel during surgery. Abdominal size and bowel sounds need to be assessed. A nasogastric tube to low intermittent suction is recommended. Once the patient is discharged to the floor, blood pressure must be taken frequently. Oral antihypertensive medications may be given for several days after the surgery. The usual hospital stay is 7 to 10 days.

References

Doyle J. Renovascular hypertension. Crit Care Quart 1985; 8(2):51–59.

Hudak C, Lohr T, Gallo B. Critical care nursing. Philadelphia: JB Lippincott, 1982:318.

Kenner C, Guzzetta C, Dossey B. Critical care nursing. Boston: Little, Brown, 1981:873.

Taylor D. Renal hypertension. Nursing 83 1983; 13:44–45.

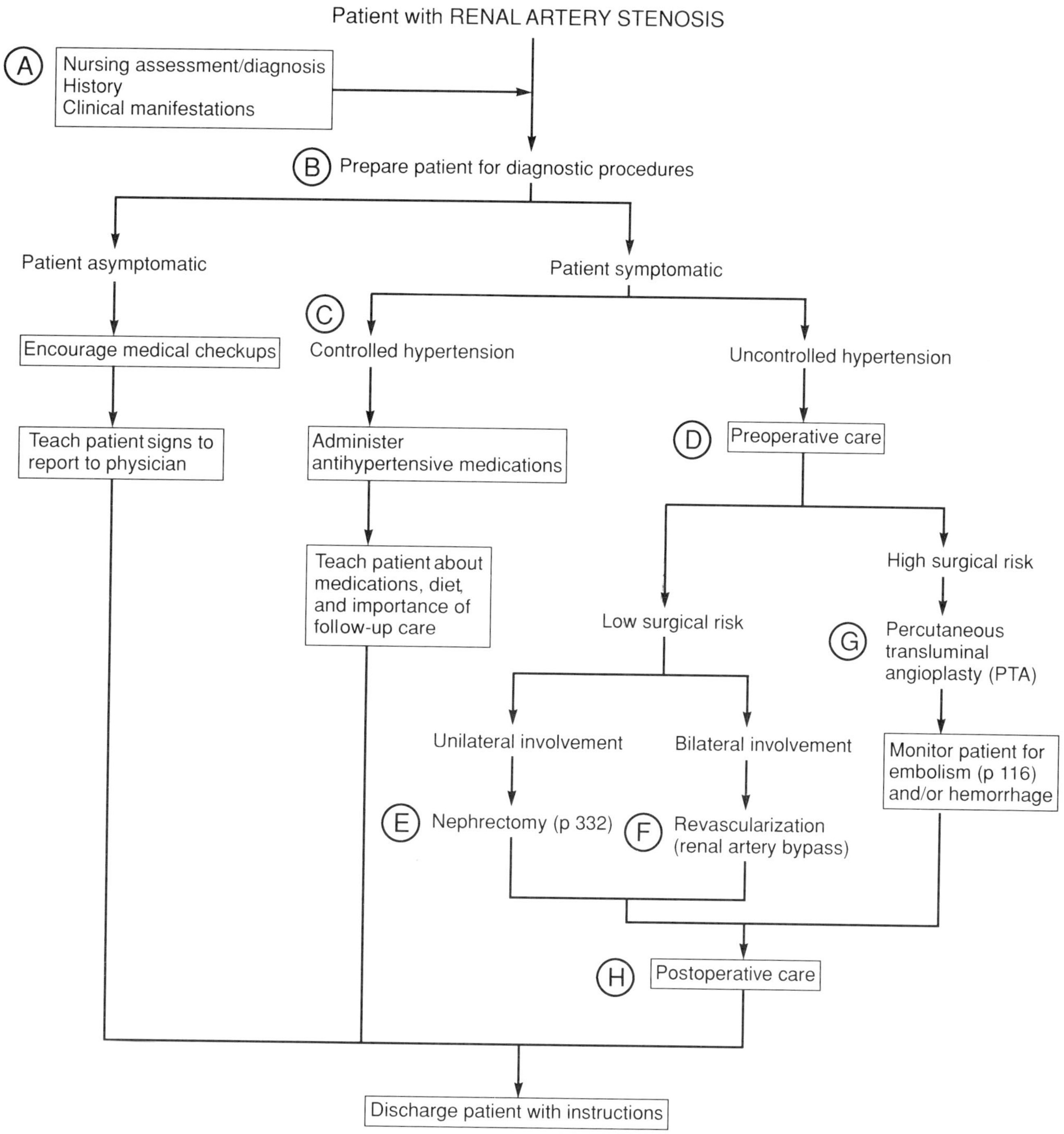
Patient with RENAL ARTERY STENOSIS
A
Nursing assessment/diagnosis
History
Clinical manifestations
B
Prepare patient for diagnostic procedures
Patient asymptomatic
Patient symptomatic
C
Encourage medical checkups
Controlled hypertension
Uncontrolled hypertension
Teach patient signs to report to physician
Administer antihypertensive medications
D
Preoperative care
Teach patient about medications, diet, and importance of follow-up care
High surgical risk
Low surgical risk
G
Percutaneous transluminal angioplasty (PTA)
Unilateral involvement
Bilateral involvement
Monitor patient for embolism (p 116) and/or hemorrhage
E
Nephrectomy (p 332)
F
Revascularization (renal artery bypass)
H
Postoperative care
Discharge patient with instructions

PERITONEAL DIALYSIS

Kathleen H. Toto

Peritoneal dialysis (PD) (Fig. 1) utilizes the peritoneum's generous blood supply, surface area, and space as a semipermeable membrane for exchange. PD is indicated for the treatment of acute renal failure, in patients without access to hemodialysis, and in hemodynamically unstable patients. It is also indicated for chronic renal failure, drug intoxication, volume overload, electrolyte imbalances (especially hyperkalemia [p 196]) and uremia (elevated blood urea nitrogen). Contraindications to PD include multiple abdominal adhesions, ileus, severe abdominal trauma, recent abdominal surgery or an aortic graft, peritonitis, and hypovolemia.

A. The nursing assessment includes physical assessment, baseline vital signs, evaluation of laboratory data, and a complete history (see Acute Renal Failure [p 314] and Chronic Renal Failure [p 318]).

B. The equipment needed can be conveniently assembled on a peritoneal dialysis cart (Table 1). Preassembled kits are available.

TABLE 1 Equipment Required for Peritoneal Dialysis

Lidocaine and suture (for insertion only)
Dialysate solution
Administration set (tubing and drainage bag)
Peritoneal dialysis tray and catheter (for insertion only)
Betadine solution
Sterile gloves
4 × 4 gauze pads
Adhesive tape
Precut dressings
Connection shields
K-pad
Betadine scrub brush
Sterile cup
Peritoneal dialysis flow sheet
Timer

C. Before beginning PD on the hospitalized chronic ambulatory peritoneal dialysis (CAPD) patient, assess the catheter site carefully for signs of infection. Peritonitis is a common complication of the indwelling PD catheter. Signs of localized infection include redness and/or purulent drainage around the catheter entry site and tenderness and pain in the lower abdomen. Notify the physician if any of these signs are present.

D. In acute situations, the patient and family require a thorough explanation of the procedure. They should be told that a catheter will be placed in the lower abdomen and that fluid will be instilled and drained as a continuous procedure to remove fluid and toxins until the kidneys have recovered (Fig. 1). When the fluid is instilled, the patient feels "full" and uncomfortable. The patient should be instructed that repositioning may increase comfort and that any pain should be reported. Complete bedrest is not necessary.

E. Before insertion of a temporary Silastic PD catheter, the patient's bladder must be emptied by voiding or catheterization to prevent perforation.

F. Insertion of a PD catheter is a sterile procedure requiring a sterile scrub and sterile garb. All individuals in the room should wear masks, including the patient. The skin is prepped with Betadine, and a local anesthetic is given. The catheter is inserted 1 to 2 cm below the umbilicus. After placement of the catheter, the skin is sutured around the catheter to reduce dialysate leakage and peritoneal infection. The site is dressed with sterile 4 × 4 pads or a precut dressing and taped occlusively and securely. A "test run" may be done to assess catheter placement. The drainage is assessed for stool, gross blood, or urine, which would indicate incorrect placement of the catheter.

G. Dialysate is ordered on the basis of the patient's volume and electrolyte status. The dialysate solution is available in 1- and 2-liter volumes, in a wide range of glucose concentrations from 1.5 percent to 7.0 percent. The higher the glucose concentration, the greater the amount of volume removed from the patient. Patients receiving 4.25 percent and 7.0 percent concentrations of dialysate should be monitored closely for hypovolemia. Potassium levels are closely monitored with 3.0 to 4.0 mEq per liter of potassium chloride added to each liter to prevent hypokalemia. Bicarbonate may also be added to manage metabolic acidosis. Heparin may be added to prevent fibrin accumulation in the PD catheter. Each bag should be labeled with the medications added, the exchange number, the time, and the nurse's initials. Dialysate should be warmed to approximately 37°C prior to infusion.

H. The patient should be weighed prior to the initiation of PD and then twice a day after the dialysate has been drained while PD is in progress. Each kilogram of weight loss approximates 1 liter of volume removed.

I. Using sterile technique, the PD administration set is inserted into the dialysate bag, purged of air and connected to the sterile end of the PD catheter. If air is instilled into the abdominal cavity it causes referred shoulder pain. The connection is protected by a connection shield or a Betadine-soaked 4 × 4 pad. Aseptic technique must be used any time the system is broken.

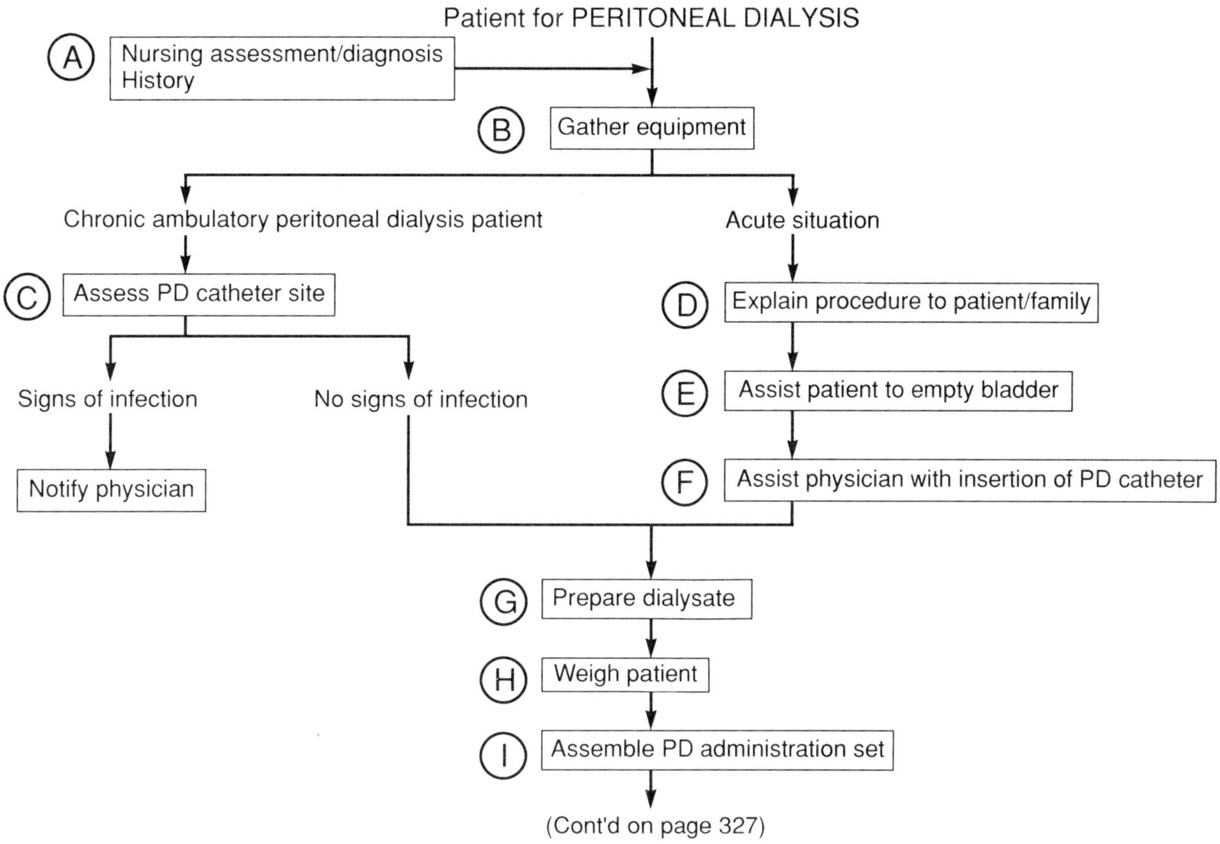
Patient for PERITONEAL DIALYSIS
A
Nursing assessment/diagnosis
History
B
Gather equipment
Chronic ambulatory peritoneal dialysis patient
Acute situation
C
Assess PD catheter site
D
Explain procedure to patient/family
Signs of infection
No signs of infection
E
Assist patient to empty bladder
Notify physician
F
Assist physician with insertion of PD catheter
G
Prepare dialysate
H
Weigh patient
I
Assemble PD administration set
(Cont'd on page 327)

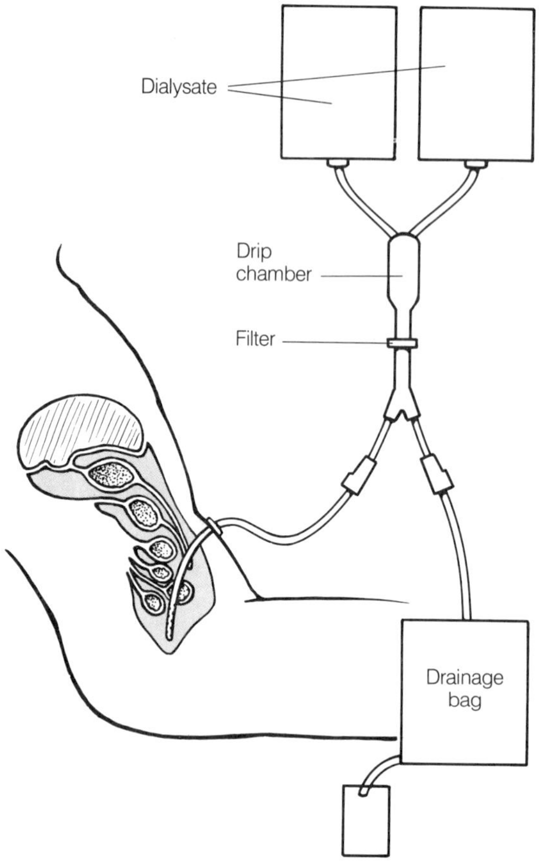

Figure 1 Peritoneal dialysis.

J. One exchange of PD includes the inflow, dwell, and drain time of the ordered volume of dialysate. The physician's order will include inflow time, dwell time, drain (outflow) time, volume and concentration of dialysate, agents to be added, and amount of volume to be removed with each exchange. Record vital signs during each cycle. Observe the patient for shortness of breath during inflow, as the diaphragm may be compressed. Elevate the head of the bed to enhance respirations. After the dialysate is instilled, all roller clamps are closed, and a timer is set for the dwell time ordered. Outflow or drainage begins after the dwell time is completed. The roller clamps at the drainage bag and near the PD catheter are opened to begin drainage for the ordered drain time. Assess and document drainage. Cloudiness may indicate peritonitis (p 138). Normally the drainage is clear and straw colored. Turn the patient from side to side to facilitate drainage. Follow universal precautions when handling the dialysate.

K. Careful recording of the exchanges is essential. The volume of dialysate outflow is subtracted from the total volume instilled, resulting in a net gain (+) or loss (−) of fluid for each exchange. A running total of net volumes (+ or −) should also be recorded. A positive fluid balance indicates volume retained by the patient. A negative fluid balance indicates volume lost by the patient. Notify the physician if the volume drained is consistently less than the volume infused. Assess the patient's electrolytes, volume status, and glucose levels regularly.

L. Change the dressing over the insertion site every 24 hours, using sterile technique and wearing a mask. Documentation should include the appearance of the site.

M. The PD administration set and drainage bag are changed once per week or any time the tubing is contaminated. Strict sterile technique should be followed. The temporary peritoneal catheter is usually changed by the physician every 3 to 4 days; new tubing is used for a new catheter.

N. Patient teaching is extremely important for the patient with renal failure. A multidisciplinary approach should be used in which physician, nursing, nutrition, and social services staff are involved.

References

American Nephrology Nurses Association. Standards of clinical practice for nephrology nursing. Pitman, NJ: Anthony J. Jannetti, 1988.

Flamenbaum W, Hamburger RJ. Nephrology: an approach to the patient with renal disease. Philadelphia: JB Lippincott, 1982.

Henkelman FP, Ostendarp CA. Nephrology nursing: perspectives of care. New York: McGraw-Hill, 1979.

Lancaster LE, ed. Core curriculum for nephrology nursing. Pitman, NJ: Anthony J. Jannetti, 1987.

Patient for PERITONEAL DIALYSIS

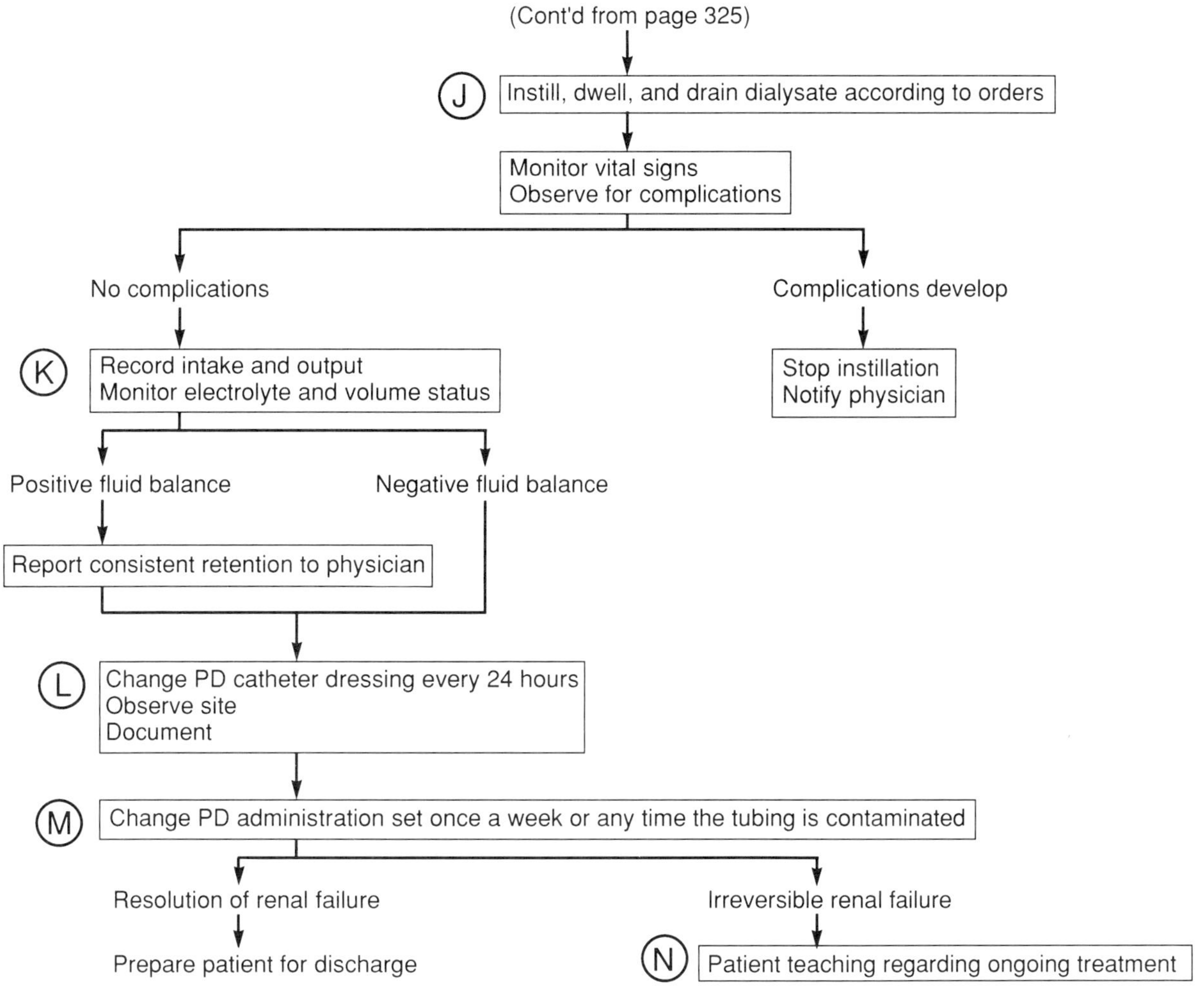

HEMODIALYSIS

Susan Nussle

The goal of hemodialysis is to correct fluid and electrolyte imbalances, remove metabolic wastes, and restore the acid-base balance of the blood in patients who have lost their renal function. Three principles are involved in dialysis: diffusion, osmosis, and ultrafiltration. These processes are accomplished by a semipermeable membrane in an artificial kidney, which filters excess fluid, electrolytes, and metabolic wastes from the blood into the dialyzing fluid. Indications for hemodialysis include acute renal failure resulting in severe fluid overload, hyperkalemia, and the clinical state of uremia; chronic renal failure; and some drug overdoses.

A. The patient presents with a history compatible with either acute or chronic renal failure. Acute renal failure is an abrupt loss of renal function (p 314). Chronic renal failure occurs when irreversible damage to both kidneys leads to progressive kidney failure and clinical signs of uremia (p 318).

B. The nursing assessment includes a complete physical assessment, in addition to evaluation of the history and vital signs. The predialysis patient may show signs of volume overload, such as peripheral edema, dyspnea, rales, progressive hypertension, jugular venous distention, and the presence of an S_3 heart sound.

C. Hemodialysis is not initiated on a patient with a systolic blood pressure less than 90 mm Hg because of the hypotensive effects of dialysis.

D. Antihypertensive medications should be held up to 4 hours before dialysis for the same reason.

E. Hyperkalemia is a common complication of renal patients and can be corrected during dialysis. Changes in the electrocardiogram are the single most important sign of hyperkalemia (p 196). These changes include: tall, peaked T waves; ST segment depression; loss of the P wave; and broadening of the QRS complex. In addition to the potassium level, the serum creatinine level is of particular importance, because high creatinine indicates the need for more aggressive dialysis. Blood work should also be done before dialysis, since laboratory values of blood drawn after dialysis are inaccurate.

F. The postdialysis patient may occasionally show signs of volume depletion, owing to excessive fluid removal during dialysis. Signs of volume depletion include orthostatic hypotension, complaints of thirst, lethargy, and dizziness. Central venous pressure readings, when appropriate, and daily weights are excellent tools for assessing fluid balance. Clinical signs of uremia are possible in both the pre- and postdialysis patient.

G. Because the patient is heparinized during dialysis, spontaneous bleeding may occur within the first 4 hours after dialysis. The most common site of bleeding is from the access site. If bleeding occurs here, place digital pressure over the bleeding site until the bleeding stops (approximately 5 minutes), and notify the physician. Other potential areas for bleeding include a wound site or the gastrointestinal tract. Because of this potential for bleeding, it is preferable to delay invasive nursing procedures, such as discontinuing an intravenous line or shaving a patient, for a few hours after dialysis if possible.

H. Disequilibrium syndrome, a rare but potential complication of dialysis, involves fluid shifts between the cerebral tissue and blood, resulting in swelling of the cerebral cells. Symptoms include increasing restlessness, headache, confusion, muscle cramping, twitching, and seizures.

I. The patient's access site should be assessed during every shift. Permanent accesses, such as arteriovenous fistulas or artificial grafts, should be auscultated for a bruit (buzzing sound) and palpated for a thrill (buzzing sensation) to ensure patency (Fig. 1). Signs of infection, such as inflammation, tenderness, or drainage from the access site, should also be assessed. Any evidence of infection at the access site is an absolute contraindication for its use in dialysis. No blood pressure measurements, intravenous lines, or needle sticks should be instituted on the access arm. A temporary access, such as a subclavian double-lumen catheter, is used solely for dialysis and should not be used by the floor nurse to infuse medications or draw blood. The nurse should ensure that a dry, occlusive dressing covers the insertion site and that there are no signs of infection present.

J. All dialysis patients should be placed on severe fluid restriction. Although specific limits vary according to the urine output, generally patients are restricted to 1,000 to 1,500 ml every 24 hours. An average weight gain between dialysis treatments is 1 pound per day.

K. Discharge planning varies according to the type of renal failure. The acute renal failure patient who does not need maintenance dialysis requires teaching related to the nature of the disease and the medication. The chronic renal failure patient who remains on maintenance dialysis requires information on basic hemodialysis principles and procedures. In addition, instructions regarding medications, access care, and diet and fluid restrictions should be given. The importance of follow-up care with a physician is stressed with all patients.

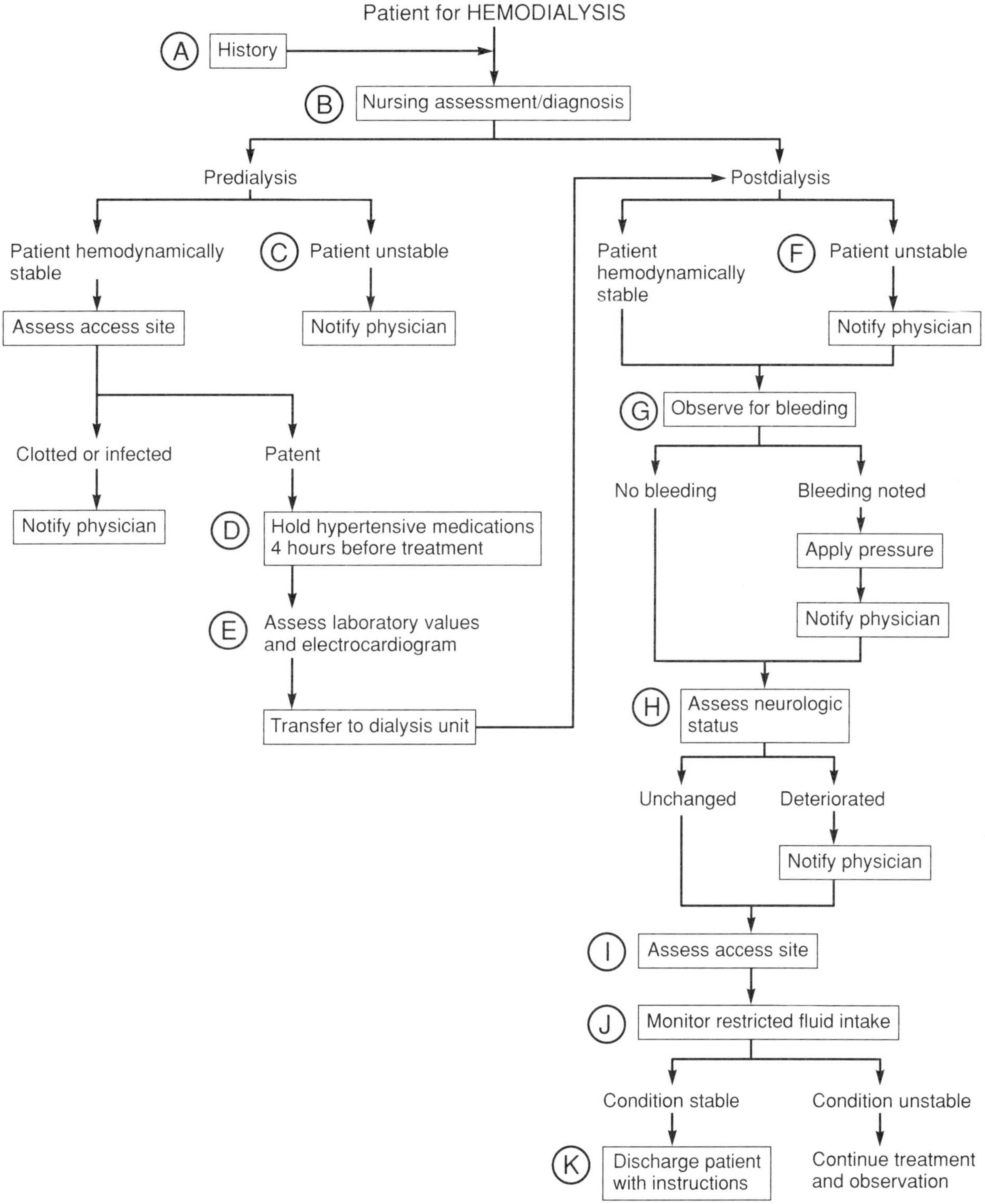
Patient for HEMODIALYSIS
A
History
B
Nursing assessment/diagnosis
Predialysis
Patient hemodynamically stable
C
Patient unstable
Assess access site
Notify physician
Clotted or infected
Patent
Notify physician
D
Hold hypertensive medications 4 hours before treatment
E
Assess laboratory values and electrocardiogram
Transfer to dialysis unit
Postdialysis
Patient hemodynamically stable
F
Patient unstable
Notify physician
G
Observe for bleeding
No bleeding
Bleeding noted
Apply pressure
Notify physician
H
Assess neurologic status
Unchanged
Deteriorated
Notify physician
I
Assess access site
J
Monitor restricted fluid intake
Condition stable
Condition unstable
K
Discharge patient with instructions
Continue treatment and observation

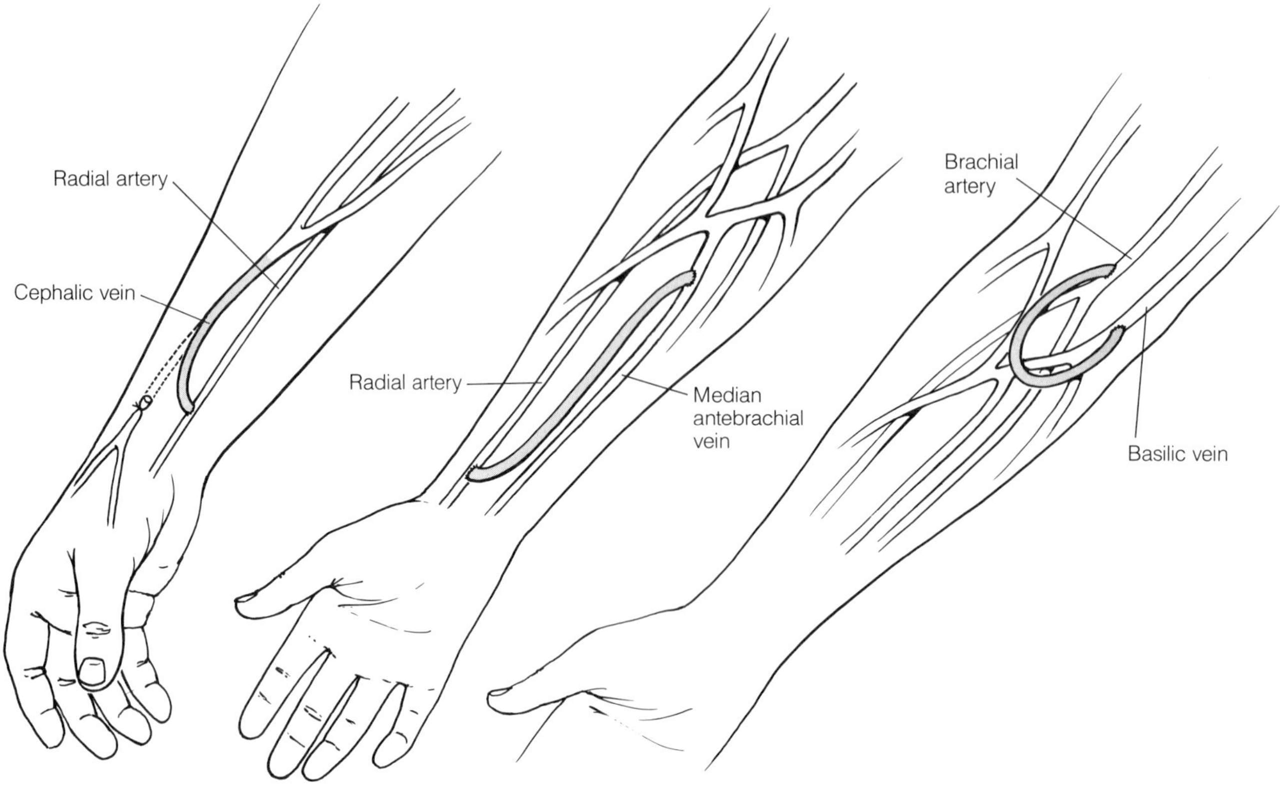

Figure 1 Access for hemodialysis. *A*, Arteriovenous fistula. *B*, Straight graft. *C*, Looped graft.

References

Gutch CF, Stones MH. Review of hemodialysis for nurses and dialysis personnel. 4th ed. St. Louis: CV Mosby, 1983.

Lancaster LE. Core curriculum for nephrology nursing. Pitman, NJ: Anthony J. Jannetti, 1987.

Lancaster LE. The patient with end stage renal disease. New York: John Wiley, 1984.

Lewis SM. Acute and chronic renal failure. In: Carroll DP, Boynton SD, Bradley JW, eds. Medical-surgical nursing. New York: McGraw-Hill, 1983:1109–1140.

NEPHRECTOMY

Leslie C. Hussey

A. Nephrectomy is the removal of a kidney. Most often, the incision for a nephrectomy is made on the right or left flank below the 12th rib. The renal pedicle, which contains the artery and vein, is clamped and divided. The ureter is also clamped. A nephrectomy is usually performed as a result of cancer, trauma, or a chronic problem, such as infection. Depending on the cause, the patient may have been through extensive testing, including a complete blood count, coagulation profile, electrolytes, blood urea nitrogen (BUN), and serum creatinine levels.

B. Preoperative care includes extensive teaching about the importance of turning, coughing, and deep breathing. Because the incision is made immediately below the diaphragm, these exercises will be painful, and the patient needs to be aware of their importance. Other teaching includes an explanation of drainage tubes that are usually inserted into the wound; therefore, the patient will not be able to lie on the affected side. The patient may receive a bowel preparation, and the appropriate side, abdomen, back, axilla, and anterior chest must be shaved and prepped. An indwelling catheter is inserted into the bladder the morning of surgery.

C. Postoperatively, nursing care is focused on promoting ventilation, maintaining urinary output, minimizing abdominal distention, preventing hemorrhage, and monitoring drainage tubes and dressings. As in all surgical patients, it is necessary to monitor vital signs, since abnormal vital signs or changes in vital signs often indicate a change in patient status (p 4).

D. Postoperatively, strongly encourage the patient to turn, cough, and deep breathe at least every 2 hours to prevent pulmonary complications and maintain ventilation. To encourage moving and deep breathing, administer pain medication every 3 to 4 hours for the first 2 days.

E. Monitor urine output. It should be at least 50 ml per hour. Measure output not only from the catheter, but also from the nephrostomy and cystostomy tubes, if present. Renal function is monitored by checking BUN, creatinine, and electrolyte levels.

F. Check the dressing frequently for drainage and reinforce or change it as necessary. The drainage is normally pink or dark red. Also assess the drainage in the bags connected to drainage tubes.

G. Check the patient for abdominal distention. Assess bowel sounds. Paralytic ileus is common after a nephrectomy. Often a nasogastric tube is inserted and the patient is given nothing by mouth.

H. Hemorrhage is a real danger. Report the presence of bright red blood in the urine or on the dressing immediately. Observe the patient for signs of shock (p 70).

I. The patient starts ambulating within 24 hours after surgery. Provide appropriate pain relief, and support the incision.

J. Prognosis depends on the reason for the nephrectomy. The patient may need further treatment and should understand plans for follow-up care. Lifting and strenuous activity need to be avoided for approximately 8 weeks.

References

Kneisl CR, Ames SW. Adult health nursing: a biopsychosocial approach. Reading, MA: Addison-Wesley, 1986.

Le Maitre GD, Finnegan JA. The patient in surgery: a guide for nurses. Philadelphia: WB Saunders, 1980.

Phipps WJ, Long BC, Woods NF. Medical-surgical nursing: concepts and clinical practice. 3rd ed. St. Louis: CV Mosby, 1987.

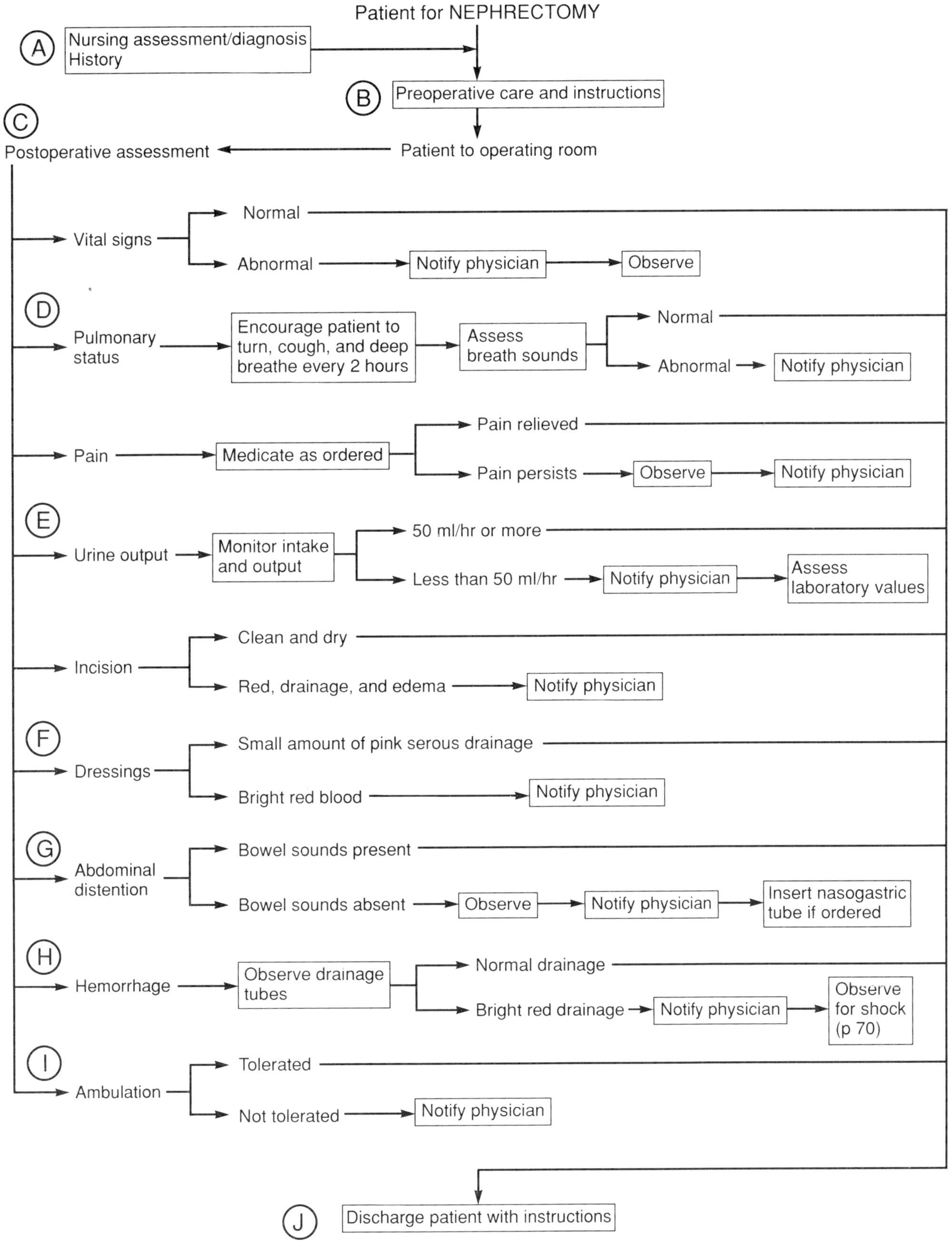
Patient for NEPHRECTOMY
A
Nursing assessment/diagnosis
History
B
Preoperative care and instructions
C
Postoperative assessment
Patient to operating room
Vital signs
Normal
Abnormal
Notify physician
Observe
D
Pulmonary status
Encourage patient to turn, cough, and deep breathe every 2 hours
Assess breath sounds
Normal
Abnormal
Notify physician
Pain
Medicate as ordered
Pain relieved
Pain persists
Observe
Notify physician
E
Urine output
Monitor intake and output
50 ml/hr or more
Less than 50 ml/hr
Notify physician
Assess laboratory values
Incision
Clean and dry
Red, drainage, and edema
Notify physician
F
Dressings
Small amount of pink serous drainage
Bright red blood
Notify physician
G
Abdominal distention
Bowel sounds present
Bowel sounds absent
Observe
Notify physician
Insert nasogastric tube if ordered
H
Hemorrhage
Observe drainage tubes
Normal drainage
Bright red drainage
Notify physician
Observe for shock (p 70)
I
Ambulation
Tolerated
Not tolerated
Notify physician
J
Discharge patient with instructions

RENAL TRANSPLANTATION

Diane M. Zintak

Renal transplantation (RT) is the surgical insertion of a human kidney from a living or cadaveric source into a patient with end-stage renal disease (ESRD), in order to replace loss of normal kidney function. If successful, it offers the individual with ESRD freedom from the constraints of conventional dialysis therapy while minimizing the physiologic complications of renal failure. With successful RT, lifestyle modifications are less restrictive, including diet, reversal of anemia, and elimination of the need for vascular access. If unsuccessful, the patient can return to dialysis or attempt a second transplant.

A. Most individuals considering RT have already started some form of dialysis (pp 324, 328). Typically a donor is sought when the patient's serum creatinine is approximately 5 mg/dl, serum blood urea nitrogen is greater than 70 mg/dl, and creatinine clearance is 15 ml per minute.

B. It is not uncommon for the RT candidate to demonstrate some degree of mental clouding because of failure of the diseased kidneys to filter blood, excrete waste products, and balance fluid and electrolytes. Other signs and symptoms frequently seen in ESRD patients include edema, hypertension, uremia, anemia, electrolyte imbalances, and serum acid accumulation.

C. Not all patients with ESRD are candidates for RT. Because of the potential complications, each patient is carefully evaluated to ensure suitability. Age is a primary concern. Individuals between 5 and 50 years of age typically present fewer risks for transplantation than younger or older patients. Thorough evaluation is conducted for preexisting conditions such as active chronic infection, malignancy, and abnormalities of the metabolic, cardiovascular, gastrointestinal, and genitourinary systems. Findings may indicate medical intervention before the patient is accepted for RT. Surgical preparation may include a splenectomy (p 370) to help decrease the body's natural defense mechanisms and a nephrectomy (p 332) if the kidneys are infected or are contributing to uncontrolled hypertension (p 80). Psychiatric evaluations are also completed and available psychosocial support factors are identified in order to determine likelihood of patient compliance during the postoperative regimen.

D. Transplant candidates may receive a kidney from a close blood relative (living related donor) who has normally functioning kidneys and no underlying disease, or a kidney may be obtained from a deceased, unrelated individual (cadaver donor) who is free of infection and cancer and does not have a history of renal disease or hypertension. In either case, it is essential to match donor and recipient tissue proteins for ABO type and human leukocyte antigen (HLA) compatibility; a mixed lymphocyte culture or white cell crossmatch is also done. The living donor may schedule the transplant at any mutually convenient time, but transplant from a cadaver must be done within 72 hours of the donor's death, or the kidney will deteriorate.

E. Nursing goals during the preoperative period aim to promote the patient's optimal physical readiness for the RT and patient understanding of expectations during and after the procedure. Screening tests may be repeated to ensure the patient remains free of infection and other underlying conditions. Assessment of vital signs, weight, fluid and electrolyte balance, complete blood count (CBC), chest film, electrocardiography (ECG), and urinalysis and urine culture are done. Detailed preoperative teaching includes information about the surgical procedure and placement of tubes and catheters, activity level, diet, pulmonary hygiene, and analgesia to be used during the immediate postoperative period.

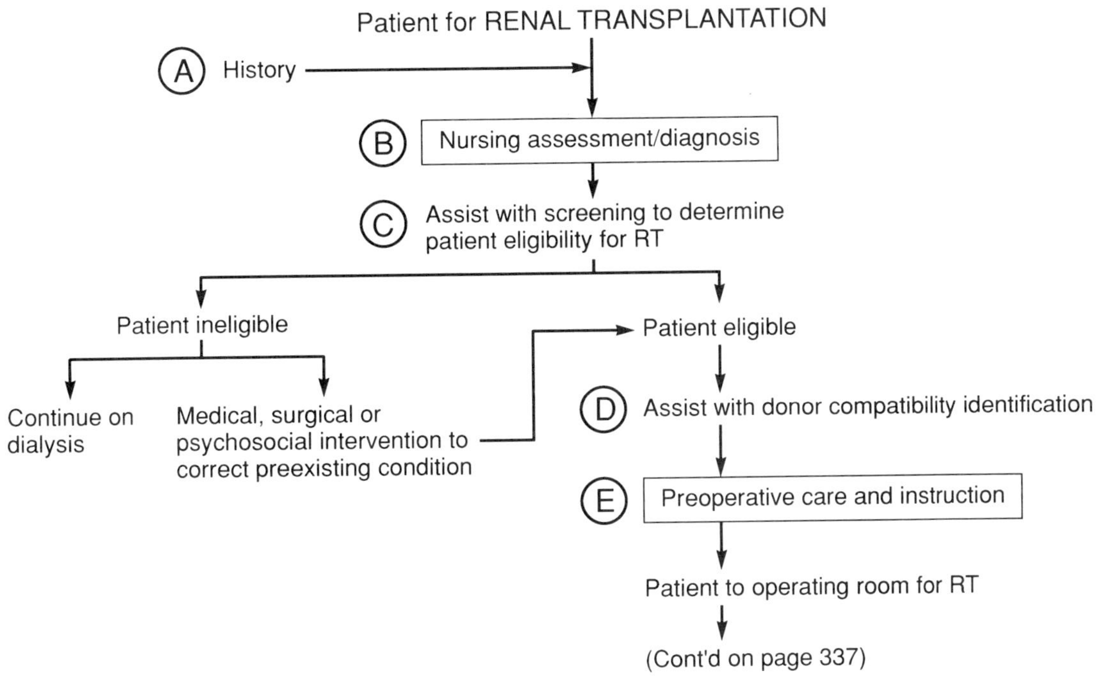
Patient for RENAL TRANSPLANTATION
A
History
B
Nursing assessment/diagnosis
C
Assist with screening to determine patient eligibility for RT
Patient ineligible
Continue on dialysis
Medical, surgical or psychosocial intervention to correct preexisting condition
Patient eligible
D
Assist with donor compatibility identification
E
Preoperative care and instruction
Patient to operating room for RT
(Cont'd on page 337)

F. Continuous assessment is required during the first 24 to 48 hours after RT to maintain fluid and electrolyte balance, promote adequate levels of urine output, prevent infection, and recognize signs of rejection.

G. Fluid and electrolyte management is a critical area of concern. The nurse must frequently assess the patient's fluid status postoperatively. Close monitoring of serum electrolytes is necessary, especially if anuria or oliguria is present. Intravenous (IV) fluid replacement based on hourly urine volume is needed if the patient is NPO, in order to promote diuresis, prevent dehydration, and avoid fluid overload. Urine output must be closely monitored via a Foley catheter. Decrease or cessation of output may indicate an obstructed catheter, hypovolemia, fluid retention, or complications such as acute tubular necrosis or accelerated rejection.

H. Closely monitor vital signs, central venous pressure (CVP), and intake and output, auscultating lung sounds, and observing for the development of edema.

I. Graft rejection occurs because the immune system attacks transplanted tissue as a foreign substance introduced into the body. Immunosuppressant drugs are always given to RT patients; however, 50 percent of all RT patients develop symptoms of rejection. Acute rejection may occur as early as 7 to 14 days postoperatively or as late as a year or more after transplant. Signs and symptoms of acute rejection reflect increasingly impaired renal function: decreased urine output; elevated blood pressure and temperature; weight gain due to fluid retention; proteinuria; increased serum creatinine, BUN, and potassium levels; and tenderness or swelling over the graft site. Renal biopsy confirms rejection. If caught early, acute rejection can usually be reversed. Chronic rejection necessitates removal of the transplanted kidney.

J. Immunosuppressant drugs protect patients from rejection, but make them extremely vulnerable to infection. Meticulous care must be given to the surgical wound, IV sites, urinary catheter, and skin lesions. Patients must avoid contact with any person who has a cold or active infection. Since steroids tend to mask signs of infection, patients must be monitored closely for subtle changes that may indicate the presence of infection. Prompt identification and diagnosis of infections with the initiation of appropriate treatment is essential.

K. If there are no complications, patients are discharged with specific diet, medication, and outpatient follow-up instructions. Patients must be able to identify signs and symptoms of rejection and must know when and how to contact the physician.

References

Gusack EB, Tatum HK. Nursing care of the kidney transplant recipient. In: Schoengrund L, Balzer P, eds. Renal problems in critical care. New York: John Wiley & Sons, 1985:191–206.

Richard CJ, ed. Comprehensive nephrology nursing. Boston: Little, Brown, 1986.

Rivers R. Nursing the kidney transplant patient. RN 1987; 50:46–53.

Ruse LA. Nursing care of the renal transplant patient. In: Richard CJ, ed. Comprehensive nephrology nursing. Boston: Little, Brown, 1986:424–440.

Patient for RENAL TRANSPLANTATION

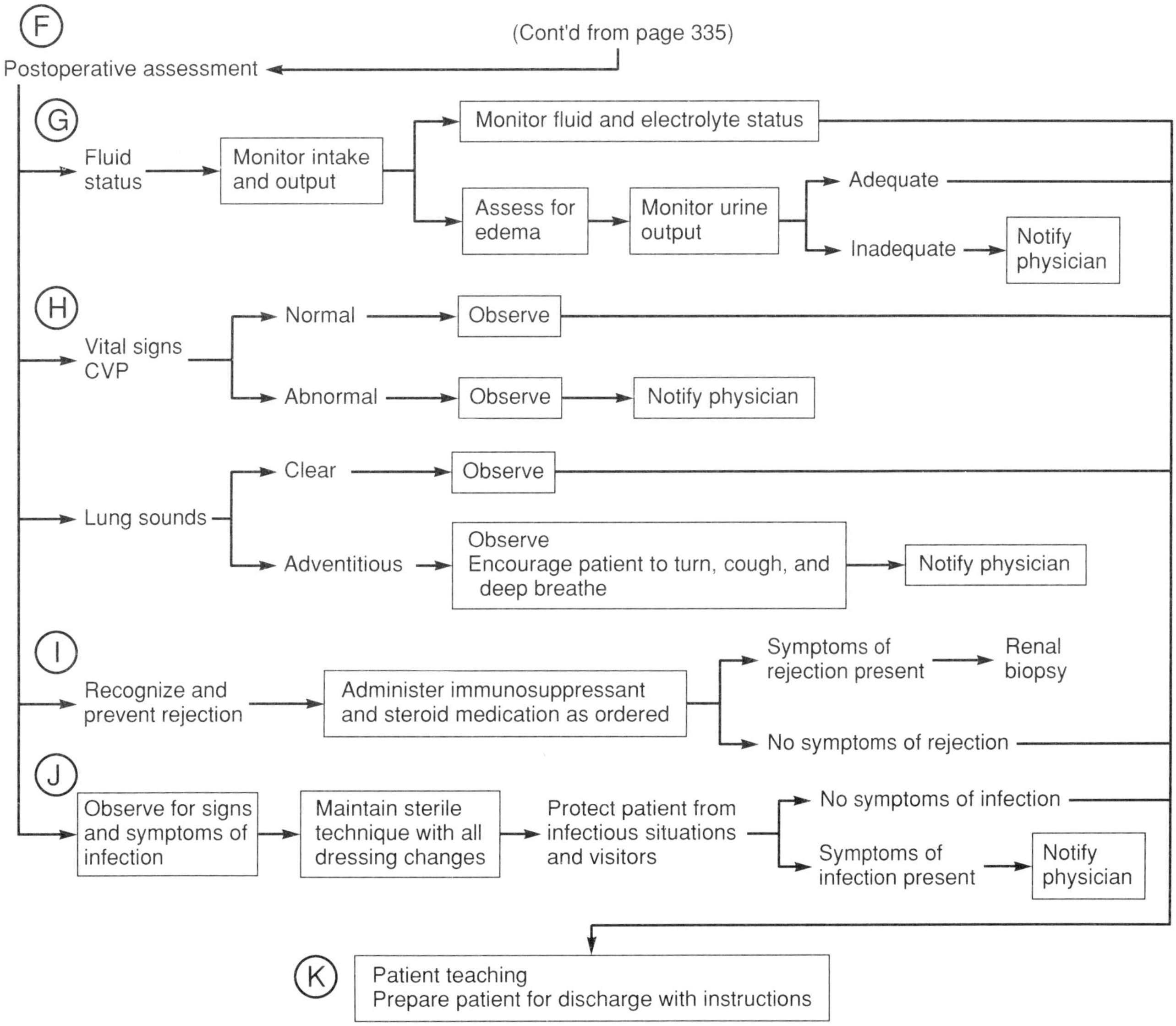

HEMATOLYMPHATIC SYSTEM

ANEMIA DUE TO BLOOD LOSS

Nina McIntosh

A. Anemia resulting from blood loss may be caused by either acute or chronic problems. Acute posthemorrhagic anemia develops as a result of the rapid loss of large quantities of erythrocytes during a hemorrhage caused by trauma, complications of surgery, or diseases that disrupt vascular integrity. A sudden reduction in the total blood volume may lead to hypovolemic shock. If the acute loss is more gradual, the plasma volume increases; however, the number of erythrocytes available to carry oxygen is significantly diminished. Chronic blood loss anemia, which is due to bleeding peptic ulcers (p 130), gynecologic disorders (p 264), bleeding hemorrhoids (p 144), or other gastrointestinal disorders, results in continuous losses of erythrocytes and iron. Laboratory findings are the same as those for iron-deficiency anemia (p 342).

B. The clinical manifestations of anemia from blood loss are caused by the body's attempts to maintain an adequate blood volume and meet oxygen requirements. It is important to understand that clinical symptoms are valuable indicators of the degree of blood volume loss, since laboratory data may not reflect the severity of hemorrhage for 2 to 3 days.

C. The nurse must assess the patient for pain, which may be localized or referred. Internal hemorrhage may cause pain because of tissue distention, organ displacement, and nerve compression.

D. The blood volume must be replaced to prevent the development of shock. Once the source of hemorrhage is found and stopped, the body can begin to manufacture the needed red cells. It is important to provide rest for the patient and supportive measures to prevent complications.

E. Minor blood loss may result in postural hypotension and tachycardia with exertion. Vital signs, drainage tubes, and dressings should be evaluated frequently to assist in finding the source of hemorrhage.

F. Patients who experience a blood loss of approximately 40 percent or more begin to experience signs of shock (p 70). This is a *life-threatening* situation. Intravenous fluid and blood product replacement is a certainty, and proper techniques must be followed. Hypoxia should be treated with oxygen at a rate ordered by the physician. Transfer to the intensive care unit (ICU) may be indicated for stabilization.

G. Once the source of hemorrhage is identified, blood loss controlled, and fluid and blood volume replaced, the anemia should begin to correct itself. Low levels of erythrocytes, hemoglobin, and hematocrit usually reflect the blood loss about 2 or 3 days after the blood loss.

H. When blood is lost, iron is also lost and must be replaced. The patient may need supplemental iron, since the iron supply affects bone marrow production of erythrocytes and dietary sources of iron will probably not be adquate to maintain iron supply after acute blood loss.

I. Discharge planning includes instruction related to stress management, adequate rest, and dietary intake of iron. The patient is also instructed to report symptoms of recurrent bleeding.

References

Brunner LS, Suddarth DS. The Lippincott manual of nursing practice. 4th ed. Philadelphia: JB Lippincott, 1986.

Lewis SM, Collier IC. Medical surgical nursing: assessment and management of clinical problems. New York: McGraw-Hill, 1983.

Thompson J, McFarland G, Hirsch J, Tucker S, Bowers A. Clinical nursing. St. Louis: CV Mosby, 1986.

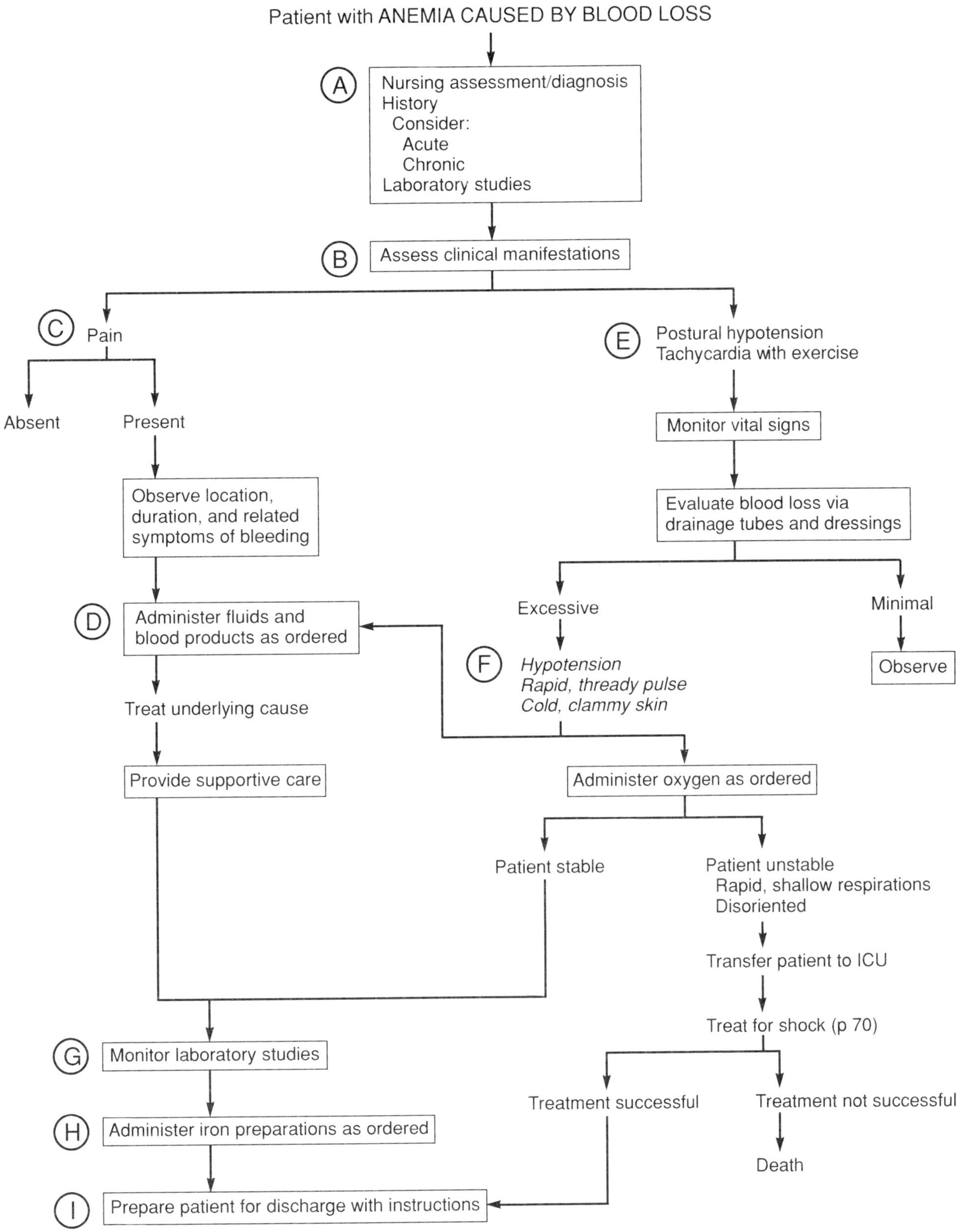
Patient with ANEMIA CAUSED BY BLOOD LOSS
A
Nursing assessment/diagnosis
History
Consider:
Acute
Chronic
Laboratory studies
B
Assess clinical manifestations
C
Pain
Absent
Present
Observe location, duration, and related symptoms of bleeding
D
Administer fluids and blood products as ordered
Treat underlying cause
Provide supportive care
E
Postural hypotension
Tachycardia with exercise
Monitor vital signs
Evaluate blood loss via drainage tubes and dressings
Excessive
Minimal
Observe
F
Hypotension
Rapid, thready pulse
Cold, clammy skin
Administer oxygen as ordered
Patient stable
Patient unstable
Rapid, shallow respirations
Disoriented
Transfer patient to ICU
Treat for shock (p 70)
Treatment successful
Treatment not successful
Death
G
Monitor laboratory studies
H
Administer iron preparations as ordered
I
Prepare patient for discharge with instructions

ANEMIA DUE TO DECREASED ERYTHROCYTE PRODUCTION

Nina McIntosh

The balance of red cell production with red cell destruction and loss is necessary to ensure that adequate numbers of erythrocytes are available. This delicate balance can be disrupted when red blood cell production is inhibited by decreased hemoglobin synthesis, defective nuclear cytoplasm, or diminished availability of erythrocyte precursors.

A. Many patients with these types of anemias are asymptomatic. As the disease becomes chronic, the patient may display general manifestations of anemia, such as pallor, nausea and vomiting, weakness, fatigue, mouth and tongue sores, and a predisposition to infections. Since some types of anemia are genetic, it is important to obtain a family history.

B. Extensive laboratory tests are conducted to determine the type and cause of the anemia. Blood samples are obtained for complete blood count (CBC), peripheral smear, reticulocyte count, serum iron, total iron binding capacity, and other tests as indicated. A gastric analysis is done when pernicious anemia is suspected. Since a nasogastric tube is inserted for this procedure, it is important to educate the patient prior to the procedure to decrease anxiety and discomfort. Another diagnostic assessment for pernicious anemia is the Schilling's test, in which radioactive vitamin B_{12} is given to the patient, and the amount excreted in the urine is measured. Bone marrow examination (p 368) may be done for any anemic state. The procedure must be explained and the patient alerted to anticipate a feeling of pressure and/or pain.

C. Iron deficiency anemia, characterized by an inadequate supply of iron needed to synthesize hemoglobin because of inadequate absorption or excessive loss of iron, is the most prevalent anemia. Usually, the iron intake is increased by supplemental doses of oral iron. Since iron is best absorbed in an acidic environment, it should be given about an hour before meals. Undiluted liquid iron may stain the patient's teeth. In some situations, parenteral iron is indicated. Because intramuscular solutions of iron may stain the skin, separate needles should be used to draw up and inject the medication. Iron should be given deep intramuscularly, using the Z-track technique. Dietary teaching, with emphasis on foods high in iron, is very important. Compliance with dietary and drug therapy needs to be emphasized, since the recovery period may last 2 to 3 months.

D. Thalassemia is a disease of inadequate production of normal hemoglobin due to abnormal hemoglobin synthesis. It is a genetic disorder found in members of ethnic groups originating near the Mediterranean Sea. Care for these patients is usually supportive, based on the symptoms exhibited. Transfusions are given on a monthly, bimonthly, or "as needed" basis.

E. Pernicious anemia is progressive, caused by a lack of intrinsic factor essential for the absorption of vitamin B_{12}. It is the most prevalent type of B_{12} deficiency in the United States and is predominantly seen in adults over 60 years of age. The patient can be maintained on monthly injections of vitamin B_{12}. Patients should be instructed to prevent injuries due to diminished sensations of heat and pain resulting from neurologic impairment. They must understand the importance of compliance with treatment and follow-up.

F. Folic acid is required for DNA synthesis, which leads to red cell formation and maturation. Folic acid deficiency is most commonly caused by poor nutrition, malabsorption syndromes, and drugs that impede the absorption and use of folic acid. The primary treatment is replacement therapy given in oral doses. The duration of treatment depends on the cause of the deficiency. Dietary teaching must include good general nutrition and identification of foods high in folic acid.

G. Aplastic anemia is characterized by a decrease in the number of circulating erythrocytes and is caused by failure of the bone marrow to produce adequate numbers of erythrocytes. The patient presenting with hypoxia should be given oxygen and encouraged to rest as much as possible. The nursing care is primarily supportive until the causative agent can be removed. The patient must be observed carefully to prevent complications from infection or hemorrhage. The physician should be notified immediately if any symptoms or changes occur in the patient. Blood products are usually administered until bone marrow production is restored. Regardless of the diagnosis and management, aplastic anemia is fatal in about 75 percent of patients.

H. Patients should be instructed to live a lifestyle that balances activity with rest. Skin cleanliness is important and because of poor circulation, extremities should be protected from injury. Patients should be counseled about adequate nutrition and the need to avoid situations that place them at high risk for infection.

References

Brunner LS, Suddarth DS. The Lippincott manual of nursing practice. 3rd ed. Philadelphia: JB Lippincott, 1982.

Lewis SM, Collier IC. Medical-surgical nursing: assessment and management of clinical problems. New York: McGraw-Hill, 1983.

Thompson J, McFarland G, Hirsch J, Tucker S, Bowers A. Clinical nursing. St. Louis: CV Mosby, 1986.

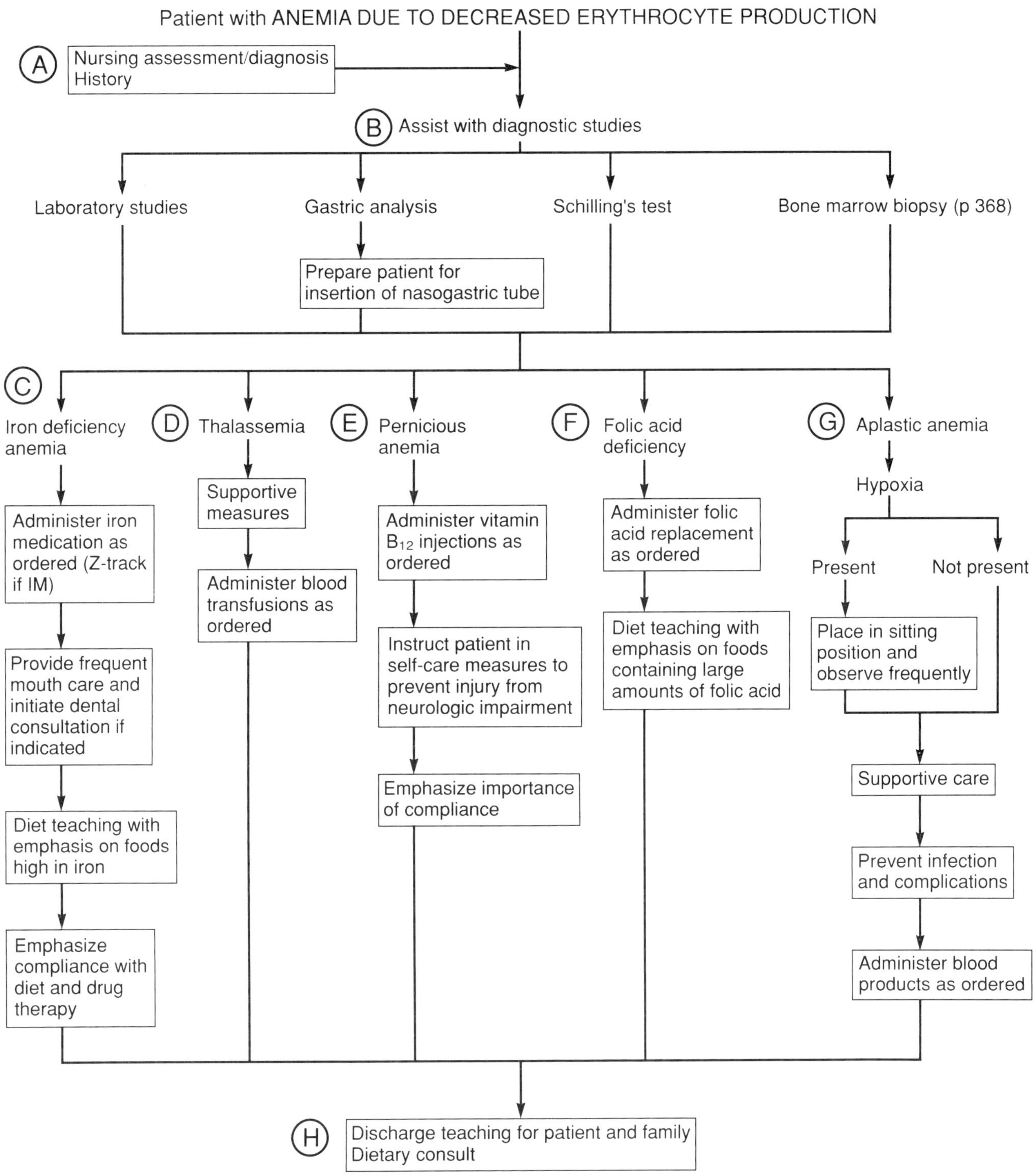

Patient with ANEMIA DUE TO DECREASED ERYTHROCYTE PRODUCTION
A
Nursing assessment/diagnosis
History
B
Assist with diagnostic studies
Laboratory studies
Gastric analysis
Prepare patient for insertion of nasogastric tube
Schilling's test
Bone marrow biopsy (p 368)
C
Iron deficiency anemia
Administer iron medication as ordered (Z-track if IM)
Provide frequent mouth care and initiate dental consultation if indicated
Diet teaching with emphasis on foods high in iron
Emphasize compliance with diet and drug therapy
D
Thalassemia
Supportive measures
Administer blood transfusions as ordered
E
Pernicious anemia
Administer vitamin B12 injections as ordered
Instruct patient in self-care measures to prevent injury from neurologic impairment
Emphasize importance of compliance
F
Folic acid deficiency
Administer folic acid replacement as ordered
Diet teaching with emphasis on foods containing large amounts of folic acid
G
Aplastic anemia
Hypoxia
Present
Not present
Place in sitting position and observe frequently
Supportive care
Prevent infection and complications
Administer blood products as ordered
H
Discharge teaching for patient and family
Dietary consult

ANEMIA DUE TO HEMOLYSIS

Nina McIntosh

Hemolysis is the destruction of red blood cells at a rate higher than the rate of production. Hemolysis may occur because of problems intrinsic or extrinsic to the red blood cells. Intrinsic hemolytic anemias are usually hereditary and result from defects in the red blood cells themselves. These defects can be due to abnormal hemoglobin (e.g., sickle cells), enzyme deficiencies that alter glycolysis (glucose-6-phosphate dehydrogenase [G6PD] deficiency), or cell membrane abnormalities. Extrinsic hemolytic anemias are acquired. The red cells are normal, but damage is caused by external factors such as antibodies, toxins, or mechanical injury.

A. The patient with hemolytic anemia manifests the general symptoms of anemia. Mild forms may exist without symptoms. However, patients with more severe forms may exhibit symptoms from exertional dyspnea and palpitations to tachycardia, pallor, jaundice, nausea, vomiting, fatigue, and dyspnea or orthopnea. Hemolytic anemias may cause enlargement of the spleen and liver. Since many of the hemolytic anemias are hereditary, it is very important to assess the family history for anemia.

B. Extensive laboratory studies include blood samples for complete blood count (CBC), reticulocyte count, peripheral smear, sickle cell preparation, hemoglobin electrophoresis, serum assays of G6PD levels, and others as indicated. Intravenous pyelography (IVP) may be done to evaluate the kidneys, and radiographs of the bones may indicate skeletal changes.

C. Individuals with sickle cell anemia have a severe form of hemolytic anemia. Because there is no treatment specific for the disease, medical care is essentially supportive. Management is usually directed toward alleviating the symptoms due to complications of the disease. Oxygen may be given to alter hypoxia and control sickling. Rest is needed to reduce metabolic requirements. Fluids and electrolytes are given to reduce blood viscosity and maintain renal function. Sedatives and analgesics are used to treat the pain. Supportive care includes mouth and skin care, positioning for comfort, and precautions taken to prevent further complications.

D. Because sickle cell disease is hereditary, genetic counseling is the only form of prevention. All family members should be screened to detect those individuals who have sickle cell trait. It is important for the patient and family to understand the implications of this hereditary disease as well as receive the support and understanding needed to cope with it.

E. Long-term care for patients with sickle cell anemia involves patient education. Individuals and their families must understand the basic disease process and the reasons for supportive care and follow-up. Patients should be instructed in ways to avoid sickle cell crises, such as avoiding high altitudes and dehydration. They must also understand the extreme importance of seeking medical attention quickly when any problems or complications arise.

F. G6PD deficiency is a genetic disorder common in blacks and individuals with a Mediterranean heritage that affects the red cell's ability to resist oxidative damage. Oxidative drugs and foods increase the red cell's metabolic needs; however, the G6PD deficiency interferes with glucose metabolism and leads to damage of older cells. Hemolytic episodes are triggered by viral and bacterial infections, drugs, and toxins. Managing the hemolysis in G6PD deficiency is accomplished by removing the cause of the hemolytic reaction. The patient should be encouraged to rest, maintain adequate hydration, and assess kidney function. Hemolytic disorders can be prevented by treating infections promptly.

G. In acquired hemolytic anemia, physical destruction of red cells results from traumatic events causing disruption of the cell membrane (e.g., heart-lung bypass and prosthetic heart valves) and extreme force pushing blood through abnormal vessels (e.g., burned vessels, diabetes). Antibodies may destroy red cells by the mechanisms involved in antigen-antibody reactions. Infectious agents and toxins may also cause hemolysis. Treatment and management of acquired hemolytic anemia consist primarily of general supportive care until the causative agent can be eliminated or at least becomes less injurious to the erythrocytes.

H. Patients with hemolytic anemias are discharged home with specific instructions about activity, medications, and continued treatment as necessary.

References

Brunner LS, Suddarth DS. The Lippincott manual of nursing practice. 4th ed. Philadelphia: JB Lippincott, 1986.

Lewis SM, Collier IC. Medical surgical nursing: assessment and management of clinical problems. New York: McGraw-Hill, 1983.

Thompson J, McFarland G, Hirsch J, Tucker S, Bowers A. Clinical nursing. St. Louis: CV Mosby, 1986.

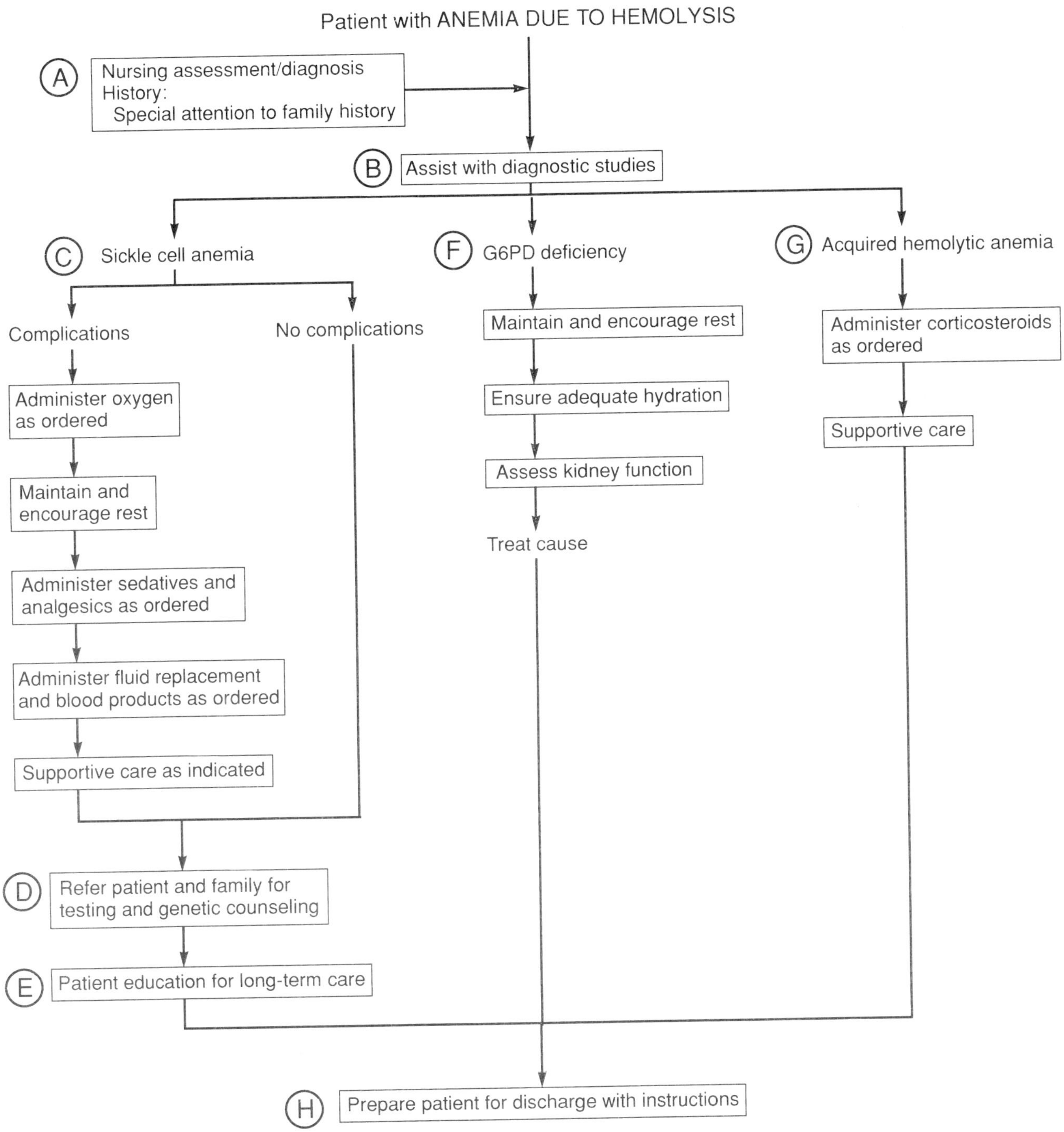

Patient with ANEMIA DUE TO HEMOLYSIS
A
Nursing assessment/diagnosis
History:
Special attention to family history
B
Assist with diagnostic studies
C
Sickle cell anemia
Complications
No complications
Administer oxygen as ordered
Maintain and encourage rest
Administer sedatives and analgesics as ordered
Administer fluid replacement and blood products as ordered
Supportive care as indicated
D
Refer patient and family for testing and genetic counseling
E
Patient education for long-term care
F
G6PD deficiency
Maintain and encourage rest
Ensure adequate hydration
Assess kidney function
Treat cause
G
Acquired hemolytic anemia
Administer corticosteroids as ordered
Supportive care
H
Prepare patient for discharge with instructions

ACUTE LEUKEMIA

Mary Beth Mardjetko

Leukemia is a malignant disease of the blood-forming tissues. Abnormal white blood cells (WBCs), unable to perform their infection-fighting roles, fill the bone marrow and blood stream. Leukemia cells crowd the bone marrow, spill into the circulating blood, and infiltrate vital organs, e.g., liver, lungs, and central nervous system. Patients with acute lymphocytic leukemia (ALL) have an abnormal increase of immature lymphocytes in their blood and bone marrow. Patients with acute nonlymphocytic leukemia (ANLL) may have immature forms of any of the other hematopoietic cells.

A. With acute leukemia, symptom onset usually occurs over a brief time and reflects the replacement of normal bone marrow with abnormal cells. Fever and "flu"-like symptoms may be the initial signs. The lymph nodes, spleen, and liver become infiltrated with WBCs and may be enlarged. Bone or joint pain, paleness, weakness, tendency to bleed or bruise easily, and frequent infections are associated symptoms. Therefore, patients should be asked to describe the time frame in which symptoms developed and the symptoms they experienced, and answer specific questions about any bleeding episodes or infections. The most common clinical manifestations are related to pancytopenia.

B. Anemia (pp 340, 342) is a quantitative or qualitative deficiency in circulating red blood cells (RBCs) with a decreased oxygen carrying capacity. Signs and symptoms may include tachycardia, dyspnea, hypotension, pallor, weakness, palpitations, headache, and lightheadedness. Nursing measures are aimed at conservation of energy and prevention of tissue hypoxia.

C. Neutropenia is defined as an absolute neutrophil count less than 500/mm^3 blood. The patient's entire body should be assessed daily for sites of infection, with special attention to the mouth and mucous membranes and the perirectal area. Fever, redness, and pain may be the only signs. Nursing measures include reporting any signs of infection. Temperatures should be taken every 4 hours and as needed, and broad-spectrum antibiotics immediately instituted for fevers of 38.5°C (101.3°F). Neutropenic precautions should be instituted, including a private room; meticulous handwashing; limited exposure to crowds, children, pets, plants, and raw fruits and vegetables; scrupulous personal hygiene; and avoiding use of rectal or vaginal thermometers and suppositories.

D. Thrombocytopenia is defined as a platelet count less than 150,000/mm^3 blood. However, significant risk of bleeding does not occur from thrombocytopenia alone until the count is 20,000. Patients should be assessed for petechiae, purpura, and ecchymosis. Bleeding precautions should be instituted, including no salicylates, no intramuscular injections, and avoiding dangerous activities, Valsalva maneuvers, and straight razors. A protective environment to prevent falls is essential. Patients should use soft toothbrushes. Ongoing monitoring of stools and urine for occult blood should be done. Assessing patients for signs of intracranial bleeding (headache, changes in level of consciousness, seizures) should be routine. Platelet transfusions are ordered when the blood count falls below 20,000 or if bleeding occurs. Controlling bleeding with local measures is paramount.

E. The diagnosis of acute leukemia is usually straightforward. A bone marrow biopsy (p 368) is needed to assess the extent of involvement. Peripheral blood studies include hematocrit, WBC count with differential, and platelet count. Blood chemistries are essential and include electrolytes, uric acid, blood urea nitrogen (BUN), and coagulation profile. A lumbar puncture, chest film, and transfusion work-up with HLA typing is completed. Patients routinely have long-term central lines placed and require postoperative care for these. Extensive dental examinations are needed.

F. Intensive chemotherapy (p 408) should begin as soon as the diagnosis is established. Many different chemotherapeutic agents may be used. ANLL is initially treated with Ara-C and daunorubicin; ALL initially is treated with vincristine, prednisone, and an antracycline. The goal of therapy is to destroy all leukemia cells and the leukemic clone; in the process, the normal bone marrow cells are destroyed. This places the patient at extreme risk because of the pancytopenia that may last from 4 to 6 weeks.

G. Patient education is paramount. It must include the disease process, side effects of drugs and measures to minimize these, the risks involved in therapy, and the precautions instituted for pancytopenia.

H. Patients need supportive care for side effects of chemotherapy (pp 366, 410).

I. Emotional support of these patients and families is essential. They are usually hospitalized for several weeks, which greatly affects their families. Further, they are faced with a life-threatening illness and treatment and experience a variety of emotional reactions. Referrals to social workers, psychologists, and chaplains should be made as needed.

References

DeVita V, Hellman S, Rosenberg S. Cancer principles and practice of oncology. Philadelphia: JB Lippincott, 1985.

Larson R, Kaminar L, Westbrook C, Daly K. Leukemia: progress through research. Unpublished paper, 1988.

Ziegfeld C. Core curriculum for oncology nursing. Philadelphia: WB Saunders, 1987.

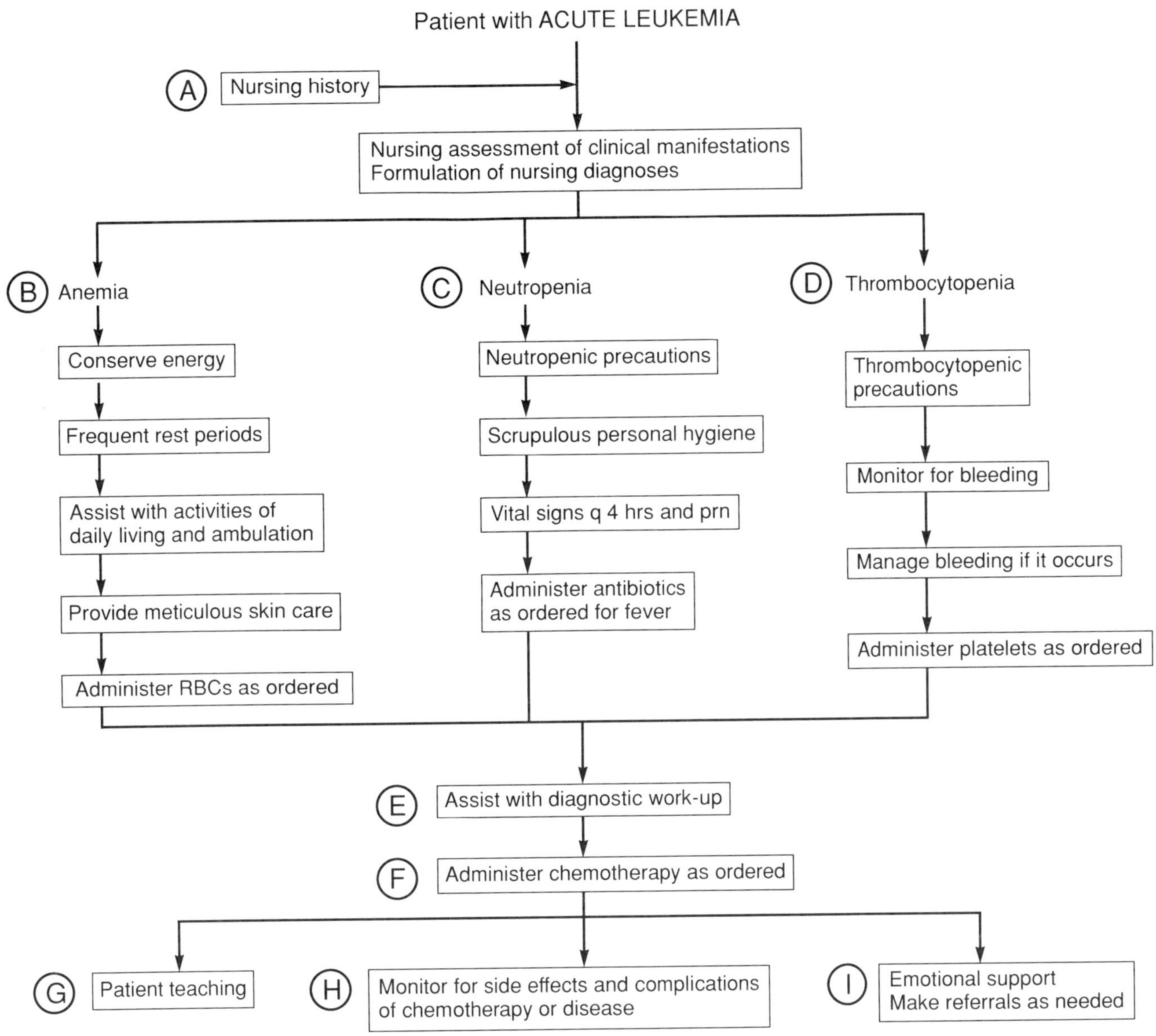
Patient with ACUTE LEUKEMIA
A
Nursing history
Nursing assessment of clinical manifestations
Formulation of nursing diagnoses
B
Anemia
Conserve energy
Frequent rest periods
Assist with activities of daily living and ambulation
Provide meticulous skin care
Administer RBCs as ordered
C
Neutropenia
Neutropenic precautions
Scrupulous personal hygiene
Vital signs q 4 hrs and prn
Administer antibiotics as ordered for fever
D
Thrombocytopenia
Thrombocytopenic precautions
Monitor for bleeding
Manage bleeding if it occurs
Administer platelets as ordered
E
Assist with diagnostic work-up
F
Administer chemotherapy as ordered
G
Patient teaching
H
Monitor for side effects and complications of chemotherapy or disease
I
Emotional support
Make referrals as needed

DISSEMINATED INTRAVASCULAR COAGULATION

Mary E. Mancini
Susan J. Smith

Disseminated intravascular coagulation (DIC) is an abnormality of coagulation that results when the clotting system is activated in all or part of the vascular tree and where both thrombosis and hemorrhage occur together.

DIC occurs as a secondary process or complication of another disorder, a complete history is important in assessing the underlying condition. DIC may result from problems that activate the intrinsic coagulation pathway (septic shock, infections, prolonged extracorporeal circulation, amniotic fluid and fat emboli, antigen-antibody complexes as seen in hemolytic transfusion reactions, acute hypoxia, and adult respiratory distress syndrome) or the extrinsic coagulation pathway (shock, sepsis, malignant tumors, abruptio placenta, missed abortion, burns, diabetic ketoacidosis, renal disease, snake bite, and heat stroke).

A. The overall results are (1) loss of fibrinogen as it is used during coagulation and by the action of plasmin on the clots; (2) loss of clotting factors as they are used in the coagulation process; (3) decreased platelet count as they are activated, aggregate, and leave the circulation; and (4) increased fibrin splint products (FSPs) as clots are digested by plasmin.

B. Nursing assessment should focus on signs and symptoms of impaired tissue and organ perfusion; changes in level of consciousness; decreased urinary output; cardiac arrhythmias; pallor; cyanosis; leg, gingival, and mucosal ulcers; occult and overt bleeding; oozing from any puncture or incision sites; bleeding from mucous membranes; purpura; hemorrhagic bullae; wound hematomas; ecchymosis; petechiae; abdominal distention; dull, persistent abdominal pain; occult or overt blood in stool, urine, or emesis; hematemesis; respiratory failure and hypoxia; dyspnea; cyanosis even with a high FIO_2; rales; wheezing; pleural friction rubs; fatigue; weakness; orthopnea; tachycardia; tachypnea; and infection.

C. Diagnostic studies show prolonged prothrombin time, prolonged activated partial thromboplastin time, increased thromboplastin time, decreased platelet count, decreased fibrinogen, elevated FSPs, and strongly positive protamine sulfate.

D. Early recognition and control of bleeding is essential as the physician begins treatment of the underlying condition. Nursing assessment includes observing all puncture sites, incisions, wounds, and skin for signs of bleeding. Test urine, stools, and emesis for occult blood. Observe for signs of internal bleeding.

E. If bleeding occurs, apply local pressure, cold compresses, and topical hemostatic agents such as Gelfoam, fibrin foam, or thrombin. Avoid disturbing any clots that are present.

F. If needle sticks cannot be avoided, use small-gauge needles, and apply pressure to bleeding sites until bleeding subsides.

G. Allow adequate rest periods by maintaining bedrest. Avoid vigorous rubbing or massage. Reposition the patient frequently to avoid pressure areas. Use an air mattress or egg crate mattress as indicated. Pad siderails or other bed parts that may induce bruising or bleeding.

H. Evaluate the extent of the hemorrhage. Carefully monitor signs of hypoxia, and bleeding from the respiratory and gastrointestinal tracts and the kidneys. Monitor coagulation panels.

I. Ventilatory support may be required if respiratory failure develops. Obtain, interpret, and keep the physician informed of arterial blood gas (ABG) results.

J. Be aware of drug interactions, especially anticoagulants. Monitor heparin therapy, obtain coagulation studies, and report results to the physician. Administer blood components as ordered. In the acute phase these may include whole blood, packed cells, leukocyte-poor blood, platelets, fresh frozen plasma, cryoprecipitate, albumin, plasma protein fraction, or plasma expanders. During transfusions, observe the patient for transfusion reactions or fluid overload.

K. Provide social and emotional support for both patient and family. Support appropriate coping strategies.

L. Continued bleeding may require transfer to the intensive care unit (ICU).

M. Monitor coagulation studies for resolving DIC and return to normal. Observe for resolution of the underlying condition associated with DIC. Assess oxygenation status, including vital signs and ABGs.

N. Provide intake of nutrients, vitamins, calories, fluids, and electrolytes to meet calculated daily requirements and to achieve weight gain or maintenance.

O. Prevent crippling deformities from hemarthrosis including total bedrest, ice packs, analgesics, passive range of motion as soon as bleeding stops, and avoidance of weight bearing until swelling resolves and muscle strength returns.

P. The discharge plan should be individualized and should include an accurate description of activity, dietary, and medication regimens; a description of the signs and symptoms requiring medical attention; information about prevention of injury or recurrence of the underlying disease condition that precipitated DIC (if appropriate); and information about the date, time, and place for follow-up care.

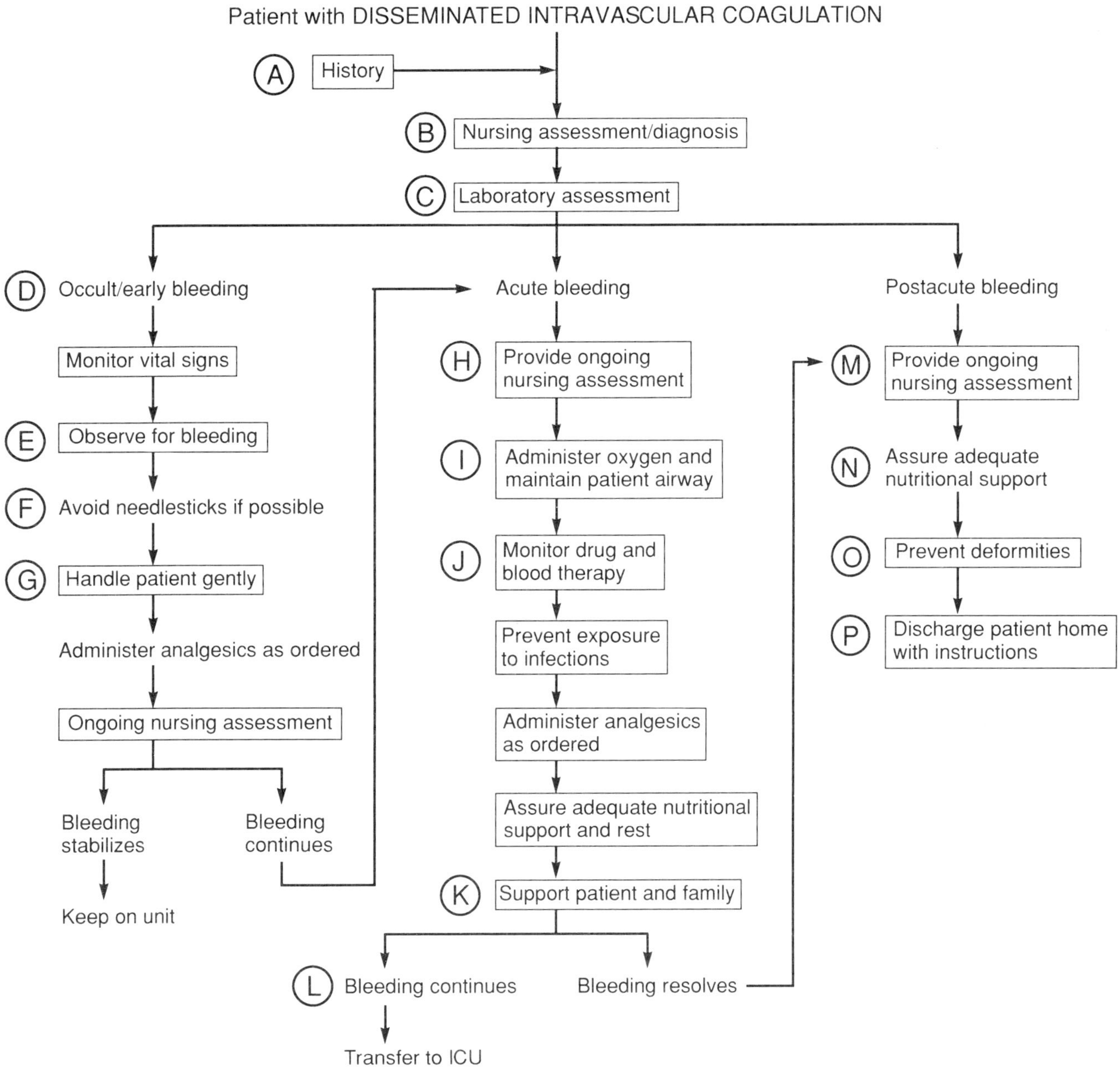

References

Alspach JG, Williams SM. Core curriculum for critical care nursing. Philadelphia: WB Saunders, 1985.

Ampel LL, Marshall S, Caprini JA. Etiology, diagnosis, and treatment of recovery room bleeding/hemorrhage. Heart Lung 1985; 14:556–561.

Babior BM, Stossel TP. Hematology: a pathophysiologic approach. New York: Churchill Livingstone, 1984:209–216.

Griffin JP. Be prepared for the bleeding patient. Nursing '86 1986; 16(6):34–42.

Moorhouse MF, Geissler AC, Doenges ME. Critical care plans: guidelines for patient care. Philadelphia: FA Davis, 1987:319–328.

HEMOPHILIA

Nina McIntosh

Hemophilia is an inherited, congenital blood dyscrasia that is characterized by reduced clotting activity of specific coagulation factors. It appears in males but is transmitted by females. Hemophilia had been considered primarily a disease of childhood because early death usually resulted from complications. Advances in treatment now enable hemophiliacs to live into adulthood.

A. There are significant clinical manifestations that suggest the presence of hemophilia. The patient may experience slow, persistent, prolonged bleeding from minor trauma and small cuts or delayed bleeding after minor injuries (the delay may be several hours or days). Uncontrolled hemorrhage can follow dental extractions or irritation of the gums with a toothbrush. The patient may experience epistaxis following a facial blow or gastrointestinal bleeding from ulcers and gastritis. Hematuria may be caused by genitourinary trauma or splenic rupture resulting from falls or abdominal trauma. Ecchymoses and subcutaneous hematomas are common. Hemarthrosis (bleeding into the joints) causes pain, swelling, and limitation of movement. These manifestations are especially important when seen in children, since the disease may not yet be diagnosed. In adults, these developments indicate that the hemophilia is poorly controlled. All of the clinical manifestations relate to bleeding, and any bleeding episode in hemophiliacs may result in death from hemorrhage.

B. Laboratory studies are used to determine the type of hemophilia present. Specific assays are performed to identify the clotting factor deficiency within the intrinsic system. The partial thromboplastin time is prolonged. When venipuncture is performed, it is imperative to apply direct pressure to the area for 5 minutes and observe the patient closely for further signs of prolonged bleeding.

C. Acute management of hemophilia is related primarily to controlling bleeding. Stop topical bleeding as quickly as possible by applying direct pressure or ice and packing the area with Gelfoam or fibrin foam. Administer the blood component ordered to raise the patient's level of the deficient coagulation factor. When joint bleeding occurs, it is important to rest the involved joint totally to prevent crippling injuries. The joint may be packed in ice, and analgesics are needed to reduce the severe pain. As soon as bleeding has stopped, it is important to encourage mobilization of the affected area through range-of-motion exercises and physical therapy.

D. The nurse must also continuously assess the environment for potential hazards. Young children should be placed in padded cribs, and all toys should be inspected for sharp or rough edges.

E. The patient should be assessed continuously for life-threatening complications, such as airway obstruction from hemorrhage into the neck and pharynx or intracranial bleeding.

F. Chronic management is a primary consideration for hemophiliacs because the disease follows an incurable, chronic course. The quality and length of life may be significantly affected by the patient's knowledge of the disease and how to live with it. The patient and family can be referred to the local chapter of the National Hemophilia Society to encourage association with other individuals who are dealing with the same types of problems.

G. Hemophiliacs must be taught to recognize disease-related problems and to learn which can be handled at home and which require hospitalization. Daily oral hygiene must be performed without causing trauma to the soft tissues. The patient must also learn to prevent injuries when doing routine household chores or participating in noncontact sports. All hemophiliacs should wear a Medic-Alert tag to ensure that health care providers are informed in case of an accident. *Note:* Patients with hemophilia should *never* take aspirin because it affects platelet function and prolongs bleeding time.

H. Patients should be given information about routine follow-up care, and their compliance must be assessed. A home-care referral may be indicated for further teaching and assessment. Home care programs can also teach parents and children to administer plasma therapy at home when a hemorrhage episode begins. Genetic counseling and family planning services should be offered to the family.

References

Brunner LS, Suddarth DS. The Lippincott manual of nursing practice. 3rd ed. Philadelphia: JB Lippincott, 1982.

Lewis SM, Collier IC. Medical-surgical nursing: assessment and management of clinical problems. New York: McGraw-Hill, 1983.

Nathan D, Oski F, eds. Hematology of infancy and childhood. Philadelphia: WB Saunders, 1974.

Oremland EK. Work dynamics in family care of hemophiliac children. Soc Sci Med 1988; 26:467–475.

Warren B. Maintaining the hemophiliac at home and school. Nursing 1974; 4:73–76.

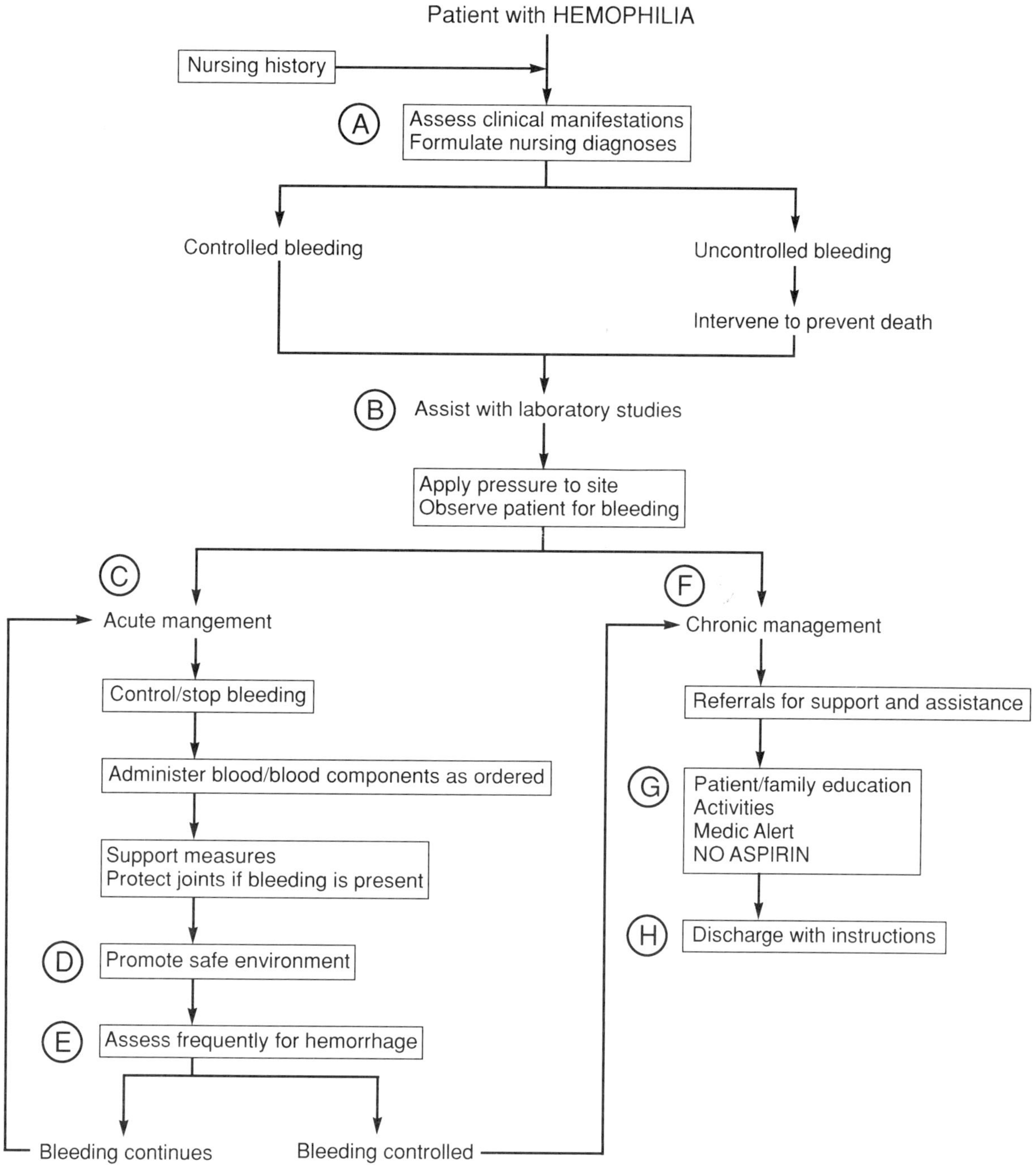
Patient with HEMOPHILIA
Nursing history
A
Assess clinical manifestations
Formulate nursing diagnoses
Controlled bleeding
Uncontrolled bleeding
Intervene to prevent death
B
Assist with laboratory studies
Apply pressure to site
Observe patient for bleeding
C
Acute mangement
Control/stop bleeding
Administer blood/blood components as ordered
Support measures
Protect joints if bleeding is present
D
Promote safe environment
E
Assess frequently for hemorrhage
Bleeding continues
Bleeding controlled
F
Chronic management
Referrals for support and assistance
G
Patient/family education
Activities
Medic Alert
NO ASPIRIN
H
Discharge with instructions

SYSTEMIC LUPUS ERYTHEMATOSUS

Joy Gorzeman

Systemic lupus erythematosus (SLE) is a chronic, autoimmune, inflammatory disease that affects many body systems. Etiology is unknown, but is thought to include genetic and viral factors. SLE should not be confused with discoid lupus erythematosus, which is a chronic eruption of the skin with no threat to life. SLE is most commonly seen in young women of child-bearing age.

A. Early clinical manifestations vary, depending on which organ systems are involved. Early symptoms may include fever, fatigue, weakness, and weight loss. These symptoms may begin abruptly or develop over time. Other common clinical features include a characteristic "butterfly rash" on the face, alopecia, and ulcerations on the mucous membranes of the mouth. Most SLE patients complain of articular symptoms and have rheumatoid arthritis (p 212). Additional clinical problems of the SLE patient may include pleurisy (p 106), carditis (p 76), generalized adenopathy, and nephritis (p 308) (the most common cause of death). Behavioral changes, convulsions, and other central nervous system (CNS) signs and symptoms are associated with severe SLE. It is important to obtain a detailed medication history, because certain drugs may cause a drug-induced form of SLE.

B. The American Rheumatism Association has developed a list of criteria for the diagnosis of SLE. Four of the following must be present:

   1. Butterfly rash (facial erythema)
   2. Discoid lupus
   3. Raynaud's phenomenon
   4. Alopecia
   5. Photosensitivity
   6. Oral or nasopharyngeal ulcers
   7. Arthritis without deformity
   8. Positive LE cell test
   9. Chronic false positive serology for syphilis
   10. Proteinuria (3.5 g per day)
   11. Cellular casts
   12. Pleuritis and/or pericarditis
   13. CNS symptoms
   14. Cytopenia.

C. Positive laboratory findings will include multiple serum protein abnormalities. A positive ANA test (presence of antinuclear antibodies) and/or LE cell factor in the serum are the most closely associated with SLE. Leukopenia with a normal differential count and elevated erythrocyte sedimentation rate is common during active disease.

D. If the history indicates that SLE may be drug-induced, discontinue the suspected drug. Symptoms should reverse within several weeks.

E. Treatment for SLE is individualized, based on the severity of the disease and current clinical manifestations. Mild disease is treated with high levels of salicylates. If pain or fever is not controlled with salicylates, indomethacin is also given. Other nonsteroidal anti-inflammatory agents may be useful for patients with gastritis. If the disease is not controlled with these medications, an antimalaria drug may be added.

F. Severe disease requires immediate corticosteroid therapy. In addition to medication, other comfort measures such as application of heat to sore joints should be used. In both mild and severe cases, after the inflammatory process is controlled, the minimal dose of corticosteroid or other agents needed to suppress tissue inflammation, must be determined.

G. Patients with SLE must be under medical supervision. They should report any change in condition or new symptoms to the physician. Intercurrent infections should be treated vigorously. Urinalysis should be done every 4 to 6 months to detect early renal involvement. Patients taking antimalarial drugs need ophthalmologic examinations every 4 months to check for retinal degeneration. Surgical procedures and pregnancy may cause exacerbation of disease and require close medical care. SLE patients should be advised to avoid stress, fatigue, and sun exposure. Emotional support is essential as the patient adjusts to living with a chronic illness. National arthritis and lupus support groups are available.

References

Berkow R, ed. The Merck manual of diagnosis and therapy. 15th ed. Rahway, NJ: Merck, Sharp and Dohme Research Laboratories, 1987.

Brunner LS, Suddarth DS. The Lippincott manual of nursing practice. 4th ed. Philadelphia: JB Lippincott, 1986.

Price SA, Wilson LM. Pathophysiology: clinical concepts of disease processes. 2nd ed. New York: McGraw-Hill, 1982.

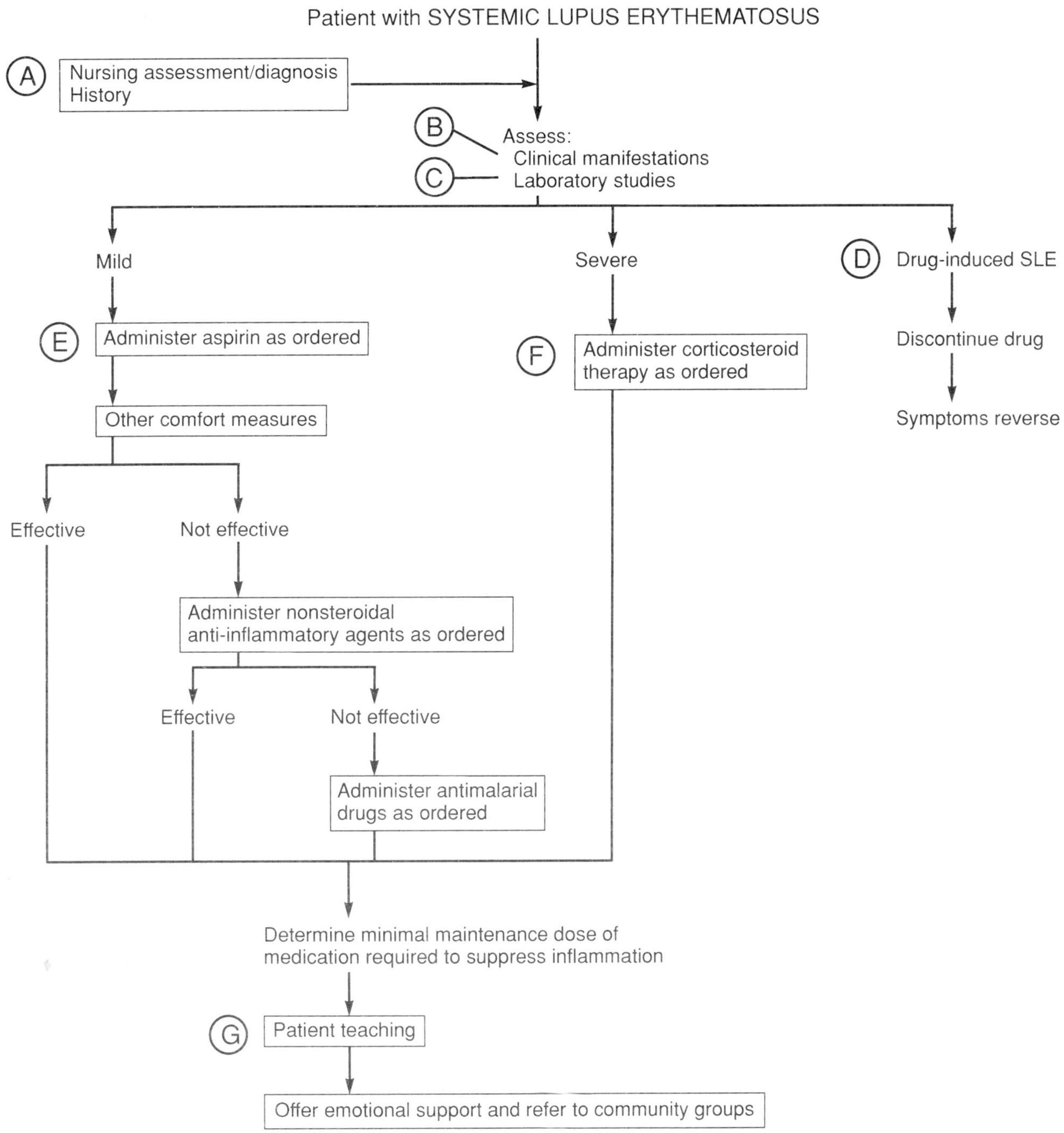
Patient with SYSTEMIC LUPUS ERYTHEMATOSUS
A
Nursing assessment/diagnosis
History
B
C
Assess:
Clinical manifestations
Laboratory studies
Mild
Severe
D
Drug-induced SLE
E
Administer aspirin as ordered
F
Administer corticosteroid therapy as ordered
Discontinue drug
Symptoms reverse
Other comfort measures
Effective
Not effective
Administer nonsteroidal anti-inflammatory agents as ordered
Effective
Not effective
Administer antimalarial drugs as ordered
Determine minimal maintenance dose of medication required to suppress inflammation
G
Patient teaching
Offer emotional support and refer to community groups

ACQUIRED IMMUNODEFICIENCY SYNDROME

Jan Metro-Emmert

Acquired immunodeficiency syndrome (AIDS) is a relatively new disease to the United States, first documented in 1981. The syndrome is caused by exposure to a retrovirus, human immunodeficiency virus (HIV-III). The HIV-III is a bloodborne virus infecting its host either by directly accessing the bloodstream or via semen during sexual intercourse. Minute tears in the mucosa of the vagina, rectum, mouth, or penis provide access to the bloodstream. HIV-III infects the T4 cells of the immune system, suppressing their activity. HIV victims may enter the health care system at any stage of the disease process. At present, there is no cure for AIDS.

A. Individuals at high risk for acquiring and transmitting HIV-III include intravenous drug abusers, hemophiliacs, those who engage in unsafe sexual practices, sexual partners of infected or high-risk persons, and children born to infected mothers.

B. Tests used to identify HIV antibodies are the enzyme-linked immunosorbent assay (ELISA) and the Western blot. Other tests are used to diagnose AIDS-related syndromes and opportunistic diseases throughout the course of the disease. Universal precautions should be utilized in handling any blood or body secretions.

C. Patients are classified for treatment using the six-stage Walter Reed Classification System based on the degree of immune system impairment (T4 cell count and function), generalized symptoms, responses to skin tests, and presence of infections. Symptoms range from mild (Stages 0 to I) and easily managed; to moderate (Stages II to IV), necessitating outpatient treatment; to severe (Stages V to VI) requiring hospitalization. A comprehensive nursing assessment is essential to planning appropriate care for each level of clinical manifestation.

D. After exposure, individuals are counseled regarding infection and the possibility of being infectious to others. Seroconversion (antibody formation) can occur 2 weeks to 1 year after exposure. Transient symptoms such as fever, malaise, fatigue, lymphadenopathy, skin rash, headache, and encephalopathy may occur. Nursing interventions are directed to prevention of transmission, maintenance of health status, and identification of disease progression.

E. Lymphadenopathy occurring in two or more areas and lasting more than 3 months without a diagnostic cause is often the first clinical indication that the immune system has been compromised (Stage II). These manifestations may begin as early as 6 months after exposure and may persist for 3 to 5 years. Individuals are typically well during this stage.

F. Diagnostic testing reveals a decrease in the T4 cell count to less than 400 (800 is normal) in Stage III. Within 18 months, skin tests indicate impairment of cell-mediated immunity (Stage IV). Stages III and IV may persist for several years. Periodic outpatient assessment and symptomatic treatment are recommended.

G. Severe constitutional symptoms, infections, and opportunistic diseases requiring intermittent inpatient management typify Stages V and VI. Examination shows fever, extreme fatigue, chronic diarrhea, unexplained weight loss, and night sweats. Nursing care focuses on reducing fever, providing rest, instituting universal precautions, restoring nutritional and hydration status, and providing meticulous skin care.

H. Many opportunistic infections, rare cancers, and central nervous system impairment are common to Stage VI. Assessment for infections such as hairy leukoplakia, thrush, vaginal infections, and chronic herpes simplex is essential. Infections may be viral, protozoal, bacterial, or fungal. Medications needed to treat these infections carry many adverse side effects such as hepatotoxicity, nephrotoxicity, bone marrow depression, and nausea and vomiting. It is essential that the nurse be knowledgeable about the medications and implement appropriate measures such as monitoring laboratory studies, maintaining hydration, checking vital signs, and administering medications with meals if compatible with food. Kaposi's sarcoma is a cancer of the blood vessels, manifested as purplish blotches initially on the lower legs and ankles, later appearing in the trunk and upper arms. Lesions in the lining of the gastrointestinal tract and heart may cause bleeding and abnormal heart sounds. *Pneumocystis carinii* pneumonia is insidious and recurrent. Prophylactic treatment with pentamidine is common. Nursing management is similar to that for other types of pneumonia (p 104). A type of dementia, characterized by alterations in thought processes and motor function, may progress to total loss of mobility and ability to communicate.

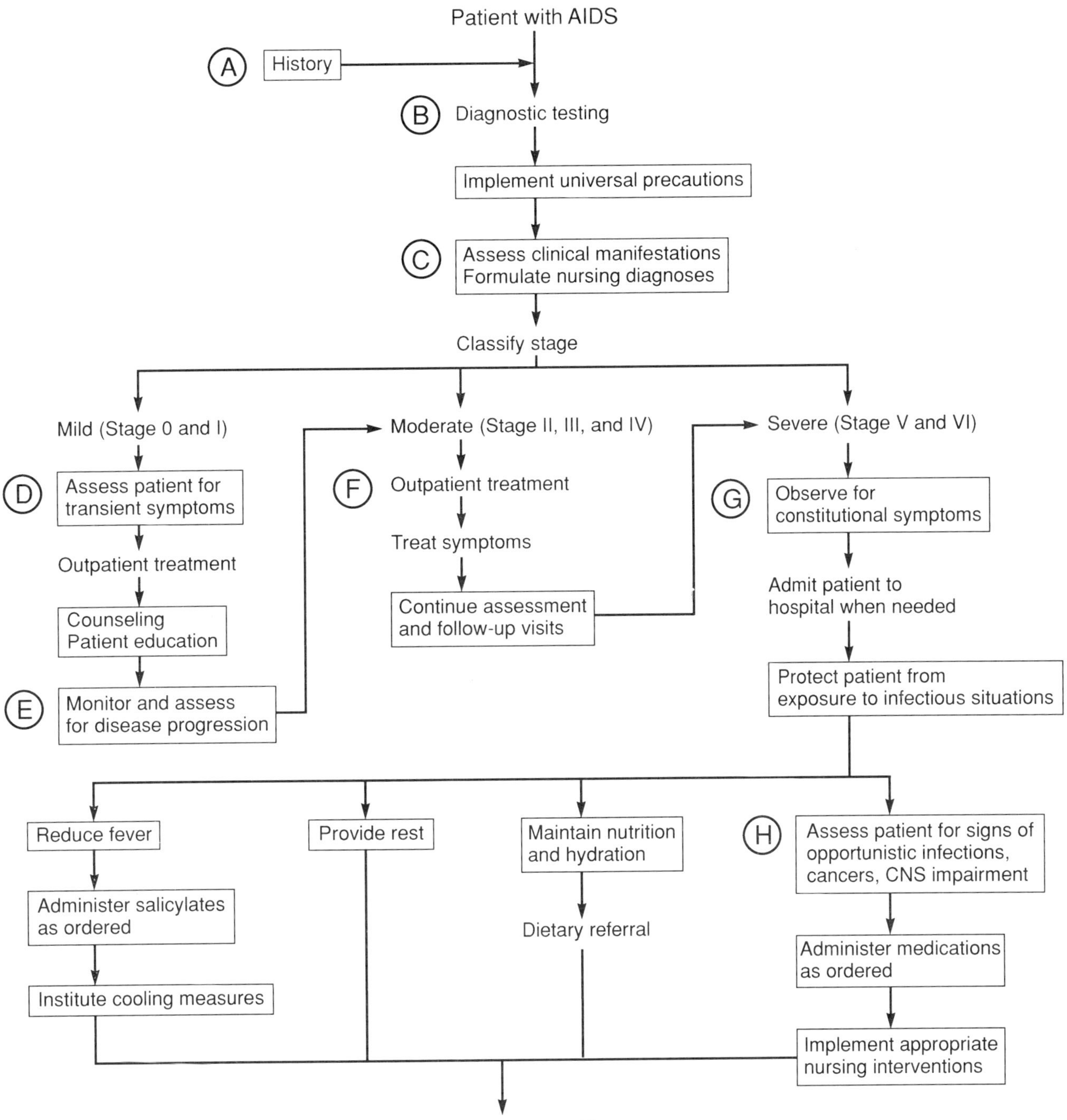

(Cont'd on page 357)

I. The social isolation felt by the patient with AIDS is superimposed on the losses of health, job, love, relationships, self-esteem, and ultimately life. Depression and anticipatory grief are common. Referral to a psychiatric liaison nurse or other health care professionals may be indicated.

J. The patient with AIDS averages two to three hospitalizations each year. Discharge planning is essential to preserve the patient's current health status. Education is essential and should include nutrition counseling, medications, indications of new health problems, and precautions to avoid transmission of HIV or other infections to others. Patients should be instructed to avoid exposure to potential pathogens, and specifically not to clean bird cages or cat boxes (toxoplasmosis, microbacteriosis) and the refrigerator or bathroom (fungi, molds). Instruct patients to avoid eating unwashed, unpeeled vegetables and foods with high bacterial counts (unpasteurized milk, raw meat, fish, or eggs). Referrals to support groups, home health agencies, psychological and/or spiritual counseling and hospice are an integral part of the discharge plan.

K. With the compromised state of the patient, each infection could be fatal. The nurse must be prepared to deal with the patient's potential death and the bereavement of the survivors. Patients with AIDS may be left to die alone because the significant others are unable to accept the disease or give support. Facilitate the grieving process, help the patient to die with dignity, and ensure that the patient does not die alone. Referrals to bereavement counselors and support groups may assist survivors.

References

Barrick B. Caring for AIDS patients: a challenge you can meet. Nursing 1988; 18(11):50–60.

Grady C, ed. AIDS. Nurs Clin North Am 1988; 23:683–862.

Redfield RR, Burke DS. HIV infection: the clinical picture. Sci Am 1988; October:90–98.

Rheifer WG, Houseman C. Bereavement and AIDS. J Psychosoc Nurs 1988; 26(10):21–25.

U.S. Department of Health and Human Services. Update: universal precautions for prevention of transmission of human immunodeficiency virus, hepatitis B virus, and other bloodborne pathogens in health settings. MMWR 1989; 24:377–382.

Weber JN, Weiss RA. HIV infection: the cellular picture. Sci Am 1988; October:101–109.

Patient with AIDS

(Cont'd from page 355)

↓

(I) Provide emotional support

↓

Make referral to psychiatric liaison nurse if needed

↓

(J) Prepare patient for discharge as appropriate
- Instruct regarding diet, medications, precautions
- Referral to home health, hospice

↓

(K) Assist patient and significant others in preparing for patient's imminent death

MONONUCLEOSIS

Jan Metro-Emmert

Mononucleosis can apply to any infectious disease in which there is an elevated number of circulating mononuclear cells. Most frequently, however, the term "mono" refers to an acute infection of the lymphatic system caused by Epstein-Barr virus (EBV). The susceptible population is typically young adults 15 to 30 years of age who are without antibodies; females are affected twice as often as males. Antibody-positive people are carriers. The sources of infection are nasopharyngeal secretions and blood. Kissing and eating and drinking from contaminated utensils can spread this disease. It is also transmitted through blood transfusions.

A. Diagnosis is made from hematologic studies, the heterophile, and the clinical symptoms. The hematologic profile reveals an elevated white blood cell count (10,000 to 20,000) with a differential of 50 percent mononuclear cells and 10 percent atypical Downey cells. Neutrophils may be decreased, and thrombocytopenia is present in 50 percent of patients. The heterophile is positive for Paul-Bunnell-Davidson (P-B-D) agglutinin tests, and the Epstein-Barr antibody titer is elevated.

B. The clinical picture reflects the immune response of the host. The prodromal period lasts 4 to 5 days. Symptoms include malaise, fatigue, fever, headache, sore throat, and cervical lymphadenopathy. The fever persists for 10 to 14 days and is often above 39.5° C (103.1°F). During the first week a sore throat develops. Also present is palatal enanthem petechiae (which makes mononucleosis indistinguishable from streptococcal pharyngitis). Lymph node enlargement is more pronounced in the anterior and posterior cervical nodes. They are palpable and very tender, often causing neck pain. Other nodes that may be enlarged include the axillary, posterior auricular, submandibular, and inguinal. Splenomegaly (the spleen often two to three times its normal size) occurs in 50 percent of patients and peaks during the second and third weeks, giving rise to left upper quadrant pain. Hepatomegaly occurs in 10 percent of patients during the first 2 weeks of illness and may result in abnormal liver function tests and jaundice. A transient erythematous maculopapular rash (similar to rubella) can occur on the trunk and extremities. Bilateral supraorbital edema may also be an early clinical finding.

C. The patient is not usually hospitalized unless severe splenomegaly and hepatomegaly with enzyme elevations are present. Treatment is supportive. Nursing interventions focus on providing comfort, relieving symptoms, and preventing complications. For fever with its accompanying chills and myalgia, salicylates, plenty of fluids, and cool sponge baths are indicated. If fever persists or spikes, be alert for complications, such as meningitis, encephalitis (p 30), myocarditis or pericarditis (p 76), and notify the physician. Teach the family to isolate the patient (if at home) from infectious sources.

D. Neck pain can be eased by using salicylates, warm compresses (or cool if preferred), and positioning for comfort. This symptom is relieved as the size of the nodes recedes.

E. Interventions for relief of sore throat include warm saline gargles, mild analgesic lozenges, ice collar, moist inhalations, liquid or soft diet, limiting conversation, and good oral hygiene. If soreness continues, suspect streptococcal pharyngitis or Vincent's angina. The physician should be notified and preparations made for a throat culture. Antibiotics may be indicated. If respiratory exchange is compromised, other complications such as obstructive tonsillitis or airway obstruction via membrane formation may be present. Both of these necessitiate surgical intervention. Fortunately, these complications are rare.

F. Abdominal discomfort is directly related to splenic enlargement. Activity should be limited, especially during the second and third weeks of the disease when peak enlargement occurs. If the patient is at home, contact sports must be prohibited because of the risk of splenic rupture. The patient and the family should be taught the signs of rupture—severe abdominal pain, shoulder pain, shock (p 70)—and report them to the physician immediately. Corticosteroids may be ordered if both splenomegaly and hepatomegaly have occurred.

G. Fatigue is the most ubiquitous sign of mononucleosis. It is characteristic of the acute stage and may persist long into the convalescent stage of the disease. Bed rest, spacing daily activities, limiting visitors, small frequent feedings, decreasing sensory input, and frequent rest periods all serve to minimize energy output and allow time for rest and sleep. Inform the family that fatigue may persist after other symptoms are resolved; they must be prepared to limit activities and allow for rest when at home.

H. Infectious mononucleosis is a self-limiting disease. Acute symptoms subside within 4 to 6 weeks. However, marked fatigue can continue for several months. Full recovery is the norm even for patients who develop complications.

I. There are three chronic forms of mononucleosis. The most common is chronic viral fatigue syndrome. Symptoms similar to those of the acute form may persist for a year or more. Because of the severe fatigue, often lasting for years, drastic alterations in the patient's lifestyle may be necessary.

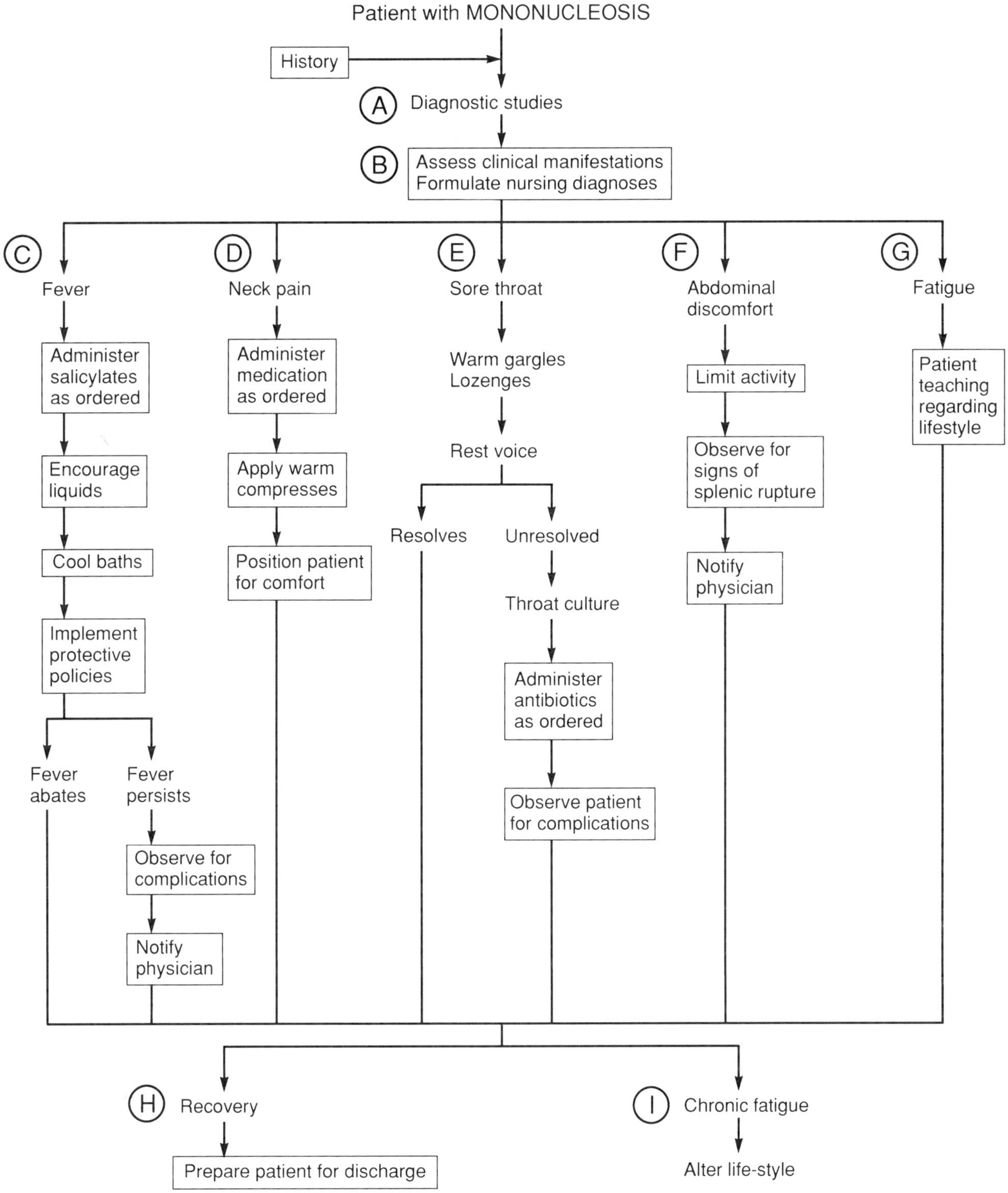

References

Brunner LS, Suddarth DS. Textbook of medical-surgical nursing. 6th ed. Philadelphia: JB Lippincott, 1988.

Komstogg SL. Chronic mononucleosis syndromes. Hosp Pract 1987; 22(5):71–75.

Laia JA. Infectious mononucleosis. In: Wyngaarden JB, Smith LH, eds. Cecil textbook of medicine. 17th ed. Philadelphia: WB Saunders, 1985.

Sabetta JR. Infectious mononucleosis. Hosp Med 1984; 20(3):109–119.

CYTOMEGALOVIRUS (CMV)

Nancy A. Young

A member of the herpesvirus group, the cytomegalovirus can cause both acquired and congenital infections referred to as cytomegalic inclusion disease (CID). The virus passes between humans through any close contact, and can be found in blood, urine, saliva, cervical mucus, semen, tears, and breast milk. CMV produces a chronic persistent infection that may recur over many years. Although generally an innocuous virus in adults and children, it may cause morbidity and mortality in the developing fetus.

A. The nurse should take a thorough history from the patient and perform a physical assessment. Sequelae from this viral disease vary significantly. The immunocompetent person experiences an asymptomatic or mild mononucleosis-type illness, whereas the immunosuppressed individual and the neonate may exhibit more severe symptoms. Nursing care depends on the symptoms of the particular patient.

B. Older children could acquire CMV iatrogenically by blood transfusion or possibly by contact in daycare centers; however, they usually remain asymptomatic. Normal adults may experience an illness that mimics mononucleosis (p 358), with malaise, fever, adenopathy, hepatosplenomegaly, and sore throat.

C. Immunosuppressed patients experience a higher incidence of morbidity and mortality from CMV. Patients with acquired immunodeficiency syndrome (AIDS) (p 354) and those who have undergone transplantation and chemotherapy suffer most frequently from acute primary infections and reactivation of the virus. The resulting interstitial pneumonia (p 104) can be mild or fulminant, producing pulmonary insufficiency and/or death.

D. A healthy mother can harbor the CMV in her urinary and/or genital tract, and transmit it to the fetus across the placenta or during childbirth as the fetus passes through the cervix. Fetal infection may result in extensive intrauterine tissue damage incompatible with life, or the neonate may survive with or without brain damage. Infected neonates may be small for gestational age and suffer from microcephaly, intracerebral calcification, hypoplasticity, and hemolysis leading to anemia, hyperbilirubinemia, petechiae, and ecchymosis. Although some infants infected with CMV die shortly after birth, subclinical infections in the newborn can produce mental retardation, auditory and visual deficits, and learning disabilities that may not materialize until childhood. Infants can acquire and harbor the virus through breastfeeding and remain asymptomatic.

E. Discharge instructions vary depending on the patient. Prevention of the infection should be promoted, considering the ineffectiveness of current therapies. Those who have a compromised immune system should avoid known viral carriers. Parents of nonsymptomatic infants who have been infected should receive information about indicators of long-term complications of the virus to assure early intervention.

References

Jordan MC. Infectious diseases. 3rd ed. Philadelphia: Harper & Row, 1983.

Olds S, London M, Ladeqig P. Maternal-newborn nursing. 2nd ed. Menlo Park, CA: Addison-Wesley, 1984.

Sinnott JT, Cancio MR. Cytomegalovirus. Infect Control 1987; 8(2):79–81.

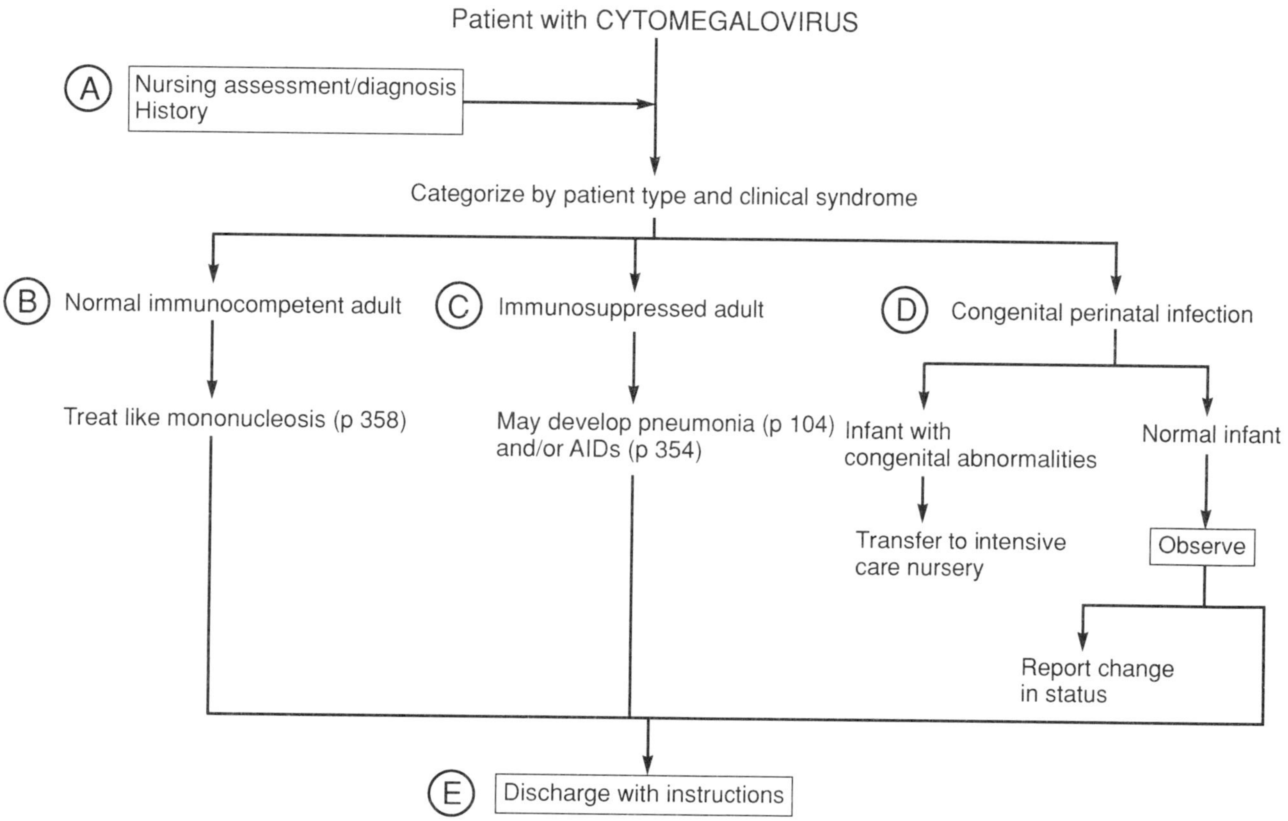
Patient with CYTOMEGALOVIRUS
A
Nursing assessment/diagnosis
History
Categorize by patient type and clinical syndrome
B
Normal immunocompetent adult
C
Immunosuppressed adult
D
Congenital perinatal infection
Treat like mononucleosis (p 358)
May develop pneumonia (p 104)
and/or AIDs (p 354)
Infant with
congenital abnormalities
Normal infant
Transfer to intensive
care nursery
Observe
Report change
in status
E
Discharge with instructions

MULTIPLE MYELOMA

Jan Metro-Emmert

A. Multiple myeloma is a neoplastic disease. The tumor originates in the hematopoietic portion of the bone marrow. Plasma cells begin to proliferate, infiltrate the bone, produce osteolytic lesions, and crowd the bone marrow, which inhibits red blood cell (RBC) and platelet production. The tumors are multiple in nature and attack many sites simultaneously: bones, lymph nodes, liver, spleen, and kidneys. The disease is particularly insidious in that it has a prolonged (5 to 20 years) presymptomatic period, which is characterized by recurrent infections, especially pneumonias (p 104). Once symptoms of bone involvement manifest, the disease is rapidly progressive and fatal, usually within 2 to 4 years. It occurs in blacks twice as frequently as in Caucasians and in men three times as often as in women. The age at onset ranges from 40 to 70 years.

B. Bone pain is the initial symptom in 90 percent of the patients and persists, often with increasing severity, as the disease progresses. The pain is increased by movement, coughing, deep breathing, straining, and muscle spasms.

C. The diagnostic workup confirms these conditions. The patient should never be NPO for any diagnostic test, because the risk is high that dehydration will precipitate acute renal failure. Radiography shows bone destruction, especially in the pelvis, vertebrae, and ribs. The skull also shows the "punched-out" lesions of myeloma. Bone destruction is manifest in hypercalcemia (p 188) and results in alteration of renal concentration, which leads to renal failure (p 314). Bone-marrow aspiration (p 368) reveals an abnormal number and immaturity of plasma cells. There is also decreased production of RBCs and platelets. The peripheral blood samples show anemia (p 342), decreased platelet count, and a high globulin concentration. Urinalysis reveals the diagnostic Bence-Jones protein, which severely damages the kidney tubules and results in renal failure. Since the immunoglobulins are abnormal, the patient has an increased risk of acquiring infections.

D. Treatment is symptomatic and palliative. Radiotherapy is used to reduce tumor size and control pain. Chemotherapy (alkylating agents and corticosteroids) achieves remission in 50 percent of patients. Combination VACP (vincristine, doxorubicin [Adriamycin], cyclophosphamide, and prednisone) is repeated every 3 weeks (p 408).

E. Nursing focuses on relieving pain, observing for and preventing complications (pathologic fractures, hypercalcemia, renal failure, anemia, bleeding, infections), and providing supportive, compassionate care. Pain presents a unique challenge in that a patient with multiple myeloma must not be immobile because this further exacerbates demineralization. Analgesia and devices to aid mobility are primary interventions. Braces, splints, slings, and surgery (fixation, laminectomy) allow for support, reduce pain, and improve mobilization. The patient must exercise according to his fullest ability. Patient and family teaching should emphasize the importance of this often painful therapy.

F. Pathologic fractures (p 230) can occur with minimal trauma. A sudden, localized pain should be evaluated for this complication. If fractures of the vertebrae occur, the spinal cord may be compressed, resulting in paralysis.

G. Anemia is medically controlled with transfusions of RBCs. Nursing care focuses on rest, nutrition, and conserving the patient's energy.

H. Because of platelet depression and the effects of radiation and chemotherapy, the nurse must monitor the patient for bleeding. Purpura, bleeding gums, epistaxis, or more severe bleeding episodes may occur. Hemorrhagic shock is a possibility.

I. Recognizing signs of hypercalcemia and attempting to prevent the complications is priority. The patient should receive 3,000 to 4,000 ml of fluid per day. His output should be no less than 1,500 ml. Maintaining this balance helps to prevent dehydration, dilute the calcium, and flush it through the kidney tubules, as well as preventing renal damage from the precipitation of excess plasma protein.

J. Fever, malaise, weakness, and irritability may herald the onset of infection. Careful assessment of lung sounds can detect pneumonia. Teaching includes the avoidance of potentially infectious situations.

K. Emotional support is especially important because the patient and family are coping not only with chronic pain but also with a terminal illness often accompanied by severe disability. The nurse provides patient and family teaching to keep information accurate and promote communication, assesses the ability of the patient and family to cope, and gives supportive, compassionate nursing care. Referrals to other health care providers may be indicated.

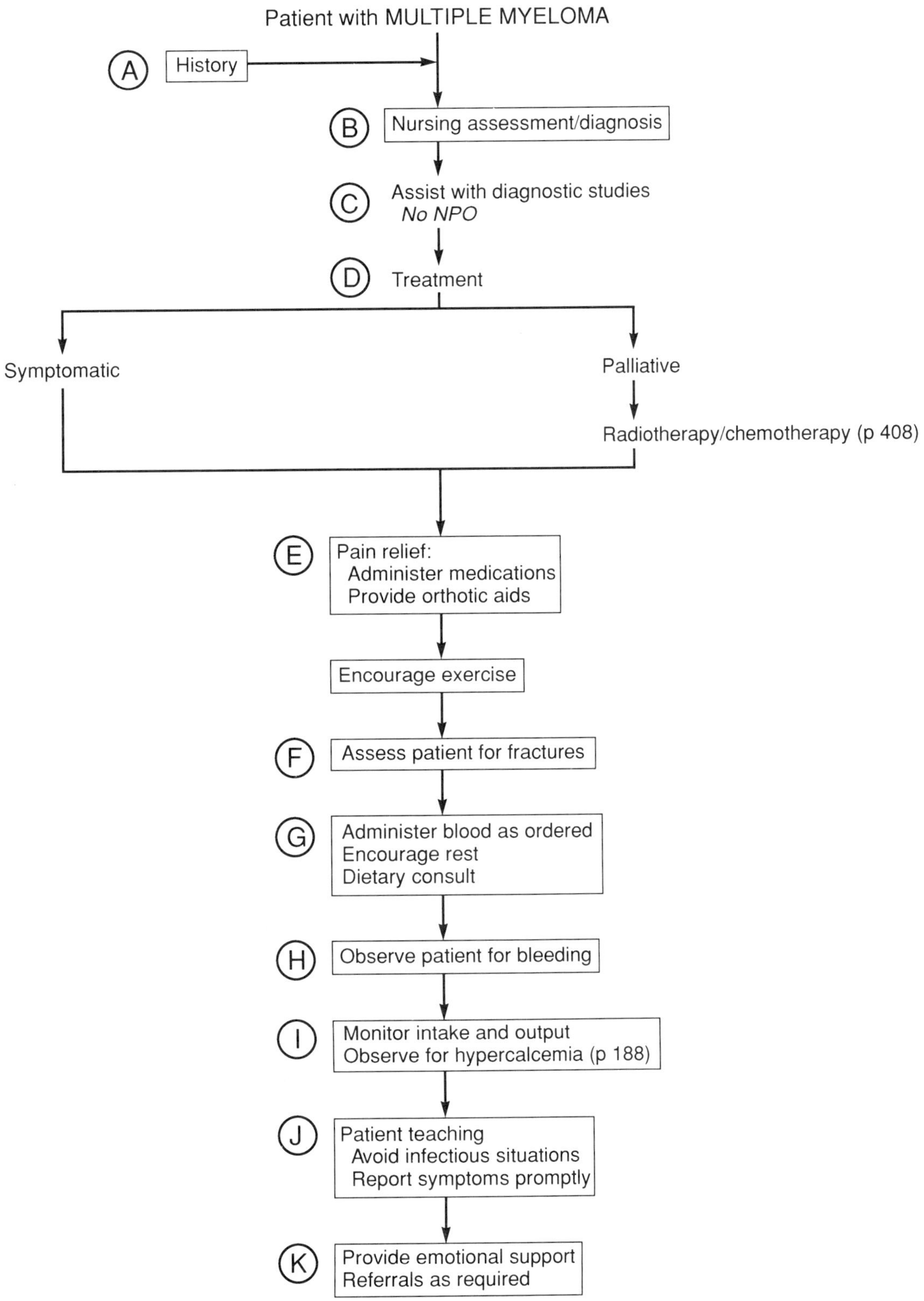

References

Farrant C. Multiple myeloma: controlling pain, prolonging survival. RN 1987; January:38–42.

Luckmann J, Sorensen KC. Medical-surgical nursing. 3rd ed. Philadelphia: WB Saunders, 1987.

Hamilton HK. Neoplastic disorders. Springhouse, PA: Nursing '85 Books, 1985.

Shackelford P. Multiple myeloma. Orthop Nurs 1985; 4(5):61–64.

Schema of clinical features in multiple myeloma. Hosp Med 1986; 22(7):114–116.

HODGKIN'S DISEASE

Leslie Hussey

Hodgkin's disease is a malignant disorder characterized by lymph gland, spleen, and liver enlargement that can progress to all parts of the body. Hodgkin's disease occurs in people of all ages, but has a higher incidence in the 20- to 40-year age group, occurring in males twice as often as females. The etiology of Hodgkin's disease is unknown.

A. The patient with Hodgkin's disease first presents with painless enlargement of the lymph nodes, usually the cervical nodes. Other early signs and symptoms include severe pruritus, intermittent fever, splenomegaly, and weakness. As the disease progresses, the patient may experience night sweats, weight loss, fever, and lymph node pain after ingesting alcohol. Depending on the stage of the disease, the patient could have facial edema, jaundice, nerve pain, anemia, increased susceptibility to infection, and pulmonary symptoms, i.e., cough, dyspnea, chest pain, pleural effusion, and cyanosis.

B. Diagnostic testing includes a complete blood count (CBC), sedimentation rate, serum albumin, globulin and alkaline phosphatase, creatinine, and uric acid levels. Radiologic testing includes chest films, computed to mographic (CT) scans, and bipedal lymphangiography. The lymph node biopsy is by far the most definitive diagnostic test for Hodgkin's disease. Reed-Sternberg cells are the classic and key characteristic in diagnosing Hodgkin's disease. These cells are atypical, giant, and anucleated.

C. The severity of Hodgkin's disease is described by stages. Staging is important because it not only determines treatment but also prognosis (see Table 1).

D. Radiation therapy is the primary treatment for Hodgkin's disease in stages I, II, and IIIA. A chemotherapy (p 408) regimen is the treatment of choice for stages IIIB and IV. Radiation and chemotherapy are used together in some patients to improve prognosis.

E. Nursing care of the patient with Hodgkin's disease focuses on psychosocial support and education. The prognosis for all phases is quite good and the patient can be encouraged to hope. Explain all procedures thoroughly. Include the family and/or significant others. Patients between 20 and 40 years of age may have concerns about childbearing. Individualized counseling must be done. Sperm banking may be considered.

F. Physical nursing care is symptomatic. Acetylsalicylic acid (aspirin) may be given for headache and general discomfort. Warm gargles may relieve a sore throat. Antiemetics should be administered to relieve nausea and vomiting. Itching may be relieved by administering antipruritic drugs.

G. If the patient is dyspneic, place him in Fowler's position. Oxygen should be administered as needed.

TABLE 1 Staging Classifications for Hodgkin's Disease

Stage	*Definition of Involvement*
I	Single lymph node area
IE	Single extralymphatic organ or site
II	Two or more lymph node areas on the same side of the diaphragm
IIE	Two or more lymph node areas on the same side of the diaphragm and localized involvement of an extralymphatic organ or site
III	Lymph node areas on both sides of the diaphragm
IIIE	Lymph node areas on both sides of the diaphragm and localized involvement of an extralymphatic organ or site
IIIS	Lymph node areas on both sides of the diaphragm and the spleen
IIISE	All of the stage III conditions
IV	Disseminated involvement of one or more extralymphatic organs or sites with or without lymph node involvement
A	Absence > of fever, night sweats, and/or unexplained weight loss of more than 10 percent of body weight within 6 months before diagnosis
B	Presence > of fever, night sweats, and/or unexplained weight loss of more than 10 percent of body weight within 6 months before diagnosis

Note: Liver involvement and bone marrow involvement away from an involved lymph node are considered stage IV disease. (Adapted from the Ann Arbor clinical staging classification of Hodgkin's disease. In: Phipps B, Woods N. Medical-surgical nursing: concepts and clinical practice. St. Louis: CV Mosby, 1987.)

H. Some patients may experience extreme weight loss while receiving chemotherapy and/or radiation treatment. These patients should be referred for nutritional counseling.

I. While the patient is receiving treatment, laboratory studies must be monitored. If the patient is anemic, blood transfusions are ordered (p 340). Protection of the patient by reverse isolation may also be necessary.

J. Discharge teaching should include symptom management. As with other types of chronic illness, the patient will probably experience periods of remission. It is necessary for the patient to remain under medical supervision. The nurse should assist the patient and family in establishing and maintaining a support system as they adjust to living with a life-threatening disease.

References

Brunner LS, Suddarth DS. The Lippincott manual of nursing practice. 4th ed. Philadelphia: JB Lippincott, 1986.

Consalvo K, Gallagher M. Winning the battle against Hodgkin's disease. RN 1986; December: 20–25.

Kneisl CR, Ames SW. Adult health nursing: A biopsychosocial approach. Reading, MA: Addison-Wesley, 1986.

Phipps W, Long B, Woods N. Medical-surgical nursing: concepts and clinical practice. St. Louis: CV Mosby, 1987.

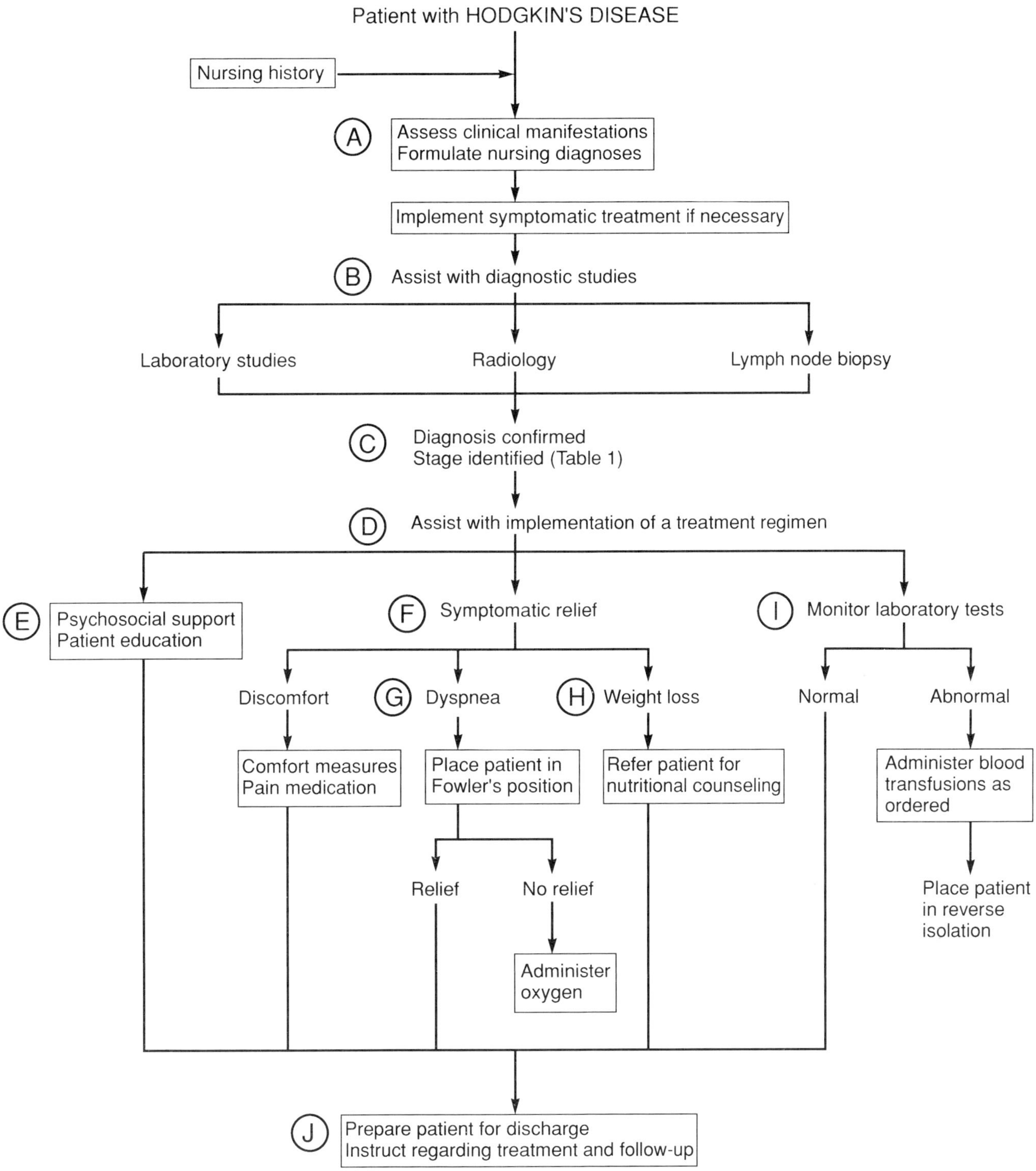
Patient with HODGKIN'S DISEASE
Nursing history
A
Assess clinical manifestations
Formulate nursing diagnoses
Implement symptomatic treatment if necessary
B
Assist with diagnostic studies
Laboratory studies
Radiology
Lymph node biopsy
C
Diagnosis confirmed
Stage identified (Table 1)
D
Assist with implementation of a treatment regimen
E
Psychosocial support
Patient education
F
Symptomatic relief
I
Monitor laboratory tests
Discomfort
G
Dyspnea
H
Weight loss
Normal
Abnormal
Comfort measures
Pain medication
Place patient in
Fowler's position
Refer patient for
nutritional counseling
Administer blood
transfusions as
ordered
Relief
No relief
Place patient
in reverse
isolation
Administer
oxygen
J
Prepare patient for discharge
Instruct regarding treatment and follow-up

NON-HODGKIN'S LYMPHOMA

Mary Beth Mardjetko

Non-Hodgkin's lymphoma (NHL) is a diverse group of malignancies of the immune system. In all types of lymphoma, lymphocytes begin growing abnormally and spread to other organs. Lymphomas display a wide spectrum of clinical morphologic, immunologic, and molecular features.

A. In most cases, patients with NHL present with painless localized or generalized lymphadenopathy. Liver and spleen enlargement or abdominal masses may be present. Nursing history should include when the patient first noticed the enlarged lymph node or nodes and which nodes were involved. Because some patients also experience fever, night sweats, fatigue, pruritus, and weight loss, these areas should be explored. The site and size of the involved lymph nodes should be assessed, as well as the potential for an obstructive complication. Vital signs and height and weight should be measured.

B. The diagnosis of NHL is confirmed by a lymph node biopsy. After diagnosis, the disease is staged to evaluate the extent of spread. This staging process usually includes chest radiography; bone marrow biopsy (p 368); liver biopsy; abdominal CT scan; lymphangiography; lumbar puncture; and laboratory tests, e.g., complete blood count (CBC), platelet count, and evaluation of liver and renal function. (See Table 1 for staging information.) Many classifications for NHL have been developed. Recently, the Working Formulation, which divides NHL into three grades—low, intermediate, and high—based on histology and survival data, was adopted for use.

C. The low-grade lymphomas account for about 35 percent of NHL. Eighty percent of patients have stage III or IV disease at the time of presentation. Many patients are asymptomatic with indolent disease progression. The initial management for this group may be only close observation until disease progression necessitates treatment. Often, these lymphomas eventually transform to a more aggressive type that requires intensive therapy. The small subset of patients with stage I and II disease should be treated with local radiation therapy.

D. Intermediate-grade lymphomas account for about 40 percent of NHL. Relatively rapid growth and dissemination are characteristic. A majority of patients present with advanced disease. Combination chemotherapy is usually recommended for this group.

E. The high-grade lymphomas account for 20 percent of NHL. These diseases tend to evolve rapidly and involve the bone marrow and central nervous system. Without intensive multidrug protocols, prognosis is poor.

TABLE 1 The Ann Arbor Staging Classification System

Stage I	Involvement of a single lymph node region or of a single extranodal organ or site (I_E)
Stage II	Involvement of two or more lymph node regions on the same side of the diaphragm, or localized involvement of an extranodal organ or site (II_E) and of one or more lymph node regions on the same side of the diaphragm
Stage III	Involvement of lymph node regions on both sides of the diaphragm, which may also be accompanied by localized involvement of an extranodal organ or site (III_E) or spleen (III_S) or both (III_{SE})
Stage IV	Diffuse or disseminated involvement of one or more distant extranodal organs with or without associated lymph node involvement

Fever greater than 38°C, night sweats, and/or weight loss greater than 10% of body weight in the 6 months preceding admission are defined as systemic symptoms and denoted by the suffix letter B. Asymptomatic patients are denoted by the suffix letter A. Biopsy-documented involvement of stage IV sites is identified by the following symbol: marrow—M; liver—H; lung—L; pleura—P; bone—O; skin—D.

American Cancer Society. Malignant lymphomas. Publication #76–2M–3355–PE. In: Ultmann J., Stein R. Non-Hodgkins lymphomas: an approach to staging and therapy. New York: American Cancer Society, 1975.

F. Several cycles of combinations of chemotherapeutic agents are used for NHL. Successful combination chemotherapy requires several criteria: (1) Each drug must have the capacity to act against the tumor; (2) the drugs should work in different ways on the tumor; and (3) the drugs should have different toxicities so maximal doses of each can be given.

G. Before therapy begins, the patient must understand the possible side effects and toxicities that may occur and the measures that will be instituted to minimize or prevent them.

H. Chemotherapeutic agents have systemic effects that can produce life-threatening complications (p 408). It is essential that ongoing, multisystem assessment of these patients be instituted. Most side effects result from the action of the agent on normal cells. Rapidly growing cells are most commonly involved, i.e., cells of the bone marrow, gastrointestinal tract, hair follicles, and gonads. Therefore, potential side effects includes bone marrow suppression, mucositis, diarrhea or constipation, nausea, vomiting, anorexia, alopecia, sexual dysfunction, and a variety of psychological reactions. Nursing care is similar to that for Hodgkin's disease (p 364) and multiple myeloma (p 362).

I. Psychological support during this time is essential. Referral to community agencies for additional assistance may be necessary.

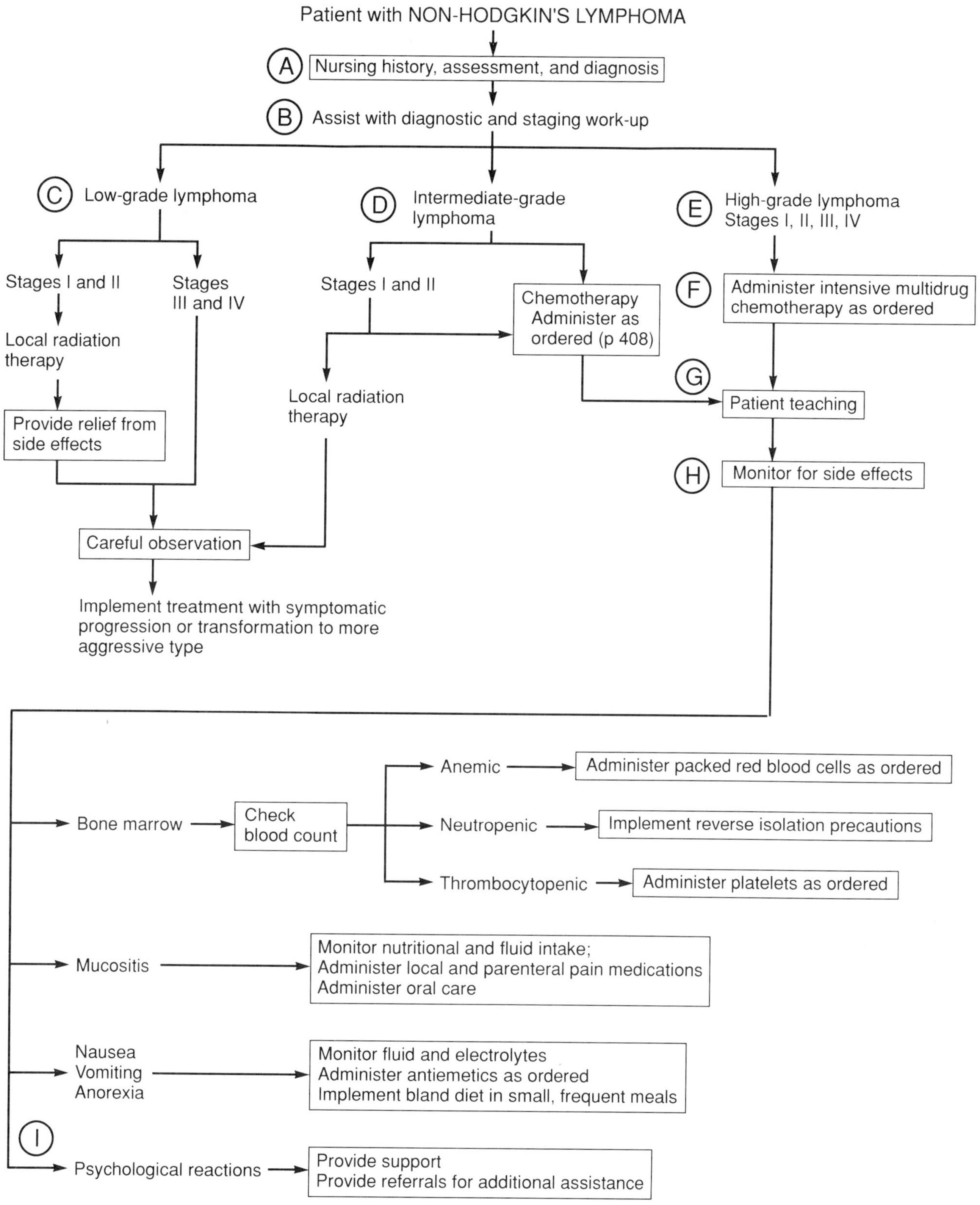

References

DeVita V. Hematologic malignancies. Non-Hodgkin's lymphomas. Hosp Pract 1986; 21:103–118.

Horning S. Non-Hodgkin's lymphoma. Mediguide to oncology. 1988; 8(2):1–5.

Ziegfeld C. Core curriculum for oncology nursing. Philadelphia: WB Saunders, 1987.

BONE MARROW ASPIRATION

Lynne Tier

Bone marrow aspiration is commonly done to diagnose conditions such as oat cell carcinoma (p 122), leukemia (p 346), Hodgkin's disease (p 364), and other lymphomas (p 366). Biopsies may also be done concurrently to stage disease and/or monitor the patient's response to treatment. Sites for the procedure include the posterior superior iliac crest, anterior iliac crest, or sternum.

A. A complete nursing history and assessment reveals the following actual or potential nursing diagnoses: lack of knowledge related to the procedure; anxiety related to the procedure and its results; alteration in comfort (pain) related to the procedure; and decreased cardiac output related to possible complications, e.g., bleeding and infection.

B. Checking diagnostic data, specifically coagulation studies, before the procedure helps to anticipate possible bleeding after the procedure. Checking the state of the patient's immune system may be necessary to determine if safeguards such as masks need to be used to protect compromised patients.

C. Although the physician usually explains the procedure, the nurse reinforces the information so that the patient can cooperate as much as possible. The patient may feel more comfortable about expressing fears and concerns to the nurse. Teaching should include postprocedure comfort measures (see G), length of procedure, type of anesthetic (local), and sensation of pressure or pulling. Ensure that a signed consent is obtained before the procedure is begun.

D. Assess vital signs to monitor the patient's general condition and to alert staff about the patient's anxiety related to the procedure (elevated pulse and blood pressure). The preprocedural assessment gives a baseline value for the postprocedure comparison.

E. Preparation includes notifying laboratory or specific personnel involved in the procedure. Assemble a bone marrow aspiration tray, sterile gloves, antiseptic solution, local anesthetic agent, dressing supplies, and possibly pain medication.

F. Gentle reassurance and touch comforts the patient during the procedure. A mild sedative may be given.

G. Besides the local infiltration of the aspiration site by the physician, other comfort measures can be used. If the iliac crest site is used, ice massage to the crest on the opposite side decreases the discomfort felt during the procedure. Massage of pressure points on the patient's foot has been found to decrease greatly the patient's perception of pain during the procedure.

H. If the patient has coagulopathy, bleeding is a common complication. Vital signs must be frequently monitored and the puncture site frequently observed.

I. Allow the patient an opportunity to discuss the procedure if needed. Document patient condition as well as specific comfort measures used during the procedure.

References

Bair T. Diagnostic procedures. In: Perry AG, Potter PA, eds. Clinical nursing skills and techniques: basic, intermediate and advanced. St. Louis: CV Mosby, 1986:1218–1258.

Brunner LS, Suddarth DS. Textbook of medical-surgical nursing. 6th ed. Philadelphia: JB Lippincott, 1988.

DeCrosta T. Relieving pain: four noninvasive ways you should know more about. Nursing Life 1984; 4(2):28–33.

Markus S. Bone marrow aspiration and biopsy. In: Hamilton HK, ed. Procedures. Springhouse, PA: Springhouse Corporation, 1983:190–193.

Strickland E. Counterpressure during bone marrow aspiration and biopsy. Oncol Nurs Forum 1987; 14(5):103–104.

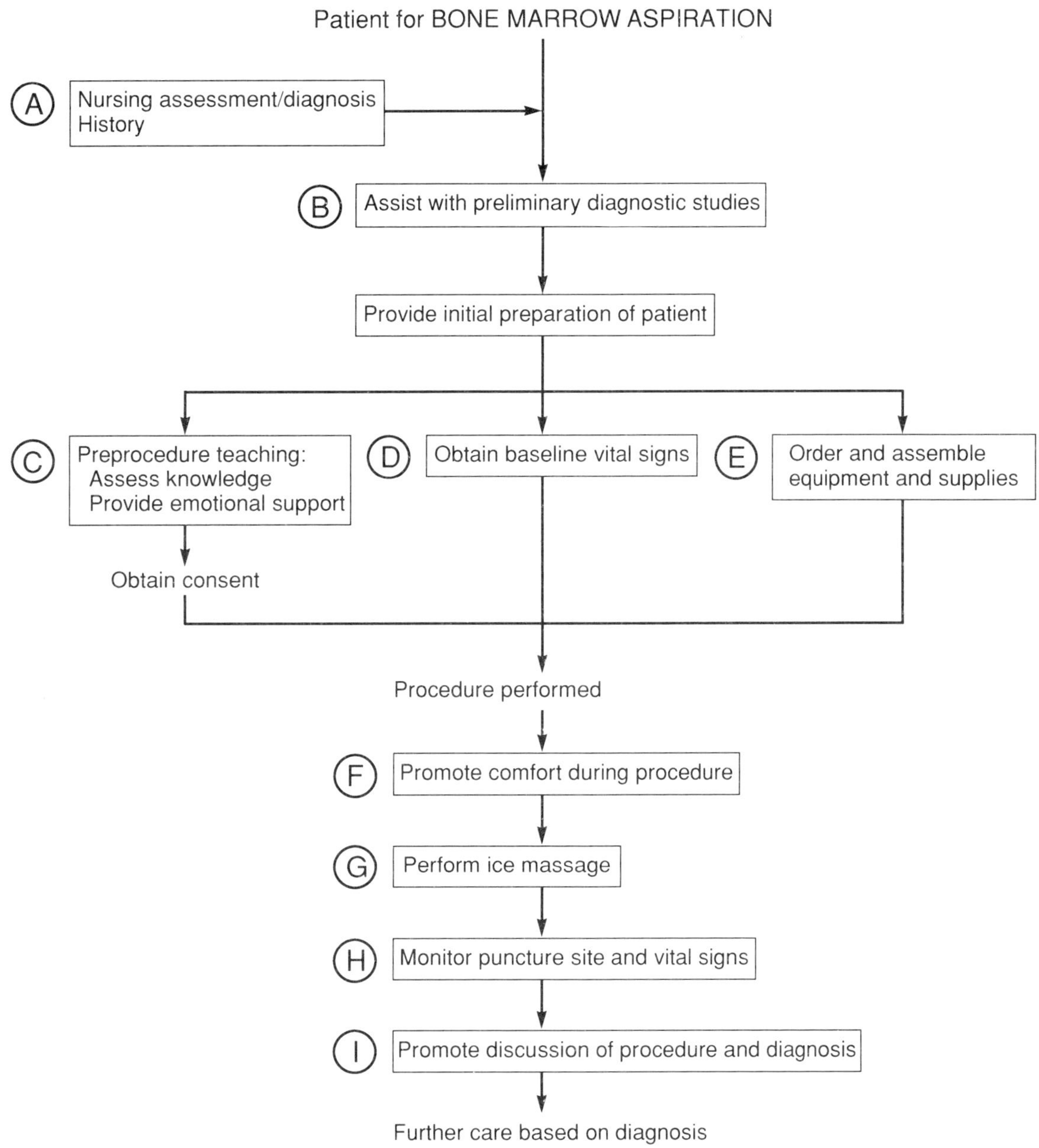
Patient for BONE MARROW ASPIRATION
A
Nursing assessment/diagnosis
History
B
Assist with preliminary diagnostic studies
Provide initial preparation of patient
C
Preprocedure teaching:
Assess knowledge
Provide emotional support
Obtain consent
D
Obtain baseline vital signs
E
Order and assemble equipment and supplies
Procedure performed
F
Promote comfort during procedure
G
Perform ice massage
H
Monitor puncture site and vital signs
I
Promote discussion of procedure and diagnosis
Further care based on diagnosis

SPLENECTOMY

Leslie C. Hussey

The spleen performs several important functions: purifying the blood, producing and storing red blood cells, removing red blood cells from the blood stream at the end of their lifespan, and producing lympohocytes, plasma cells, and antibodies.

A. Removal of the spleen is performed only in life-threatening situations, but the adult can function normally after removal. A splenectomy is most often the result of rupture owing to trauma or hypersplenism (overactivity of the spleen).

B. The trauma patient may present with upper abdominal and left shoulder pain. Hemorrhage and shock (p 70) are a major concern. Other manifestations include pallor, hypotension, and a rapid, thready pulse. The abdomen is tender to palpation, especially on the left side and over ribs 10 and 11. There may be left rectus muscle rigidity. Bowel sounds may be diminished or absent.

C. The patient may have a history of splenomegaly and prior treatment for a chronic illness such as leukemia (p 346) or Hodgkin's disease (p 364).

D. Preoperative nursing care includes accurate assessment and quick intervention should shock and hemorrhage ensue. It is vitally important to watch for falling hematocrit levels, a loss or change in sensorium, increasing anxiety or restlessness, unstable vital signs, and/or increase in the severity of abdominal pain or distention. Coagulation studies are done and the patient is cross-matched for 4 to 6 units of blood. Whole blood is administered preoperatively if the spleen has ruptured. A nasogastric tube and intravenous line are also inserted preoperatively. Depending on the reason for surgery, the patient may or may not be psychologically prepared for the procedure.

E. Postoperatively, the patient must be observed for hemorrhage and shock, the most common complications following splenectomy. Monitor the patient closely for unexplained changes in condition. If changes occur in the patient's level of consciousness or vital signs, notify the physician. An elevated temperature up to 38.3°C (101°F) is common following a splenectomy and is not considered a reliable indicator of infection, which increases the importance of observing the patient for symptoms of possible complications.

F. The platelet count may be three to five times normal (thrombocytosis) the first 2 weeks postoperatively, thus increasing the risk of thrombosis. Daily platelet counts should be monitored.

G. Observe the patient for abdominal distention and discomfort. Other organs of the abdomen such as the stomach and intestines, may expand to compensate for the space left when the spleen has been removed. Abdominal binders should be applied snugly to minimize distention and increase comfort. However, abdominal distention may also indicate hemorrhage.

H. Splenectomy patients are susceptible to pulmonary complications, especially left lower-lobe pneumonia (p 104). Turning, coughing, and deep breathing help minimize the chance of pulmonary complications.

I. Other postoperative assessment includes nursing management similar to that for other abdominal surgical procedures. Observe the dressings for drainage. Drains are not usually inserted. The nasogastric tube is connected to low intermittent suction.

J. On discharge, instruct the patient to avoid situations in which exposure to infection is possible. Advise the patient to contact the physician if a febrile illness is contracted.

References

Kneisl CR, Ames SW. Adult health nursing: a biopsychosocial approach. Reading, MA: Addison-Wesley, 1986.

Le Maitre GD, Finnegan JA. The patient in surgery: a guide for nurses. Philadelphia: WB Saunders, 1980.

Phipps WJ, Long BC, Woods NF. Medical-surgical nursing: concepts and clinical practice. 3rd ed. St. Louis: CV Mosby, 1987.

Ulrich SP, Canale SW, Wendell SA. Preventing postsplenectomy complications. Nursing 87 1987; 17(3):98, 100.

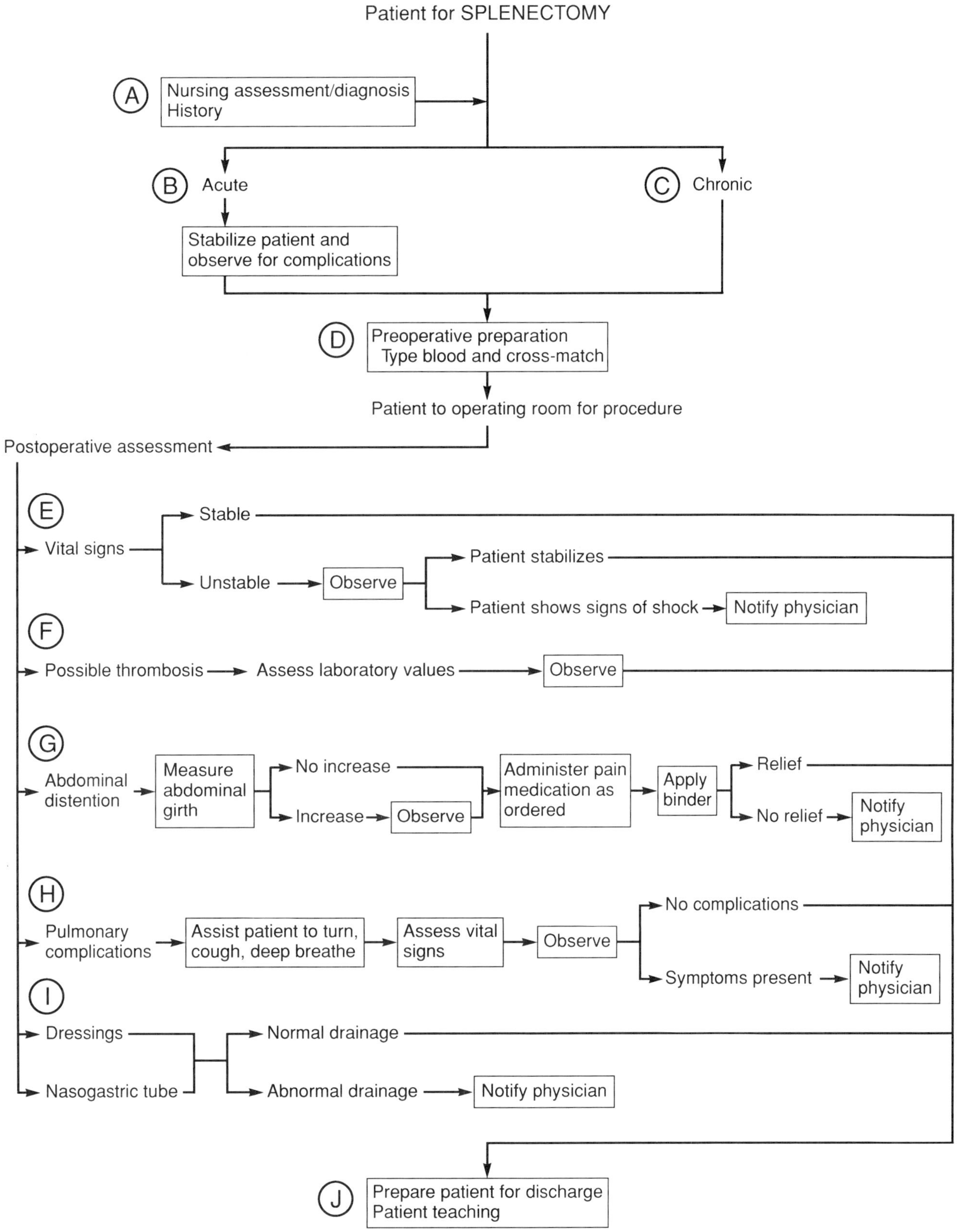
Patient for SPLENECTOMY
A
Nursing assessment/diagnosis
History
B
Acute
C
Chronic
Stabilize patient and
observe for complications
D
Preoperative preparation
Type blood and cross-match
Patient to operating room for procedure
Postoperative assessment
E
Vital signs
Stable
Unstable
Observe
Patient stabilizes
Patient shows signs of shock
Notify physician
F
Possible thrombosis
Assess laboratory values
Observe
G
Abdominal distention
Measure abdominal girth
No increase
Increase
Observe
Administer pain medication as ordered
Apply binder
Relief
No relief
Notify physician
H
Pulmonary complications
Assist patient to turn, cough, deep breathe
Assess vital signs
Observe
No complications
Symptoms present
Notify physician
I
Dressings
Nasogastric tube
Normal drainage
Abnormal drainage
Notify physician
J
Prepare patient for discharge
Patient teaching

THE EYE

GLAUCOMA

Joy Gorzeman

A. Glaucoma is a condition in which the intraocular pressure is increased. This pressure is related to the input and outflow of aqueous humor. Over time the increased pressure results in optic nerve degeneration and causes visual impairment. If untreated, glaucoma frequently results in blindness. Glaucoma is an insidious disease that impairs vision without the person's being aware of it. The only way to identify glaucoma before permanent damage occurs to the eye is by routine examinations that include tonometer measurements and visual field testing. These procedures should be a part of an annual eye examination in persons who are 40 years of age or older and in those with a family history of glaucoma, since the condition is hereditary.

B. There are three classifications of glaucoma: narrow angle (closed-angle), wide angle (open-angle), and congenital. Contributing factors may be genetic or secondary to disease, injury, or neoplasia. The most common form is open-angle glaucoma, which is hereditary.

C. Open-angle glaucoma may cause fatigue or a slight ache in the eyes, but is usually painless and progresses insidiously. This type of glaucoma is usually bilateral. Over the years, the patient may notice foggy vision and diminished accommodation. Peripheral vision is also gradually lost. Decreased visual acuity that cannot be corrected by glasses and other late symptoms occur only after severe, irreversible damage has been done.

D. The treatment of choice for open-angle glaucoma is medical. Useful vision can usually be preserved in patients if glaucoma is diagnosed early and controlled with medication. Miotics are given to contract the ciliary muscle, which lowers intraocular pressure, thus facilitating aqueous outflow. Other medications (eyedrops) may be given to decrease the rate of aqueous humor production.

E. Laser therapy or surgery is done as a last resort, if medical treatment is not successful. The appropriate laser or surgical procedure (iridotomy) is done to create an opening or filter system to allow aqueous humor to flow through and reduce the pressure (p 378).

F. Closed-angle glaucoma is most often a unilateral, acute condition and is considered a *medical emergency*. The intraocular pressure rises rapidly, causing the patient to experience severe pain in and around the eye. The patient also sees colored halos around lights, and vision is diminished. Nausea and vomiting may occur. The eye may be red and the pupil mildly dilated and nonreactive. Without treatment, blindness will result within 3 to 5 days.

G. Although surgery is the only option, the first step of treatment in closed-angle glaucoma is to decrease the intraocular pressure by administering miotics and carbonic anhydrase inhibitors (restrict the action of the enzyme necessary to produce aqueous humor). Pain medication should also be given.

H. After the pressure is decreased (ideally within 6 hours), surgery is performed to facilitate filtering of aqueous humor and relief of intraocular tension. Surgery on the other eye is often performed later as a preventive measure.

I. Patients with glaucoma must be advised of the importance of following their doctor's orders. Each case is different, so advice about medications, fluid intake, and activity varies from patient to patient. It is of utmost importance that the patient be informed about medications, the need to use them faithfully, the side effects of medication, and when to notify the physician. The patient with glaucoma should wear a medical ID tag, so that medication would be continued in an unforeseen situation. The patient with glaucoma should avoid stress and exertion and must remain under a doctor's care for regular eye examinations.

References

Brunner LS, Suddarth DS. The Lippincott manual of nursing practice. 4th ed. Philadelphia: JB Lippincott, 1986.

Luckmann J, Sorensen KC. Medical-surgical nursing: a psychophysiologic approach. Philadelphia: WB Saunders, 1980.

Thompson JM, McFarland GK, Hirsch JE, Tucker SM, Bowers AC. Clinical nursing. St Louis: CV Mosby, 1986.

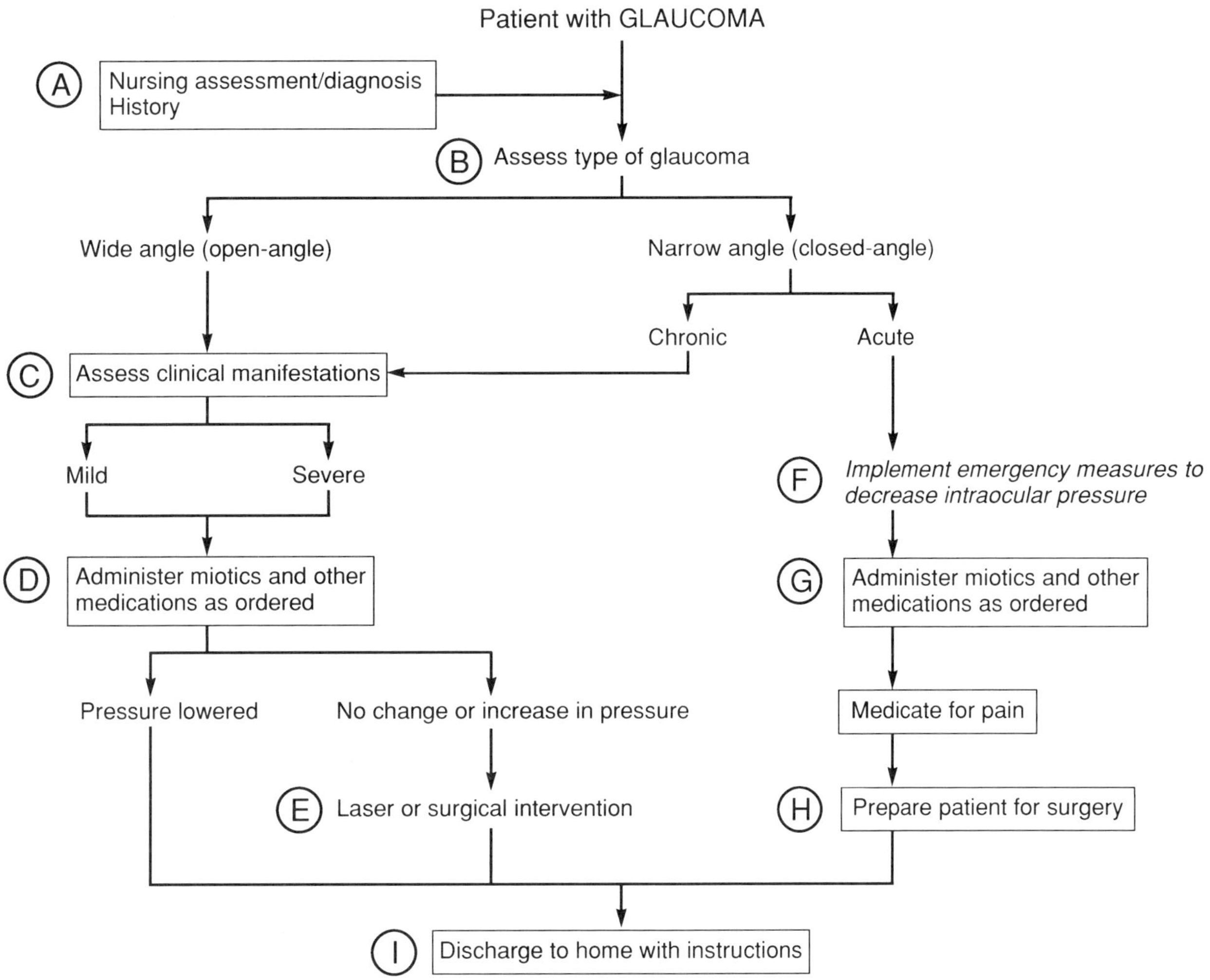
Patient with GLAUCOMA
A
Nursing assessment/diagnosis
History
B
Assess type of glaucoma
Wide angle (open-angle)
Narrow angle (closed-angle)
Chronic
Acute
C
Assess clinical manifestations
Mild
Severe
F
Implement emergency measures to decrease intraocular pressure
D
Administer miotics and other medications as ordered
G
Administer miotics and other medications as ordered
Pressure lowered
No change or increase in pressure
Medicate for pain
E
Laser or surgical intervention
H
Prepare patient for surgery
I
Discharge to home with instructions

CATARACTS

Susan Cauley

A cataract is opacity or clouding of the crystalline lens, which is normally transparent. It is not a "growth over the eye," as it is sometimes described. There are two groups of cataracts, developmental and degenerative. They usually occur in both eyes, but the progression varies in each eye. Cataracts are the leading cause of blindness in the United States. Cataract extraction (p 380) is not usually recommended if the corrected vision with glasses is better than 20/60 in either eye.

A. Nursing assessment should include a complete assessment of all systems, with special attention to visual acuity. A complete history is taken to determine the onset of the symptoms. Patients may present with the complaint of progressively worsened blurred vision.

B. Instruct the patient about the importance of keeping pathways clear to ensure safe ambulation. The patient will receive eye drops or other medications that require careful instructions to ensure that they are administered correctly. The patient also needs to be instructed to wear prescription glasses.

C. Follow-up appointments are important. Instruct patients to keep regular appointments and call their physicians if vision becomes worse.

References

Brunner LS, Suddarth DS. The Lippincott manual of nursing practice. 4th ed. Philadelphia: JB Lippincott, 1986.

Lewis SM, Collier IC. Medical-surgical nursing: assessment and management of clinical problems. 2nd ed. New York: McGraw-Hill, 1987.

Luckmann J, Sorensen KC. Medical-surgical nursing: a psychophysiologic approach. 3rd ed. WB Saunders, 1987.

Smith JF, Delbert PN. Ophthalmologic nursing. Boston: Little, Brown, 1980.

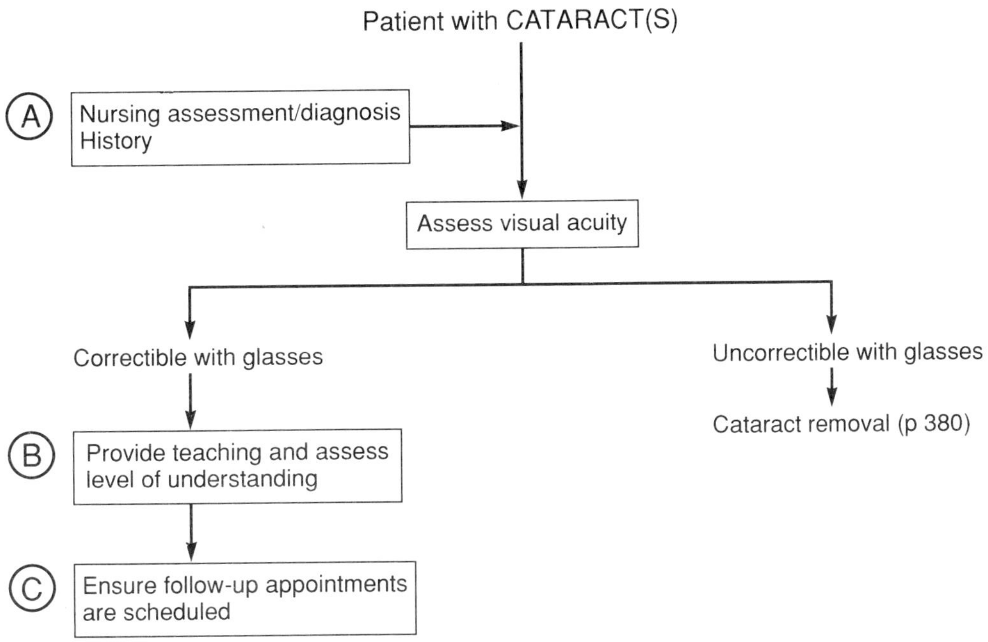
Patient with CATARACT(S)
A
Nursing assessment/diagnosis
History
Assess visual acuity
Correctible with glasses
Uncorrectible with glasses
Cataract removal (p 380)
B
Provide teaching and assess level of understanding
C
Ensure follow-up appointments are scheduled

LASER THERAPY

ManJa Lee

The term "laser" is the acronym *l*ight *a*mplification by the *s*timulated *e*mission of *r*adiation. Laser irradiation is an electromagnetic wave with properties similar to those of normal "white" light, but is different from "white" light in the manner in which it is generated and converted into optical energy. This intense beam of light can be precisely focused to deliver high energy levels to a small area. The lasers used most often in medical fields are carbon dioxide (CO_2), argon (AR), and neodymium: yttrium-aluminum-garnet (Nd:YAG) lasers. By selecting the appropriate wavelength and intensity of laser light, a surgeon can perform a variety of operations (see Table 1).

Lasers provide noncontact surgery and a dry field. The laser also acts as a hemostatic agent and reduces mechanical trauma. The patient has less postoperative edema, pain, scarring, and trauma, which results in a faster recovery and lower costs. However, laser surgery has risks and complications such as massive bleeding, perforation, gas embolism, overdistention, fever, sepsis, and pain. Danger of combustion and fire and dissemination of viable cells are other risks to consider. Laser exposure to other than the intended operative sites must be reported through the appropriate channels. Laser surgery may be done on an inpatient or outpatient basis.

TABLE 1 Surgical Uses of Laser

Open blocked coronary arteries
Repair cardiac valves*
Prevent dental caries and minor buccal surgery*
Remove skin tumors, lesions, necrotic tissue
Treat laryngeal polyps and tracheal strictures or stenosis
Remove gastrointestinal ulcers, tumors, and polyps
Treat endometriosis, cervical neoplasia
Remove solid brain tumors
Reattach retinas
Remove cataracts
Perform joint arthroscopy*
Remove bunions
Perform thoracotomy
Perform photoradiation of lung tumors*
Treat urinary tract stones and tumors

* Experimental

A. Careful psychological and physical assessment of a patient contributes to the successful outcome of care. The physical assessment is important to positioning, laser application, and preparation of appropriate laser ancillary equipment for perioperative nursing care.

B. For many patients the word "laser" may have frightening connotations. To allay fears, the physician provides basic information about lasers and reasons why the laser is the treatment of choice. The nurse provides reassurance and allows the patient to verbalize stress and anxiety.

C. The planning phase of the nursing process involves providing for the patient's comfort and safety and preparing needed equipment. The safety guideline must be reviewed by the surgical team at this time.

D. The nurse should be prepared with positioning aids and other comfort and safety measures for the patient. Providing the proper protective eyewear is imperative, not only for the patient but also for the surgical team.

E. The preparation of needed equipment includes gathering the laser itself, the delivery systems (i.e., handpiece, fibers, microscope), other ancillary equipment, and routine supplies for the procedures. Usually, laser procedures require blackened instruments to prevent accidental reflection of the laser beam to other organs.

F. The laser must be tested to prevent malfunction or unnecessary delays during the procedure.

G. The implementation phase of patient care includes admission of the patient to the operating room, preparation of surgical instruments and laser equipment, positioning the patient, skin preparation, and draping preparation. Safety precautions vary according to the laser in use, the operating room environment, and the patient and health care professionals involved in the case. The most important safety factors for the patient are preventing eye injury by covering the eyes with moist gauzes or appropriate glasses and protecting the surrounding tissues from potential damage. When the laser is used near the patient's airway, a noncombustible (i.e., protected red rubber or specific metal) endotracheal tube is used and wet towels are placed around the surgical field to prevent an accidental fire. In the operating room, "Laser In Use" signs are posted, and a smoke evacuator is required whenever a smoke plume may be generated. The laser should be kept secured with a key and must be operated only by qualified personnel according to policies.

H. The most crucial nursing activities during laser surgery involve patient safety, laser operation, accurate documentation, and proper maintenance of equipment for future use.

I. Effective discharge planning such as a follow-up schedule and patient/family education contribute to positive surgical experiences. A simple written postoperative instruction sheet can assist the patient during recovery.

References

Dixon JA, ed. Surgical application of lasers. Chicago: Year Book Medical Publishers, 1983.

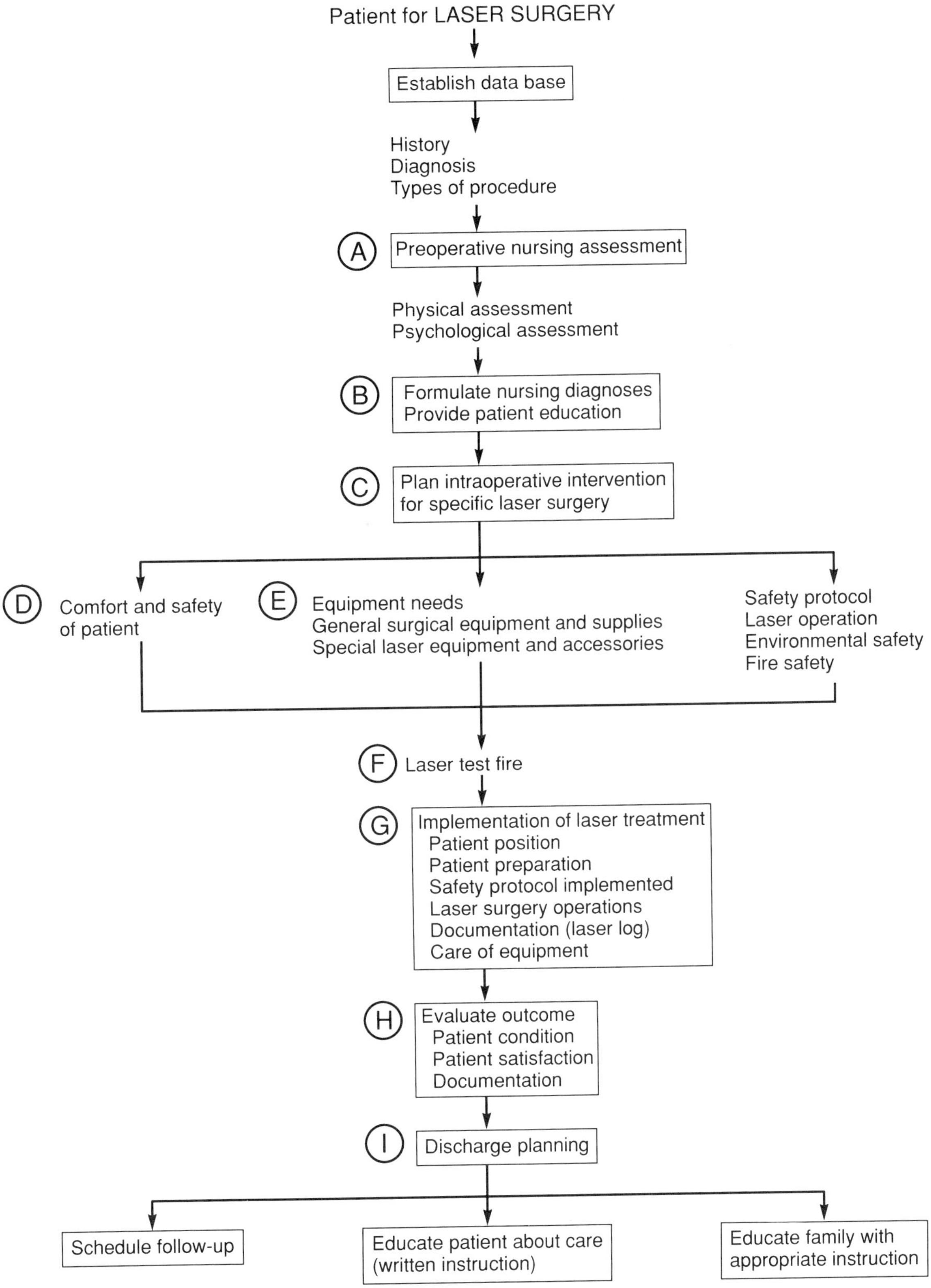

Gruendemann BJ, Meeker MH. Alexander's care of the patient in surgery. 8th ed. St. Louis: CV Mosby, 1987:170.

Huether SE. How lasers work. AORN 1987; 28:207.

Pfister J, Kneedler J. A guide to lasers in the OR. Aurora, CO: Education Design, 1983.

Zacherl A. Perioperative CO_2 laser nursing responsibilities. Laser Nurs 1987; 2(1):5–12.

CATARACT REMOVAL

Susan Cauley

Cataract removal is indicated when the patient's vision interferes with normal activities. There are two major methods of extracting the lens. *Intracapsular extraction* is done if the whole lens, including the capsule, is removed. *Extracapsular extraction* is done if the lens material is removed, leaving the lens capsule. Extracapsular extraction is the procedure of choice. This procedure is followed by intraocular lens insertion. Most extractions are done in day surgery under local anesthesia, with patients not staying overnight unless complications occur.

A. The nursing assessment includes a full systems assessment. Since most clients for cataract extraction are elderly, a thorough history that addresses chronic diseases or other health problems must be taken (p 412). It is also important to assess the home situation and the availability of significant others to assist the patient after discharge. Visual acuity is assessed, especially in the unoperated eye.

B. Preoperative nursing care includes promoting comfort, physical preparation, and patient teaching. Encourage the patient to voice fears about eye surgery. Mydriatic eye drops are given to dilate the pupil. Some patients may require hyperosmolar drugs to reduce intraocular pressure. The patient should be instructed to request assistance with ambulation after surgery. It is also important to provide instruction about taking deep breaths, moving extremities, and not squeezing eyelids tightly closed. Eyelids should be closed slowly.

C. Postoperative nursing care includes full systems assessment (p 4). Comfort, safety, and the avoidance of internal and external pressure to the eye are addressed. The patient will have an eye patch in place and usually a shield. Both should be left intact, and the eye patch is assessed for drainage.

D. The patient is encouraged to lie on the unoperated side. The head of the bed is elevated 45 degrees. Antiemetic drugs may be necessary if the patient complains of nausea. Nausea may lead to vomiting and result in increased intraocular pressure.

E. The patient may experience pressure rather than pain in the operated eye. Analgesics are administered as ordered. Sudden pain in the eye may indicate complications.

F. If there are no complications, the patient is discharged with specific instructions. The main points to be addressed include patient safety and the importance of wearing the eye shield or glasses at all times to protect the eye. Heavy lifting and scratching the eye should also be avoided. Some patients may experience a scratchy feeling or mild pain in the eye. They should take analgesics as prescribed. Careful instruction about instillation of eye drops is given and follow-up appointments are arranged.

References

Brunner LS, Suddarth DS. The Lippincott manual of nursing practice. 4th ed. Philadelphia: JB Lippincott, 1986.

Lewis SM, Collier IC. Medical-surgical nursing: assessment and management of clinical problems. 2nd ed. New York: McGraw-Hill, 1987.

Luckmann J, Sorensen KC. Medical-surgical nursing: a psychophysiologic approach. Philadelphia: WB Saunders, 1987.

Smith JF, Delbert PN. Ophthalmologic nursing. Boston: Little, Brown, 1980.

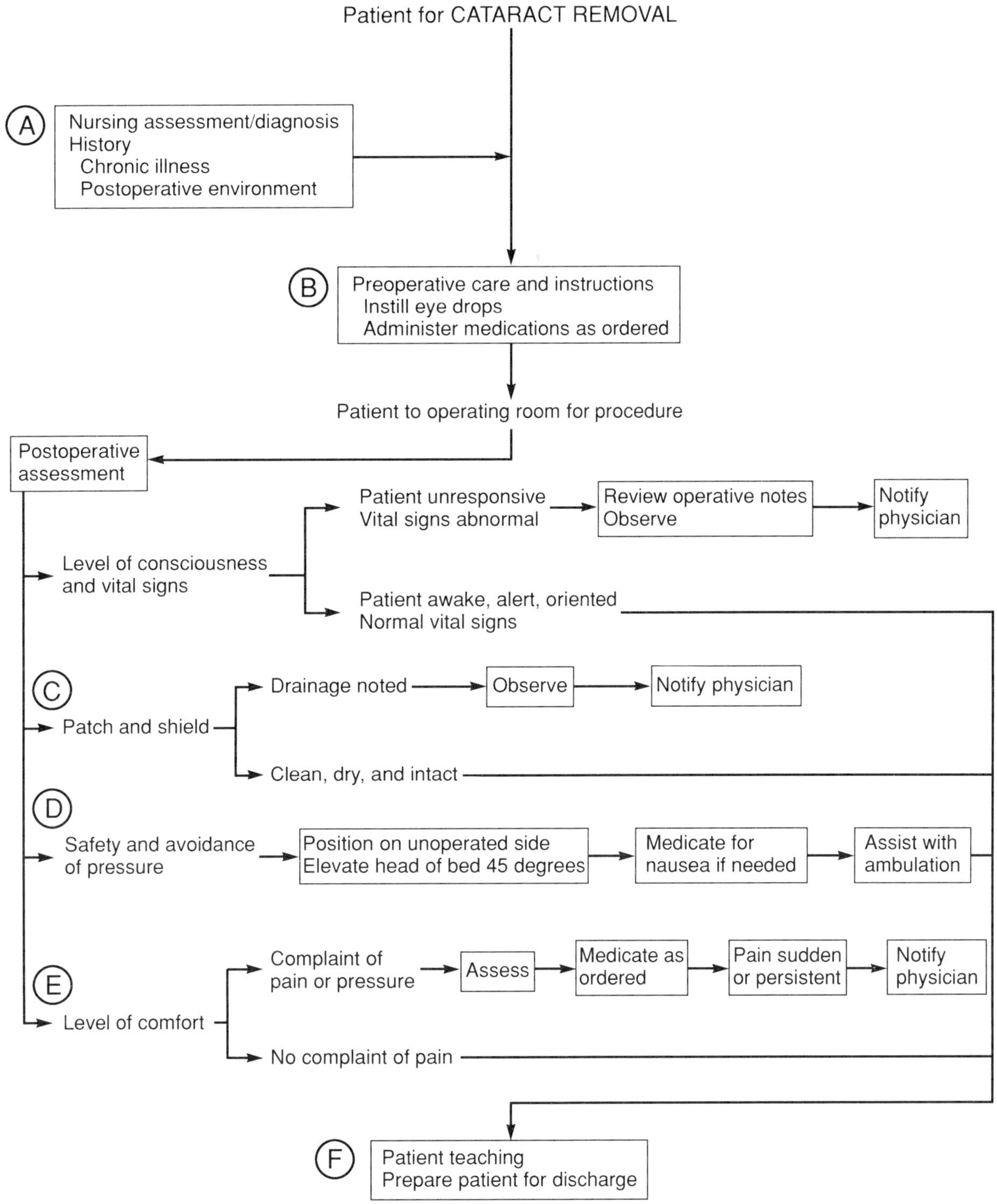

Patient for CATARACT REMOVAL
A
Nursing assessment/diagnosis
History
Chronic illness
Postoperative environment
B
Preoperative care and instructions
Instill eye drops
Administer medications as ordered
Patient to operating room for procedure
Postoperative assessment
Level of consciousness and vital signs
Patient unresponsive
Vital signs abnormal
Review operative notes
Observe
Notify physician
Patient awake, alert, oriented
Normal vital signs
C
Patch and shield
Drainage noted
Observe
Notify physician
Clean, dry, and intact
D
Safety and avoidance of pressure
Position on unoperated side
Elevate head of bed 45 degrees
Medicate for nausea if needed
Assist with ambulation
E
Level of comfort
Complaint of pain or pressure
Assess
Medicate as ordered
Pain sudden or persistent
Notify physician
No complaint of pain
F
Patient teaching
Prepare patient for discharge

RETINAL DETACHMENT AND REPAIR

Susan Cauley

Retinal detachment is the separation of the two layers of the retina. Fluid enters between the two layers and causes permanent loss of vision unless surgery is performed. There are many causes of retinal detachment, the most common being a tear or hole in the retina caused by trauma.

A. The nursing assessment includes a complete physical assessment and queries about emotional support. Patients may present with a chief complaint of the appearance of flashing lights lasting a few seconds, followed by the sudden appearance of moving spots. The patient may also complain of visual loss or blurred vision in the affected eye. Retinal detachment may occur suddenly or slowly. Surgical correction is necessary; retinal detachments do not heal themselves.

B. Preoperative care includes physical preparation (p 2) as well as an explanation of the surgical procedure and the postoperative course. Inform the patient and significant other that both eyes may be patched postoperatively. The patient should be cautioned to avoid straining and rubbing or touching the eyes and to lie flat on the back. Sedatives may be offered to promote comfort and relaxation. Emotional needs and fears about blindness must be addressed.

C. Postoperative assessment should include vital signs and routine assessment (p 4). An eye patch is usually in place for 12 to 24 hours. Eye drops are administered as ordered.

D. Positioning is important for patients after eye surgery. Unless other instructions are given, the patient may lie on the unoperated side or supine. The patient is usually allowed to ambulate with assistance after recovering from anesthesia.

E. Administer pain medication as needed. If nausea occurs, administer antiemetics as ordered. Vomiting should be avoided, because it increases intraocular pressure. The patient should be encouraged to deep breathe, but coughing is contraindicated.

F. If there are no complications, the patient is discharged after 2 to 5 days. The patient is instructed that reading may be difficult because of the use of dilating drops and that rapid eye movement should be avoided. The eyes should be rested, and long periods of reading or watching television should be avoided. Analgesics are ordered for discomfort. It is important to give careful instruction about the instillation of eye drops. Eye patches may be worn after discharge if ordered by the physician. The patient should be cautioned against straining or jarring the head. Driving is usually restricted for 3 to 6 weeks. Signs of repeat retinal detachment are reviewed with the patient. The importance of follow-up appointments is explained.

References

Brunner LS, Suddarth DS. The Lippincott manual of nursing practice. 3rd ed. Philadelphia: JB Lippincott, 1982.

Lewis SM, Collier IC. Medical-surgical nursing: assessment and management of clinical problems. 2nd ed. New York: McGraw-Hill, 1987.

Luckmann J, Sorensen KC. Medical-surgical nursing: a psychophysiologic approach. 3rd ed. Philadelphia: WB Saunders, 1987.

Smith JF, Delbert PN. Ophthalmologic nursing. Boston: Little, Brown, 1980.

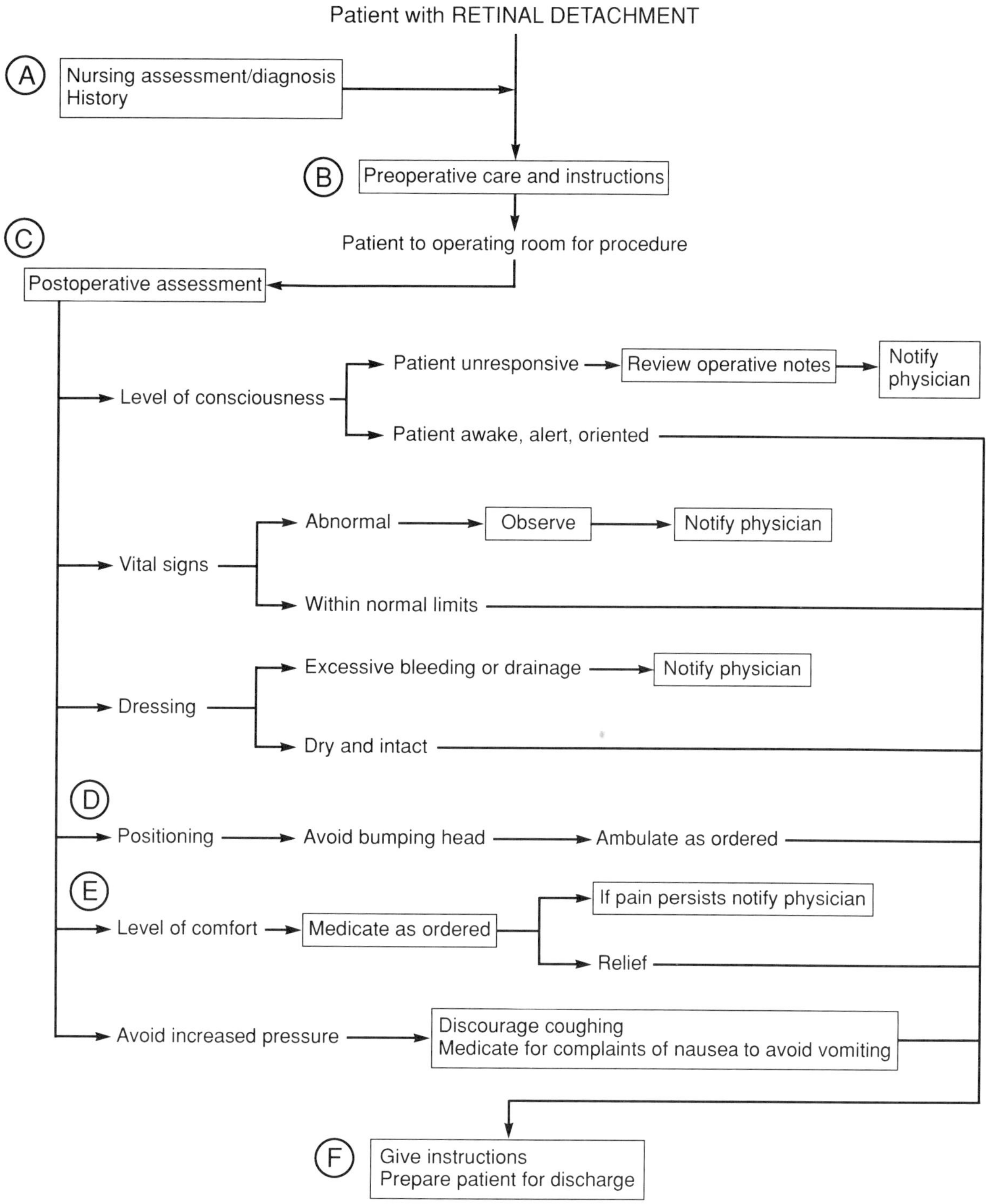
Patient with RETINAL DETACHMENT
A
Nursing assessment/diagnosis
History
B
Preoperative care and instructions
Patient to operating room for procedure
C
Postoperative assessment
Level of consciousness
Patient unresponsive
Review operative notes
Notify physician
Patient awake, alert, oriented
Vital signs
Abnormal
Observe
Notify physician
Within normal limits
Dressing
Excessive bleeding or drainage
Notify physician
Dry and intact
D
Positioning
Avoid bumping head
Ambulate as ordered
E
Level of comfort
Medicate as ordered
If pain persists notify physician
Relief
Avoid increased pressure
Discourage coughing
Medicate for complaints of nausea to avoid vomiting
F
Give instructions
Prepare patient for discharge

CORNEAL TRANSPLANT

Leslie C. Hussey

Corneal transplant (keratoplasty) is a surgical procedure in which the central portion of the cornea is removed and replaced with one obtained from a cadaver. Corneas are removed from cadavers within 6 hours of death and frozen in eye banks to retain transparency. Transplantation should be done within 48 hours of removal of the cornea from the cadaver. Patients of all ages undergo corneal transplantation because of decreased vision due to injury, burn, infection, congenital deformities, or corneal degeneration. Defective corneas are the leading cause of blindness worldwide.

A. The host patient must be in good general health and be able to take care of the new cornea very carefully for the first 12 to 24 months to increase the chances of success. Other conditions such as glaucoma (p 374) may interfere with or prevent a corneal transplant.

B. There are two types of corneal transplant: full-thickness (FT; penetrating) and partial-thickness (LT; lamellar). The lamellar type may be done on an outpatient basis. Preoperative nursing care varies with the type of anesthesia used. General or local anesthesia may be chosen by the surgeon, however, local anesthesia is more common. Explain the intense follow-up care and need to keep intraocular and external pressure on the operated eye at a safe level. Wash the patient's face with an antibacterial soap. Instill prophylactic antibiotic eyedrops (such as gentamicin) every hour for 3 hours the night before surgery and again just before surgery in the morning. Instill a miotic, such as pilocarpine hydrochloride, to constrict the pupil and lengthen and flatten the iris to prevent damage during surgery. An intravenous hyperosmotic agent, such as mannitol, may be used to decrease intraocular pressure (IOP) and soften the eye. Morphine sulfate or diazepam (Valium) may be given to decrease the patient's anxiety.

C. If local anesthesia is used, the patient is awake, but drowsy, during surgery. Immediately after transplantation, an antibiotic ointment is instilled into the eye, the eye is patched, and an eye shield is taped over the pads for added protection.

D. Postoperatively, the patient lies on the back or unoperated side. Activity depends on the type of graft. Nursing care for patients requiring longer bedrest (full-thickness grafts) includes measures to prevent pulmonary and circulatory complications.

E. Instruct the patient that activities that increase IOP should be avoided, because increased IOP places stress on the suture line. These activities include heavy lifting; straining, especially during a bowel movement; excessive fluid intake; vomiting; bending over; lifting; strenuous activity; and emotional stress. The patient should avoid sudden turning of the head, minimize activities or irritants that may cause sneezing (dusting, scented flowers, pepper), and avoid sleeping on the affected side during the convalescent period.

F. The eye patch stays on for 24 hours and is changed daily, using strict aseptic technique. The pad is secured tightly to prevent movement and consequent scratching of the eye. Some physicians recommend patching both eyes to avoid "twin movement." The patient must not touch the dressing. Pain medication may be needed during the early postoperative period. Unrelieved pain should be reported, since it may indicate a dressing that is too tight, a slipped graft, hemorrhage, infection, or postoperative glaucoma.

G. Topical antibiotics (prevent infection), steroids (decrease risk of rejection), and cycloplegics (paralyze the ciliary muscle) are usually instilled after corneal transplants, according to physician preference. The patient must be taught the proper technique for instilling eyedrops, which can determine successful grafting. The lower lid is pulled down to form a pocket; the patient looks up and inserts one drop into the pocket. The nozzle of the bottle should not touch the eye (the nose may be used to balance the patient's hand). After the drop is in, the eye is closed gently for 5 minutes to enhance absorption.

H. Patient instructions about care and follow-up medical treatment are extremely important. Pain or discomfort in the eye lasting more than 4 to 6 hours should be reported to the physician. In addition, redness, sensitivity to glare, and decreased vision must be reported, since they may indicate rejection of the cornea. Reinforce previous teaching about activity limitations.

References

Brunner LS, Suddarth DS. The Lippincott manual of nursing practice. 3rd ed. Philadelphia: JB Lippincott, 1982:676–677.

Kneisl C, Ames S. Adult health nursing: a biopsychosocial approach. Reading, MA: Addison-Wesley, 1986.

Tooke MC, Elders J, Johnson DE. Corneal transplantation. Am J Nurs 1986; 86(6):685–687.

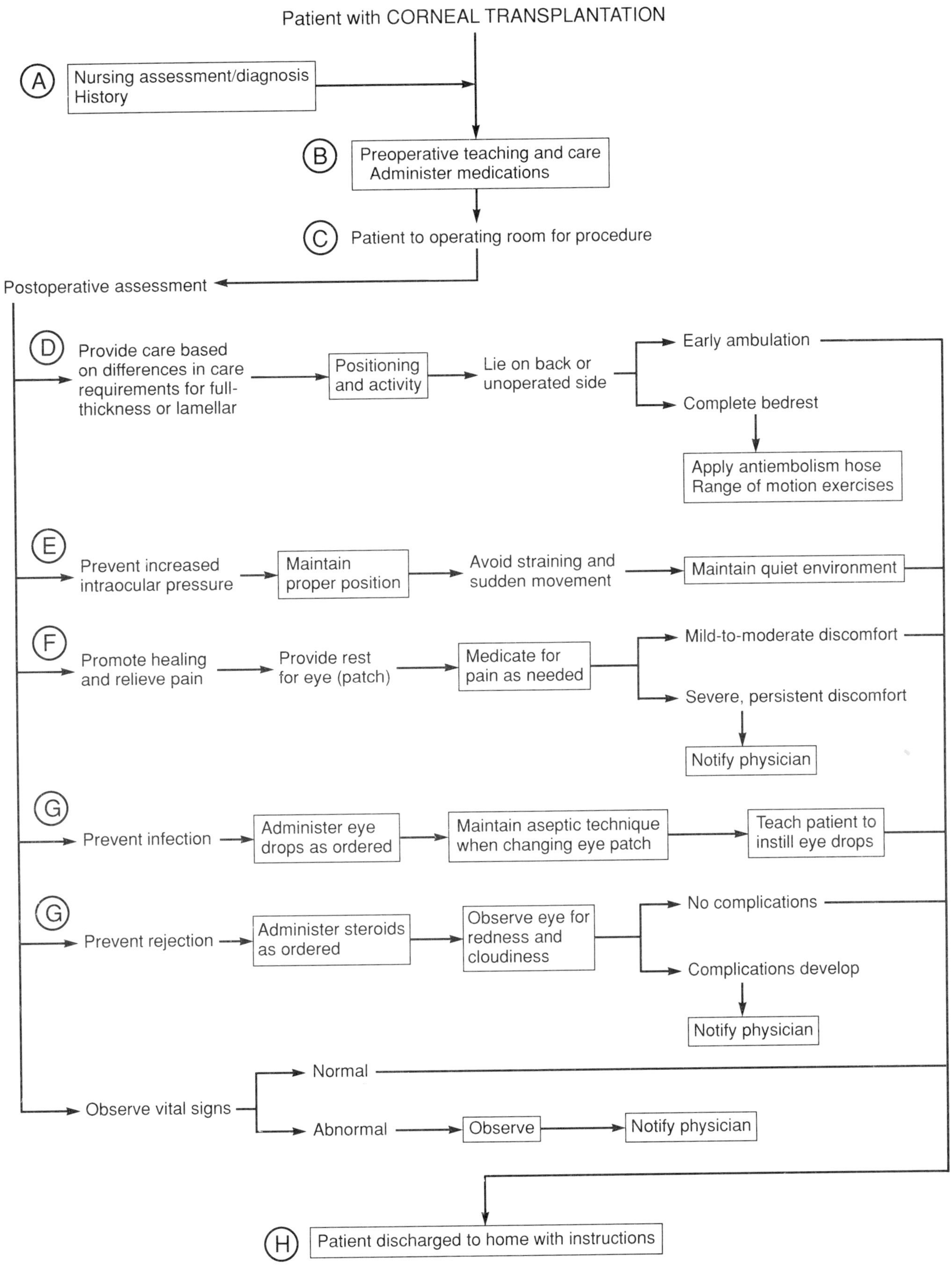
Patient with CORNEAL TRANSPLANTATION
A
Nursing assessment/diagnosis
History
B
Preoperative teaching and care
Administer medications
C
Patient to operating room for procedure
Postoperative assessment
D
Provide care based on differences in care requirements for full-thickness or lamellar
Positioning and activity
Lie on back or unoperated side
Early ambulation
Complete bedrest
Apply antiembolism hose
Range of motion exercises
E
Prevent increased intraocular pressure
Maintain proper position
Avoid straining and sudden movement
Maintain quiet environment
F
Promote healing and relieve pain
Provide rest for eye (patch)
Medicate for pain as needed
Mild-to-moderate discomfort
Severe, persistent discomfort
Notify physician
G
Prevent infection
Administer eye drops as ordered
Maintain aseptic technique when changing eye patch
Teach patient to instill eye drops
G
Prevent rejection
Administer steroids as ordered
Observe eye for redness and cloudiness
No complications
Complications develop
Notify physician
Observe vital signs
Normal
Abnormal
Observe
Notify physician
H
Patient discharged to home with instructions

ENUCLEATION

Susan Cauley

Enucleation is the surgical removal of the eyeball. Indications for enucleation include injury, infection, painful blind eye, malignancy of the eye, and absolute glaucoma (p 374). Enucleation may be done with general or local anesthesia. The surgery includes severing the extraocular muscles close to the globe. The muscles may be sutured over a round plastic or Teflon globe.

A. Nursing assessment includes full systems assessment. A complete history is taken to determine the reason for the enucleation.

B. Preoperative instruction includes a basic explanation of the procedure, physical preparation, and emotional support. Some patients may have antibiotics ordered if the enucleation is necessary because of infection or injury.

C. Postoperative assessment includes routine assessment and vital signs (p 4). The nursing care is directed at preventing complications or further injury and promoting wound healing.

D. The patient has a pressure dressing for 24 to 48 hours and may also have a conformer placed in the socket until a prosthesis can be fitted. Report excessive bleeding to the physician immediately.

E. Pain medication should be administered as needed. Increased pain may be a sign of complications and should be assessed by a physician immediately.

F. Encourage the patient to verbalize concerns about altered body image or change in appearance. It is important to provide honest answers to questions. Explain that a prosthesis may be fitted in about 1 month.

G. The patient is usually allowed out of bed with no restrictions on the first postoperative day.

H. If there are no complications, the patient is discharged with specific instructions. An eye patch may be worn until a prosthesis is fitted. The patient who experiences fever or increased pain is instructed to notify the physician. The importance of returning for follow-up care is stressed.

References

Brunner LS, Suddarth DS. The Lippincott manual of nursing practice. 4th ed. Philadelphia: JB Lippincott, 1986.

Lewis SM, Collier IC. Medical-surgical nursing: assessment and management of clinical problems. 2nd ed. New York: McGraw-Hill, 1987.

Luckmann J, Sorensen KC. Medical-surgical nursing: a psychophysiologic approach. 3rd ed. Philadelphia: WB Saunders, 1987.

Smith JF, Delbert PN. Ophthalmologic nursing. Boston: Little, Brown, 1980.

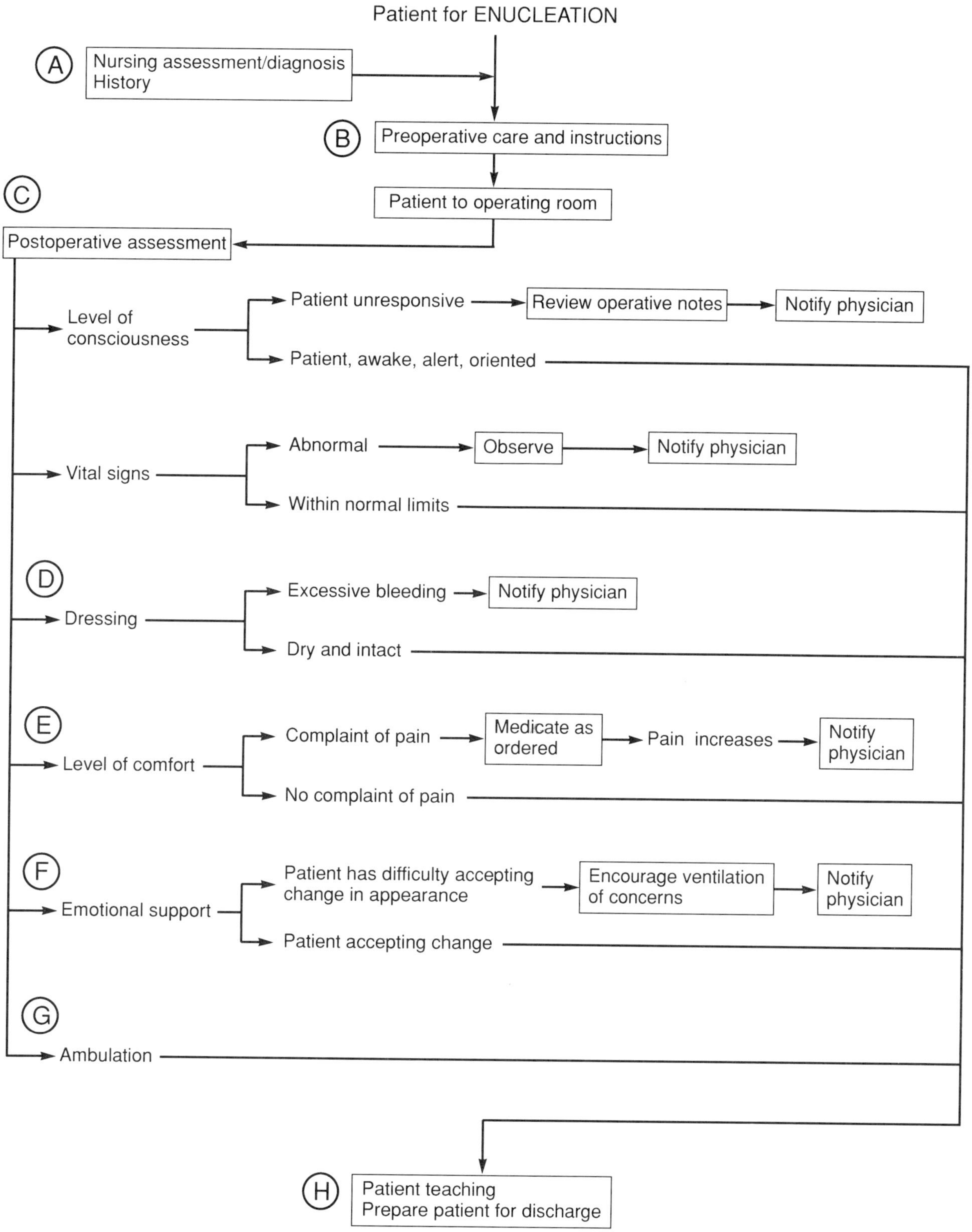
Patient for ENUCLEATION
A
Nursing assessment/diagnosis
History
B
Preoperative care and instructions
Patient to operating room
C
Postoperative assessment
Level of consciousness
Patient unresponsive
Review operative notes
Notify physician
Patient, awake, alert, oriented
Vital signs
Abnormal
Observe
Notify physician
Within normal limits
D
Dressing
Excessive bleeding
Notify physician
Dry and intact
E
Level of comfort
Complaint of pain
Medicate as ordered
Pain increases
Notify physician
No complaint of pain
F
Emotional support
Patient has difficulty accepting change in appearance
Encourage ventilation of concerns
Notify physician
Patient accepting change
G
Ambulation
H
Patient teaching
Prepare patient for discharge

EAR, NOSE, AND THROAT

EPISTAXIS

Karen O'Brien

A. Patients experiencing epistaxis are often anxious. Thus, reassurance and comfort measures are important. Assess the patient for active bleeding, which may not be obvious because posterior bleeding drains into the back of the throat. Carefully check the patient's vital signs, which may signal early hypovolemia or indicate underlying causes. Rapid, acute bleeding or abnormalities in vital signs, such as hypotension, must be dealt with immediately. Try to determine the cause of epistaxis. Past medical history, recent injury, and onset of bleeding must be explored. Epistaxis may be precipitated by trauma to the nose, allergies leading to drying of the mucous membrane, or hypertension (p 80). Other causes to consider include drug use, especially cocaine; bleeding disorders; neoplasm; or rheumatic fever.

B. Identification of the bleeding site determines specific treatment. Bleeding from the anterior septum is the most common cause of epistaxis. Anterior bleeding sites are usually identified by blood oozing from the nostrils, which is usually easily controlled unless the site is the anterior thyroid artery. Bleeding from this site is usually caused by facial trauma and is difficult to control because it is rapid and the source is high and posterior. The elderly often experience posterior epistaxis. Bleeding is profuse but may be difficult to monitor because large amounts run into the back of the throat. Bleeding control is also difficult because the posterior location of the bleeding site prevents visualization.

C. Initial attempts to control bleeding should involve having the patient apply pressure to the soft lobar portions of the nose for at least 10 minutes. Some patients prefer the mechanical pressure of two tongue blades taped together and clipped onto the nose. Patients should be instructed to lean forward to decrease the amount of swallowed blood. A vasoconstricting nasal spray may also be helpful.

D. If direct pressure fails to stop the bleeding, attempt to visualize the bleeding site, using a head mirror, nasal speculum, and suction. Apply electrocautery or a silver nitrate stick to the source when observed.

E. Should attempts to visualize the bleeding site fail, pack the nose, especially for posterior epistaxis. Pass a catheter through the nose into the oropharynx, attach a lubricated nasal pack to the end of the catheter, and guide it back through the oropharynx, around the soft palate, and into the nasal pharynx. This pack is kept in place for 2 to 4 days.

F. If posterior nasal packing depresses the soft palate and causes airway resistance, CO_2 retention, and hypoxia, place the patient in a semi-Fowler's position and give supplemental oxygen. Nursing observations include level of consciousness, respiratory efforts, breath sounds, arterial blood gases, and vital signs. A blood-saturated nasal packing is a perfect medium for bacteria and may cause infection, which may be treated with antibiotics. If the packing obstructs the eustachian tubes, otitis media may develop. Assess the patient for signs of an ear infection. Swallowed blood may cause nausea.

G. Nasal packing is uncomfortable for the patient. Provide reassurance and remind the patient to breathe through the mouth while the packing is in place. Pain medication may be required, but respiratory depressants should be used sparingly. Frequent mouth care and the use of room deodorizers help to minimize the foul odors associated with nasal packing.

H. Surgical repair is not commonly required for the treatment of epistaxis because less drastic measures are generally successful. However, surgical ligation is usually indicated for repair of the interior maxillary artery or ethmoid artery. Arterial bleeding may be treated by using the nasal balloon.

I. In adults, severe epistaxis may cause up to 1 L of blood loss per hour. Observe the patient for continued bleeding through orthostatic vital signs, serial hemoglobin and hematocrit, skin color, temperature, and capillary refill. After an acute bleeding episode, transfusion may be necessary.

J. Once bleeding is controlled, treat underlying diseases. Control hypertension through diet and medication. Vitamin K replacement may be required to treat deficiencies, and anticoagulant therapy may require adjustment. More severe pathology such as neoplasm or blood dyscrasias such as leukemia (p 346), hemophilia (p 350), and anemia (p 340) may be identified.

K. Patient education begins with prevention of recurrence, which is individualized according to etiology. General guidelines include avoiding vigorous exercise for 2 to 3 days after discharge and avoiding hot or spicy foods, because they cause vasodilation. Patients should avoid nasal trauma such as picking and forceful blowing and prevent drying of mucous membranes through humidification and lubrication. Remind the patient to remain calm and apply manual pressure should bleeding resume. Discharge instructions include follow-up, especially if a treatable cause of epistaxis has been identified.

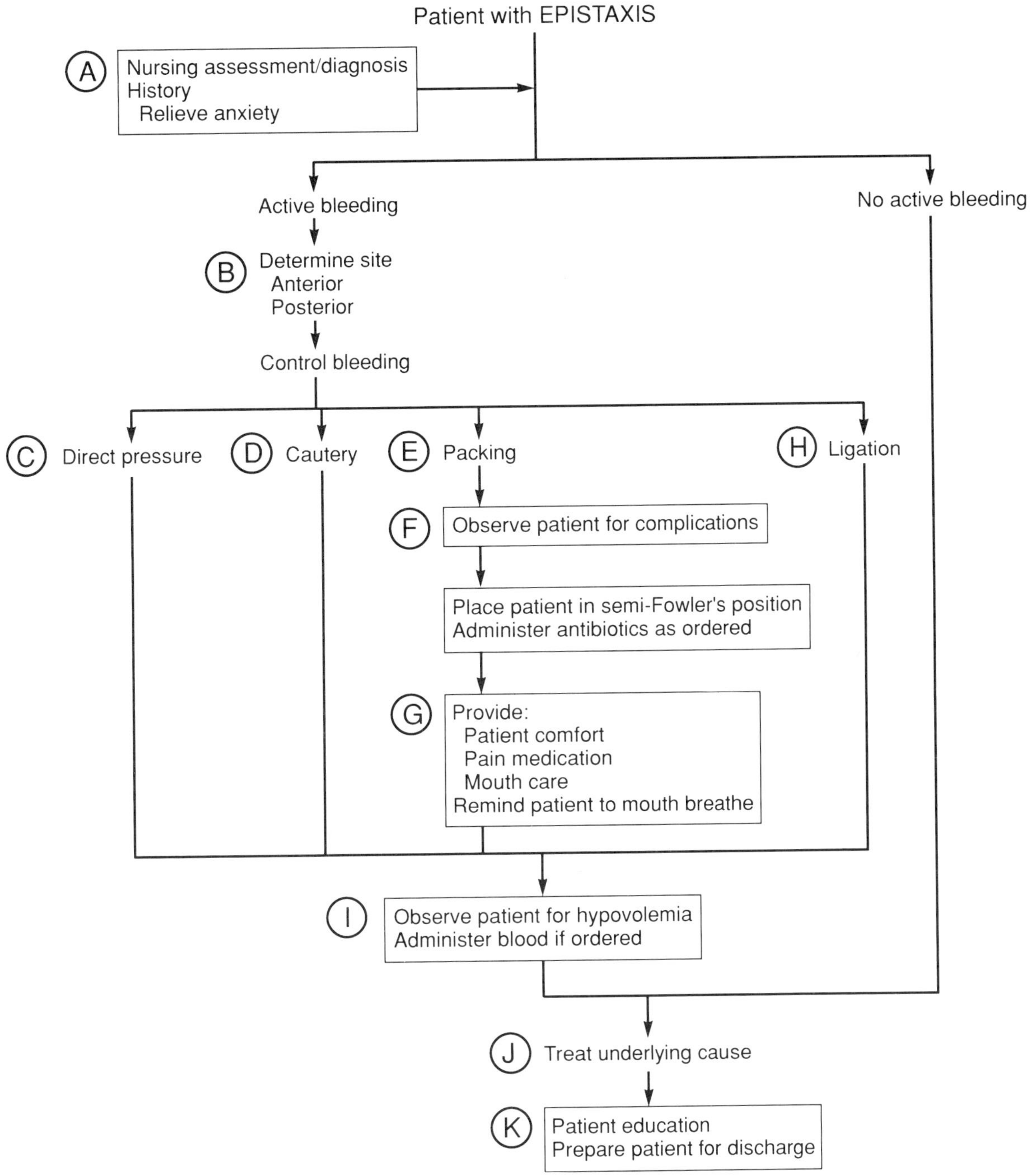

References

Abelson TI, Witt WJ. Otolaryngologic procedures. In: Roberts JR, Hedges JR, eds. Clinical procedures in emergency medicine. Philadelphia: WB Saunders, 1985: 916.

Brunner LS, Suddarth DS. The Lippincott manual of nursing practice. 3rd ed. Philadelphia: JB Lippincott, 1982.

Hamilton H. Diseases. Horsham, PA: Intermed Communications, 1982.

Johnson JT, Rood SR. Epistaxis management. Postgrad Med 1981; 70:231.

LARYNGEAL CANCER

Leslie Rach

Laryngeal cancer accounts for approximately 2 percent of all cases of cancer in the United States. Eighty to 90 percent of laryngeal cancers occur in males over 50 years of age. Early detection and treatment prevents the disfiguring and disabling effects of later treatment. Glottic tumors are confined to the vocal cords and have the best prognosis because they are usually detected early. The prognosis for supraglottic and subglottic tumors is not as good.

A. Clinical manifestations alert the patient to a problem. Hoarseness or voice change and tenderness are usually the first signs of laryngeal cancer. Hoarseness lasting 2 weeks or longer and sore throat that lasts 6 weeks or longer should be investigated. Later manifestations include palpable lump in the throat or neck, foul breath, dysphagia, dyspnea, blood-tinged sputum, or frank bleeding.

B. The nursing assessment and history are needed to establish a baseline for postprocedure comparison and to identify potential nursing problems. Assessment includes airway patency, vital signs, pain, and a full physical assessment. The history targets tobacco and alcohol use and exposure to industrial chemicals. Initially, the most outstanding potential problem is airway patency. Assessment also includes an evaluation of patient knowledge and feelings about the potential diagnosis. Reassurance, honesty, and reinforcement of fact help allay fears and knowledge deficits.

C. Diagnostic procedures include a gentle physical examination of the throat and neck. Palpation of lymph nodes may indicate metastasis. Visualization by laryngoscope (direct or indirect laryngoscopy) locates the tumor and determines the region and depth. Radiologic studies include chest and neck films, laryngography, and computed tomographic (CT) scan. These help determine the extent and metastasis of the tumor. A biopsy may be done to determine whether the tumor is malignant or benign.

D. Patient teaching begins with admission. Evaluate the patient's ability to absorb information before beginning. The nurse must adjust the level of teaching to the patient's educational and cultural background. Encourage the family and/or significant other to participate. Provide an environment conducive to learning, i.e., quiet, relaxed, nonthreatening. Encourage openness and questions. Clarify and reinforce the teaching done by the physician. Establish a way to communicate if the patient cannot speak and surgery is a possibility. Magic slates or flash cards work well. Give direct and brief answers. A laryngectomy support group may be mentioned at this time and a group member may be asked to see the patient to provide hope and encouragement.

E. Benign growths may be removed if painful or if they interfere with normal function of larynx. No change in voice results.

F. If the tumor proves malignant, surgery is generally planned. The entire health care team must be involved in preoperative planning. Surgical options vary from endoscopic removal of an in situ lesion to a total laryngectomy (p 396). The type of surgery depends on the site, stage of tumor, age of the client, and degree of regional neck involvement. Oncology specialists determine the need for radiation preoperatively and/or postoperatively and chemotherapy. Most commonly, radiation follows surgery to combat malignant cells left after the bulk of the tumor has been removed. Metastasis is likely if the tumor is supraglottic or subglottic, because later detection is usual since the voice does not change and these areas are more vascular than the glottic region.

G. Rehabilitation includes physical therapy, speech therapy, and nursing care. The effects of radiation and chemotherapy (p 408) may weaken the patient beyond usual postoperative weakness. Rehabilitation is a long process and demands that the patient receive support and encouragement the entire time. Include the family and/or significant other in the rehabilitation phase. Teaching must begin early because these patients need a great deal of information.

H. Discharge teaching should reinforce previous teaching. Follow-up care must be stressed prior to discharge, and support groups play an important role at this time. Patients leave the familiar and accepting atmosphere of the hospital and go into society where people may be repelled by disfigurement. Family acceptance and support is essential. These patients go on to lead normal and productive lives.

References

Anderson KL. Neoplastic disorders related to respiratory function. In: Patrick ML, Woods SL, Craven RF, Rokosky JS, Bruno PM, eds. Medical-surgical nursing—pathophysiological concepts. Philadelphia: JB Lippincott, 1986:419–426.

Brunner LS, Suddarth DS. The Lippincott manual of nursing practice. 4th ed. Philadelphia: JB Lippincott, 1986.

McCormick KB. Neurological trauma. In: Lewis SM, Collier IC, eds. Medical-surgical nursing: assessment and management of clinical problems. 2nd ed. New York: McGraw-Hill, 1987:958–962.

Saunders WH. Nursing care in eye, ear, nose and throat disorders. 4th ed. St. Louis: CV Mosby, 1979.

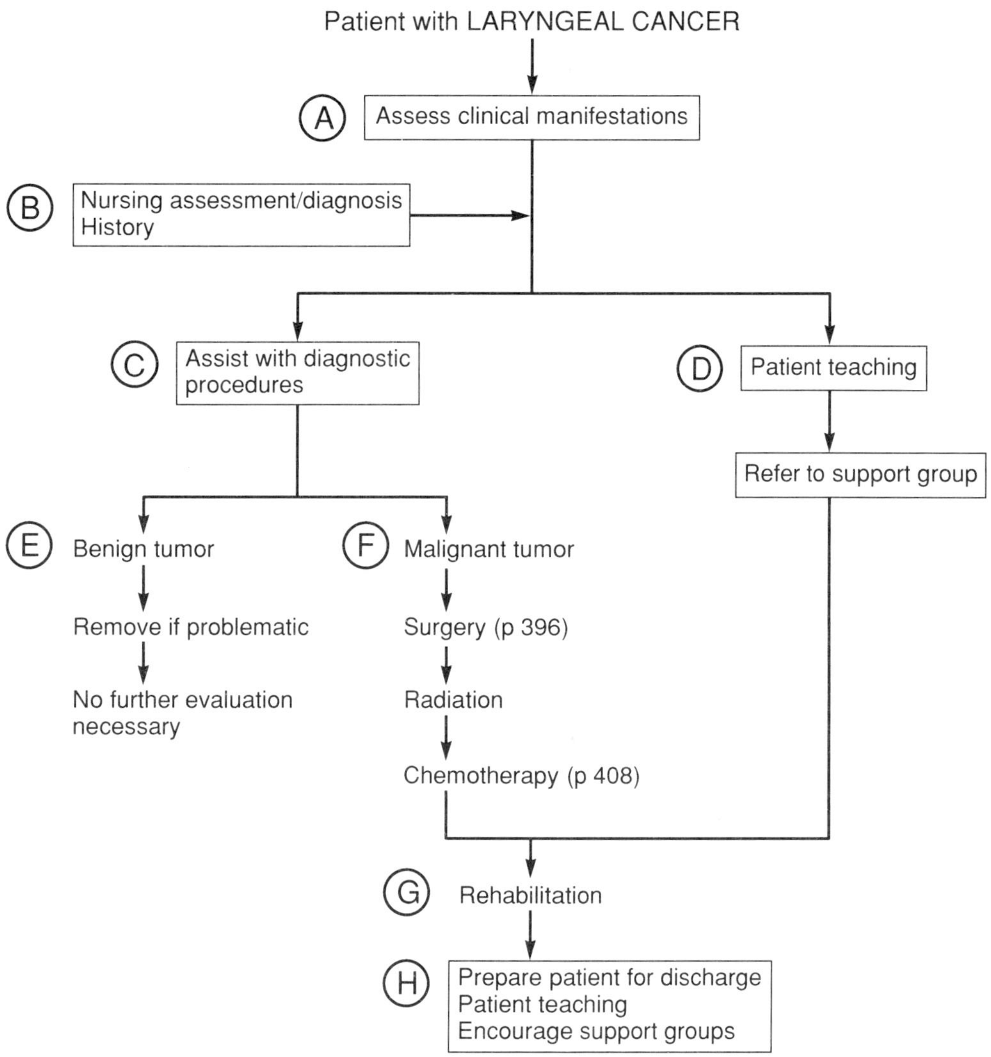
Patient with LARYNGEAL CANCER
A
Assess clinical manifestations
B
Nursing assessment/diagnosis
History
C
Assist with diagnostic procedures
D
Patient teaching
Refer to support group
E
Benign tumor
Remove if problematic
No further evaluation necessary
F
Malignant tumor
Surgery (p 396)
Radiation
Chemotherapy (p 408)
G
Rehabilitation
H
Prepare patient for discharge
Patient teaching
Encourage support groups

HEAD AND NECK CANCER

Leslie Rach

Six percent of all cases of cancer in the United States involve the upper aerodigestive tract, i.e., the head and neck. These modest numbers do not express, however, the gravity of incidence. Often, the tumor interferes with nutrition, communication, and appearance in a way not easily concealed. Therapy is prolonged, expensive, radical, and often leads to psychological and physical sequelae. The larynx is the most common site (p 392). Other sites include the oral cavity, salivary glands, and pharynx.

A. Nursing assessment and history are needed to establish a database for complications and to identify problems. Assessment includes, but should not be limited to, airway patency, swallowing ability, pain, identification of palpable or visual lumps in neck or head, and vital signs. History includes tobacco use, i.e., pipe, cigar, cigarettes, and chewing tobacco. Tobacco use is the greatest cause of head and neck cancers. Alcohol consumption is also causative. Together these two factors place a patient at highest risk. Other factors to be considered include familial traits and diet.

B. Clinical manifestations vary according to the site and include a sore or swelling that does not heal in the oral cavity, pain with swallowing, pain referred to the ear, hoarseness, or bloody drainage from the nose.

C. Diagnostic work-up starts with a slow, gentle physical examination by the physician in a quiet, unhurried atmosphere. The patient must be relaxed and quiet because the nodes are deep within tissue and muscle. The physician palpates the neck and head beginning at the sternal notch and working upward. Examination of the carotid artery may cause decreased pulse and blood pressure. Since older patients may develop slight faintness or sudden syncope and collapse, palpation must not be done on both sides at once. Indirect laryngoscopy often gives more information than direct laryngoscopy. Visualizing the tumor is necessary to determine the method of treatment. Contrast-enhanced computerized tomographic (CT) scan and radiology are used in conjunction with the history and physical. Unfortunately, unless the lesion is large or disrupts normal anatomy, the CT scan and radiographs may be inconclusive.

D. Interventions may include surgery to remove the main body of the tumor, radiation to arrest the cancer cell deposits, and chemotherapy (p 408) to combat metastasis. The treatment regimen is patient specific. The recovery plan must be interdisciplinary and be communicated to all members of the health care team. Treatments may be used independently or in combination, including any or all interventions.

E. Patient emotional status centers on concerns of treatment, altered body image, and the future. Fear of disfigurement caused by treatment is common. Honesty and sensitivity while encouraging verbalization of these fears helps the patient to understand and deal with them and establish attainable goals. Early referral for psychological evaluation and intervention may be helpful.

F. The postprocedure goal is to return the individual to an optimal level of function as quickly as possible. The patient cannot accept responsibility for recovery until he has accepted the diagnosis and treatment, which may include a changed body image that he may find repulsive. Pain may also delay progress. Medication is administered as ordered to keep the patient comfortable. The procedure of choice is usually surgery. Postoperative care includes constant observation and ensuring a patent airway. If the patient had preoperative radiation, bleeding and hemorrhage are strong possibilities.

G. Rehabilitation may include speech therapy, occupational therapy, or physical therapy. Returning the patient to the optimal level of functioning, mentally and physically, is the goal of therapy.

H. Follow-up care must be agreed upon prior to discharge. Discharge teaching begins on admission and includes good oral hygiene. Small, slow feedings are recommended. Tube feedings or parenteral nutrition may be required for patients with extensive surgery. Encourage increased protein intake for proper wound healing. If the patient is receiving chemotherapy, some if not most foods may cause nausea and vomiting. Consult with a dietitian prior to discharge. Support groups can help the patient and family adjust to a changed lifestyle and physical appearance.

References

Devita VT, Hellman S, Rosenberg SA. Cancer: principles and practice of oncology. Vol 1. Philadelphia: JB Lippincott, 1985.

Marvin J. Reconstructive problems. In: Patrick ML, ed. Medical-surgical nursing: pathophysiological concepts. Philadelphia: JB Lippincott, 1986:1450.

Oettgen HF. Cancer-achievements, challenges, and prospects for the 1980's. In: Burchenal JH, ed. International Symposium on Cancer. Vol 2. New York: Grune & Stratton, 1981:551–561.

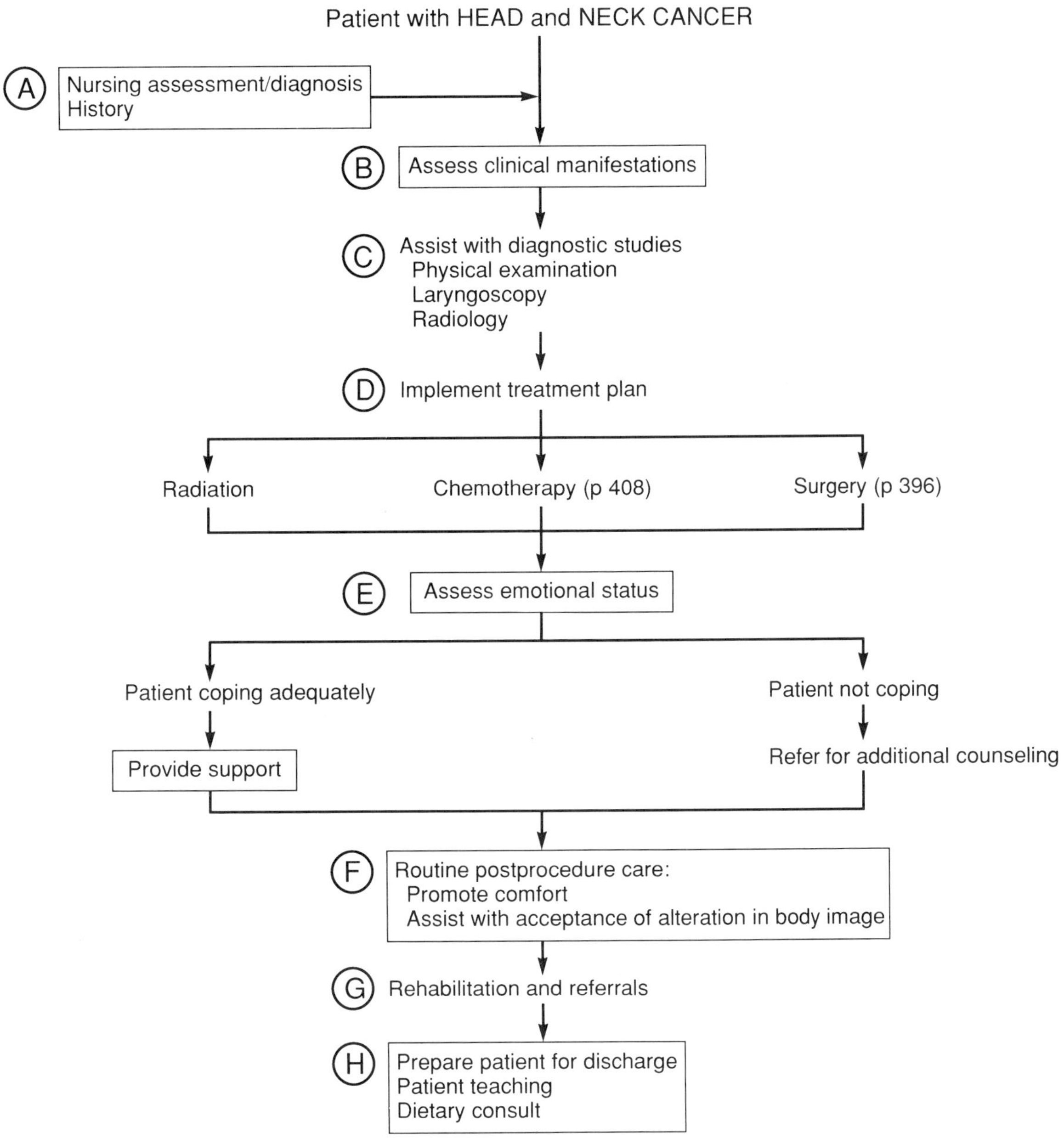
Patient with HEAD and NECK CANCER
A
Nursing assessment/diagnosis
History
B
Assess clinical manifestations
C
Assist with diagnostic studies
Physical examination
Laryngoscopy
Radiology
D
Implement treatment plan
Radiation
Chemotherapy (p 408)
Surgery (p 396)
E
Assess emotional status
Patient coping adequately
Provide support
Patient not coping
Refer for additional counseling
F
Routine postprocedure care:
Promote comfort
Assist with acceptance of alteration in body image
G
Rehabilitation and referrals
H
Prepare patient for discharge
Patient teaching
Dietary consult

LARYNGECTOMY AND RADICAL NECK DISSECTION

Leslie Rach
Joy Gorzeman

Procedures required to remove tumors of the upper respiratory tract range from endoscopic removal to total laryngectomy with permanent tracheostomy. Radical neck dissection is required when the tumor is in the epiglottis or false vocal cords and if metastasis to cervical lymph nodes has occurred. This procedure involves removal of the hyoid bone, epiglottis, and false cords (all structures above the glottis). Depending on the extent of the lesion, the sternocleidomastoid and other associated muscles, the internal jugular vein, the mandible, the submaxillary gland, the spinal accessory nerve, and parts of the thyroid and parathyroid gland may be removed. The patient's voice remains intact. Total laryngectomy involves removal of the hyoid bone, two or three tracheal rings, the cricoid cartilage, the entire larynx, and the strap muscles connected to the larynx. Normal speech is taken away with a total laryngectomy.

A. The preoperative assessment establishes a database for intraoperative and postoperative comparison and helps to identify potential problems. This assessment should include patency of the airway, swallowing ability, vital signs, levels of pain, causative factors (i.e., smoking), and physical and emotional preparation.

B. Preoperative care begins as soon as the decision is made to proceed with surgery. The most important aspect is helping the patient deal with anxiety. Explain hospital routines, procedures, and treatments, and answer patient questions and concerns truthfully. Provide time to discuss expectations, goals, and preoperative teaching (i.e., turning, coughing and deep breathing, NPO status, postoperative high-protein diet). Encourage the support and participation of friends and family. Explain probabilities of preoperative scrubs, medication, and review the preoperative checklist (p 2), using language the patient understands. It may help to have a laryngectomee visit and reassure the patient. However, too much information can increase anxiety. Establish a system of communication (slate or pencil and paper) to be used postoperatively.

C. The postoperative goal is to return the patient to an optimal level of function as quickly as possible. Nursing management includes maintaining a patent airway, assessing swallowing ability, monitoring dressing and wound status, ensuring the patency of drainage devices, and promoting comfort. Assess emotional status and provide supportive care. Referral to a psychiatric liaison nurse may be indicated as patients begin to cope with an altered self-image.

D. Assess patency of the airway frequently, and suction secretions carefully to avoid further injury. Swelling may compress the trachea. Encourage coughing to keep secretions mobile. Perform tracheostomy care as ordered (p 398). Keep the head of the bed elevated 45 degrees. Tracheal aspiration, which can occur up to 1 week after surgery, is a possible complication. Keeping the airway clear prevents this.

E. The wound and dressing must be inspected early and often. Hemorrhage is possible because of increased vascularity in the head and neck. Other complications include infection, air leaks under skin flaps, and necrosis of flaps. The pressure dressing should be tight but not constrictive. A Hemovac may drain 80 to 120 ml the first day; the amount decreases each day. A rare but serious complication is a ruptured carotid artery; *bright red or increased drainage should be reported immediately*. Salivary fistulas are fairly common after laryngeal surgery. Suspect a fistula if redness and swelling are noted around the incision. Pooling of secretions beneath the skin may cause fever 3 to 4 days postoperatively.

F. Assess swallowing ability early. If the epiglottis is removed, new swallowing techniques must be learned. Patients usually have a nasogastric tube for about 10 days. They may complain of a sore throat when eating is resumed. Frequent oral suctioning of tube feedings or hyperalimentation helps to prevent aspiration pneumonia. If secretions are thick, mist therapy may be helpful. Pain medication should be administered as needed.

G. Frequent oral hygiene is indicated to prevent infection because mucus and old blood provide an excellent medium for bacterial growth. Rinsing with normal saline, sterile water, or dilute hydrogen peroxide minimizes odor and unpleasant taste.

H. Occasionally complications arise, even with the most diligent care. If the neck shrinks or becomes stiff because of scar tissue, plastic surgery may be required at a later date. Removal of the spinal accessory nerve may cause the shoulder to drop, which can be corrected or prevented by physical therapy and exercise. Lower facial paralysis can result from facial nerve injury.

I. Patients are encouraged to verbalize their concerns about appearance and prognosis.

J. Patients and family must participate in the long recovery and rehabilitative process. Lifestyle changes include avoidance of cigarettes and alcohol. Physical therapy, speech therapy, occupational therapy, home health nursing, and dietary counseling are all components of rehabilitation.

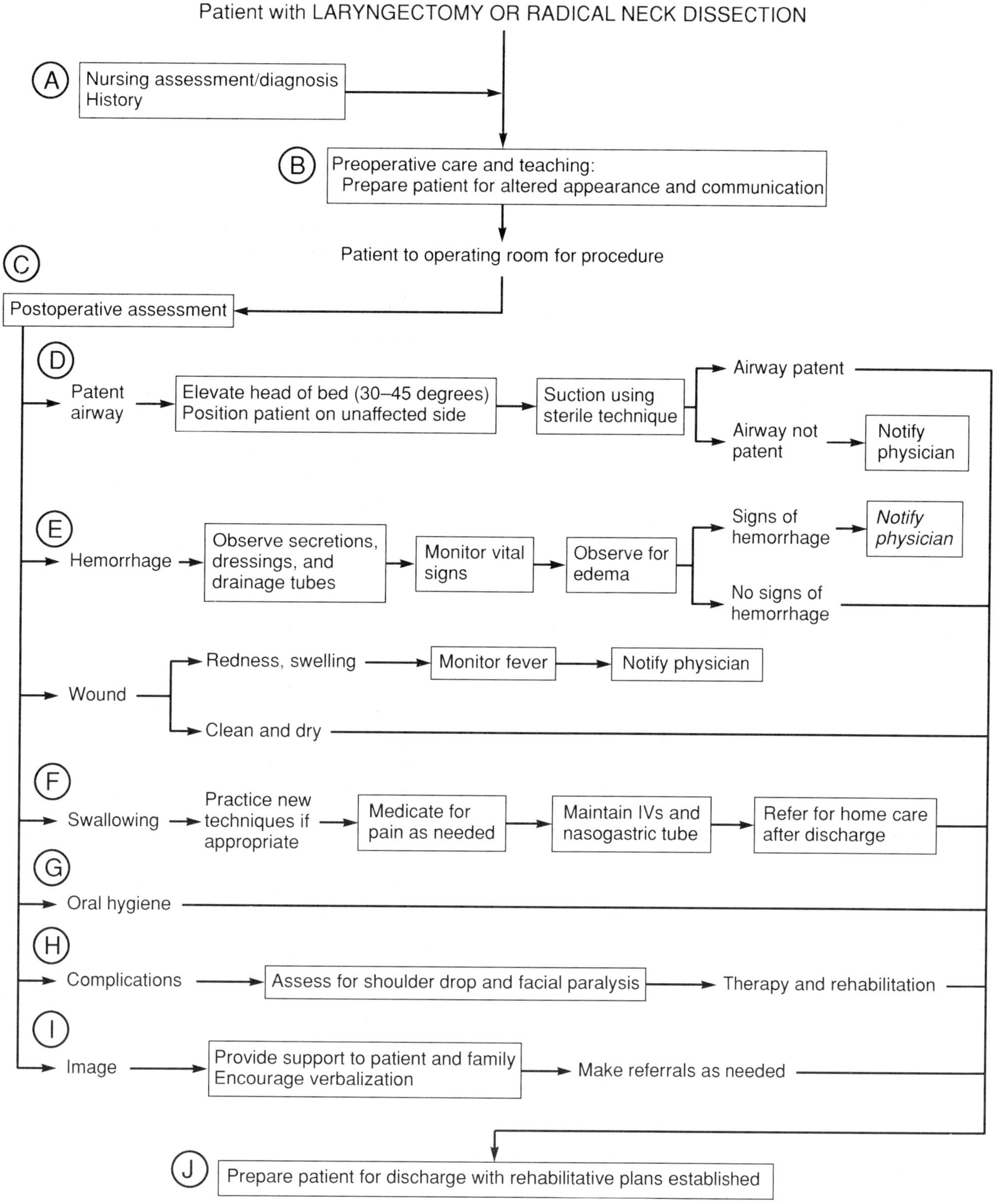

References

Biggs C. The cancer that can cost a patient his voice. RN 1987; 50(4):44–51.

Brunner LS, Suddarth DS. Textbook of medical-surgical nursing. 6th ed. Philadelphia: JB Lippincott, 1988.

McCormick KB. Neurological trauma. In: Lewis SM, Collier IC, eds. Medical-surgical nursing: assessment and management of clinical problems. 2nd ed. New York: McGraw-Hill, 1987:958–962.

Marvin J. Reconstructive problems. In: Patrick ML, ed. Medical-surgical nursing: pathophysiological concepts. Philadelphia: JB Lippincott, 1986:419–426.

TRACHEOTOMY AND TRACHEOSTOMY

Michelle Cornish

A. A tracheotomy is an incision made into the trachea through the neck below the larynx. It is performed to gain access to the airway below a blockage by a foreign body, tumor, or edema of the glottis or to permit long-term mechanical ventilation. Should the blockage persist, a tube is inserted into the opening to create a tracheostomy to relieve airway obstruction. It may be temporary or permanent. In an emergency any available instrument may be used as a dilator, even the barrel of a ballpoint pen with the inner portion removed. If respirations return to normal, the incision can be closed.

B. Assess the patient's condition. Symptoms that indicate a compromised airway are stridor, wheezing, intercostal muscle retraction, flared nares, inability to speak, and tachycardia, accompanied by signs of hypoxia. The patient may be cyanotic, agitated progressing to lethargic, and eventually comatose. Auscultation of lungs reveals limited air movement or possibly no air movement at all.

C. Diagnostic studies include measurement of arterial blood gases (ABGs) to assess respiratory status and chest films. Baseline complete blood count (CBC), clotting studies, and electrolytes are helpful, but not necessary, prior to an emergency tracheotomy.

D. Monitor the patient for arrhythmias, an indication of hypoxemia.

E. Provide the patient with oxygen. Cool humidified oxygen is best because it helps decrease existing edema. If necessary, provide initial oxygenation through an Ambu-Bag with 100 percent oxygen.

F. Preparing the patient for the procedure is essential because patients are extremely apprehensive. Explain the basic purpose and procedure in understandable terms and obtain a written consent. Reassure patients that they will not asphyxiate and that a communication method will be established. Newer fenestrated tracheostomy tubes allow patients to speak with a tracheostomy tube in place.

G. In addition to setting up all the equipment (see hospital policy) that the physician uses to perform the tracheostomy, supplies for suctioning during and after the procedure are needed. Tracheostomy tube position is secured by twill tapes. A back-up tracheostomy tube and obturator should be at the bedside.

H. After the tracheostomy, the patient should have repeat ABGs. Vital signs must be monitored every 15 minutes initially to assess for signs of hypoxia and fluid loss. Compare breath sounds to the baseline data. Notify the physician of signs of increasing respiratory distress.

I. Perform suctioning with sterile technique as needed to maintain a patent airway and prevent hypoxemia and pneumonia (p 104), which are caused by the accumulation of secretions. A fresh tracheostomy may bleed, so suctioning should be done cautiously. Warn the patient that the suctioning may cause coughing and gagging.

J. Ongoing assessment includes taking vital signs every 2 hours to assess for an elevated temperature. Report changes in the appearance of secretions to the physician, and send a specimen to the lab for culture and sensitivity. Regularly replace all equipment to reduce the risk of infection. Tracheostomy care with dressing change should be done every 8 hours, and more frequently if secretions are excessive or if the dressing gets wet.

K. Patients can be taught to suction themselves if the tracheostomy is to be long-term or permanent. They can also perform tracheostomy care with proper instruction. Encourage frequent coughing and deep breathing to maintain a clear airway. The nurse should also instruct the patient in how to remain mobile.

L. Patients with a tracheostomy are frustrated at their inability to talk. Be understanding and supportive and assist in finding a method of communication that is comfortable. Provide pen and paper, picture cards, magic slate, or a small chalkboard. Be patient and remember to talk in a normal tone.

M. Patients who are to be discharged with a tracheostomy must be instructed in tracheostomy care methods and suctioning technique. Provide patients with a list of resources in the community that sell supplies and make arrangements for a visiting nurse. Start teaching early so that patients can practice until comfortable performing self-care. Stress the importance of adhering to the prescribed medical regimen and follow-up.

References

Boyda MS. Problems affecting oxygen-carbon dioxide exchange and respiration. In: Brunner LS, Suddarth DS, eds. Medical-surgical nursing. 6th ed. Philadelphia: JB Lippincott, 1988:432–433, 436.

Potter D. Emergencies. Horsham, PA: Intermed Communications, 1985:114–167.

Robinson S, Russo P. Providing respiratory care. Horsham, PA: Intermed Communications, 1982:45–55.

Sheehy S, Barber J. Emergency nursing: principles and practice. St. Louis: CV Mosby, 1985: 146.

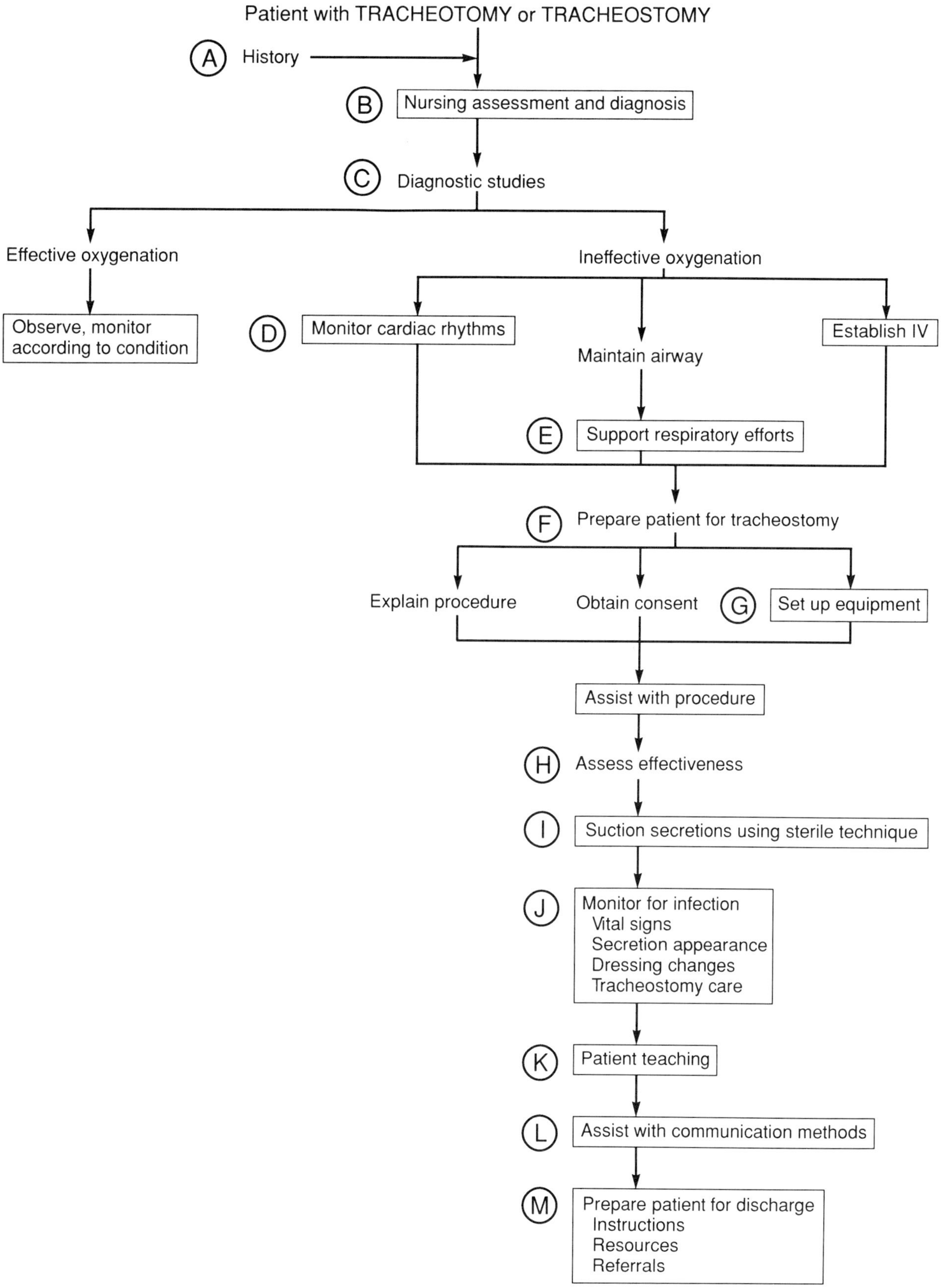
Patient with TRACHEOTOMY or TRACHEOSTOMY
A History
B Nursing assessment and diagnosis
C Diagnostic studies
Effective oxygenation
Observe, monitor according to condition
Ineffective oxygenation
D Monitor cardiac rhythms
Maintain airway
Establish IV
E Support respiratory efforts
F Prepare patient for tracheostomy
Explain procedure
Obtain consent
G Set up equipment
Assist with procedure
H Assess effectiveness
I Suction secretions using sterile technique
J Monitor for infection
Vital signs
Secretion appearance
Dressing changes
Tracheostomy care
K Patient teaching
L Assist with communication methods
M Prepare patient for discharge
Instructions
Resources
Referrals

SPECIAL CONSIDERATIONS

Alcoholism
Substance Abuse
Pain Management
Chemotherapy
The Geriatric Patient

ALCOHOLISM

Cecile A. Lengacher

Alcoholism is usually treated in a facility staffed for that purpose. However, patients with medical or surgical problems may also be alcoholic, which has a real impact on nursing care. Alcoholism is a progressive illness characterized by acute and chronic physiologic and behavioral manifestations in the progression of the illness. Alcoholism is a disease that is considered to have a psychogenic origin and then progresses into a physiologic dependency.

A. Alcoholics often use drink to resolve or lessen tension. Alcohol acts like an anesthetic; however, when the effect of alcohol wears off, the alcoholic's emotions range through tension, relief, and guilt. An alcoholic goes through four stages: the prealcoholic phase, early alcoholic phase, addiction phase, and chronic phase.

B. In order to develop a workable treatment plan the nurse must be able to differentiate between acute and chronic manifestations of the disease process. Acute behavioral manifestations include morning drinking, irresponsible behavior (missed work), rationalization for drinking, and personality changes such as being hostile, demanding, resentful, lonely, intolerant, paranoid, depressed, lacking in self-respect, and feeling worthless. The patient will resist treatment.

C. Initial nursing care is related to reducing anxiety. Strategies include orientation to reality, therapeutic communication, prevention of injury, and promotion of rest.

D. Physiologic manifestations include acute withdrawal symptoms such as tremors, weakness, tachycardia, increased blood pressure, and motor seizures.

E. Treatment is symptomatic, with careful monitoring of vital signs, cardiopulmonary status, hydration, and nutritional intake. The patient may need assistance with self-care. One of the goals of care is to have the patient retain control of behavior as well as physical care.

F. Chronic alcoholism is characterized behaviorally by episodes of binge "holiday" drinking, paranoia, and social withdrawal. Physiologic complications resulting from chronic alcoholism are Wernicke's syndrome (a condition of old age marked by loss of memory and disorientation), Korsakoff's syndrome (disorientation, muttering delirium, insomnia, illusions, hallucinations, and painful extremities), liver damage, hepatitis (p 150), cirrhosis (p 146), gastritis, gastric ulcers (p 130), pancreatitis (p 148), cardiomyopathy, adrenocortical insufficiency and central nervous system dysfunction, and organic brain syndrome.

G. Hospitalization usually prohibits the supply of alcohol, and these patients may go through withdrawal that may culminate in delirium tremens (DTs). Treatment of the physiologic problems related to withdrawal are essential to the patient's survival. Manifestations of DTs are agitation, tremors, autonomic hyperactivity, seizures, fever, visual hallucinations, and delusions. DTs is a *medical emergency* that can result in death.

H. Referrals to a psychiatric liaison nurse may be indicated to assist the patient and family in developing functional coping mechanisms and/or a plan of action. Alcoholics need to admit that they have a problem, and confrontation of that problem by the family and treatment team is vital. Treatment must be ongoing because relapses occur. Patients should enter an alcoholic treatment program, which includes Alcoholics Anonymous (AA) and may include Antabuse therapy.

References

Lewis S, McDowell W, Messner R, Gregory R, Brown J. Alcoholism: the problem behind the problem. J Soc Gastrointest Assist 1985; Fall:9–13.

Benner M. Mental health and psychiatric nursing: a study and learning tool. Springhouse, PA: Springhouse Corporation, 1988.

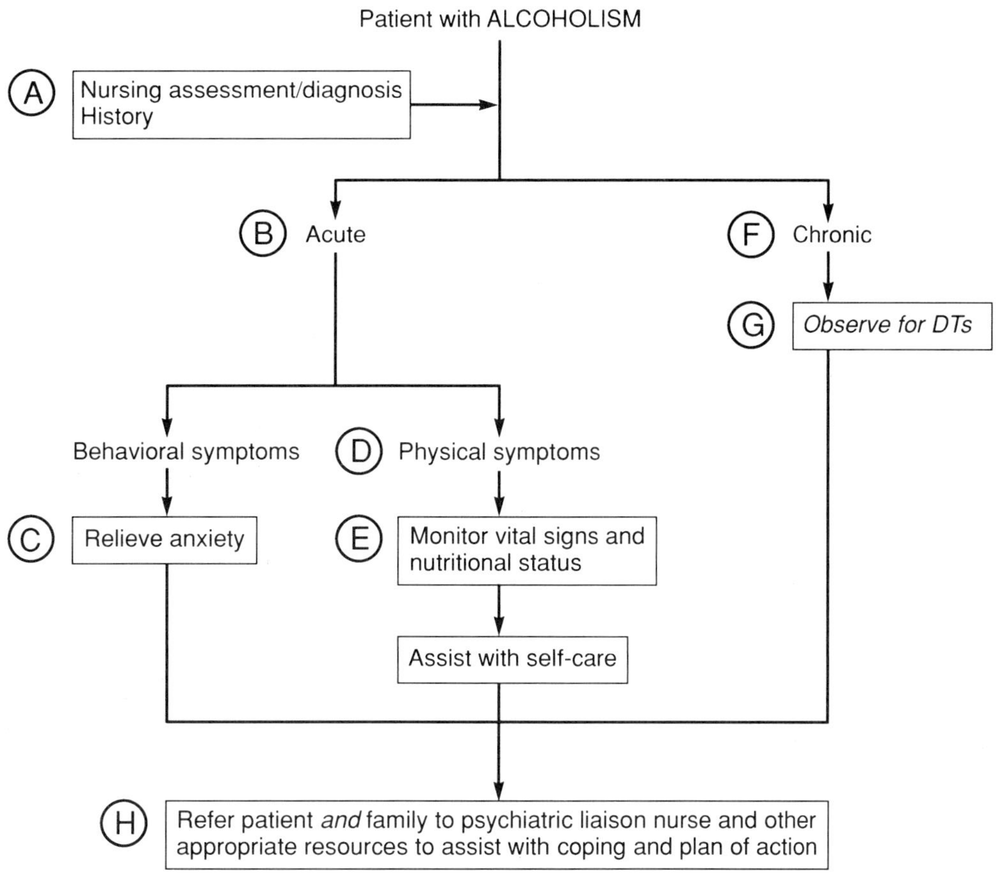
Patient with ALCOHOLISM
A
Nursing assessment/diagnosis
History
B
Acute
F
Chronic
G
Observe for DTs
Behavioral symptoms
D
Physical symptoms
C
Relieve anxiety
E
Monitor vital signs and nutritional status
Assist with self-care
H
Refer patient *and* family to psychiatric liaison nurse and other appropriate resources to assist with coping and plan of action

SUBSTANCE ABUSE

Bonita M. Garvey

Although the youthful drug abuser has been the focus of public attention, drug abuse can occur at any age. Abuse is the overuse and/or continuing use of drugs for other than legitimate medical reasons. Dependency refers to physiologic and psychological desire or need to continue taking the drug, increasing the dose. Drug abuse may involve a single drug or multiple agents. A severe financial, marital, employment, or medical crisis is often the precipitating event that precedes the search for care. Often these individuals are seen in the hospital setting undergoing treatment for an unrelated illness or injury.

A. A detailed history is crucial because denial often prevents full recognition of a chemical dependency. Since patterns of drug use vary widely, it is important to assess in detail the specific nature and extent of drug use. Family members or significant others may provide data regarding time frames and observed changes in behavior patterns: sleep-wake cycle, choice of friends and associates, mood, direction of school work or work performance, truthfulness, and attitudes. Obtain information related to accidents, chronic absences from school or work, family discord, violent behavior, memory lapses, seizures, poor dietary intake, or loss of driver's license due to drug abuse. Patient history includes questions to determine pattern, amount, and recent use of drugs. Ask about drug use to handle stress or escape from life's problems; unsuccessful attempts to decrease or stop use of the substance; trouble with the law or arrest because of drug use; avoidance of people or places that do not support drug use; neglect of responsibilities; and expressions of concern about drug use from friends, family, or employer.

B. Basic laboratory evaluation includes complete blood analysis to identify electrolyte imbalance, nutritional anemia, or other abnormalities. Blood cultures could identify blood stream infections acquired from the use of group needles and syringes. Diagnostic studies also include a drug screen, usually using a urine sample. This test establishes that a suspected drug or its metabolite is present in the specimen. Only after the same drug has been detected by two separate techniques is a sample reported as positive.

C. Appropriate nursing management depends on the diagnoses derived from a thorough assessment and physical examination. Depending on the type of substance abuse under consideration, a wide spectrum of physical symptoms is possible, and almost any organ system may be involved. Subjective symptoms might include insomnia, exhaustion, loss of appetite, dryness of mouth or excess salivation, nausea and vomiting, weight loss, a craving for sweets, increased appetite, constipation, impotence or amenorrhea, depression, panic or anxiety states, dizziness, nosebleeds, headaches, or chest pain. Objective symptoms might include altered level of consciousness, depressed respirations, convulsions, confusion, illusions and hallucinations, pupil constriction or dilation, slurred speech, drunken behavior without alcohol odor, staggering gait, poor perception of time and distance, hyperactive reflexes, increased alertness, or excitation. Other general symptoms might include fever; increased pulse rate and blood pressure; unusual breath odor; bloodshot or watery eyes; runny nose; congested lungs; tremors; skin rashes; recent needle marks or pigmented, linear "track" markings along the course of superficial veins of arms, legs, penis, and between toes; abscesses or depressed, scarred skin areas; jaundice; flushed face and neck; discoloration of fingers (thumb and forefinger); flat affect; and malnourished and/or unkempt personal appearance.

D. A combination of accurate, thorough history, laboratory, and physical evaluation is necessary to assess and clarify the specific problem. Some agencies use an addiction severity index (ASI) that produces a problem severity profile of the patient, which indicates specific areas needing intervention. Deviations may range widely depending on type of drug being abused, its source, the dose, the way it is used, degree of psychological dependence, and social-behavioral factors, such as age and personality. A manipulative teenager may be "acting out" hostilities toward family members, an elderly person may be experiencing an overreaction to a certain combination of prescription drugs, or a middle-aged person may be using drugs to deal with temporary or ongoing stresses. In these cases, counseling or adjusting the medications may be the only intervention necessary. Follow-up is an important deterrent to future abuse.

E. Referral sources for minor substance abuse problems may include Employee Assistance Programs (EAPs), physicians, hospitals, and clergy. The National Council on Drug Abuse is a useful information source.

F. For more complex problems, professional help may be found at drug abuse treatment centers or from therapists, addiction counselors, and community mental health centers. Family members and significant others often benefit from therapy themselves. Various self-

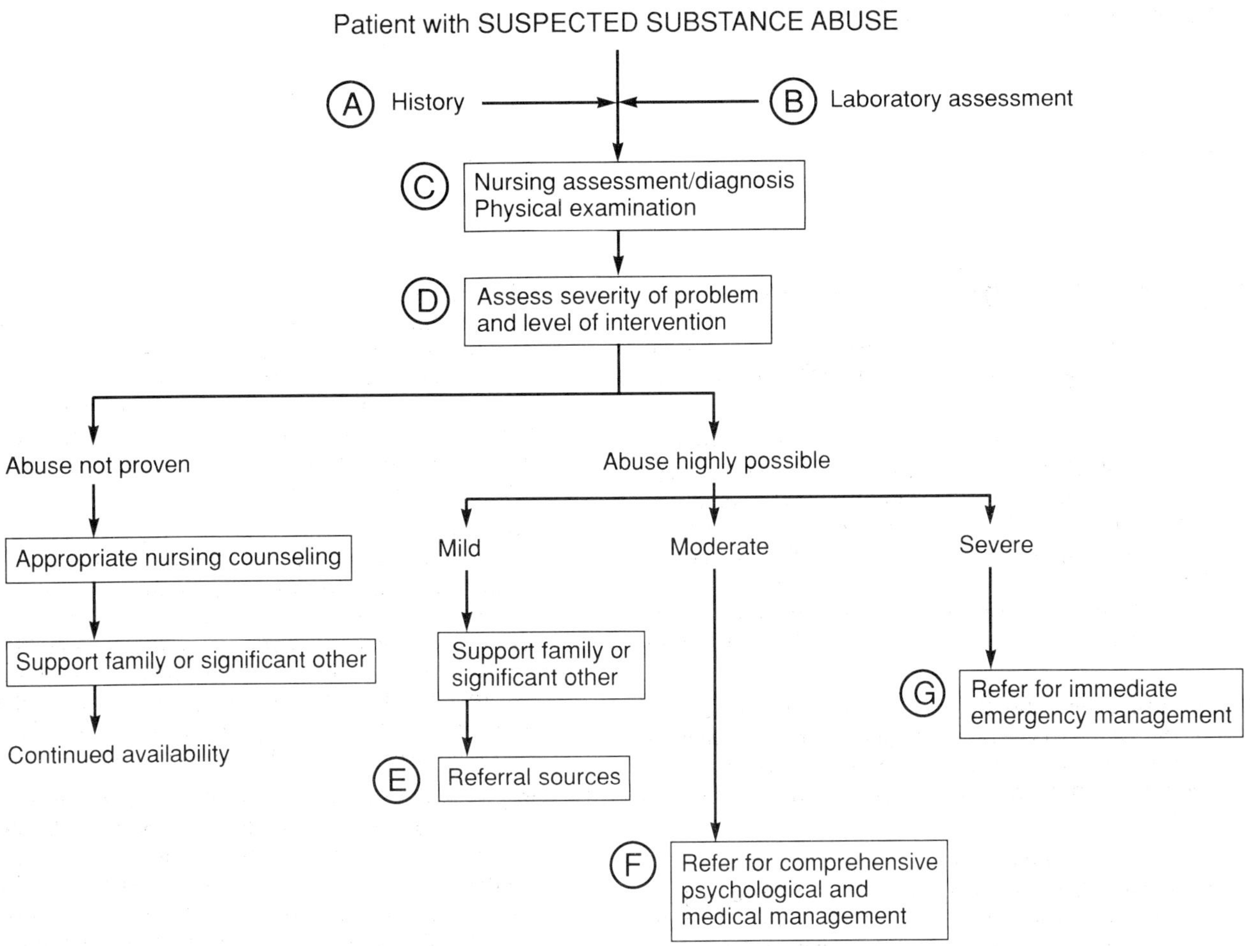

help groups such as Narcotics and Cocaine Anonymous or Alcoholics Anonymous are also available.

G. Severe drug abuse may require emergency management to protect the client (and others) from possible violent behavior, toxic side effects of substances used, and/or withdrawal. Patients may require transfer to specialized chemical treatment units for appropriate care. Managing the patient's anxiety and agitation by decreasing stimulation (dark, quiet, nonthreatening environment), reassuring the patient in a soft, nonthreatening manner, and cautious reality orientation is necessary until transfer can be arranged.

References

Chemical dependency: is there a problem? Daly City, CA: Krames Communications, 1987.

Cohen S. The substance abuse problems. New York: Haworth Press, 1981.

Doenges ME, Jeffries C, Moorhouse MF. Nursing care plans. Philadelphia: FA Davis, 1984.

U.S. Department of Health and Human Services. Sedative-hypnotics: marijuana; inhalants; opiates. Washington, DC: Alcohol, Drug Abuse, and Mental Health Administration, 1984.

PAIN MANAGEMENT

Barbara Kalo

Most medical-surgical problems are associated with pain, and it is the most common symptom for which patients seek relief. To manage the pain is to remove the primary cause. It is the nurse's responsibility to increase the patient's comfort and assist with relief of pain.

A. Taking a complete history of the pain aids in making an accurate diagnosis. Because pain is subjective, evaluation relies on careful questioning of the patient. The history of pain includes chronology, nature, location, radiation, aggravating factors, and alleviating factors. Observable signs of pain include increased blood pressure, pulse and respiratory rate, dilated pupils, perspiration, moaning, grimacing, and rubbing the painful area.

B. Assessing the patient's pain includes observing nonverbal cues and the psychological factors that may be causing the pain. It is important that the nurse not make judgments about the degree of pain being experienced by the patient.

C. Determining whether the pain is acute or chronic is necessary. Acute pain is an intense epidose of pain which can last seconds or 6 months. Usually it is the result of organic disease or injury, with pain decreasing as healing occurs.

D. Providing comfort measures may offer relief from pain before the administration of drugs. Some comfort measures are pillows, repositioning, adjusting environmental temperature, elevating extremities (unless contraindicated), heat, massage, and exercise.

E. It is preferable to diagnose the cause before analgesics are given, because they may mask the symptoms. The nurse must know the actions and the side effects of the medications that are given. Oral analgesics are preferred; however, for moderate to severe pain the most common analgesics are intramuscular narcotics. Intravenous or rectal routes may be used for patients who are nauseated or on fluid restrictions or who need immediate relief.

F. Chronic pain is often obscure, and several techniques may be applied in place of continued doses of analgesics. Explanations and teaching are necessary. Some of the techniques that may require the nurse's assistance are operant conditioning, visual imagery, biofeedback, progressive relaxation, distraction, placebo, transcutaneous electrical nerve stimulation (TENS), hypnosis, and acupuncture.

G. Recent developments in pain management include the intraspinal infusion of narcotics or local anesthetics, implantable devices for continuous analgesia, and patient-controlled analgesia. In these methods, frequent small doses of narcotic analgesics can be administered to achieve efficient control of continuous severe pain. Patients receiving intraspinal analgesia must be observed for respiratory depression. Narcan should be readily available to reverse side effects.

H. In preparation for discharge, the patient is instructed about the action of the medication and the side effects. Referral to a community health nurse for continued evaluation and management of the pain control program may be required when invasive methods are used. Hospice programs provide care and symptomatic relief to dying patients.

References

Krupp MA, Chatton MJ, Werdegar D, eds. Current medical diagnosis and treatment. Los Altos, CA: Lange, 1985.

Lewis SM, Collier IC. Medical-surgical nursing: assessment and management of clinical problems. New York: McGraw-Hill, 1983.

McCaffery M. The person experiencing pain. In: Brunner LS, Suddarth DS, eds. Textbook of medical-surgical nursing. 6th ed. Philadelphia: JB Lippincott, 1988:244–261.

Nichols BS. Pain: transmission and theories. Nurse Review. Springhouse, PA: Nursing 86 Books, 1986:143–156.

Thompson JM, McFarland GK, Hirsch JE, Tucker SM, Bowers AC. Clinical nursing. St. Louis: CV Mosby, 1986.

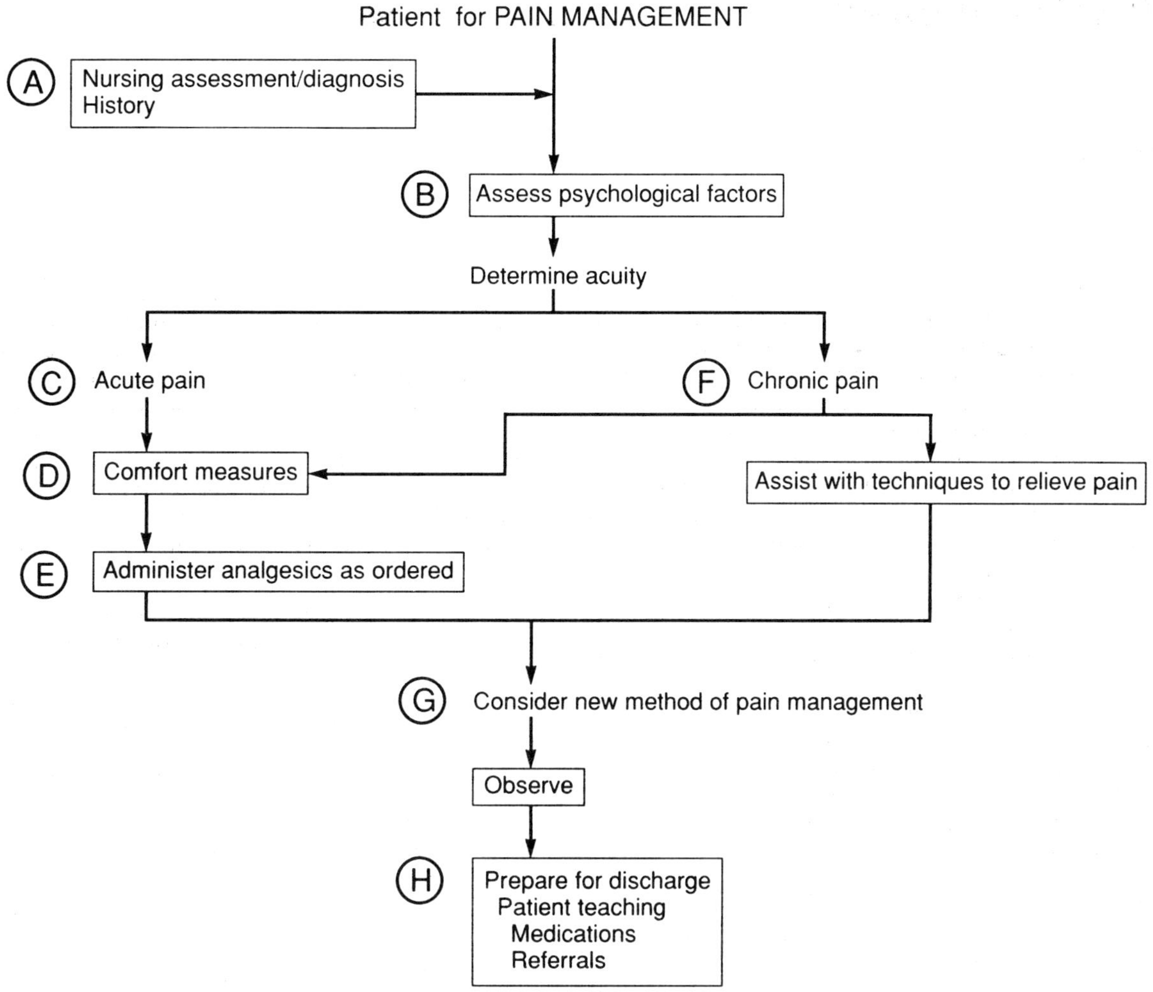
Patient for PAIN MANAGEMENT
A
Nursing assessment/diagnosis
History
B
Assess psychological factors
Determine acuity
C
Acute pain
F
Chronic pain
D
Comfort measures
Assist with techniques to relieve pain
E
Administer analgesics as ordered
G
Consider new method of pain management
Observe
H
Prepare for discharge
Patient teaching
Medications
Referrals

CHEMOTHERAPY

Marsha Cloak

Cancer chemotherapy, the use of drugs to treat cancer, has become an important component of the treatment regimen, resulting in cures and long-term control of many types of cancer. Twelve types of cancer are now considered curable with chemotherapy. Chemotherapy has a systemic effect as opposed to the localized effect of surgery or radiation. Most chemotherapeutic agents work by interrupting cell division and/or altering DNA synthesis. They are classified into six categories (see Table 1). When chemotherapeutic agents are used to treat cancer, four goals are sought: cure, control of the disease, increased survival, and improved quality of life. Adjuvant chemotherapy is given after surgery and/or radiation have freed the patient of any clinically detectable tumor, anticipating the biologic nature of certain malignancies to metastasize early in the course of disease. Palliation is a goal of chemotherapy when the tumor is so widespread that control or cure is not possible. The objective is to diminish the tumor mass in order to reduce side effects, such as pain or obstruction. The most significant disadvantage of chemotherapy is that the drugs cannot differentiate between malignant and normal cells, and so damage both. However, because of the high percentage of malignant cells that are reproducing, the toxic effect is greater to the malignant cells. Side effects of chemotherapy may affect every body system (see Table 2). The severity of the side effects is determined by the specific agent, dosage, route and schedule of administration, combination of agents given, prior therapy received, and the patient's physical condition and individual reaction.

The nurse plays a vital role in the management of the patient receiving cancer chemotherapy. Responsibilities encompass administration of the therapy, patient assessment, symptom control, and patient teaching. The nurse must know each agent's side effects, special precautions and their implications, acceptable dosage, rationale for therapy, and proper method of administration. Since the most common method of administering chemotherapy is the intravenous route, the nurse must be skilled in intravenous technique. With advancing technology in intravenous administration the nurse must be familiar with the utilization of central venous access devices and large- and small-volume infusion pumps. Other methods of administering cancer chemotherapy include oral, subcutaneous, intramuscular, intra-arterial, hepatic arterial, intraperitoneal, and intrathecal.

A. Prior to chemotherapy administration, a thorough patient assessment must be conducted to determine the patient's physical status, acceptable laboratory values, presence of symptoms that contraindicate administering the therapy, and the patient's psychological status.

B. A key role of the nurse after the assessment is to implement measures to prevent and/or reduce the severity of the side effects. For each potential side effect the patient may experience, an individualized plan of care must be developed and implemented. (See Baird S. Decision making in oncology nursing. Toronto: BC Decker, 1988.)

C. The patient and family must have a thorough understanding of the rationale for the therapy, the schedule of administration, the potential side effects, self-care measures that will prevent and/or reduce the severity of the side effects, and when to notify the physician or nurse. Providing this information relieves fears of the unknown and reduces the patient's anxiety level, which helps to reduce some side effects and, most important, makes the patient an active participant in the process and allows some sense of control.

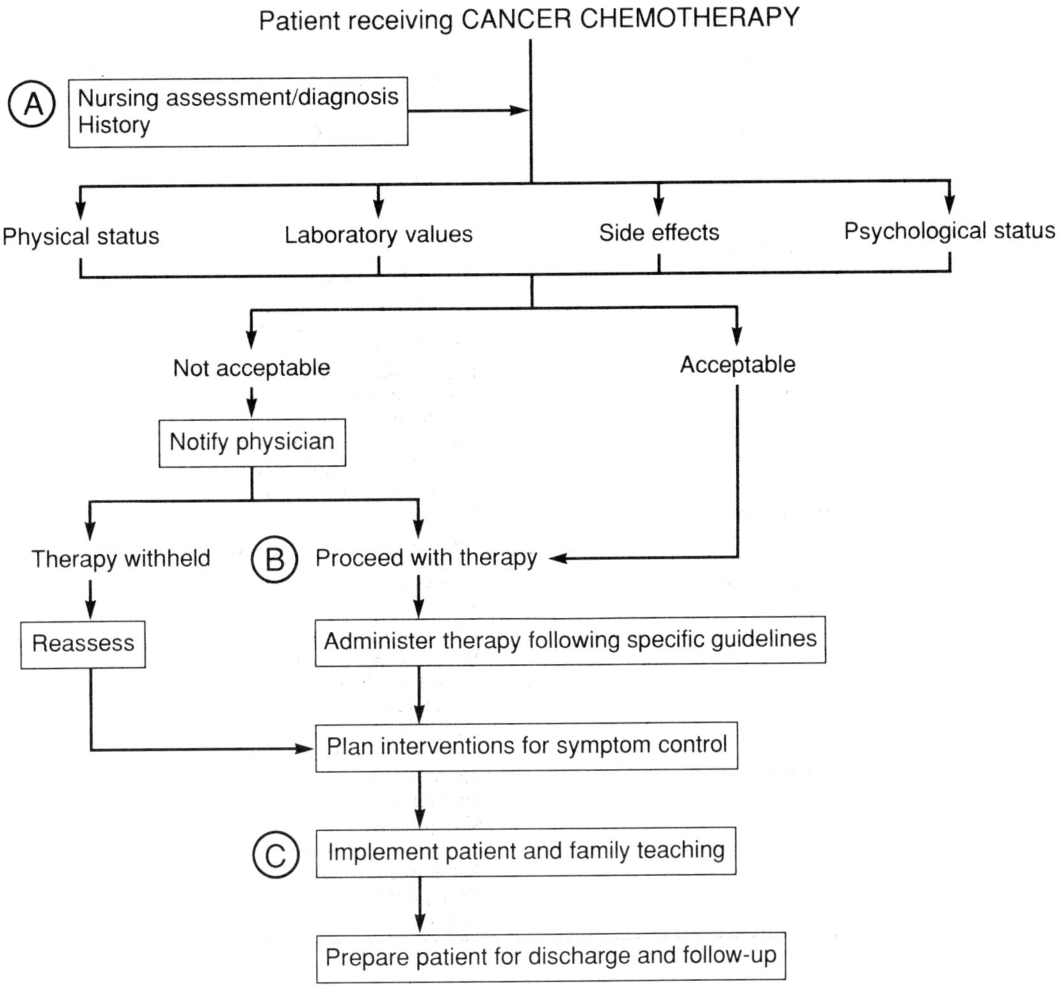

TABLE 1 Categories of Chemotherapeutic Agents

Alkylating Agents
- Alkeran (melphalan)
- BiCNU (carmustine)
- CeeNu (lomustine)
- Cytoxan (cyclophosphamide)
- DTIC (dacarbazine)
- Leukeran (chlorambucil)
- Mustargen (mechlorethamine hydrochloride)
- Myleran (busulfan)
- Platinol (cisplatin)
- Thiotepa (thiotepa)
- Zanosar (streptozocin)

Antitumor Antibiotics
- Adriamycin (doxorubicin hydrochloride)
- Blenoxane (bleomycin sulfate)
- Cerubidine (daunorubicin hydrochloride)
- Cosmegen (dactinomycin)
- Mutamycin (mitomycin)

Antimetabolites
- Cytosar-U (cytarabine)
- Fluorouracil (fluorouracil)
- Methotrexate (methotrexate sodium)
- Purinethol (mercaptopurine)
- Thioguanine (thioguanine)

Vinca Alkaloids (mitotic inhibitors)
- Oncovin (vincristine)
- Velban (vinblastine sulfate)
- VePesid (etoposide)

Hormones
- Emcyt (estramustine phosphate sodium)
- Lupron (leuprolide acetate)
- Megace (megestrol acetate)
- Nolvadex (tamoxifen citrate)
- Teslac (testolactone)

Miscellaneous Agents
- Elspar (asparaginase)
- Hydrea (hydroxyurea)
- Matulane (procarbazine hydrochloride)

TABLE 2 Side Effects of Chemotherapeutic Agents

Body Systems	*Side Effects*
Hematolymphatic	Leukopenia Thrombocytopenia Anemia
Gastrointestinal	Nausea Vomiting Anorexia Stomatitis Diarrhea
Genitourinary	Cystitis Acute renal tubular necrosis
Cardiac	Transient ECG changes Cardiomyopathy Hypotension
Hepatic	Transient enzyme elevations Permanent cirrhosis
Neurologic	Peripheral neuropathies Cranial nerve dysfunction Autonomic dysfunction
Pulmonary	Fibrosis Edema Infiltrates
Integumentary	Alopecia Acne Hyperpigmentation Vesicant extravasation Photosensitivity Dry texture Dermatitis Radiation recall
Reproductive	Azoospermia Impotence Mutagenicity Ovarian suppression Amenorrhea Menopause Vaginitis

References

Baird S. Decision making in oncology nursing. Toronto: BC Decker, 1988.

Brager BL, Yasko J. Care of the client receiving chemotherapy. Reston, VA: Reston Publishing, 1984.

Dorr RT, Fritz WL. Cancer chemotherapy handbook. New York: Elsevier-North Holland, 1980.

Krakoff IH. Cancer chemotherapeutic agents. CA—A Cancer Journal for Clinicians 1987; 37:93–105.

THE GERIATRIC PATIENT

Barbara Kalo
Carol Bowdoin

Aging is a normal process, and the gradual biological changes that occur are influenced by hereditary and environmental factors. Proper health care and continued socialization is important for the elderly to function in society. It has been noted that 80 percent of patients over 80 years of age function well and live independently. Nursing care must be individualized based on a patient's past experiences and needs.

A. Taking an elderly client's history requires sensitivity, patience, and an understanding that there is decreased function of one or more organ systems. At this time, note whether hearing or speech is impaired and whether there are disturbances in orientation to person, place, and time. Depression or anxiety may be observed. A thorough review of chronic disease and current therapy, including medications, is necessary.

B. A head-to-toe assessment of the geriatric patient is important. The aged are vulnerable to disease because of decreased physiologic reserve and less effective body defense mechanisms. Identify patients who are at high risk for deterioration. Neurologically, a slower psychomotor performance and slower reflexes will be noticed. Pupil size will be decreased, presbyopia will be present, and the lens may be opaque and discolored.

C. Respirations may be shallow, or labored breathing may be noted if a respiratory disease is present. Shortness of breath may be noted after exertion. Assist the patient to maintain positions that maximize lung expansion. Assess breath sounds in the immobile patient to detect congestion.

D. Circulatory diseases are the most common disorders in this age group. The geriatric patient will have decreases in cardiac output, response of the heart rate to stress, and elasticity of peripheral vessels. Assessing the apical and radial pulse rate and peripheral pulses is necessary to evaluate cardiovascular status. Foot problems are common. Avoid prolonged sitting or inactivity, because dependent edema and emboli may develop in the lower extremities. Change positions gradually to prevent orthostatic hypotension and vertigo.

E. Digestion slows down, resulting in intolerance of various foods. Many patients may be on special diets for health problems. Elimination may be a problem because of a decrease in colon motility, fluid intake, cultural practices, state of health, lack of exercise, use of laxatives, and nutritional intake. Eating habits should be discussed. In the hospital, maintaining hydration and "home routine" facilitates adequate elimination. If patients need help to meet daily nutrition requirements at home, assistance programs such as "Meals on Wheels" can be arranged.

F. Urgency or obstruction of urine flow may be noted. Common dysfunctions are prostatic hypertrophy (p 300) in males and structural prolapse in females. Postmenopausal bleeding may indicate neoplastic disease and should be evaluated. There is drying and atrophy of the vaginal mucosa and a slower sexual response in both sexes. Urinary bladder infections are common; increasing fluid intake and taking meticulous care of urinary catheters may decrease the frequency of infection.

G. Geriatric skin is drier and exhibits less turgor. There is a decrease in subcutaneous fat, an increase in wrinkling, and atrophy of sweat glands. Avoid frequent use of hot water and soap or other drying agents. Lubricate the skin with lotions that trap moisture. Use care when removing adhesive tape to prevent trauma to fragile skin.

H. The geriatric client may complain about the inability to get adequate rest. Sleep often is interrupted and dreamless; elderly patients require frequent naps to make up lost deep sleep. Rest is enhanced by moderate activity, occasional short naps, and a reduction in caffeine intake before bedtime.

I. Evaluation of the patient's sensory acuity, vision, hearing, and pain response is important. The elderly may require additional lighting, especially at night, to prevent injury. The older patient may feel cold and require extra covers or higher room temperature for comfort. Extra care is necessary when applying heat or cold, because sensitivity to pain is decreased.

J. Socioeconomic circumstances may be revealed during the history taking. It is important to understand the problems encountered for the elderly to remain independent. Nursing care focuses on promoting, maintaining, and restoring independence and health. Psychological problems may be identified and a psychiatric consult indicated.

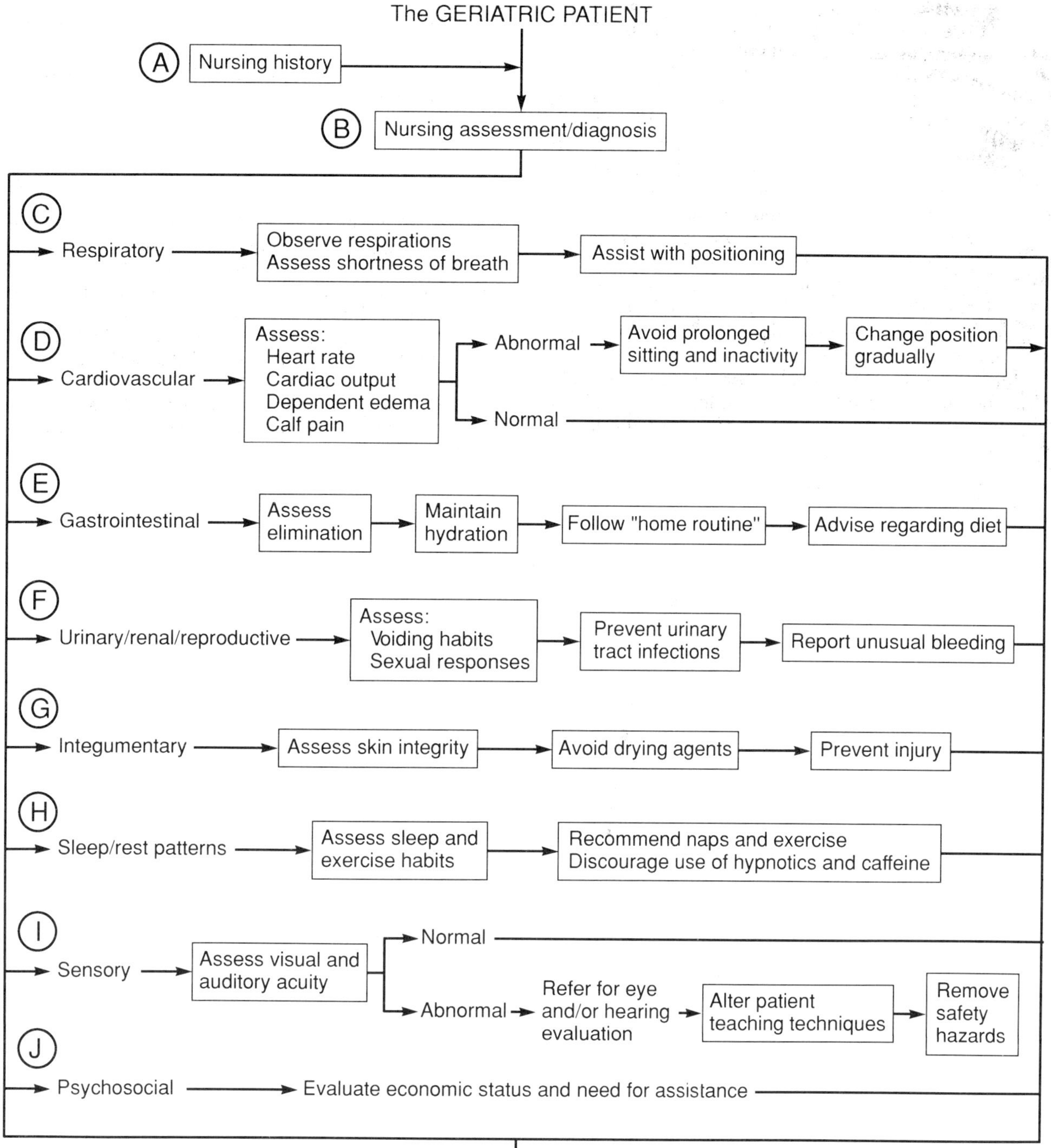

(Cont'd on page 415)

K. Teaching the geriatric patient about the aging process and how it affects specific medical problems is done on an individual basis. Promote a positive approach. Provide adequate, nonglare lighting, sharp colors, and large print when teaching elderly patients with sensory impairment. Speak in a clear, low-pitched voice. Teaching sessions should be short, concise, and concrete. Provide written instructions that can be reviewed at home. The short-term memory may be poor and elderly patients often get instructions confused. Review all medications during the hospital stay and again at time of discharge. Dietary instructions are important for the elderly. A dietary regimen may be important in controlling a serious medical problem. Elderly patients should be taught methods to conserve their health but still be socially and mentally active. Family should be included in teaching when possible. Home accident prevention is an important part of patient and family education.

L. Routine health checks are essential to identify disease at the early stage. With a thorough history and complete assessment, appropriate community resources may be utilized.

References

Bowdoin C. Application of the Orem self-care theory in the acute care geriatric setting. Unpublished graduate paper. Arlington, VA: Marymount College of Virginia, 1984.

Brunner LS, Suddarth DS. Textbook of medical-surgical nursing. 6th ed. Philadelphia: JB Lippincott, 1988.

Feigenbaum LZ. Geriatrics. In: Krupp MA, Chatton MJ, Werdegar D, eds. Current medical diagnosis and treatment. Los Altos, CA: Lange, 1985:18–25.

Lewis SM, Collier IC. Medical surgical nursing: assessment and management of clinical problems. New York: McGraw-Hill, 1983.

(Cont'd from page 413)

- Serious abnormalities noted
  - Notify physician
    Make referrals if indicated
    - Implement appropriate interventions
- No serious abnormalities noted
  - (K) Patient teaching about lifestyle and aging process
    - (L) Routine health checks

APPENDIX

NANDA NURSING DIAGNOSES GROUPED ACCORDING TO THE UNITARY PERSON FRAMEWORK*

EXCHANGING: MUTUAL GIVING AND RECEIVING

Altered nutrition: more than body requirements
Altered nutrition: less than body requirements
Altered nutrition: potential for more than body requirements
Potential for infection
Potential for altered body temperature
Hypothermia
Hyperthermia
Ineffective thermoregulation
Dysreflexia
Constipation
Perceived constipation
Colonic constipation
Diarrhea
Bowel incontinence
Altered patterns of urinary elimination
Stress incontinence
Reflex incontinence
Urge incontinence
Functional incontinence
Total incontinence
Urinary retention
Altered tissue perfusion (renal, cerebral, cardiopulmonary, gastrointestinal, peripheral)
Fluid volume excess
Fluid volume deficit: actual
Fluid volume deficit: potential
Decreased cardiac output
Impaired gas exchange
Ineffective airway clearance
Ineffective breathing pattern
Potential for injury
Potential for suffocation
Potential for poisoning
Potential for trauma
Potential for aspiration
Potential for disuse syndrome
Impaired tissue integrity
Altered oral mucous membrane
Impaired skin integrity
Potential impaired skin integrity

COMMUNICATING: SENDING MESSAGES

Alterations in verbal communication

RELATING: ESTABLISHING BONDS

Impaired social interaction
Social isolation
Altered role performance
Altered parenting
Potential altered parenting
Sexual dysfunction
Altered family processes
Parental role conflict
Altered sexuality patterns

VALUING: ASSIGNING OF RELATIVE WORTH

Spiritual distress (of human spirit)

CHOOSING: SELECTION OF ALTERNATIVES

Ineffective individual coping
Impaired adjustment
Defensive coping
Ineffective denial
Ineffective family coping: disabling
Ineffective family coping: compromised
Family coping: Potential for growth
Noncompliance (specify)
Decisional conflict (specify)
Health-seeking behavior

MOVING: ACTIVITY

Impaired physical mobility
Activity intolerance
Fatigue
Potential activity intolerance
Sleep pattern disturbance
Diversional activity deficit
Impaired home maintenance management
Altered health maintenance
Feeding self-care deficit
Impaired swallowing

* The Unitary Framework describes nine human response patterns that are necessary for health maintenance. This list does not include all possible nursing problems. The nurse should synthesize available data and formulate an appropriate diagnostic label.

Adapted from Taxonomy I (Revised). St. Louis: North American Nursing Diagnosis Association (NANDA), 1988.

Ineffective breastfeeding
Bathing/hygiene self-care deficit
Dressing/grooming self-care deficit
Toileting self-care deficit
Altered growth and development

PERCEIVING: RECEPTION OF INFORMATION

Body image disturbance
Self-esteem disturbance
Chronic low self-esteem
Situational low self-esteem
Personal identity disturbance
Sensory/perceptual alterations (visual, auditory, kinesthetic, gustatory, tactile, olfactory)
Unilateral neglect
Hopelessness
Powerlessness

KNOWING: MEANING ASSOCIATED WITH INFORMATION

Knowledge deficit (specify)
Alterations in learning
Altered thought processes

FEEDING: SUBJECTIVE AWARENESS OF INFORMATION

Pain
Chronic pain
Dysfunctional grieving
Anticipatory grieving
Potential for violence: self-directed or directed at others
Post-trauma response
Rape-trauma syndrome
Rape-trauma: compound reaction
Rape-trauma: silent reaction
Anxiety
Fear

INDEX